COMPLICATIONS IN ENDOVASCULAR SURGERY

COMPLICATIONS IN ENDOVASCULAR SURGERY

Peri-Procedural Prevention and Treatment

EDITORS

MACIEJ L. DRYJSKI, MD, PhD, FACS, DFSVS

Professor and Vice Chairman,
Department of Surgery, Jacobs School of
Medicine & Biomedical Sciences,
University at Buffalo
Director, Vascular and Endovascular
Surgery, Kaleida Health,
Buffalo, New York

LINDA M. HARRIS, MD, FACS, DFSVS

Professor of Surgery
Program Director Vascular Surgery
Residency and Fellowship
Jacobs School of Medicine & Biomedical
Sciences, University at Buffalo
Buffalo, New York

ASSOCIATE EDITORS

Hasan Dosluoglu
Jason Lee
Elad Levy
Gustavo Oderich
Joseph Dante Raffetto
Timothy Resch

ELSEVIER

ELSEVIER
1600 John F. Kennedy Blvd.
Ste 1800
Philadelphia, PA 19103-2899

COMPLICATIONS IN ENDOVASCULAR SURGERY, FIRST EDITION ISBN: 978-0-323-55448-0

Library of Congress Control Number 2020941977

Content Strategist: Jessica McCool
Content Development Specialist: Deborah Poulson
Publishing Services Manager: Shereen Jameel
Project Manager: Rukmani Krishnan
Design Direction: Bridget Hoette

Printed in The United States of America

Last digit is the print number: 9 8 7 6 5 4 3 2

We would like to dedicate this book to our patients and our families.

Maciej L. Dryjski
Linda M. Harris

LIST OF CONTRIBUTORS

Karl Abi-Aad, MD
Resident, Department of Surgery
SUNY Upstate Medical Center
New York, New York

Shadi Abu-Halimah, MD, FACS
Associate Professor of Surgery
Division of Vascular and Endovascular surgery
West Virginia University, Charleston Division
Charleston, West Virginia

Ali F. AbuRahma, MD, FRCS, FACS, RVT, RPVI
Professor of Surgery
Chief, Vascular & Endovascular Surgery
West Virginia University - Charleston Division
Charleston, West Virginia

Yogesh Acharya, MD, MSc, FAcadMEd, AFAMEE
Research Fellow
Western Vascular Institute and Galway Clinic
Royal College of Surgeons in Ireland and National University of Ireland
Galway affiliated Hospital
Doughiska
Galway, Ireland

Paul Anain, MD
Chair, Vascular Surgery at Catholic Health System/Trinity Vascular
Buffalo, New York

Hanaa Dakour Aridi, MD
Vascular Surgery Resident
Indiana University School of Medicine
Indianapolis, Indiana

Giuseppe Asciutto, MD, PhD
Associate Professor
Department of Clinical Science
Lund University, Sweden
Managing Director
Department of Vascular and Endovascular Surgery
Münster University Hospital
Münster, Germany

Gursant S. Atwal, MD
Clinical Assistant
Professor of Neurosurgery
University of Illinois at Chicago
Chicago, Illinois

Efthymios D. Avgerinos, MD, PhD, MSc
Associate Professor of Surgery
Division of Vascular Surgery
University of Pittsburgh Medical Center
Pittsburgh, Pennsylvania

Micheal T. Ayad, MD, RPVI, FACS
Associate Division Chief
Co-Director Vascular Lab
Division of Vascular and Endovascular Surgery
Mount Sinai Medical Center
Miami Beach, Florida

Jeffrey S. Beecher, DO
Director
Cerebrovascular and Endovascular Neurosurgery
New Hanover Regional Medical Center
Wilmington, North Carolina

Bernard R. Bendok, MD, MSCI
William J. Charles H Mayo Professor
Chair of Neurological Surgery
Mayo Clinic
Phoenix, Arizona

Clayton J. Brinster, MD, FACS
Senior Staff Surgeon
Vascular Surgery Section
Ochsner Clinic
New Orleans, Louisiana

Andrew J. Cantos, MD
Assistant Professor of Imaging
Department of Imaging Sciences
University of Rochester
Strong Memorial Hospital
Rochester, New York

Jeffrey P. Carpenter, MD
Professor and Chairman
Department of Surgery
Cooper Medical School of Rowan University
Vice President for Perioperative Services and Chief of Surgery
Cooper University Health Care
Camden, New Jersey

Rabih A. Chaer, MD, MSc
Professor of Surgery
Division of Vascular Surgery
University of Pittsburgh Medical Center
Pittsburgh, Pennsylvania

Jason Chang, MD
Vascular Fellow
Maimonides Medical Center
Brooklyn, New York

Gregory S. Cherr, MD
Professor of Surgery
Associate Dean for GME
Designated Institutional Officer
University at Buffalo
Jacobs School of Medicine and Biomedical Sciences
Buffalo, New York

Tracy J. Cheun, MD
Research Fellow
Division of Vascular and Endovascular Surgery
University of Texas Health San Antonio
San Antonio, Texas

Timothy A. M. Chuter, MD
Professor Emeritus
Department of Surgery
University of California
San Francisco, California

Richard Curl, MD
Clinical Professor of Surgery
Jacobs School of Medicine & Biomedical Sciences, SUNY at Buffalo
Buffalo, New York

Michael D. Dake, MD, FSIR, FCIRSE
Senior Vice President, UA Health Sciences
Professor, Department of Medical Imaging
Professor, Department of Surgery
Professor, Department of Medicine
University of Arizona
Tucson, Arizona

R. Clement Darling, III, MD
Professor of Surgery
Albany Medical College
Chief, Division of Vascular Surgery, Albany Medical Center Hospital
Director, The Institute for Vascular Health and Disease
Albany Med Vascular
Albany, New York

Mark G. Davies, MD, PhD, MBA
Professor and Chief
Division of Vascular and Endovascular Surgery
Director, South Texas Center for Vascular Care
Director, South Texas Aortic Center
Director, Center for Quality
Effectiveness and Outcomes in Cardiovascular Diseases
University of Texas Health San Antonio
San Antonio, Texas

Dolly Thakkar Doshi, MD, FVIR
Consultant Interventional Radiologist
Doshi Nursing Home and Fortis Hospital
Mumbai, Maharashtra, India

Hasan H. Dosluoglu, MD, FACS
Professor of Surgery
Chief of Vascular Surgery
Jacobs School of Medicine and Biomedical Sciences
State University of New York at Buffalo;
Chief of Surgery and Vascular Surgery
VA Western NY Healthcare System
Buffalo, New York

Ashwini D'Souza, MSc
Research Assistant
Department of Vascular and Endovascular Surgery
Galway Clinic
Royal College of Surgeons in Ireland and National University of Ireland
Galway affiliated Hospital, Doughiska
Galway, Ireland

Maciej L. Dryjski, MD, PhD, FACS, DFSVS
Professor and Vice Chairman
Department of Surgery
Jacobs School of Medicine & Biomedical Sciences, University at Buffalo
Director, Vascular and Endovascular Surgery
Kaleida Health
Buffalo, New York

Jeffrey B. Edwards, MD
Resident Physician
Division of Vascular Surgery
University of South Florida Morsani College of Medicine
Tampa, Florida

Quirine L. Eijkenboom, BS
Medical Scholar
Department Of Dermatology and Allergy
Ludwig-Maximilian University
Munich, Germany

Gianluca Faggioli, MD, PhD
Full Professor of Vascular Surgery
Director, Fellowship Program in Vascular Surgery
Alma Mater Studiorum - University of Bologna
Bologna, Italy

Mark A. Farber, MD, FACS
Chief, Division of Vascular Surgery
Director, UNC Aortic Network
Professor of Surgery and Radiology
Department of Surgery
University of North Carolina
Chapel Hill, North Carolina

Joseph B. Farnsworth, PA-C MMS, MBMS
Department of Neurological Surgery
Neurovascular, Neuroncology and Skullbase Program
Mayo Clinic
Phoenix, Arizona

Vernard S. Fennell, MD, MSc
Cerebrovascular and Endovascular Neurosurgery
Capital Institute for Neurosciences
Pennington, NJ

Jared T. Feyko, DO
Vascular Surgeon
Cardiothoracic and Vascular Surgical Associates
Jacksonville, Florida

Tanya R. Flohr, MD
Department of Surgery
University of Maryland
Baltimore, Maryland

Danielle Fontenot, MD
Vascular Surgery Resident
USF Health Morsani School of Medicine
Tampa, Florida

Enrico Gallitto, MD, PhD
Vascular Surgeon, Metropolitan Unit of Vascular Surgery
Alma Mater Sutudiorum - University of Bologna
Bologna, Italy

Mauro Gargiulo, MD, PhD
Full Professor of Vascular Surgery
Chief, Metropolitan Unit of Vascular Surgery
Alma Mater Studiorum - University of Bologna
Bologna, Italy

David L. Gillespie, MD, RVT, FACS
Professor of Surgery
Uniformed Services University
Department of Vascular and Endovascular Surgery
Cape Cod Hospital
Hyannis, Massachusetts

Catherine C. Go, MD
Vascular Surgery Resident
University of Pittsburgh Medical Center
Pittsburgh, Pennsylvania

Michael R. Hall, MD
Major, USAF, USAFSAM
Visiting Assistant Professor of Surgery
University of Maryland School of Medicine
Department of Surgery, Division of Vascular Surgery
Baltimore, Maryland

Linda M. Harris, MD, FACS, DFSVS
Professor of Surgery
Program Director Vascular Surgery Residency and Fellowship
Jacobs School of Medicine & Biomedical Sciences, University at Buffalo
Buffalo, New York

Jeffrey C. Hnath, MD
Assistant Professor of Surgery
Albany Medical College/Albany Medical Center Hospital
Albany, New York

Niamh Hynes, MD, MMSc, ChM, FRSCI, FEBVS
Senior Vascular and Endovascular Surgery Fellow
Department of Vascular and Endovascular Surgery
Galway Clinic
Royal College of Surgeons in Ireland and National University of Ireland
Galway Affiliated Hospital
Doughiska
Galway, Ireland

Karl A. Illig, MD
Vascular Surgeon
Dialysis Access Institute
Orangeburg, South Carolina

Lalithapriya Jayakumar, MD
Assistant Professor
Division of Vascular and Endovascular Surgery
University of Texas Health San Antonio
San Antonio, Texas

Samir R. Kapadia, MD
Chairman
Department of Cardiovascular Medicine
Professor, Lerner College of Medicine
Cleveland Clinic
Cleveland, Ohio

Jussi M. Kärkkäinen, MD, PhD
Consultant, Vascular Surgery
Heart Center, Kuopio University Hospital
Kuopio, Finland

Piotr M. Kasprzak, MD
Professor and Senior Expert
Department of Vascular Surgery
University Medical Center
Regensburg, Germany

Edel P. Kavanagh, MSc, PhD
Research Associate
Department of Vascular and Endovascular Surgery
Galway Clinic
Royal College of Surgeons in Ireland and National University of Ireland
Galway affiliated Hospital
Doughiska
Galway, Ireland

Sikandar Z. Khan, MD
Clinical Assistant Professor of Surgery
Jacobs School of Medicine & Biomedical Sciences
SUNY at Buffalo
Buffalo, New York

Zachary W. Kostun, MD
Vascular Health Partners
Community Care Physicians, P.C.
Latham, New York

Dimitrios Koudoumas, MD, PhD
Division of Vascular Surgery
Jacobs School of Medicine and Biomedical Sciences
State University of New York at Buffalo
Buffalo, New York

Chandan Krishna, MD
Assistant Professor of Neurosurgery
Senior Associate Consultant, Department of Neurological Surgery
Mayo Clinic
Phoenix, Arizona

Amar Krishnaswamy, MD
Section Head
Interventional Cardiology
Director, Sones Cardiac Catheterization Laboratories
Program Director, Interventional Cardiology Fellowship
Cleveland Clinic
Cleveland, Ohio

Brajesh K. Lal, MD, FACS
Department of Vascular Surgery
University of Maryland Medical School
Baltimore, Maryland;
Department of Biomedical Engineering
University of Maryland
College Park, Maryland

Evan D. Lehrman, MD, FSIR
Assistant Professor
Clinical Radiology
University of California
San Francisco, California

Elad I. Levy, MD, MBA, FACS, FAHA
L. Nelson Hopkins Chair of Neurological Surgery and Professor of Neurosurgery and Radiology
Jacobs School of Medicine and Biomedical Sciences at the University at Buffalo
Buffalo, New York

Patric Liang, MD
Integrated Vascular Surgery Resident
Department of Surgery
Division of Vascular and Endovascular Surgery
Beth Israel Deaconess Medical Center;
Harvard Medical School
Boston, Massachusetts

Jaims Lim, MD
Neurosurgery Resident
Department of Neurosurgery
Jacobs School of Medicine and Biomedical Sciences at the University at Buffalo;
Department of Neurosurgery
Gates Vascular Institute at Kaleida Health
Buffalo, New York

Mahmoud B. Malas, MD, MHS, RPVI, FACS
Professor In Residence
Vice Chair of Surgery For Clinical Research
Chief Division Vascular and Endovascular Surgery
University of California San Diego, Health System
San Diego, California

Luke Marone, MD, DFSVS
Professor of Surgery and Radiology
Co-Director Heart and Vascular Institute
Chief Division of Vascular and Endovascular Surgery
West Virginia University
Morgantown, West Virginia

James F. McKinsey, MD, FACS
Mount Sinai Endowed Professor of Vascular Surgery and Interventional Radiology
Systems Chief of Aortic Intervention
Mount Sinai Health Systems
New York, New York

Katherine K. McMackin, MD
Vascular Integrated Resident
Department of Surgery
Cooper University Hospital
Camden, New Jersey

Manish Mehta, MD, MPH
Director
Vascular Health Partners
Community Care Physicians, P.C.
President/CEO, Center for Vascular Awareness, Inc.
Latham, New York

George H. Meier, MD
Attending Surgeon
CHI Franciscan Healthcare
Silverdale, Washington

Ross Milner, MD, FACS
Professor of Surgery
Section of Vascular Surgery and Endovascular Therapy
Co-Director, Center for Aortic Diseases
The University of Chicago Medicine & Biological Science
Chicago, Illinois

Brittany C. Montross, MD
Clinical Assistant Professor of Surgery
University at Buffalo
Jacobs School of Medicine and Biomedical Sciences
Buffalo, New York

John F. Morrison, MD
Neurosurgeon
Morrison Clinic
Delray Beach, Florida

Nicolas J. Mouawad, MD, MPH, MBA, FSVS, FACS, FRCS, RPVI
Chief and Medical Director
Vascular & Endovascular Surgery
McLaren Health System – Bay Region
Bay City, Michigan

Albeir Y. Mousa, MD, FACS, DFSVS, CWS, MBA, MPH, RPVI
Professor
Department of Surgery
Vascular and Endovascular Surgery Division
West Virginia University
Charleston, West Virginia

Gustavo S. Oderich, MD
Chair, Division of Vascular and Endovascular Surgery
Professor of Surgery
Program Director, Vascular and Endovascular Surgery Integrated Residency and Fellowship
Program Director, Advanced Endovascular Aortic Fellowship
The University of Texas Health Science Center
Houston, Texas

Thomas F.X. O'Donnell, MD
Vascular Fellow
Beth Israel Deaconess Medical Center
Massachusetts General Hospital
Boston, Massachusetts

Kyriakos Oikonomou, MD
Associate Professor and Deputy Chief
Department of Vascular Surgery
University Medical Center
Regensburg, Germany

Christine Ou, DO
Vascular Surgeon
Sentara RHM Hospital
Harrisonburg, Virginia

Jean M. Panneton, MD, FRCSC, FACS
Professor of Surgery
Division Chief of Vascular Surgery
Director of Vascular Surgery Fellowship and Integrated Residency Programs at Eastern Virginia Medical School
Norfolk, Virginia

Devi P. Patra, MBBS, MCh, MRCSED
Neurosurgery Resident
Mayo Clinic
Phoenix, Arizona

Karin Pfister, MD
Professor and Chief
Department of Vascular Surgery
University Medical Center
Regensburg, Germany

Rodolfo Pini, MD, PhD
Vascular Surgeon, Metropolitan Unit of Vascular Surgery
Alma Mater Sutudiorum - University of Bologna
Bologna, Italy

Richard J. Powell, MD
Chief, Section of Vascular Surgery
Dartmouth Hitchcock Medical Center
Lebanon, New Hampshire
Professor of Surgery and Radiology
Dartmouth Geisel School of Medicine
Hanover, New Hampshire

Joseph D. Raffetto, MD
Chief of Vascular Surgery
Department of Surgery
Division of Vascular Surgery
VA Boston Healthcare System
West Roxbury, Massachusetts
Associate Professor of Surgery
Harvard Medical School
Brigham and Women's Hospital
Boston, Massachusetts

Andre R. Ramdon, MBBS
Vascular Fellow
Albany Medical Center Hospital
Albany, New York

Animesh Rathore, MD
Assistant Professor
Eastern Virginia Medical School
Norfolk, Virginia

Reid Ravin, MD
Assistant Professor Surgery, Departments of Surgery and Radiology at the Icahn School of Medicine at Mount Sinai
New York, New York

Amy B. Reed, MD, DFSVS, RPVI
Director, M Health Fairview Vascular Services
Professor and Chief, Vascular and Endovascular Surgery
University of Minnesota
Minneapolis, Minnesota

Brendon Reilly, MD, RPVI
Division of Vascular Surgery
Jacobs School of Medicine and Biomedical Sciences
State University of New York at Buffalo
Buffalo, New York

Timothy Resch, MD, PhD
Consultant Vascular Surgeon, Rigshospitalet, Copenhagen, Denmark
Associate Professor, Lund University
Lund, Sweden

Robert Rhee, MD
Chief of Vascular Surgery
Maimonides Medical Center
Brooklyn, New York

Mariel Rivero, MD
Assistant Professor of Surgery
Jacobs School of Medicine and Biomedical Sciences
State University at Buffalo
VA Western NY Healthcare System
Buffalo, New York

Mithun G. Sattur, MD, MBBS, MCh, FEBNS
Department of Neurosurgery
Division of Neuroendovascular Surgery
Medical University of South Carolina
Charleston, South Carolina

Marc L. Schermerhorn, MD, FACS
George H. A. Clowes Jr. Professor of Surgery
Harvard Medical School
Chief, Vascular and Endovascular Surgery
Beth Israel Deaconess Medical Center
Harvard Medical School
Boston, Massachusetts

Hakeem J. Shakir, MD
Neurosurgery
SSM Health
Oklahoma City
Ohlahoma

Murray L. Shames, MD, DFSVS, FACS
Professor and Chief Division of Vascular Surgery
Vice-Chair of Clinical Operations, Department of Surgery
USF Health Morsani School of Medicine
Co-Director Tampa General Hospital Heart and Vascular Institute
Tampa, Florida

Michael Shih, MD
Assistant Professor of Surgery
Division of Vascular Surgery
UT Southwestern Medical Center
Dallas, Texas

Daniel M. Shivapour, MD
Fellow in Interventional Cardiology
Department of Cardiovascular Medicine
Cleveland Clinic
Cleveland, Ohio

Adnan H. Siddiqui, MD, PhD, FACS, FAHA
Professor of Neurosurgery and Radiology
Jacobs School of Medicine and Biomedical Sciences
University at Buffalo, State University of New York;
Gates Vascular Institute at Kaleida Health
Buffalo, New York

Kenneth V. Snyder, MD, PhD, FACS, FAANS
Associate Professor
Departments of Neurosurgery and Neurology
Jacobs School of Medicine and Biomedical Sciences at the University at Buffalo
State University of New York;
Department of Neurosurgery
Gates Vascular Institute at Kaleida Health
Buffalo, New York

Andrea Stella, MD
Full Professor of Vascular Surgery
Alma Mater Studiorum - University of Bologna
Bologna, Italy

Michael C. Stoner, MD, FACS, DFSVS
Professor and Chief
Vascular Surgery University of Rochester
Rochester, New York

Sherif Sultan, MCh, MD, FRCS, FACS, PhD
Professor
Department of Vascular and Endovascular Surgery
Western Vascular Institute and
Galway Clinic
Royal College of Surgeons in and National University of Ireland
Galway affiliated Hospital
Doughiska
Galway, Ireland

Michael Sywak, MD, DABS
Vascular and Endovascular Surgeon
Cookeville Regional Medical Center
Cookeville, Tennessee

Tiziano Tallarita, MD
Consultant, Vascular and Endovascular Surgery
Department of CardioVascular Surgery
Mayo Clinic Health System
Eau Claire, Wisconsin

Tze-Woei Tan, MD, MPH, FACS
Associate Professor
Division of Vascular Surgery
University of Arizona
Tucson, Arizona

Emanuel R. Tenorio, MD, PhD
Aortic Research Fellow
Department of Cardiothoracic and Vascular Surgery
The University of Texas Health Science Center at Houston
Houston, Texas

Matthew J. TerBush, MD
Clinical Assistant Professor
UPMC Hamot Medical Center
Erie, Pennsylvania

Fucheng Tian, MD
Department of Neurological Surgery
The First Affiliated Hospital of Harbin Medical University
Harbin, China

Kenneth Tran, MD
Resident
Division of Vascular Surgery
Stanford University School of Medicine
Stanford, California

Brant W. Ullery, MD, FACS, FSVS
Medical Director
Vascular and Endovascular Surgery
Providence Heart and Vascular Institute
Portland, Oregon

Kunal Vakharia, MD
Fellow
Mayo Clinic
Rochester, Minnesota

David L. Waldman, MD, PhD
Professor of Imaging and Surgery
Department of Imaging Sciences
University of Rochester
Strong Memorial Hospital
Rochester, New York

Sophie Wang, MD
Integrated Vascular Surgery Resident
Department of Surgery
Division of Vascular and Endovascular Surgery
Beth Israel Deaconess Medical Center
Harvard Medical School
Boston, Massachusetts

Joshua L. Weintraub, MD, FSIR
Executive Vice Chair
Director, Vascular and Interventional Radiology
Professor of Radiology (in Surgery) at CUIMC
Columbia University Irving Medical Center
New York Presbyterian Hospital
New York, New York

Matthew E. Welz, MS
Department of Neurological Surgery
Mayo Clinic
Phoenix, Arizona

Karen Woo, MD, MS
Associate Professor of Surgery
Division of Vascular Surgery and Endovascular Therapy
Department of Surgery
David Geffen School of Medicine
University of California Los Angeles
Los Angeles, California

Mathew Wooster, MD
Assistant Professor of Surgery
Division of Vascular Surgery
Medical University of South Carolina
Charleston, South Carolina

Winona Wu, MD
Integrated Vascular Surgery Resident
Department of Surgery
Division of Vascular and Endovascular Surgery
Beth Israel Deaconess Medical Center;
Harvard Medical School
Boston, Massachusetts

Michael Yacoub, MD, FACS, RPVI
Assistant Professor of Surgery
Vascular and Endovascular Therapy
University of Florida
Gainesville, Florida

Nikolaos Zacharias, MD, FSVS, FACS
Clinical Assistant Professor of Surgery
Section of Vascular Surgery
Dartmouth-Hitchcock Medical Center
Dartmouth Geisel School of Medicine
Lebanon, New Hampshire

Wayne W. Zhang, MD, FACS
Professor of Surgery
Division of Vascular and Endovascular Surgery
University of Washington
Puget Sound VA Healthcare System
Seattle, Washington

FOREWORD

Much has been written about the advantages of endovascular treatments for various vascular lesions. Some of these writings have dealt with the limitations of endovascular treatments. Other articles have dealt with specific complications of endovascular methods of therapy. However, there is no current textbook that systematically reviews complications of endovascular treatments, how to prevent them and how to manage them. The authors of the present volume fill this gap.

They begin with a discussion of various vascular access methods, what can go wrong with them, what complications can occur, and how to prevent and treat them.

Then, in a systematic way, they examine the many endovascular treatments used in all the important vascular beds exclusive of the coronary circulation. They describe the complications of the standard and newer endovascular treatments used within these vascular beds, methods to prevent these complications, and how to treat them when they do occur. Transcatheter aortic valve replacement (TAVR) and complications of various forms of angiography are also briefly discussed.

Excellence in administering any form of manipulative treatment requires the ability to deal with the unexpected, including complications. The methods described will allow the endovascular therapist not only to avoid many problems but also to recognize others early so they can be resolved effectively. Adverse outcomes and litigation can thereby be minimized. Because of these assets, this unique book will be invaluable for any physician or surgeon practicing endovascular interventions. It is a "must have" volume for all those involved in endovascular treatments.

Frank J. Veith, MD

CONTENTS

INTRODUCTION

In the past several decades there has been a revolution in the way we practice vascular surgery, with endovascular interventions becoming first-line therapy for most vascular beds. Consequently, there has been an explosion in technology, with a constant influx of new devices and interventions. It is not always possible even for experienced providers to be completely familiar with the potential complications that can occur while employing new technology and utilizing new devices. Manufacturing companies frequently provide a clinical specialist as technical support; however, physicians cannot solely rely on these representatives to always be available or knowledgeable about all of the potential difficulties that can occur. This book addresses the management of a wide range of periprocedural complications, with a secondary focus on device-specific issues. In addition, it provides streamlined guidance in the event an intraprocedural complication occurs, thus averting greater long-term issues. Both common and uncommon complications are discussed in detail, featuring the firsthand expertise of over 50 renowned interventionalists, and in-depth information provided by device manufacturers. The availability of this volume as an e-book allows it to be accessed from mobile devices during procedures to serve as a troubleshooting guide in the field.

Many of us are familiar with Morbidity and Mortality conferences. These originated in Boston under the auspices of Ernest Codman, who promulgated the meetings in order to identify mistakes in care and to improve the treatment of future patients. While we all wish we were infallible, it is clear that as we continue to push boundaries in vascular disease, particularly involving new technology, we will sometimes encounter unexpected complications. As Winston Churchill once said, "All men make mistakes, but only wise men learn from their mistakes." By gathering some of the best and brightest minds' wisdom and experience, our goal is to decrease the risk of truly serious adverse events during endovascular intervention.

Maciej L. Dryjski
Linda M. Harris

Access Complications

Michael Yacoub, MD, FACS, RPVI and Ali F. AbuRahma, MD, FRCS, FACS, RVT, RPVI

INTRODUCTION

The common femoral artery (CFA) is considered the most frequently used percutaneous arterial access site.[1] Multiple methods are used as a landmark for entry, including pulse palpation, fluoroscopic guidance, and ultrasound-guided puncture to achieve arterial access. Many access-related complications can occur, and some are life and limb threatening, such as retroperitoneal hemorrhage or arterial occlusion. Older studies have reported femoral access site complication rates ranging from 2% to 17% in patients undergoing diagnostic and interventional procedures.[2–4] A more recent study has shown femoral access complications of 1.8% for diagnostic and 4% for interventional procedures.[5] Arterial sheath placement into the CFA, and not the deep or superficial femoral artery (SFA), has been shown to decrease access complications. The purpose of this chapter is to discuss the common complications caused by femoral artery access and their management.

RISK FACTORS

Vascular access site complications are the most frequent cause of complications during peripheral vascular and coronary interventions. Risk factors for access complications can be divided into physiological (patient related) and anatomical (procedure related). Physiological risk factors include female gender, body mass index, older age, peripheral vascular disease, renal failure, and low platelet count.[6–8] Anatomical related factors include previous catheterization, high doses of anticoagulation and prolonged anticoagulation, use of thrombolytic agents, use of GP IIb/IIIa inhibitors, larger arterial sheaths, concomitant venous sheaths, prolonged sheath placement, and prolonged procedure duration.[6–8]

Identifying patients with these risk factors is a crucial step in planning the appropriate access site and technique to decrease the incidence of access complications. Most of these complications are preventable by following a good patient selection process, utilizing a thorough history and physical examination and a good access technique. History of prior interventions, previous groin complications, use of closure devices, prior groin radiation, and use of anticoagulation should be documented prior to the procedure. A thorough physical examination, including inspection of the groin for any signs of infection, scars from previous surgeries, and palpation of the femoral pulse, will minimize surprises on the day of the procedure and will decrease the risk of complications.

IDEAL PUNCTURE SITE

The CFA is defined as the continuation of the external iliac artery from the level of the inguinal ligament to its bifurcation into the profunda femoris artery and the SFA. It is relatively large, less involved with atherosclerosis, and compressible against the underlying head of the femur. The ideal site of femoral arterial puncture is at the CFA at a point approximately 1 cm lateral to the most medial aspect of the middle of the femoral head (Fig. 1.1). Caudal punctures usually result in more tendencies for sheath insertion below the bifurcation into the SFA or the profunda femoral artery. These vessels don't have the underlying bony structure, resulting in increased incidents of bleeding, hematoma, and pseudoaneurysm (PSA) formation.[9,10] The inferior epigastric artery courses toward the inguinal ligament, then turns upwards in a U-shape configuration. The lowest point of the inferior epigastric artery corresponds to the inguinal ligament. Any arterial puncture above the level of the lowest point of inferior epigastric artery is associated with a significant increase in the risk of retroperitoneal hemorrhage.[6]

Despite agreement on the optimal location for artery puncture, there is a large variation in the landmarks utilized to identify the puncture site. The most commonly used landmarks are the inguinal skin crease, maximal pulsation, and bony landmarks.[11] The inguinal skin crease is located 3 cm below the inguinal ligament in 95% of cases and

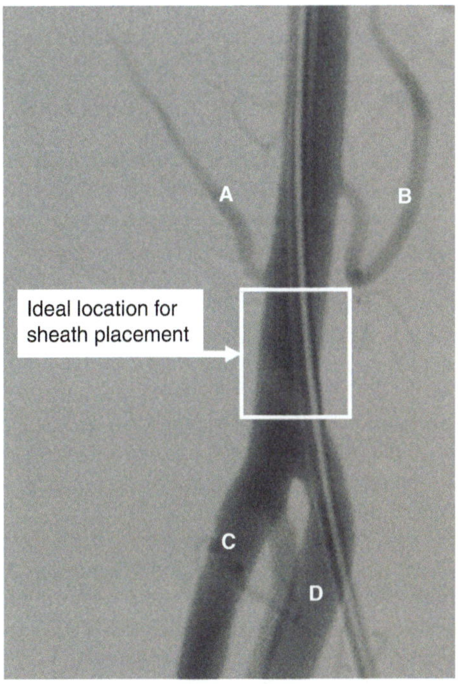

Fig. 1.1 Right common femoral artery angiogram in an ipsilateral oblique view. The square outlines the area of the CFA that is ideal for sheath placement. The arteries are labeled as follows: (A) deep circumflex iliac artery, (B) inferior epigastric artery, (C) profunda femoris artery, and (D) superficial femoral artery.

(From Bates MC, Campbell JE. Technical issues in coronary and peripheral procedures. In: Lanzer P, ed. *Pan Vascular Medicine*, Berlin Heidelberg: Springer-Verlag; 2015: 1465, Chapter 47, Fig. 5.)

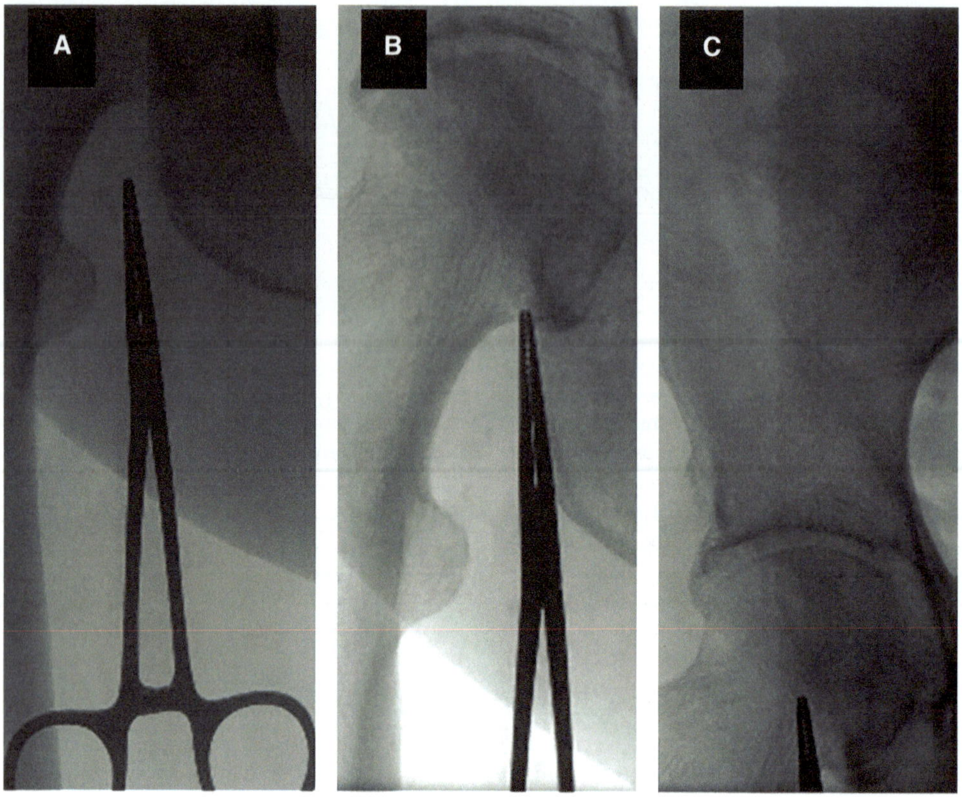

Fig. 1.2 The fluoroscopic images demonstrate parallax in a single obese patient (note the hemostats did not change position on the surface of the patient), with the center of the field of view changing from below the femoral head (A), mid-femoral head (B), and above the femoral head (C). This figure demonstrates the importance of placing the x-ray source as near to the center of the field of view as possible to limit the effect of parallax.

(From Bates MC, Campbell JE. Technical issues in coronary and peripheral procedures. In: Lanzer P, ed. *PanVascular Medicine*, Berlin Heidelberg: Springer-Verlag; 2015: 1466, Chapter 47, Fig. 7.)

doesn't correlate with its location.[12] It is the least reliable method and should be avoided. The point of maximum pulse can often be obscured by obesity, prior hematoma, or scarring from previous surgery; this makes it less reliable.

The anatomic relationship of the CFA to the underlying femoral head is relatively constant. Garrett et al. found that the CFA overlies the femoral head in 92% of cases. They also concluded that the femoral head has a consistent relationship to the CFA, and localization using fluoroscopy is a useful landmark.[13] However, there are critical issues that must be considered in the application of this technique, including the impact of parallax. Placing a hemostat on an obese patient to identify the femur head may be misleading, and correction of the parallax is important prior to arterial cannulation (Fig. 1.2).

During the past decade, real-time ultrasound guidance has gained popularity among angiographers. It allows the user to visualize, in real time, the needle as it enters the ideal point in the mid-CFA. The Femoral Arterial Access with Ultrasound Trial (FAUST) randomized patients to fluoroscopic- versus ultrasound-guided puncture.[14] This study showed no significant difference in successful CFA cannulation rates between the fluoroscopic group versus the ultrasound-guided group. However, in the subgroup of patients with a high bifurcation, there was a significant difference in favor of ultrasound. Ultrasound guidance also improved the first-pass success rate, reduced the number of attempts, decreased inadvertent venipuncture, reduced median time to access, and decreased subsequent vascular complications. Visualizing the tip of the needle entering the mid portion of the CFA is a very critical step when using real-time ultrasound guidance. Failure to perform this step adequately can result in a higher puncture rate by "losing sight" of the needle tip that transverses the tissue in a cephalad trajectory.

Most physicians in the authors' institution prefer a combined approach. First, the femur head is identified by fluoroscopy. Then, real-time ultrasound guidance is used to identify the CFA bifurcation. The tip of the puncturing needle has to be identified in the middle of the CFA prior to advancing the wire and placing the sheath. If the CFA can't be safely identified using ultrasound guidance, a fluoroscopy-assisted technique using a Doppler needle (SMART needle) is used. The CFA is identified using fluoroscopy and the artery is punctured using the Doppler needle. This allows the operators to identify the CFA waveform, which reduces inadvertent venous and arterial branch punctures.

GROIN HEMATOMA AND PSEUDOANEURYSM

Etiology and Clinical Presentation

Bleeding complications from a femoral artery access and sheath insertion have a wide range of clinical manifestations, ranging from localized hematoma to life-threatening hemorrhage. Failure of the arteriotomy to completely seal or dislodgment of the formed clot results in a hematoma formation. A PSA is a hematoma with evidence of arterial flow on duplex ultrasound. It has a sac and a neck that track to a nonsealed arteriotomy. The term "pseudo" refers to the sac being surrounded by soft tissue, lacking arterial wall. The reported incidence of femoral artery pseudoaneurysms ranges from 0.2% to 2.9%.[15] Multiple patient-related and procedure-related factors have been identified. Patient-specific factors include body mass index, female gender, degree of arterial calcifications, and preprocedural platelet counts. Procedure-specific risk factors include the urgency of the procedure, site of arterial cannulation, size of the sheath, combined arterial and venous access, procedural antiplatelet medication use, and anticoagulation.[6–8]

PSA is a result of inadequate compression of the blood vessel following sheath removal or failure of a closure device to adequately close the arteriotomy. Identifying the femoral head using fluoroscopy, even when ultrasound is used for access, will decrease the incidence of high or low accesses and prevent inadequate compression. Identifying patients at high risk is crucial in avoiding multiple attempts to obtain access and decreasing the incidence of access complications and PSA formation. Making sure the operating room staff are well trained and capable of performing manual compression will aid in decreasing the overall complication rate. If using closure devices, proper selection and deployment are crucial in decreasing bleeding complications.

The clinical presentation of PSAs is determined by their size. Groin pain, discoloration, and pulsatile mass are manifestations of small PSAs. Larger PSAs can present with compression symptoms, including nerve compression, resulting in neuropathy, compression of adjacent vein causing deep vein thrombosis (DVT), or skin compression causing necrosis. The first step in diagnosing PSA is to perform a thorough physical exam. A pulsatile mass with a systolic bruit is evident on examination, with or without skin manifestations. Limb swelling may also be present. It is caused by an underlying hematoma or PSA compression of the femoral vein that rarely results in DVT. Kent et al. reported that physical examination was extremely accurate, with a sensitivity of 83% and a specificity of 100%.[16]

Diagnosis and Management

Groin Hematoma

Arterial duplex is the study of choice for the diagnosis of patients with a groin complication after CFA access. It is considered the primary study for size monitoring for conservative treatment. It is also used for direct manual compression and thrombin injection, if a nonsurgical approach is considered. Duplex imaging using B-mode identifies hematomas as a hypoechoic mass and measures their size. The color flow imaging is used to assess flow to differentiate a hematoma from a PSA. Color flow will demonstrate the classic "yin–yang" shape as arterial blood leaves the arteriotomy and reflects back into the artery. Doppler waveform analysis should also be performed to rule out the presence of concomitant arteriovenous fistulae, presenting with a low resistance pattern with a diastolic flow component.

Groin hematomas can occur acutely in the angiography suite or in the recovery room immediately after the procedure. These hematomas can be a marker for an underlying catastrophe (retroperitoneal bleed or arterial rupture). Direct manual compression on the access site is the first step in management. The patient's vitals should be monitored to identify any hemodynamic instability requiring fluid resuscitation and blood products' administration. All intravenous and oral anticoagulants should be discontinued. Laboratory assessment of coagulation factors, platelets, and hemoglobin should be done every 4–6 hours until corrected. CT angiography may be required if retroperitoneal bleeding or active extravasation is suspected.

Asymptomatic groin hematomas should be observed with serial physical exams to assess their growth or resolution, and a duplex ultrasound should be obtained to rule out PSA formation. Most of these hematomas resolve spontaneously and rarely require surgical intervention. Symptomatic hematomas and patients with hemodynamic instability require open groin exploration and evacuation. The femoral vessels should be inspected and the arteriotomy should be primarily repaired. CFA endarterectomy may be required if the artery is significantly diseased.

Pseudoaneurysm

The management of PSA has evolved during the past decade. Multiple approaches have been used including observation, ultrasound-guided compression, ultrasound-guided thrombin injection, and, rarely, open surgical repair.

Observation

Observation plays an important role in the treatment of iatrogenic PSAs, and it's reserved for small asymptomatic PSAs (<3 cm in diameter). Multiple studies have reported successful thrombosis of PSAs with conservative management. Kresowik et al. treated seven PSAs conservatively, ranging in size from 1.3 to 3.5 cm.[17] These PSAs were monitored weekly with serial duplex examinations, and all of them spontaneously thrombosed within 4 weeks from the initial diagnosis. Kent et al.[16] reported that one-third of observed femoral pseudoaneurysms required repair. Nine of 16 pseudoaneurysms spontaneously thrombosed, and the size of these PSAs did not correlate to the number of patients who required repair. Three of the seven patients who required repair were taking anticoagulation medications, which led the authors to recommended PSA repair in patients who require anticoagulation.

Toursarkissian et al. have the largest and most quoted study in the literature.[18] They observed 147 patients with PSAs with a maximum diameter <3 cm. The main exclusions for enrollment were the need for immediate surgical intervention or the use of anticoagulants. Intervention was avoided in 89% of patients, with a mean time to thrombosis of 23 days.[18]

Ultrasound-Guided Compression

Fellmeth et al. reported the first minimal invasive treatment for iatrogenic PSAs in the 1990s. They reported a >90% success rate with ultrasound guided compression, encouraging a nonsurgical approach as the first line of management. The procedure is done by placing the ultrasound probe on the groin with direct visualization of the neck of the PSA. Pressure is applied to the probe to eliminate flow through the PSA neck, with maintenance of arterial flow in the femoral artery and continued evaluation at 5- to 10-minute intervals to assess arrest of flow into the PSA sac. Limitations of this technique include patient discomfort, frequent need for sedative administration for patient comfort, and operator fatigue. In a series of 219 PSAs, the highly statistically significant predictors of failure of ultrasound-guided compression were ongoing anticoagulation and length of aneurysm neck (<10 mm), with a success rate of 71% versus >93%, respectively.[19]

Duplex-Guided Thrombin Injection

Cope and Zeit described the initial technique 25 years ago.[20] Duplex-guided thrombin injection (DGTI) has replaced ultrasound-guided compression as the initial therapy of choice, secondary to the speed of thrombosis, reduction in pain associated with the procedure, and improved success in most series. The procedure is performed under the guidance of B-mode imaging by injecting thrombin directly into the PSA sac. Color Doppler mode is used to assess the PSA thrombosis while the thrombin is being injected. The most significant complication of the procedure is thrombosis of the femoral artery or vein as a result of direct injection of thrombin into these vessels. This can be avoided by visualizing the tip of the needle in the PSA sac prior to thrombin injection, and injection of small amounts of thrombin under color flow imaging to avoid spillover into the arterial system. The patency of the femoral vessels has to be confirmed at the end of the procedure, which can be accomplished using color Doppler mode and by performing a pulse exam.

The largest nonrandomized study directly comparing ultrasound-guided compression and DGTI was reported by Khoury et al.[21] One hundred eighty-nine patients were treated using compression and 131 using DGTI; the success rate favored DGTI (96%) over ultrasound-guided compression (75%). The primary reason for compression failure was pain with compression or deep PSAs that did not allow for adequate compression. DGTI failures were primarily related to intraarterial injection of PSAs <2.5 cm and those with short necks. In the authors' experience of >200 DGTI, we had one patient with acute limb ischemia. This patient presented immediately after the injection procedure with CFA occlusion and underwent successful open surgical thrombectomy.

It appears from the aggregate of retrospective studies that symptomatic and large (>3 cm) PSAs are more effectively treated with DGTI. DGTI should be avoided in asymptomatic patients with a PSA sac <1 cm and PSAs with short necks. These patients should be treated with ultrasound-guided compression or open surgical approach if compression fails.

RETROPERITONEAL HEMORRHAGE

Retroperitoneal hemorrhage is a result of a poor access technique that fails to identify the CFA, causing unsafe cannulation and sheath insertion. High punctures, cephalad to the lowest portion of the inferior epigastric artery, increase the risk of developing retroperitoneal hemorrhage. A puncture at this location is difficult to compress because there is no bony structure (i.e., the femoral head). In addition, the retroperitoneum is a large cavity and can accommodate large amounts of blood, which can result in hemodynamic instability in some patients. Retroperitoneal hemorrhage is rare, but can be life-threatening. High suspicion and early diagnosis are keys to decreasing morbidity and mortality.

Clinical Presentation and Diagnosis

This diagnosis is readily made on clinical presentation and manifests as unexplained hypotension or vagal reaction, either during the procedure or immediately after CFA sheath removal. If the patient complains of vague back pain or abdominal pain after a CFA access procedure, this should raise suspicions of retroperitoneal hemorrhage. A large retroperitoneal bleed may compress the femoral nerve, causing neuropathy. The physical exam is usually unremarkable; however, patients may present with abdominal fullness and flank ecchymosis (Grey Turner sign). Computed tomography (CT) is the diagnostic test of choice, and the use of contrast can aid in identifying the source of bleeding and guiding treatment. Patients with active retroperitoneal hemorrhage can present with continuous dropping of hematocrit and hemodynamic instability. These patients should be stabilized prior to obtaining a CT scan.

Management

Retroperitoneal hemorrhage can be managed conservatively in most cases by aggressive fluid resuscitation, correction of coagulopathy, and transfusion of packer red blood cells to maintain hematocrit. The patient should be placed on bed rest and undergo serial abdominal exams. Serial laboratory tests, including hemoglobin, platelets, and serum creatinine, should be obtained every 4–6 hours. Indications for surgical intervention include hemodynamic instability, continuous drop in hematocrit, and intractable pain and neuropathy. Patients with signs of hemodynamic instability, who respond appropriately to fluid resuscitation, should be evaluated by CT angiography to identify the source of bleeding. Hypotensive patients who are unresponsive to fluid resuscitation should undergo emergent surgical intervention. Both open and endovascular approaches have been described to manage patients with retroperitoneal hemorrhage. There are no randomized trials to guide the treatment strategies for retroperitoneal hemorrhage, and the evidence is based on small cohort series or isolated case reports. In the authors' institution, most physicians prefer an endovascular approach, and open surgery is used only if the bleeding cannot be controlled. A contralateral CFA access is obtained and an angiogram of the iliac and femoral vessels is performed to identify the bleeding source. Hemostasis can be achieved by prolonged balloon inflation at the arteriotomy site or placement of a cover stent. If use of a covered stent is planned, care should be taken not to undersize the graft, as this will lead to continued extravasation. If extravasation from a branch vessel is identified, coil embolization of this vessel can be easily performed. If bleeding can't be controlled using an endovascular approach, retroperitoneal exploration is performed to identify and control the bleeding source.

ARTERIOVENOUS FISTULA

Iatrogenic arteriovenous fistula (AVF), a communication between the femoral artery and vein, following CFA access is rare. Low arterial punctures caudal to the bifurcation of the SFA and profunda femoral artery can increase the risk of AVF formations. Most AVFs are asymptomatic and are detected during physical exam by palpating a thrill or listening to a bruit. They are usually found incidentally during duplex evaluation of a groin hematoma after a CFA access. The clinical significance of an AVF may result from hemodynamically relevant left-to-right shunts. Kelm et al. investigated the clinical outcome of iatrogenic femoral AVF,[22] and found that none of their patients developed cardiac volume overload. In their study, shunt volumes were estimated in the range of 160 to 510 mL/min, which is far below the 30% of cardiac output that is required to deteriorate right heart function.

The incidence of postcatheterization AVFs varied from 0.006% to 2.28%.[16,17] Kent et al. routinely examined patients for a new femoral bruit after cardiac catheterization, followed by a duplex scan. The authors diagnosed six new AVFs in 1838 consecutive patients (0.3%).[16] Kresowik et al. used primary duplex scanning to evaluate patients for an AVF development after CFA access. They diagnosed four new AVFs in only 144 patients, resulting in an incidence of 2.8%.[17] Kelm et al. evaluated a total of 10,271 consecutive patients undergoing cardiac catheterization who were followed prospectively over 3 years and reported a 0.86% incidence of AVFs.[22] The risk factors for developing an AVF after CFA access include arterial hypertension, female gender, use of anticoagulation during the procedure, and low arterial puncture.

Diagnosis and Management

Since it is sensitive and cost effective, duplex ultrasound is the study of choice for the diagnosis of iatrogenic AVFs. A communication between the artery and vein is identified on color flow Doppler with evidence of low resistance, diastolic flow in the CFA, and arterialization of the venous signal. CT and magnetic resonance (MR) imaging play an essential role in the diagnosis of extremity AVFs; however, in most cases conventional angiography is still required for accurate lesion localization and tailoring of the surgical or endovascular treatment.

The natural history of traumatic AVFs is poorly understood and, thus, treatment strategies are controversial. Multiple options have been advocated, including observation, open repair, and an endovascular approach. Most AVFs are asymptomatic, which makes observation a safe treatment option. In fact, multiple studies have shown spontaneous resolution of the majority of iatrogenic femoral AVFs with close observation.[17,18] The authors reported no adverse outcomes of the remaining fistulae that persisted and concluded that asymptomatic patients can be managed safely by close observation. Patients who are treated with conservative management should be followed with routine physical exams and duplex surveillance. Surgical intervention is indicated for patients who develop symptoms of congestive heart failure or limb swelling; or for fistulae that show an increase in size on duplex surveillance.

Open surgical repair is performed via the standard groin exploration. Proximal and distal control of the artery and the vein is obtained and the fistula tract is identified and ligated. The artery and vein are repaired primarily or with patch angioplasty in rare occasions. In cases with a delayed diagnosis of AVF, significant enlargement of the surrounding venous structures and nerve damage can potentially cause difficulties. Recent improvements in endovascular techniques have created significant and effective alternatives to surgical treatment. Metallic coils and covered stents have been utilized frequently for endovascular treatment of AVFs. Treating AVFs with covered stents is technically easy and has been reported to have high technical success rates and low complication rates in different series. However, there is no accurate data regarding the long-term follow-up results of using covered stents in peripheral arteries.

THROMBOSIS

Local thrombosis of the CFA is a rare well-known complication after femoral access; however, it is more common in patients with preexisting CFA atherosclerotic disease and patients with previous groin reconstruction. Placing a large-diameter sheath in a small CFA can result in CFA thrombosis. Technical errors while using closure devices and local dissection during CFA access can also cause CFA thrombosis. The risk factors associated with thrombosis of the access site include peripheral vascular disease, advanced age, hypercoagulable state, small caliber vessels, and female gender.

CFA occlusion results in a sudden onset of lower extremity pain, pallor, and absence of distal pulses. The symptoms may not be sudden, if peripheral vascular disease and collateral flow are present. These patients may present with worsening claudication or a new onset of rest pain days or weeks after intervention. Acute limb ischemia, requiring immediate revascularization, may develop. An open surgical approach with CFA endarterectomy and patch angioplasty is preferred. Thromboembolectomy using a Fogarty catheter should be performed to confirm adequate in-flow and out-flow. An endovascular approach using catheter-directed thrombolysis and mechanical thrombectomy is an alternative to open surgery. Using a small sheath in high-risk patients can reduce CFA thrombosis. Appropriate anticoagulation and adequate heparinized saline flushing of the CFA sheath during the procedure is necessary to help prevent local thrombosis.

GROIN INFECTION

Groin infections after CFA access are extremely rare and have a delayed presentation of 1 to 2 weeks postoperatively. Gram-positive organisms, especially *Staphylococcus aureus*, are the predominate causes of groin abscesses and endarteritis associated with femoral arterial cannulation. Patients present with local signs of infection, including pain and erythema. Fluctuation and local discharge are present in cases with abscess formation, and fever and rigors indicate systemic involvement.

Duplex ultrasound can diagnose groin abscesses and rule out the involvement of the CFA and the presence of PSAs. CT angiography is another modality to confirm the diagnosis of groin abscesses and evaluate for arterial involvement. A complete blood count and blood cultures should be obtained in all patients to assess the level of involvement. A local infection at the access site without abscess formation responds well to oral antibiotics, while systemic involvement requires hospitalization and intravenous antibiotics. Treatment consists of operative exploration and drainage of the abscess. If the arterial wall is involved, debridement of all necrotic tissue and repair with vein patch angioplasty or interposition vein graft is necessary. In cases with significant tissue loss, coverage with a muscle flap can improve wound healing. Extraanatomic bypass (obturator bypass) should be considered in complex cases where groin reconstruction is not feasible.

REFERENCES

1. Noto TJ, Johnson LW, Krone R, et al. Cardiac catheterization 1990: a report of the registry of the Society for Cardiac Angiography and Interventions. *Cathet Cardiovasc Diagn.* 1991;24:75.
2. Pompa JJ, Satler LF, Pichard AD, et al. Vascular complications after balloon and new device angioplasty. *Circulation.* 1993;88:1569–1578.
3. Muller DW, Shamir KJ, Ellis SG, et al. Peripheral vascular complications after conventional and complex percutaneous coronary interventional procedures. *Am J Cardiol.* 1992;69:63–68.
4. Blankenship JC, Hellkamp AS, Aquirre FV, et al. Vascular access site complications after percutaneous coronary intervention with abciximab in the evaluation of c7E3 for the prevention of ischemic complications (EPIC) trial. *Am J Cardiol.* 1998;81:36–40.
5. Chandrasekar B, Doucet S, Bilodeau L, et al. Complications of cardiac catheterization in the current era: a single-center experience. *Catheter Cardiovasc Interv.* 2001;52:289–295.
6. Sherev DA, Shaw RE, Brent BN. Angiographic predictors of femoral access site complications: implication for planned percutaneous coronary intervention. *Catheter Cardiovasc Interv.* 2005;65(2):196–202.
7. Wiley JM, White CJ, Uretsky BF. Noncoronary complications of coronary intervention. *Catheter Cardiovasc Interv.* 2002;57(2):257–265.
8. Piper WD, Malenka DJ, Ryan Jr TJ, et al. Predicting vascular complications in percutaneous coronary interventions. *Am Heart J.* 2003;145(6): 1022–1029.
9. Rapoport S, Sniderman K, Morse S, et al. Pseudoaneurysm: a complication of faulty technique in femoral arterial puncture. *Radiology.* 1985;154:529–530.
10. Altin RS, Flicker S, Naidech HJ. Pseudoaneurysm and arteriovenous fistula after femoral artery catheterization: association with low femoral punctures. *Am J Roentgenol.* 1989;152:629–631.
11. Grier D, Hartnell G. Percutaneous femoral artery punctures: practice and anatomy. *Br J Radiol.* 1990;63:602–604.
12. Grossman M. How to miss the profunda femoris. *Radiology.* 1974;111:482.
13. Garrett PD, Eckart RE, Bauch TD, et al. Fluoroscopic localization of the femoral head as a landmark for common femoral artery cannulation. *Catheter Cardiovasc Interv.* 2005;65(2):205–207.
14. Seto AH, Abu-Fadel MS, Sparling JM, et al. Real-time ultrasound guidance facilitates femoral arterial access and reduces vascular complications: FAUST (Femoral Arterial Access with Ultrasound Trial). *JACC Cardiovasc Interv.* 2010;3(7):751–758.

15. Hirano Y, Ikuta S, Uehara H, et al. Diagnosis of vascular complications at the puncture site after cardiac catheterization. *J Cardiol.* 2004;43:259–265.
16. Kent KC, McArdle CR, Kennedy B, et al. A prospective study of the clinical outcome of femoral pseudoaneurysms and arteriovenous fistulas induced by arterial puncture. *J Vasc Surg.* 1993;17:125–133.
17. Kresowik TF, Khoury MD, Miller BV, et al. A prospective study of the incidence and natural history of femoral vascular complications after percutaneous transluminal coronary angioplasty. *J Vasc Surg.* 1991;13:328–336.
18. Toursarkissian B, Allen BT, Petrinec D, et al. Spontaneous closure of selected iatrogenic pseudoaneurysms and arteriovenous fistulae. *J Vasc Surg.* 1997;25:803–809.
19. Fellmeth B, Roberts AC, Bookstein JJ, et al. Postangiographic femoral artery injuries: nonsurgical repair with ultrasound guided compression. *Radiology.* 1991;178:671–675.
20. Cope C, Zeit R. Coagulation of aneurysms by direct percutaneous thrombin injection. *Am J Roentgenol.* 1986;147:383–387.
21. Khoury M, Rebecca A, Greene K, et al. Duplex scanning guided thrombin injection for the treatment of iatrogenic pseudoaneurysms. *J Vasc Surg.* 2002;35:517–521.
22. Kelm M, Perings SM, Jax T, et al. Incidence and clinical outcome of iatrogenic femoral arteriovenous fistulas: Implications for risk stratification and treatment. *JACC Cardiovasc Interv.* 2002;40(2):291–297.

2

Other Access

Christine Ou, DO, Animesh Rathore, MD and Jean M. Panneton, MD, FRCSC, FACS

INTRODUCTION

General Issues

Anatomy

While access sites such as the common femoral artery are easily accessible, sometimes alternative access may be needed as a result of the previous site being infected, scarred, or occluded. Preoperative planning by considering the patient's anatomy, vessel to be accessed, location of intended treatment, positioning of the patient for comfort, and devices needed for treatment is paramount in making the procedure safe and efficient.

Depending on the area of access and body habitus, patients may need further adjustments or retraction of extra tissue, which can be done with tape. Full exposure of the site allows the clinician the ease of access and control.

For patients with heavily scarred access sites, a small incision at the area of access may help advance the sheath through scar tissue. The use of serial dilation is also helpful. In addition, the use of stiffer wires such as Amplatz or Rosen can help with trackability and ability to push forward.

The anatomy of the access site should also be taken into consideration. The diameter of the access vessel will determine the maximum size of sheath that can be placed (Table 2.1). This will in effect determine which device can be delivered through the sheath. Vessel tortuosity can affect the placement of the sheath. It may preclude the full advancement of the sheath or the ability of the device to be able to navigate the curves and turns. If the vessel is very tortuous, use of a stiffer system (wire, guide catheter. and/or sheath) or an alternative access site should be considered.

Pathology

Within the vessel, if the area of desired access is heavily calcified or has significant atherosclerotic plaque, it is difficult and potentially dangerous to insert a sheath through this area. It can cause rupture, dissection, thrombosis, or distal embolization. Preferably, a different access site that does not include the area of stenosis or occlusion should be chosen. If the lesion is not precisely at the access site, adjuncts such as balloon angioplasty with or without stenting can be used to allow the passage of the sheaths through the stenotic vascular segments.

TABLE 2.1 **Arterial characteristics and positioning.**

Artery	Diameter	Positioning
Superficial femoral artery	6–8 mm	Supine, external rotation
Popliteal artery	4–6 mm	Supine with flexion and external rotation, prone
Pedal artery	1–3 mm	Supine
Graft	Various	Various
Radial	2–2.5 mm	Supine with wrist extension
Brachial	3–4 mm	Supine, arm extension
Axillary	4.8–8.0 mm	Abduction, external rotation, flexion of elbow

Location

The location of the intended treatment area will help determine the possible access sites. A shorter working distance from the access site to the treatment site is favorable because of better deliverability, trackability, and torque ability. For longer distances, it may be difficult to navigate devices to the location of interest and to maintain enough support in the system to be able to perform the planned interventions. For access sites in the lower extremity, a lesion at the mid superficial artery or popliteal artery can be potentially accessed from the contralateral common femoral artery, the ipsilateral common femoral artery, pedal access, or brachial access. Brachial access is unlikely to reach tibial or pedal arteries. Patients are supine for most procedures, but popliteal access requires preferentially a prone position or, less frequently, supine position with flexion and external rotation of the leg. Brachial access requires the patient's arm to be supinated and can be extended or abducted if needed (Table 2.2).

Guidance for Puncture

After choosing the appropriate site, there are various types of techniques for access. The preferred technique for obtaining access is with the use of B-mode ultrasound using the longitudinal or transverse view. The vessels are directly identified and the anterior wall is accessed under direct visualization with the needle. The benefits of ultrasound guidance are the visualization of the intended vessel and surrounding structures (adjacent vein, nerve, arterial branches, etc.).[1] With severely calcified vessels, it can also alert the operator that there may be some difficulty with initial access or that another site may need to be considered.

Alternative ways to access include direct pulse palpation combined with anatomic landmarks, fluoroscopy guidance, or the use of Doppler needle. The access needle at the surface of the artery can transmit pulsation, providing a tactile feedback to the operator indicating the access needle is upon the vessel. Alternatively, a Doppler needle will transmit arterial signals with proximity to the artery. These techniques are associated with higher incidence of access-related complication, as the vessels and branch points are not specifically identified.[2] Multiple attempts are frequently needed, with increased risk of back wall injuries as well, subsequent risks of dissections, laceration of the vessel, and bleeding complications. Also, with blind access, the needle can roll off the anterior surface of the artery and enter either the medial or lateral wall instead of the intended anterior wall. This can cause difficulty where compression with direct pressure or closure devices can be

TABLE 2.2 Comparison of access sites.

	Advantages	Disadvantages	Pitfalls	Troubleshooting
Common femoral	Antegrade and retrograde access, most common access site	Difficult in obese patients, previous history of surgery	Calcification, atherosclerotic plaque, anatomic variants	Ultrasound guidance for access, proper positioning of patient
Superficial femoral artery	Antegrade and retrograde access, large diameter, alternative site	Depth of vessel, comfort of positioning	Calcification, atherosclerotic plaque, anatomic variants, hemorrhage can be difficult to control	Ultrasound guidance, balloon occlusion during hemorrhage
Popliteal artery	Antegrade and retrograde access, alternative site	Comfort of positioning, small vessel, short distance for antegrade intervention	Calcification, atherosclerotic plaque, anatomic variants, nerve injury	Ultrasound guidance, balloon occlusion during hemorrhage
Pedal artery	Retrograde access, alternative site	Small vessel	Calcification, atherosclerotic plaque, anatomic variants, spasms	Ultrasound guidance
Graft	Large diameter	Risk of infection, scar tissue	Pseudoaneurysm, hematoma, back wall punctures	Antibiotic periop, suture closure
Radial	Alternative to transfemoral approach	Smaller vessel, spasms, hematoma, nerve injury, long distance	Ischemia to hand, embolism to carotid artery, thrombosis	Allen's test, proper positioning of hand and wrist, ultrasound guidance micropuncture set, antispasmodic
Brachial	Alternative to transfemoral approach	Smaller vessel, spasms, hematoma, nerve injury, long distance	Ischemia to hand, embolism to carotid artery, thrombosis, need for open exposure	Proper positioning of arm, ultrasound guidance micropuncture set, antispasmodic
Axillary	Alternative to transfemoral approach	Smaller vessel, spasms, hematoma, nerve injury, long distance, discomfort with positioning	Ischemia to hand, embolism to carotid artery, thrombosis	Proper positioning of arm, ultrasound guidance micropuncture set, antispasmodic

misplaced with resultant increased risk of bleeding or pseudoaneurysm formation.

Troubleshooting Access Site Complications Applicable to all Sites

Most access site complications can be treated in relatively the same manner. The most common complication is bleeding, which can happen in a wide spectrum of severity from a small hematoma to significant hemorrhage. A balloon brought to the area of injury or even proximal to the injury site can be used to occlude the vessel to temporize while the situation is assessed for more profuse bleeding. Treatment for minor injuries to a vessel include balloon occlusion or a covered stent while open repair for larger injuries.

Arteriovenous fistulas (AVF) can occur whether from initial access through the artery and the vein creating the connection or through wire work. A small AVF can resolve spontaneously or with simple compression. Larger fistulas may need intervention as this can lead to edema of the extremity, high output cardiac failure, or aneurysmal degeneration of the vessel. Exclusion of the fistula may require a covered stent or open surgical repair. When treating AV fistulas, it is critical to size the vessel correctly if endovascular repair is planned. Intravascular Ultrasound (IVUS) is ideal in this manner because an undersized stent graft will continue to permit flow behind the graft and into the fistula. The stent graft can be placed in either the artery or the vein if placement in the artery would risk coverage of critical branches, such as the profunda.

Dissections can be treated with either conservative management, balloon angioplasty, or stent placement, depending upon the extent and disturbance to flow. Initially, a small dissection may be observed or treated with prolonged inflation of a balloon. In many cases, this will resolve small dissections. A dissection that persists and interferes with flow should be further treated.

Thrombosis is another common complication. When accessing smaller arteries, heparinizing the patient prior to sheath placement is important. Use of additional medications, including vasodilators, can be considered for accessing radial arteries, as discussed later. If thrombosis occurs, treatment includes mechanical thrombectomy, pharmacomechanical thrombolysis, or open thrombectomy with or without endarterectomy to remove dissected plaque or large atheroma. Additionally, closure devices should be used with caution in smaller vessels, as many have components that remain intraarterial, and can occlude small vessels.

Pseudoaneurysms can also occur when the puncture site is not adequately sealed initially. These can be identified immediately after the procedure or several days later. A duplex ultrasound is the diagnostic investigation of choice. Cross-sectional imaging such as CT scan and MRI can also be used. Pseudoaneurysms less than 2 cm in size usually resolve spontaneously and rarely need further intervention.[3,4] Ultrasound-guided compression can be considered if it does not spontaneously resolve. For pseudoaneurysms larger than 2 cm, direct thrombin injection with ultrasound guidance is the current standard of care. However, care should be taken to assess for a small neck and the absence of AVF to have greater success and to avoid complications.[3,4] Repeat ultrasound of the area for resolution can further help to guide treatment. For pseudoaneurysms that do not resolve or have wide necks, open repair may be needed (Fig. 2.1).

Small vessels also have the potential of being occluded by the sheaths and catheters and can spasm during the procedure, causing pain and increased risk of thrombosis. This is more commonly seen in upper extremity access sites. To avoid this, intraarterial injection of vasodilator medications such as verapamil, nitroglycerin, or papaverine can be administered to the vessel. A traditional radial cocktail might include 100-200 μg of nitroglycerin, 5 mg of verapamil, and

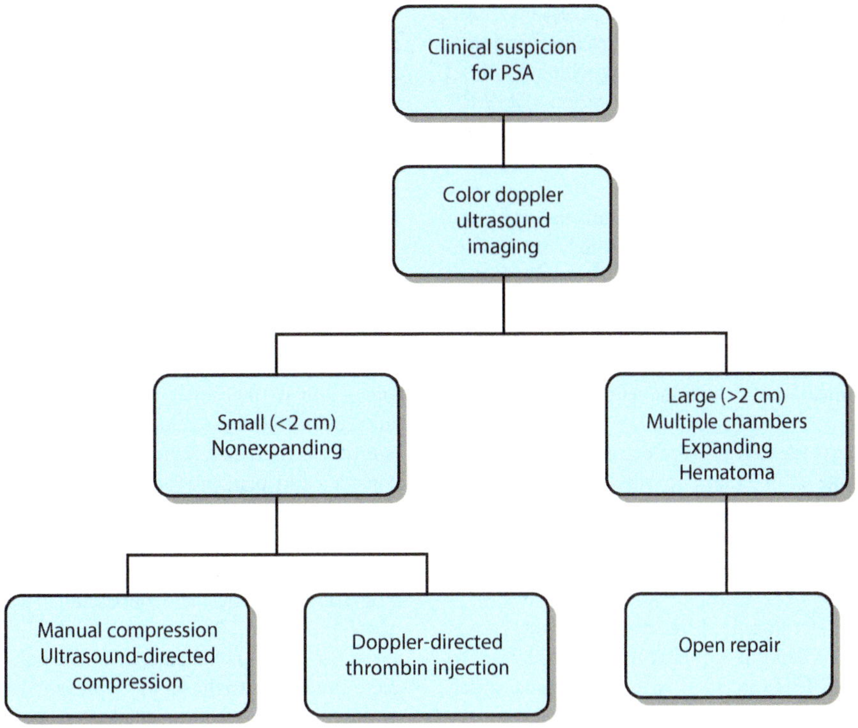

Fig. 2.1 Treatment algorithm for access site pseudoaneurysm.[3,4]

3000 units of heparin. Additional heparin is dosed per patient weight.

ACCESS-SITE-SPECIFIC ISSUES

Lower Extremity Access

Superficial Femoral Artery

Lower extremity access is most commonly achieved through the common femoral artery, which is discussed in Chapter 1. There are times, because of patient anatomy or an occluded vessel, when the access needs to be approached from the superficial femoral artery (SFA). As mentioned earlier, preoperative planning by factoring the anatomy of the patient, patient size, and consideration of the intended treatment area will help decide how to approach the case. Access to the SFA will require the patient to be supine with external rotation at the hip with partial flexion at the knee.

The vessel should be accessed with ultrasound guidance. The SFA is usually 15–70 mm from the surface and 6–8 mm in size, depending on body habitus.[5] In obese patients, the SFA can be much deeper from the surface. The SFA courses posterior to the sartorius with the femoral vein before it courses through the Hunter's canal. Access can be antegrade or retrograde. An angulation of 45 degrees with the needle can aid in correctly accessing the vessel. The sheath is then chosen to provide access for the treatment device.

Common complications for access into the SFA include pseudoaneurysm and AV fistulas. Closure of the vessel is more difficult because compression is less successful as a result of the lack of a bony surface posterior to the artery. Closure devices may be considered, but again should be used cautiously and based on vessel size. Pseudoaneurysm rates can range from 2% to 9%.[6]

Limitations include those mentioned in Table 2.2.

Popliteal Artery

Use of the popliteal artery as an access point can be challenging. The popliteal artery is often used as a retrograde access to treat proximal disease in the SFA or iliac vessels. It can be used as an antegrade access to treat tibial disease, but the ability to have enough support for the sheath is compromised by the distance of the popliteal to the tibial arteries. With the popliteal access, the patient will need to be positioned either in the supine position with external rotation and flexion of the knee or in a prone position. The prone position is the preferred position as it is easier to access and more comfortable for the patient. Ultrasound guidance is highly recommended for access as the popliteal artery is roughly 4–6 mm in size and deep in the popliteal fossa with surrounding veins and nerves.[6]

Complications of the popliteal access include those mentioned above and injury to the distal part of the sciatic nerve, the tibial nerve, or the common peroneal nerve, which can cause significant motor and sensory dysfunction of the lower extremity. This includes loss of sensation of the plantar aspect of the foot, paresthesia to the foot and toes, weakness in the posterior calf and toes, and vasomotor changes, and it potentially causes recurrent ulcerations and paralysis of the muscles of the foot leading to toe deformities.

Limitations associated with this access site include the diameter of the vessel, distance from intended treatment area, spasm and occlusion with the sheath, and comfort of the patient with positioning.

Posterior Tibial, Anterior Tibial, and Peroneal Arteries

Distal tibial access has increasingly been considered as a route when more proximal access and attempt at crossing lesions are difficult to achieve or have failed. Some rotation of the ipsilateral leg may be needed depending on the access vessel, anterior tibial, peroneal, or posterior tibial artery. Dorsalis pedis or anterior tibial access can be done with plantar flexion of the foot while posterior tibial access may need supination. The size of access will depend on whether intervention is planned from the tibial approach or merely crossing with subintimal arterial flossing using antegrade–retrograde intervention (SAFARI) technique. With this technique, microdilators and microcatheters (0.018) are placed and sheaths are entirely avoided to minimize damage to the tibial vessels.

Complications of tibial intervention other than the standard include arterial rupture or bleeding into the calf, which can lead to potential compartment syndrome if control cannot be established. If endovascular occlusion cannot be obtained, patients may require operative repair and fasciotomies. There is also the potential of direct nerve injury from puncture and nerve compression if significant hemorrhage occurs. Complications of pseudoaneurysm and hemorrhage range from 2% to 9%.[7]

Limitations of these access sites include the diameter of the vessel. Pedal vessels are an average of 1–3 mm in size.[5] Smaller sheaths (4 French), 0.018 or 0.014 catheters, and wires will be needed for procedures performed entirely from a tibial access.

Leg Grafts

Patients may have bypass grafts that need intervention at the inflow, outflow, or the distal runoff. When this occurs, it might be necessary to access directly the graft itself. This can occur with aortic grafts, which make traversing the bifurcation difficult, or when patients have severe stenosis at the orifice of the graft, which is not amenable to crossing from above. When this occurs, the bypass graft can act as an access point. Another indication for bypass graft access is to avoid an infected or heavily scarred area. If infection is present, strict sterile procedure should be observed because of the high risk of introducing infection into the bypass graft.

If accessing lower extremity graft in a retrograde fashion, the patient should be supine with the legs in an external rotation with knee flexion. Antibiotics should be administered prior to obtaining access. For grafts that are subcutaneous, it may be possible to palpate and to isolate the graft between your fingers during access, but traditionally ultrasound can help identify the graft and decrease the risk of improper access or through-and-through puncture to the graft. Access close to the proximal anastomosis is appropriate for autogenous grafts with a patent proximal anastomosis to assess fully the entirety of the graft, while avoiding damage to the native vessel or sutures. Another issue to consider is the incorporation of the graft. If the graft is well incorporated, there may be some scar tissue around it that will require slightly greater force, while a newer graft that is not yet incorporated may be more mobile and also at high risk of back-wall puncture. Care is taken to prevent any back-wall puncture especially when new grafts are being accessed as there is greater risk of hematoma formation. Once the needle is in, stiff wires can help track the sheath. If the sheath has a difficult time entering the graft, the access point may need to be serially dilated or a stiffer dilator may need to be used.

As mentioned previously with other access, hemorrhages are a common complication of graft access. Pressure can be held at the site, closure devices can also be used, and a stitch can be placed. Rupture is less of a risk with prosthetic grafts as they have increased tensile strength compared with vein conduits. Rupture is a greater risk at an anastomosis, especially in a new bypass or if an aneurysm is present at anastomotic sites. Knowing the history, bypass anatomy, and correct timing of intervention (i.e., noninfectious period) would help to tailor the intervention to the patient. A limitation of using a prosthetic graft access is the increased risk of infection. Procedural antibiotics and strict attention to sterile technique is suggested as prophylaxis.

Upper Extremity Access

Radial and Brachial Approach

The advantages for using the upper extremity access is that it is a more proximal approach and can be used when the femoral access is unavailable or the lesion is unable to be crossed from the standard approach frequently as a result of stenosis at the origin of iliac arteries, aortic bifurcated grafts, unilateral iliac occlusion, or the need for mesenteric access. This area is also a good choice when the femoral sites are infected and risk of contamination is high. Disadvantages include higher complication rates in women compared with men, 11% and 2.7% respectively, because of smaller vessel size.[8] Hematomas in this area can cause compression and potential median nerve injury. Spasm is not infrequent and can be prevented or treated with vasodilators. The angulation of the aortic arch makes it harder to track devices and sheaths. With the proximal approach, the distance to the intended area is much farther, and device, wire, and sheaths are important things to consider and plan preoperatively. In addition, depending on patient height, some lesions may not be accessible by stents, stent grafts, or even balloons.

Radial access is often used for arch or aortic intervention, neuroangiography, or cardiac catheterization. The radial artery has a diameter of about 2.5 mm.[5] Patients who need a radial artery access first need an Allen test to assess the patency of the radial and ulnar artery and complete circulation to the hand, to prevent a serious complication of hand or digit ischemia. With a radial artery approach and a radial occlusion, the ulnar artery can serve as blood flow to the hand, as long as you have first confirmed an intact palmar arch.

To access the radial artery, the patient's wrist should be positioned in hyperextension with a rolled towel underneath the wrist. Ultrasound guidance can aid in identifying the artery. The area of the artery can be anesthetized to aid in comfort and decrease spasm of the vessel with either topical or local anesthetic. Using a micro puncture needle set is recommended because of the small diameter of the vessel. Difficulty advancing the wire can indicate that the wire is not within the vessel, the wire is at a side branch, the wire is dissecting the vessel, or the artery is in spasm. Vasodilator medications can be directly injected into the vessel, once confirmation of luminal access is obtained. We recommend using a radial artery preparation that includes 100–200 μg of nitroglycerin, 5 mg of verapamil, and 3000 units of heparin. Patients should also be fully heparinized to decrease the risk of thrombosis, which can occur in 1%–10% of patients.[9] Once the wire is within the vessel, sheaths can be slowly advanced. Because of the small size of the vessel, available sheath sizes are limited.

A key limitation is the diameter of the vessel. A 7-French sheath has a 2.9 mm outer diameter, and this may be the largest sheath size amenable for access of radial artery diameters of 2.5 mm.

Neurological complication (NC) rates are similar to transfemoral access with a 0.11% risk of NC in patients undergoing percutaneous coronary interventions.[10]

The brachial artery is a common access site for patients who are unable to have a femoral access or who need a more proximal access than the radial artery. It is approximately 3–5 mm and is easily located with ultrasound guidance superior to the antecubital fossa and 5 mm from the surface.[11] The same principles used to access the radial artery can also be applied here with ultrasound access and use of antispasmodics.

Concerns for the brachial approach echo those of the radial approach. Hemorrhage can be addressed with compression. However, hematoma in this region can lead to nerve compression with long-term sequelae if not rapidly addressed. The brachial artery is difficult to compress as it is mobile. There is a greater risk of ischemia with injury or large sheaths occluding the vessel for prolonged time periods. In the brachial access approach, occlusion or embolization here can potentially cause occlusion to both the radial and ulnar artery, leading to hand ischemia. This must be addressed with thrombectomy of the artery, either angiographically or with open surgery, to reestablish blood flow. Rupture of the vessel is another potential concern that needs to be addressed as an emergency in the operating room. Perforation of the vessel can be the result of a through-and-through or back-wall access. Depending on the degree of perforation, the area may be compressed or may require operative repair. The brachial artery lies close to the median nerve, and injury or compression of the nerve from a hematoma can result in sensory loss in the arm and hand and also weakness in the arm. This neuro deficit requires urgent exploration and decompression with open repair. Dissection of the artery can occur and, depending on the length of the injury, it may be observed with conservative treatment or may require intervention if flow to the hand is compromised. Closure devices can be used and have been comparable to manual compression; however, size of the vessel must be considered in choosing appropriate closure devices (Chapter 3).[12]

As with the radial artery, the size of the brachial artery limits the size of the sheaths that can be used for access, thereby limiting the interventions that can be performed. Sheath sizes from 6 to 8 French can traditionally be used, although the larger the sheath size, the higher the risk of complications.[8] The brachial access can be limited by the length from the intended treatment area. If treating the lower extremities, the distance from the treatment area must be considered in order to plan for the sheaths and devices that need to be used.

Axillary

As for the axillary approach, this is less commonly used but is seen with placement of transcatheter heart valves and with endovascular repair of thoracoabdominal aortic aneurysms requiring an antegrade approach to deliver a branched endograft or for deployment of parallel stent grafts into the visceral vessels requiring larger sheath. Ultrasound guidance can aid in accessing the artery, which can accommodate sheath sizes >7 French. Patients can be positioned with the arm behind their head or extended out. Common complications include hematoma with a rate of 11%–14% and brachial plexus injury.[13]

Carotid Artery

The transcarotid approach has been used for both innominate and carotid intervention, as well as for transcatheter aortic valve implantation and TEVAR. This approach can be achieved most safely under local anesthesia with a small cutdown with distal common carotid artery cross clamping to assess for any neurological changes and to prevent embolization.[14,15]

It is important to understand the options for alternative access when the common femoral artery is unavailable or unsuitable as an access point for intervention. Knowing the risk and benefits of each option can aid the clinician in choosing the access point that will provide the ease, deliverability, intervention, and comfort for the patient, and will reduce complications.

REFERENCES

1. Lo R, Fokkema M, Curran T, et al. Routine use of ultrasound-guided access reduces access-site related complications after lower extremity percutaneous revascularization. *J Vasc Surg.* 2015;61(2):405–412.
2. Seto A, Abu-Fadel M, Sparling J, et al. Real-time ultrasound guidance facilitates femoral arterial access and reduces vascular complications FAUST (Femoral Arterial Access With Ultrasound Trial). *JACC Cardiov Interv.* 2010;3(7):751–758.
3. Toursarkissian B, Allen B, Petrinee D, et al. Spontaneous closure of selected iatrogenic pseudoaneurysms and arteriovenous fistulae. *J Vasc Surg.* 1997;25:803–808.
4. Mishra A, Rao A, Pimpalwar Y. Ultrasound guided percutaneous injection of thrombin: Effective technique for treatment of iatrogenic femoral pseudoaneurysm. *J Clin Diagn Res.* 2017;11(4):TC04–TC06.
5. Steigler H, Brandl R. Importance of ultrasound for diagnosing peripheral arterial disease. *Ultraschall Med.* 2009;30(4):334–371.
6. Gutzeit A, Graft N, Schoch E, et al. Ultrasound-guided antegrade femoral access: comparison between the common femoral artery and the superficial femoral artery. *Eur Radiol.* 2011;21(6):1323–1328.
7. Mustapha J, Diaz-Sandoval L, Jaff M, et al. Ultrasound-guided arterial access: outcomes among patients with peripheral artery disease and critical limb ischemia undergoing peripheral interventions. *J Invasive Cardiol.* 2016;28(6):259–264.
8. Alvarez-Tostado J, Moise M, Bena J, et al. The brachial artery: A critical access for endovascular procedures. *J Vasc Surg.* 2009;49:378–385.
9. Avidkos G, Karatasakis A, Tsoumeleas, et al. Radial artery occlusion after transradial coronary catheterization. *Cadiovasc Diagn Ther.* 2017;7(3):305–316.
10. Ratib K, Mamas M, Routledge H, et al. Influence of access site choice on incidence of neurologic complications after percutaneous coronary intervention. *Am Heart J.* 2013;165:317–324.
11. Tomiyama Y, Yoshinaga K, Fujii S, et al. Accurate quantitative measurements of brachial artery cross-sectional vascular area and vascular volume elastic modulus using automated oscillometric measurements: comparison with brachial artery ultrasound. *Hypertens Res.* 2015;38:478–484.
12. Mirza A, Steerman S, Ahanchi, et al. Analysis of vascular closure devices after transbrachial artery access. *Vasc Endovascular Surg.* 2014;48(7):466–469.
13. Schafer U, Deuschl F, Schofer N, et al. Safety and efficacy of the percutaneous transaxillary access for transcatheter aortic valve implantation using various transcatheter heart valves in 100 consecutive patients. *Int J Cardiol.* 2017;232:247–254.
14. Makaloski V, Deimling C, Mordasini, et al. Transcarotid approach for retrograde stenting of proximal innominate and common carotid artery stenosis. *Ann Vasc Surg.* 2017;43:242–248.
15. Azmoun A, Amabile N, Ramadan R, et al. Transcatheter aortic valve implantation through carotid artery access under local anaesthesia. *Eur J Cardiothorac Surg.* 2014;46(4):693–698.

3

Vascular Closure Devices for Small Arteriotomies: How to Avoid and Deal With Complications

Evan D. Lehrman, MD, FSIR and Joshua L. Weintraub, MD, FSIR

INTRODUCTION: OPTIONS FOR ACHIEVING HEMOSTASIS

Arterial access was first described by Sven Ivar Seldinger in the 1950s and is increasingly being utilized as open surgeries are replaced by minimally invasive image-guided procedures. The common femoral artery (CFA) continues to be one of the preferred sites of access for both diagnostic angiography and percutaneous interventions ranging from coronary artery stenting to aortic aneurysm repair.

Vascular closure devices (VCD) were introduced in the 1990s to help achieve hemostasis in the common femoral artery after angiography. Prior to closure devices, manual compression (MC) of the CFA between the skin and the femoral head for at least 15 minutes, followed by a mandatory 6-hour bedrest, was used to achieve hemostasis after arterial access. This technique is still considered the gold standard and can be used if a VCD fails, is contraindicated, or when the operator does not wish to leave an implant behind. The advantages of manual compression include low complication rate, no significant learning curve, and no direct cost. However, increased physician time and pain at the compression site represent drawbacks. Furthermore, MC may not be safe in select populations. Application of MC in very obese patients may not deliver the necessary pressure to achieve hemostasis at the arteriotomy. Patients with lumbar disc herniation and other musculoskeletal or nerve derangements may not be able to tolerate the 6-hour period of bedrest required to consolidate the hemostasis achieved by manual compression. With the increased use of periprocedural anticoagulant and antiplatelet medications, risk of bleeding complications after initial hemostasis with MC has increased.[1]

Advantages of vascular closure devices include immediate hemostasis, early ambulation, hemostasis despite anticoagulation/antiplatelet administration, hemostasis in high or low punctures that cannot be compressed against the femoral head, and improved comfort. Expense (which may be offset by improved workflow), clinical learning curve, and the possibility of complications during device deployment are considered drawbacks of VCD.

To date, there is little evidence that clearly dictates whether to use manual compression or a vascular closure device to achieve hemostasis. There are very few studies comparing different devices head to head in specific populations, such as coronary interventions, peripheral arterial disease interventions, interventional oncology, stroke, etc. Two meta analyses from the early 2000s looked at MC versus VCD in cardiac catheterization patients and found little if any benefit for using VCD[2,3]; however, the studies included in the analysis were heterogeneous and the MC patients usually had anticoagulation reversed, which was not the case for VCD patients. In the years since these initial meta-analyses were published, operator experience has increased while industry has produced newer generations of VCD, resulting in a decrease in VCD related complications.[4,5] A prospective randomized controlled trial published in 2014, ISAR-CLOSURE, looked at 4524 patients undergoing diagnostic coronary angiography who were randomized to an intravascular VCD (FemoSeal), an extravascular VCD (ExoSeal), or manual compression. The primary endpoint was met indicating non-inferiority of the VCDs compared with MC.[6] A Cochrane review including 52 studies and 19,192 patients was published in 2016 and concluded that there was no difference in vascular injury or mortality when VCDs were compared with MC, and there was no difference in safety or efficacy when VCDs with different mechanisms of action were compared.[7] Another systematic review published in 2015 included 34 randomized controlled trials and 14,401 patients showing overall success rate for achieving hemostasis with VCD was 95.7%.[8] There are two basic types of closure devices: active and passive. The passive devices are placed externally to replace handheld compression. Active devices deploy a variety of methods to close the arterial puncture actively.

Complications Related to Active Vascular Closure Devices

Access-site complications can occasionally be life-threatening, but even minor complications may result in longer hospital stays and increased 1-year mortality.[9] VCDs are essentially used to avoid complications related to incomplete hemostasis. Therefore, complications are often multifactorial with potential contributions from the initial access because of the location of the puncture and size of the access; anticoagulant, antiplatelet, and thrombolytic medications; and choice of closure device and technique used for deployment. These complications related to device implantation include arterial laceration, arterial thrombosis, device embolization, and infection. This chapter will discuss general steps to be taken prior to and during device deployment to protect against different types of complications followed by discussion of the nuances of several of the individual devices and how to troubleshoot them. There is no single best device; each VCD has its own unique benefits and drawbacks. Understanding how each device creates hemostasis will help the operator choose the appropriate device for a particular patient.

Access Site Considerations

Initially, rigid guidelines were used for evaluating the access vessel prior to deployment of a closure device. These guidelines included only retrograde CFA puncture below the inguinal ligament and above the takeoff of the profunda femoris artery in vessels that were at least 5 mm in diameter without atherosclerotic plaque. More recently, however, the literature has been populated with reports of safe off-label use of VCDs

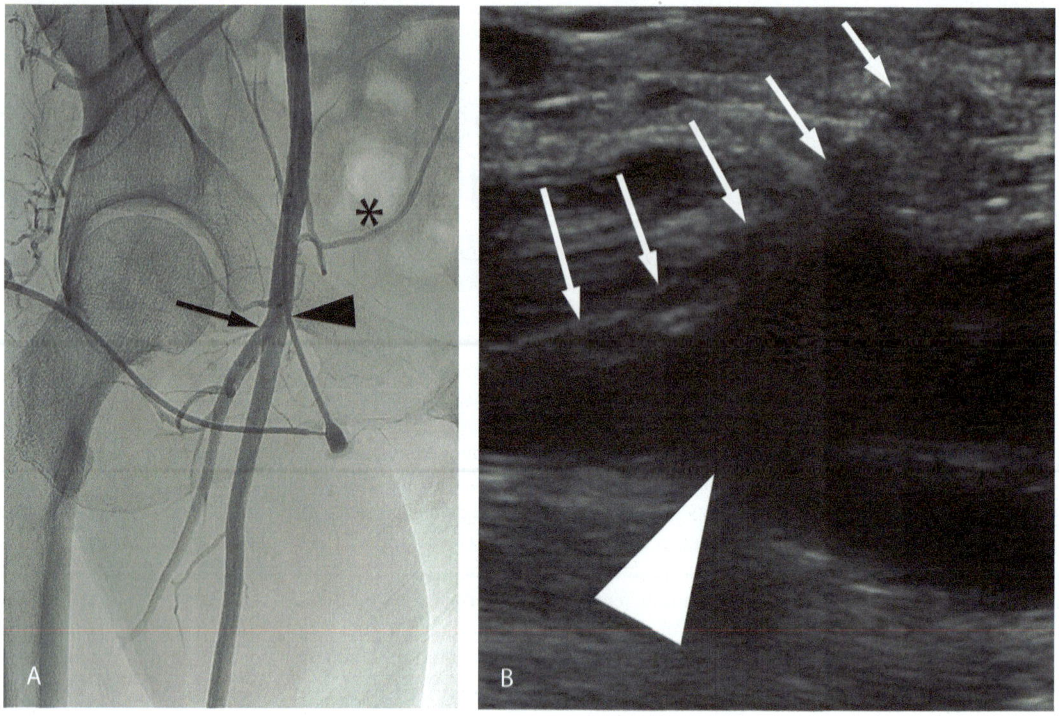

Fig. 3.1 Identifying Puncture Location. (A) Femoral angiogram performed by injecting the side arm of the sheath in a 30- to 40-degree ipsilateral oblique projection. The access site *(arrowhead)* is identified just superior to the bifurcation of the common femoral artery (CFA) *(black arrow)* into superficial femoral artery and profunda femoris artery. The oblique projection helps splay out the CFA bifurcation and identifies the puncture site relative to the bifurcation. The proximal aspect of the CFA is demarcated by the inferior epigastric artery *(asterisk)*. The caliber of the accessed artery and presence of any arterial pathology near the proposed site of vascular closure device deployment should be evaluated on this angiogram. (B) Sagittal grayscale ultrasound of the arterial access in the same patient shows the 5-French vascular sheath *(white arrows)* entering the CFA just above its bifurcation *(arrowhead)*.

in small and diseased arteries (and veins) all over the body, including high and low punctures in the groin as well as arterial access in the upper extremities. In fact, VCD deployment in the setting of unintended high puncture into the external iliac artery may prevent life-threatening hemorrhage in a situation where MC cannot be effective. Regardless of the circumstances and location of the arterial access, an angiogram should be performed through the sheath prior to its removal and deployment of the VCD. Typically, a 30-degree ipsilateral oblique projection is used so that the sheath does not directly overlap the entry vessel, helping to identify the exact site of entry (Fig. 3.1A). The angiogram helps the operator identify any potential obstacles that could interfere with successful device deployment such as calcified plaque at the arteriotomy, small vessel caliber, or nearby regions of focal stenosis or dissection.

GENERAL STEPS TO AVOIDING COMPLICATIONS WITH ACTIVE VASCULAR CLOSURE DEVICES

Ultrasound and Fluoroscopic Guidance for Arterial Access

Effective hemostasis starts with appropriate access technique. This topic was covered in detail in Chapters 1 and 2. However, studies show that using ultrasound guidance during initial femoral access results in decreased complication rates related to postprocedural hemostasis as seen in the FAUST Trial.[10] Ultrasound should be used to identify the femoral bifurcation (Fig. 3.1B), with desired access being just above the bifurcation. Fluoroscopy should be used to confirm that this location is over or inferior to the femoral head. If the patient has a high femoral bifurcation, then more inferior access into the SFA may be preferred so that manual compression can be used if a VCD fails or is not appropriate because of the patient's anatomy or vascular disease. Ultrasound should also be used to avoid puncturing directly into anterior wall CFA atherosclerotic plaque (and in particular calcified plaque) as this can lead to device failure for some VCDs. Additionally, if a patient has a recent history of VCD placement prior to the current arterial access, ultrasound should be used to identify the prior VCD placement site to avoid re-accessing the same location because this can lead to device failure and incomplete hemostasis or, rarely, embolization of VCD components.

Preparing the Tract from Skin to Vessel

A soft tissue tract is traversed for all patients receiving a VCD. In a thin patient who has never had an angiogram, this tract usually does not pose much resistance to successful VCD delivery. However, in obese patients and patients who have had prior arterial access, VCD placement, or surgery in the region of the percutaneous access, aggressive dissection of the tract may be necessary. A Kelly clamp should be passed along the sheath down to the anterior wall of the artery prior to VCD placement for scarred tissue. It is advisable to administer additional lidocaine prior to this dissection and VCD deployment to decrease patient discomfort. Effective soft tissue dissection can also help an operator understand if there is a failure in hemostasis prior to development of a large hematoma or pseudoaneurysm; pulsatile arterial blood is seen exiting the dermatotomy rather than pooling between the artery and the subcutaneous soft tissues. For obese patients, another concern is kinking of the sheath for the closure device. Consideration should be given to using stiffer sheaths, or maintaining stiff wires, when possible to facilitate delivery of the closure devices.

Avoiding Infection

All of the devices discussed in this chapter involve implanting material at the arteriotomy, and steps should be taken in every case to ensure sterile technique. VCD infection is a rare complication, but it can require surgical resection of the device and debridement of the femoral artery, with rare instances requiring resection and extra-anatomic bypass, in addition to long courses of intravenous antibiotics. The skin around the percutaneous access site should be resterilized with chlorhexidine directly prior to VCD deployment. New sterile towels should be placed around the access site and along the leg where the device will be placed prior to deployment. Sterile gloves should be changed prior to handling the device. Prophylactic antibiotic administration can be considered prior to VCD deployment, particularly if the access was maintained overnight (such as during arterial thrombolysis), in diabetic patients who have demonstrated poor wound healing, and when closing access after synthetic graft puncture.[11]

Optimizing Patient Parameters

A patient's blood pressure and coagulation status can affect the ability to achieve hemostasis. Consider antihypertensive medications such as metoprolol or hydralazine to bring blood pressure into the normal range prior to VCD deployment or MC if the clinical situation allows. Similarly, when clinically feasible, consider reversing anticoagulation prior to attempting hemostasis.

Vascular Closure Device Selection

Several vascular closure devices are commercially available. There is no consensus as to which device is most effective. Each device has its own mechanism of action and learning curve. It is not necessary to become facile with all available VCDs; one or two options are sufficient for most practices. Select devices are described in detail here.

Angio-Seal (Terumo Medical, Somerset, New Jersey)

The mechanism of closure involves an intravascular footplate and an extravascular collagen plug that are cinched tight by an intervening suture (Fig. 3.2A). First the procedural sheath is exchanged for an Angio-Seal sheath over a wire. Pulsatile blood from the extravascular portion of the dilator indicates that the sheath tip is in appropriate intravascular position (Fig. 3.2B). The wire and dilator are removed. The Angio-Seal device is advanced through the sheath until the barrels meet the sheath as indicated by a click deploying the footplate. The footplate is centered into optimal alignment by pulling back on the barrel until another click is heard and a colored indicator is revealed between the sheath and barrel. The device and sheath are then retracted along the suture until the collagen plug and tamper are exposed (Fig. 3.2C). The tamper is advanced along the suture compressing the collagen onto the arterial wall until a black indicator is exposed on the suture (Fig. 3.2D). The suture is cut at the dermatotomy and the tamper is removed.

Angio-Seal is an extremely secure form of closure and is preferred in patients on anticoagulation/antiplatelet medications in many practices.[11] Both the intravascular polymer footplate and extravascular plug are completely resorbed by 90 days. Prior to 90 days, a small lump can be palpated anterior to the vessel in thin patients, which may represent a reason to choose a different device. Re-access of the same vessel prior to 90 days after Angio-Seal deployment should occur at least one centimeter from the previous device deployment to avoid embolization of the anchor. The device is available in 6 and 8 French sizes.

Angio-Seal Deployment Tips and Troubleshooting

Avoiding intraarterial delivery of the collagen component of the Angio-Seal is paramount. The collagen is thrombogenic, and intraarterial delivery will likely result in thrombotic occlusion of the access vessel.

When initially inserting the Angio-Seal sheath, advance until pulsatile flow is seen, then retract until flow stops, then re-advance slowly until flow starts again. This prevents inserting the sheath too far into the vessel and deploying the anchor remote from the arteriotomy. If this happens, the footplate can catch on plaque away from the arteriotomy, and the collagen plug will be shuttled through into the arterial lumen.

Maintaining consistent back tension on the device and suture as the tamper is used to compact the collagen plug onto the external portion of the arterial wall is also important. This ensures that the anchor remains pulled up against the arterial wall. If there is slack in the suture during the tamping process, the anchor can drift away from the arteriotomy, allowing the plug to be driven into the lumen.

Since the footplate represents an implanted intraarterial component of the device, the device is not recommended for small CFAs (less than 5 mm) or CFAs with significant atherosclerotic plaque as the luminal diameter of the vessel could be slightly diminished postdeployment. Additionally, the device should not be used near an indwelling stent where the footplate can catch on stent interstices, potentially leading to intraarterial collagen deposition.

StarClose (Abbott Vascular, Abbott Park, Illinois)

The mechanism of closure involves a circular nitinol clip with barbs that cinch the arteriotomy closed (Fig. 3.3A). First, the procedural sheath is exchanged for a StarClose sheath over a wire. The wire and dilator are removed. The device is inserted into the sheath until a click is heard (step 1). A plunger in the back of the device is depressed which deploys intravascular locator wings (step 2) (Fig. 3.3B). The device and sheath are retracted until resistance is felt, indicating the locator wings are in proper position at the arteriotomy. A thumb advancer is slid down the device toward the access site delivering the clip to the vessel wall (and splitting the sheath) (step 3). The device is tilted up at 60–75 degrees, slight downward force is applied, and the clip is deployed by pressing a button (step 4). The intravascular locator wings are simultaneously collapsed and retracted during clip deployment. Each step has a corresponding labeled number on the device.

The clip is a permanent implant that does not incite an inflammatory response, which can make it an attractive choice for VCD in young thin patients. Immediate re-access is feasible, but the implanted clip should be avoided during subsequent ultrasound guided access. The device is 6 French.

StarClose Deployment Tips and Troubleshooting

The most common mode of failure for this device is related to incomplete tract dissection. The clip catches on soft tissue and is not fully applied onto the arterial wall. To avoid this complication, aggressive dissection of the soft tissue tract is warranted prior to StarClose use.

Occasionally, the device will appear to be "stuck" in place even though the 4-button has been pushed and the clip deployed onto the artery. A manual release needs to be performed. Care should be taken

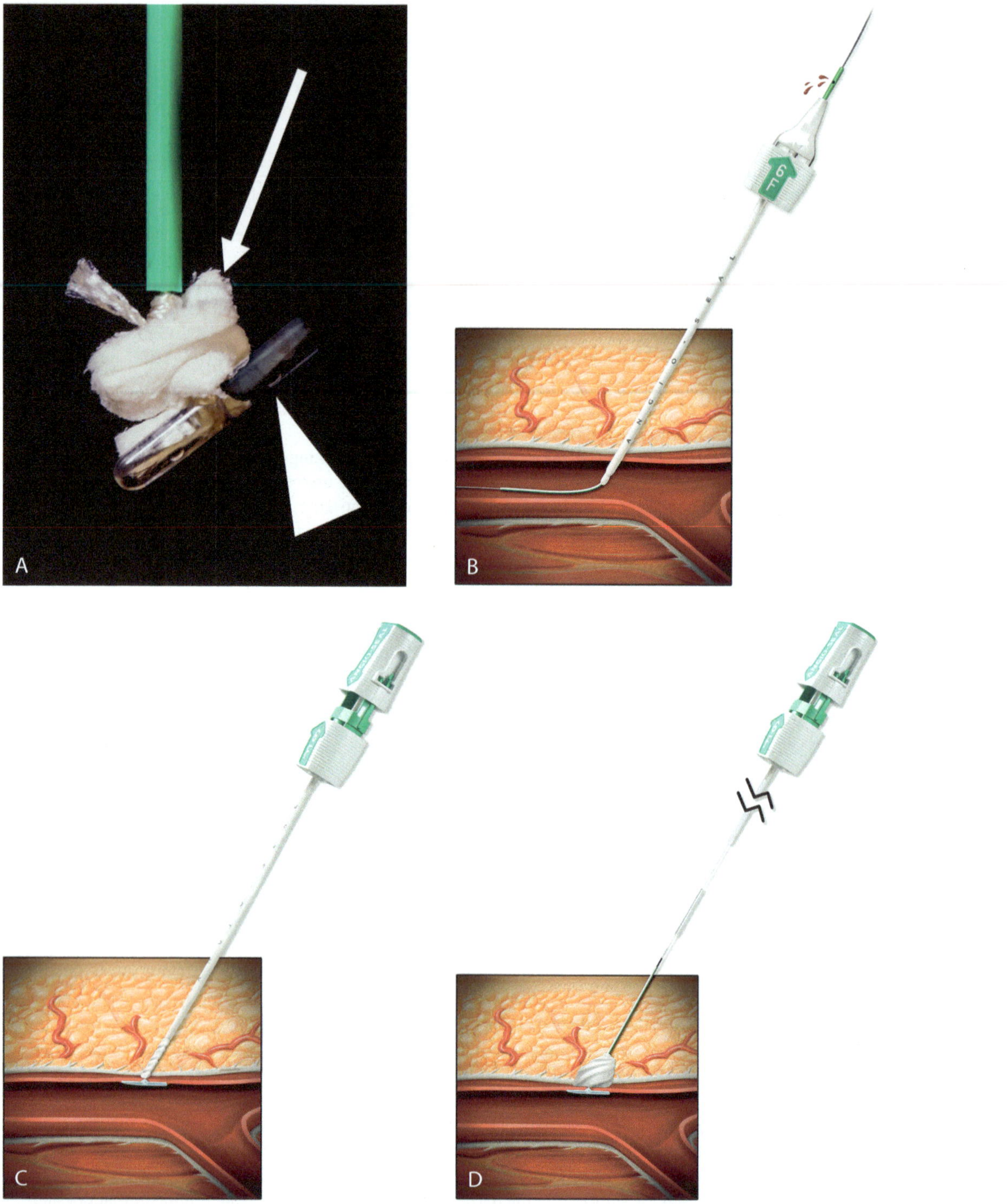

Fig. 3.2 Angio-Seal Deployment. (A) Photograph of a deployed Angioseal device showing the collagen plug (white arrow) and co-polymer footplate (arrowhead) connected by a suture. (B) Proper intravascular positioning of the tip of the Angio-Seal sheath is indicated by pulsatile blood return from the indicator port. (C) Partial deployment of the Angioseal device with intravascular footplate and extravascular collagen plug. (D) A tamper is advanced toward to arteriotomy to compact the collagen plug against the extravascular portion of the arterial wall creating a sandwich with the intravascular footplate.

(Photography credit: ANGIO-SEAL® Vascular Closure Device - ©2020 Terumo Medical Corporation. All rights reserved).

to avoid twisting the device prior to the manual release to avoid lacerating the vessel. The device should not be forcefully removed without performing the manual release as this will result in a significant arterial injury. The manual release is performed by inserting a small dilator or needle into each of two small access ports across from each other on the side of the device near the StarClose logo (Fig. 3.3C,D). The locator wings also need to be manually retracted by depressing a red switch near the back of the device (Fig. 3.3C).

"Carving" refers to a problem caused when the StarClose sheath is relaxed into a curved configuration during delivery of the clip to the

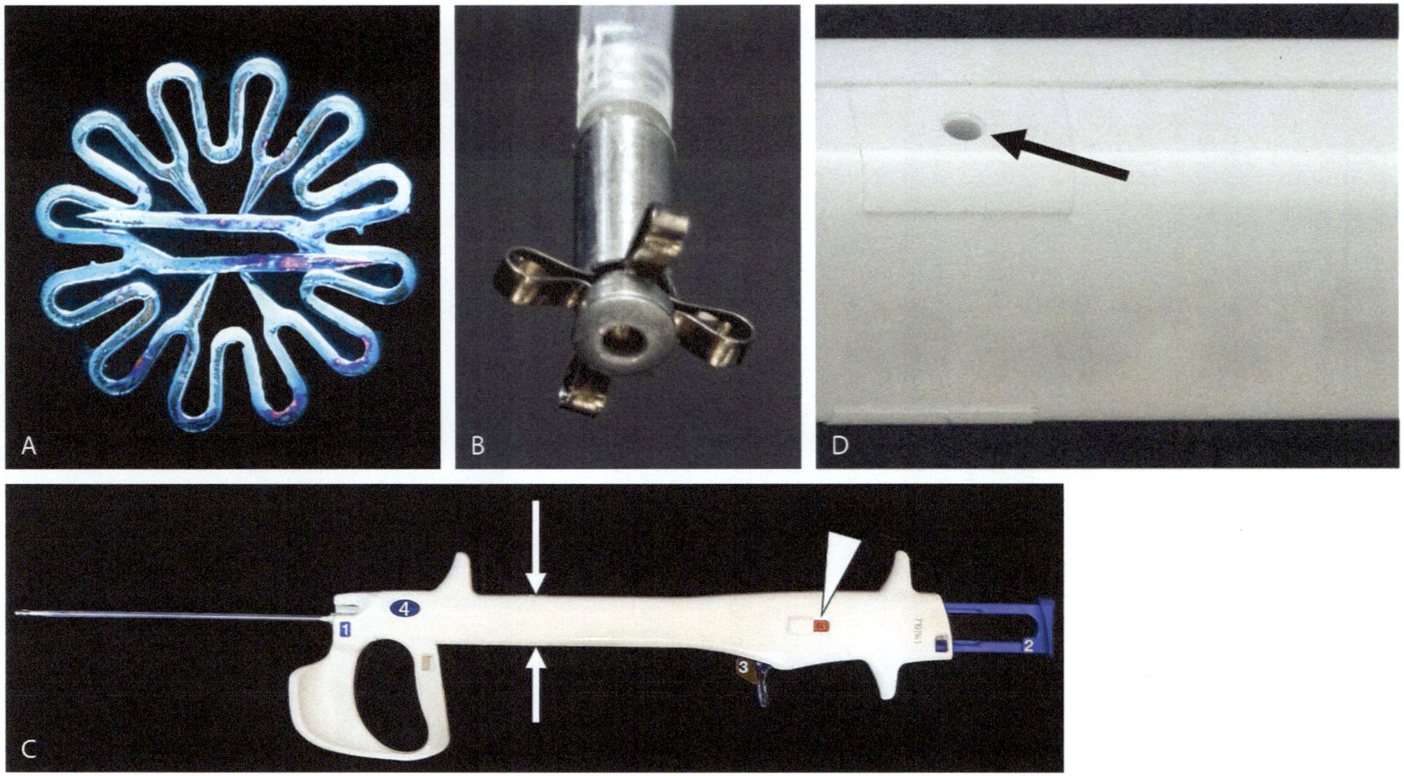

Fig. 3.3 StarClose SE Vascular Closure System. (A) Photograph of the nitinol Starclose clip. (B) Photograph of the intravascular locator wing deployed during step 2. (C) Photograph of the Starclose device showing the location of the manual release ports (arrows) and manual locator wing collapse button (arrowhead). (D) Close up of one of the manual release ports (black arrow). (Photography credit: Julio Gonzalez, RT, UCSF) StarClose SE is a trademark of Abbott or its related companies. Reproduced with permission of Abbott,

arteriotomy (step 3). This results in deformity of and damage to the sheath and ultimately failed closure. Carving can be avoided by applying back-tension to the device as the thumb advancer is shuttled toward the arteriotomy, keeping the sheath in a straightened configuration. If carving occurs, the locator wings should be released manually, the device removed, and manual compression applied.

Clip misfire or attaching to the sheath can be caused by failure to raise the device from 45 degrees to 75 degrees during deployment (step 4). At a 45-degree angle, only a small portion of the clip is able to capture the anterior wall of the artery and the arteriotomy is not completely cinched closed. MC needs to be applied in this situation. In addition to the 75-degree configuration, slight downward pressure should be applied and the 4-button held down for 5 to 10 seconds.

The primary method by which StarClose fails is superficial misfiring; intraarterial deployment is not typically considered an issue with this device.

Perclose (Abbott Vascular, Abbott Park, Illinois)

The mechanism of closure involves a braided polyester (AT model) or monofilament polypropylene (ProGlide model) suture with a preformed knot that is tightened and locked at the arteriotomy (Fig. 3.4A). The procedural sheath is exchanged for the device over a wire. The device is partially inserted until the wire-exit hole of the device reaches the dermatotomy, at which point the wire can be removed. The device is inserted further until pulsatile blood from the side port indicates intravascular tip location and a lever is flipped up deploying an intravascular footplate. The device is then retracted slightly, bringing the footplate firmly up against the anterior arterial wall. Two needles are deployed through the arterial wall to engage suture cuffs in the footplate by depressing a plunger (Fig. 3.4B). After hearing a click, the plunger is pulled out of the back of the device, revealing one blue suture tail, which can be separated from the plunger using the trimming tool on the front of the device. The footplate is then collapsed and the device partially retracted until the blue and white suture tails are seen at the dermatotomy. The sutures are harvested and set to the side. The device is then removed entirely or removed over a guidewire, while manual pressure is held to prevent bleeding from the puncture site prior to securing the suture. The knot is tightened by advancing the knot pusher over the blue suture tail and locked by pulling on the white suture tail. The suture tails are cut with the knot pusher device. Similar to StarClose, immediate re-access is feasible with Perclose, and the lack of a lump at the access site makes Perclose a good choice for young thin patients. The device is 6 French.

Perclose Deployment Tips and Troubleshooting

Guidewire access may be maintained during deployment of the device and hemostasis can be tested with the wire in place. If satisfactory hemostasis has been achieved, the wire is removed, the knot tightened and locked, and the sutures cut. If hemostasis has not been achieved, another Perclose or alternate VCD can be deployed using the guidewire to re-access the artery.

It is important to note that if the blue suture tail is not present when the plunger is pulled out of the Perclose, the device has failed. This may occur in the setting of calcified atherosclerotic plaque near the arteriotomy, whereby the path of the needle is deflected and does not engage the cuff of the suture seated in the intravascular footplate. Additionally, the angle of the device needs to be maintained throughout the plunger deployment without rotation or rocking so that the needles can properly engage the cuffs on the footplate. Fortunately, since wire access is not given up during (attempted) deployment of a Perclose, the device may be removed and an alternate closure device can be deployed or hemostasis may be achieved by manual compression.

Avoid breaking the suture during tightening by making sure not to pull medially or laterally on the suture and using slow consistent tension rather than quick jerky movements. If the suture breaks after the wire has been removed, hemostasis must be achieved by manual compression.

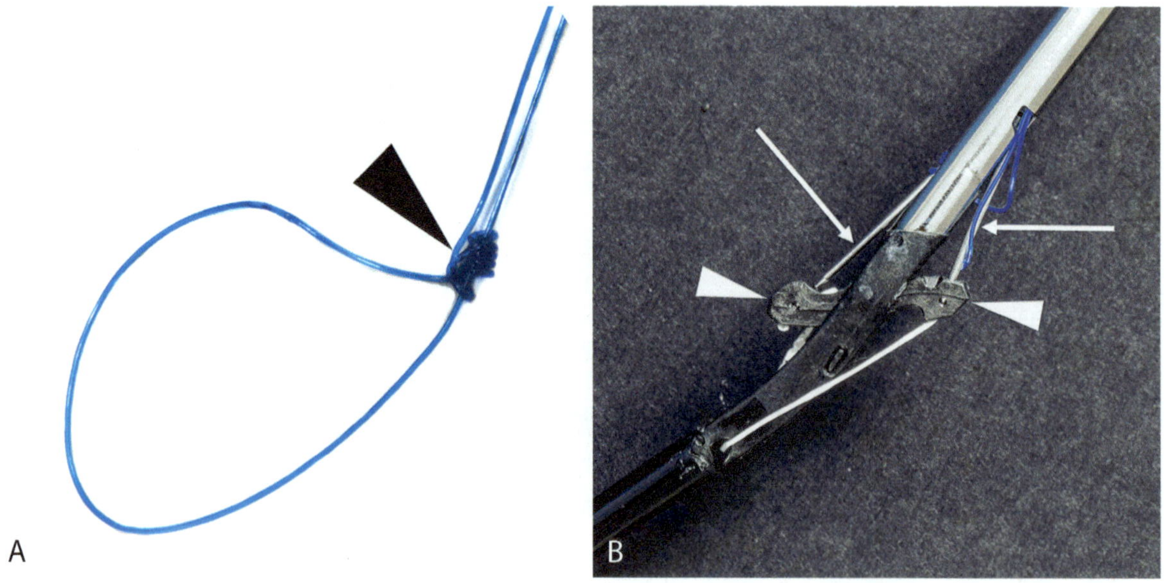

Fig. 3.4 Perclose ProGlide Device. Photograph of the deployed perclose suture loop with a pretied knot (arrowhead) that is subsequently tightened, locked, and trimmed. During deployment, two needles (white arrows) extend down from the extravascular space and dock with suture cuffs in the intravascular footplate (arrowheads) completing the loop of suture.

(Photography credit: Julio Gonzalez, RT, UCSF) Perclose ProGlide is a trademark of Abbott or its related companies. Reproduced with permission of Abbott,

The wire may also be maintained during placement of the Perclose for more tortuous vessels, until the device is more fully seated within the artery. If there is difficulty advancing the Perclose after removing the wire, the wire should be replaced and the device tracked over the wire prior to removing the wire again.

Mynx (Cardinal Health, Dublin, Ohio)

The mechanism of closure involves delivery of a polyethylene glycol (PEG) sealant plug onto the external wall of the artery that swells after interacting with blood products and extracellular fluids in the subcutaneous soft tissue tract. The second iteration of this device, the Mynx Grip features a PEG plug that adheres to the vessel wall. The newest iteration, the Mynx Ace, also employs the grip technology but requires exchange for a proprietary sheath prior to a modified deployment. For the original Mynx and the Mynx Grip, the device is inserted through the existing procedural sheath into the access artery and a small balloon is inflated. The device and sheath are pulled back until resistance is encountered, indicating that the balloon is at the arteriotomy site. The stopcock on the sheath should be opened to test for hemostasis at this point. An advancer tube is then used to shuttle the PEG plug to the external wall of the artery and tension is held for 30 seconds to allow adherence of the plug. The device is then laid down on the patient without tension for 90 seconds. The balloon is deflated entirely and removed along with the procedural sheath, leaving just the plug in place. Manual compression is held for one to three minutes after deployment to allow for continued hemostasis while the plug expands. One major advantage is the lack of intraarterial closure material. The device is available in 5 and 6/7 French sizes.

Mynx Deployment Tips and Troubleshooting

Avoid delivering the PEG sealant plug intraarterially. Fifty percent contrast may be used to inflate the balloon, making it radio-opaque during device delivery. This is useful for fluoroscopically confirming that the balloon has been retracted all the way back to the arteriotomy and is flush against the vessel wall, rather than stuck against plaque remote from the arteriotomy.

Avoid losing access in case too much back tension is applied with the balloon inflated, causing the balloon to burst. A buddy wire can be deployed adjacent to the procedural sheath prior to insertion of the Mynx device, preserving access in the case of a burst balloon. If this happens, another Mynx or alternate VCD can still be deployed.[11]

It is important to avoid intraarterial placement of the Mynx as this plug can cause an aberrant pain syndrome in addition to vessel occlusion when the plug is deployed incorrectly.

ExoSeal (Cardinal Health, Dublin, Ohio)

The mechanism of closure involves delivery of a bioabsorbable polyglycolic acid (PGA) plug into the subcutaneous soft tissue tract overlying the arteriotomy. The device is inserted through the indwelling procedural sheath until pulsatile blood is identified at the indicator port. The sheath and device are then retracted until pulsatility diminishes. An indicator window (which is tied to an intravascular nitinol ring at the end of the device) is then checked. The plug is delivered by pushing the green switch when the indicator window shows all black. The sheath and device are removed together. Manual compression is held for one to three minutes after deployment to allow for continued hemostasis while the plug expands. Similar to the Mynx device, ExoSeal does not deposit any intravascular material. The device may be used through 5–8 French sheaths. The device should not be used with sheaths longer than 12 cm.

ExoSeal Deployment Tips and Troubleshooting

Use the indicator window to understand the location of the device tip and where the plug will be delivered. In resting position, the indicator window is black and white. When the device has been retracted to the appropriate position, just external to the arteriotomy, tension on the intravascular ring will cause the indicator window to switch to all black. If the device is further retracted to a location that is too far from the arteriotomy to create hemostasis, the additional tension causes the indicator window to display black and red. If this occurs, tension should be released until the window returns to all black and the plug can be safely deployed.

Celt (Vasorum)

The Celt ACD is a second generation device, recently FDA approved in the United States and CE approved in Europe. It is intended for 5–7 French punctures but has been used for 8 and 9 French. This device allows for immediate re-access if needed. It has a very thin footplate that remains intraarterial and is biocompatible. The device requires three basic steps. It is very important to image the puncture site prior to deployment. The device is inserted through the pre-existing sheath (10–11 cm long). Once the device is near the hub of the sheath, the sheath is pulled back and clicked in to the device. The device is pulled back slightly under fluoroscopy. The handle is then rotated clockwise (step 1), opening the distal wings (Fig. 3.5). The device and attached sheath are then gently pulled back under fluoroscopic guidance, until gentle tension is felt, as the wings meet the arterial wall. The device should now be abutted against the arterial wall at the entry site. If the device appears to be too far in the vessel, it should be gently rotated and then withdrawn until tension is again felt and the device is at the access site. Gentle external compression is performed to ensure the device meets the wall of the vessel. Once the device is in the correct location, the handle is twisted counter-clockwise until it clicks, with the device held at a 90-degree angle to the puncture (step 2). This will open the external wings outside the arterial wall. The final step is to release the lever, which deploys the device. Gentle pressure can be held for a minute to ensure hemostasis.

This device can be used at bifurcations, for antegrade sticks, and in calcified or small vessels. It is not recommended for high sticks. While not FDA indicated, it has been successfully used for popliteal and brachial sticks. The smallest vessel recommended for closure with the Celt is 4 mm. The device can inadvertently be deployed intraarterially if care is not taken to identify the correct site. Most often this will result in continued bleeding, which can be handled with MC. If the entire device is deployed intraarterially, it can place the patient at risk for device embolization.

Celt Tips and Troubleshooting

Tips. If an area of stenosis or plaque is noted in the vessel above the access site, consider pulling the device back under fluoroscopy to just below the plaque prior to opening the wings. Always keep tension and maintain the device at 90 degrees when turning knob 2 to prevent deploying the outer wing intraluminally. After turning knob 2, completely relax tension and "wiggle" under fluoroscopy to confirm positioning.

Troubleshooting. If knob 1 does not click, this is usually because of a kink in the device and sheath. Flatten the angle of the sheath and manually try to pull the knob on the device back while stabilizing the device with the other hand. If this does not work, ask an assistant to

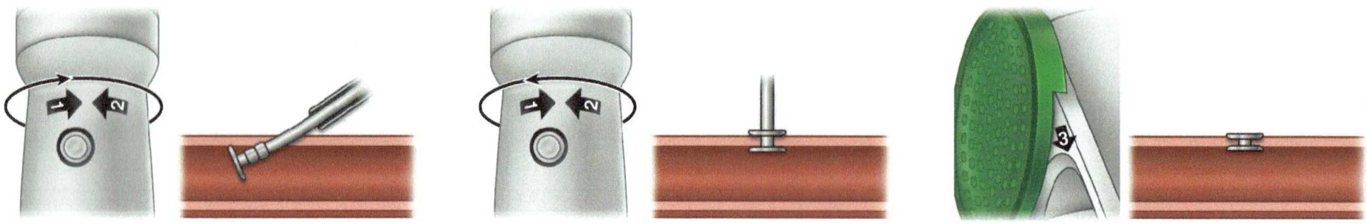

Step 1
Clockwise rotation of handle to open distal set of wings (inside puncture site)

Step 2
Anti-clockwise rotation of handle to open proximal set of wings (outside of puncture site)

Step 3
Release implant providing almost immediate hemostasis

Fig. 3.5 Celt Deployment Steps.

hold the sheath and disengage the sheath jaws on the Celt to remove it from the patient, exchange for a stiffer sheath, and use a different closure device or manual compression. If there is difficulty obtaining a 90-degree angle prior to firing the device, massage the tissue and skin down the sheath or ask an assistant to push down on both sides of the sheath. If you still cannot get to 90 degrees, a slightly smaller angle is acceptable and the knob 2 turn is then done under tension. If knob 2 does not click, decrease the angle and turn the knob until it clicks. If this does not work, maintain tension and fire the lever, and the device should release.

If significant bleeding is seen from the puncture site after relaxing the tension between the second turn and the lever, the device should be imaged under fluoroscopy with slight movement to see whether it moves easily and is therefore not attached to the vessel wall. At any point during deployment, prior to firing the final lever, the device can be pulled out as one piece and manual pressure held. The wings collapse under tension, preventing the puncture site from being enlarged. If significant bleeding occurs after completion of the procedure, manual pressure should be held. This suggests that the device is either too superficial (too much tension applied), or intraarterial. If the device is deployed intraarterially and embolizes, hemostasis should be obtained at the puncture site, then the device should be located by fluoroscopy. It can be snared with an Ensnare or trapped against the vessel wall with a stent, or simply observed if it is not impeding flow in the vessel.

DEALING WITH COMPLICATIONS

Failure of Hemostasis

Hematoma

The most important consideration when dealing with an access site hematoma is to understand whether the puncture occurred above or below the inguinal ligament. Hematomas occurring below the inguinal ligament occur in a relatively confined space at the top of the thigh and are usually self-limited. The second important consideration is whether the hematoma is still expanding or whether it is controlled with manual pressure, for those below the inguinal ligament. Because the patient may require transfusion, it is important to have a current Type and Screen and to follow serial hematocrits. If the hematoma occurs after a high puncture above the inguinal ligament, the complication can be life-threatening. Anatomically, the puncture in this situation is located in the pelvis rather than the thigh, and a large volume of blood can rapidly be lost into the peritoneum or retroperitoneum. Multiple large bore IV access sites should be secured immediately with the potential need for rapid transfusion. Closing the hole in the artery can be achieved by covered stent graft insertion from the opposite CFA or by cutdown and repair. Obese patients with large pannus can be a set up for access above the inguinal ligament and efforts must be made to tape up the pannus allowing the puncture to occur below the inguinal ligament. If a high stick is suspected at femoral sheath angiography, successful VCD deployment takes on greater importance and choice of VCD should be limited to the device with which the individual operator is most confident. Consideration should be given for devices that maintain access until confirmation of success is achieved.

Pseudoaneurysm

When hemostasis fails after arterial access, a pseudoaneurysm (PSA) can persist resulting in a pulsatile mass in the groin on physical examination. These are more common in low punctures, especially those involving the profunda or superficial femoral arteries, where there is no osseous structure behind the posterior wall. Depending on the size of the PSA, there are multiple treatment options. Small PSAs can be observed or compressed using an ultrasound probe until thrombosis occurs. Larger PSAs (>2 cm) with long narrow necks can be treated with thrombin injection. Under ultrasound guidance, a 25-gauge needle is inserted into the PSA as far away from the neck as possible. One mL of thrombin at 1000 units/mL is drawn into a 1 cc syringe and injected through the 25-gauge needle in 100–200 unit aliquots until thrombosis is visualized in real time by color Doppler ultrasound. PSA refractory to manual compression and/or thrombin injection can be treated by covered stent insertion or cutdown and repair. A final option for PSA treatment involves percutaneously accessing the PSA with a micropuncture needle and manipulating a guidewire through the hole in the artery back into the lumen of the parent artery (Fig. 3.6). If this can be achieved, one of the above-described VCD, may be used to achieve hemostasis; reports in the literature include use of StarClose and Angio-Seal for this purpose.[12] Devices that rely on creating hemostasis solely by expansion of a plug within the extravascular soft tissue tract (i.e., Mynx and ExoSeal) will not work with this technique.

Vascular Injury

Vascular Occlusion

This was a more frequent occurrence in VCDs in older patients. While this complication is very rare in modern clinical practice, femoral and pedal pulses need to be checked before and after VCD deployment in every patient to ensure that vascular occlusion has not occurred. There are several mechanisms for vessel occlusion after VCD deployment. The first mechanism involves insertion of plug material through the arteriotomy and into the vessel. Since this material is designed to achieve hemostasis, it is very thrombogenic and typically results in thrombotic occlusion of the CFA. Various device-specific tips for avoiding this problem have been discussed earlier for Angio-Seal, Mynx, and ExoSeal. Atherectomy is an endovascular option for revascularization in this setting, but surgical repair may be required. The second mechanism involves suturing the back wall of the CFA to the

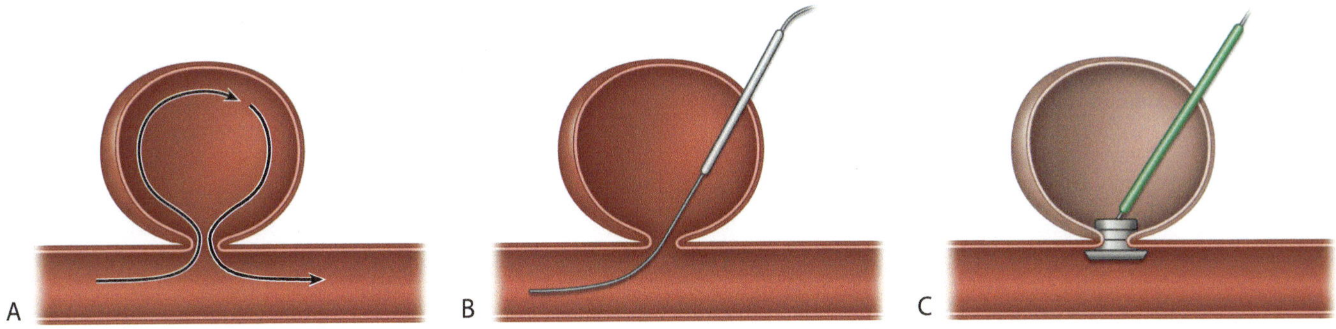

Fig. 3.6 Angio-Seal Deployment to Seal a Femoral Pseudoaneurysm. (A) Typical postcatheterization pseudoaneurysm forms after incomplete hemostasis resulting in a collection of pulsatile blood flow without overlying endothelium, contained only by the subcutaneous soft tissues and skin. (B) The pseudoaneurysm (PSA) is accessed percutaneously with a micropuncture needle (under ultrasound guidance, not pictured) and an 0.018″ guidewire is manipulated through the neck of the PSA into the parent artery. (C) The wire access is upsized to 0.035″ using a micropuncture sheath and an Angio-Seal device is deployed, sealing the neck of the PSA which then thromboses. StarClose and Perclose could also be deployed after re-accessing the femoral artery through the PSA.

front wall of the CFA with Perclose. This occurs if the footplate gets caught under back wall plaque prior to needle deployment. Treatment options include prolonged angioplasty to break the suture and open repair. Surgical bypass can also be considered in any patient with acute ischemia from arterial occlusion resulting in limb threat when flow cannot be readily restored by other techniques. A third mechanism of occlusion is with use of devices with intraarterial components in small vessels, in which the footplate may obstruct flow causing ischemia. In this case, the device should be surgically removed.

Vascular Embolization of VCD Components

This may occur several days or even weeks after successful Angio-Seal deployment if the suture holding the footplate and plug snaps. Typically, hemostasis has been achieved when this occurs, but the footplate can embolize distally resulting in focal occlusion of the popliteal or tibial arteries, which may or may not be clinically significant. Endovascular treatment options include suction thrombectomy and/or stent placement depending on the arterial anatomy involved. Surgical bypass could be considered in cases of limb threat without endovascular treatment options. Open thrombectomy may also be feasible if it is possible to get a wire or Fogarty catheter past the occluding footplate.

Arterial Injury

Laceration and dissection are extremely rare complications after VCD deployment, but may occur if an intravascular device component gets stuck and the device is forcefully removed from the vessel. If a device is stuck and the troubleshooting techniques described earlier (particularly for StarClose) are not successful in removing the device, cutdown with removal under direct visualization and repair of the vessel is warranted. Forceful removal of a VCD should never be performed.

Infection

Prevention is truly the best way to deal with this rare but serious complication and was discussed in detail earlier. It is recommended to follow strict sterile technique and reprepare all access sites prior to utilizing a VCD. Aggressive prompt medical and surgical treatments are necessary if VCD infection does occur. Typically, infected closure devices will require surgical debridement of the anterior wall of the vessel, with patch closure, primary closure, or extra-anatomic bypass, depending on the involved organism and amount of destruction.

CONCLUSIONS

The Hippocratic oath requires physicians to “first, do no harm”. This is important to remember when using closure devices because the gold standard to which they are being compared, manual compression, is quite safe. The severity of access site complications correlates with higher rates of discharge to rehabilitation/nursing facilities compared with home discharge. Patients with severe access site complications can have higher 30-day mortality, and those with moderate access site complications requiring transfusion can have elevated 1-year mortality.[9]

Patient selection is paramount in all procedures. This includes not only the initial access but also the final arterial closure. Subsets of patients (including obese patients, patients who cannot tolerate bed rest, and patients on anticoagulant/antiplatelet medications) are more likely to avoid bleeding if an appropriate VCD is successfully deployed. No single device is perfect for every patient; therefore, it is critical to understand the mechanism used by each device to achieve hemostasis. Knowing what is happening during each click or lever-pull while deploying a VCD is the first step toward successful deployment, hemostasis, healing, and eventually discharge home.

REFERENCES

1. Hon LQ, et al. Vascular closure devices: a comparative overview. *Curr Probl Diagn Radiol.* 2009;38(1):33–43.
2. Nikolsky E, et al. Vascular complications associated with arteriotomy closure devices in patients undergoing percutaneous coronary procedures: a meta-analysis. *J Am Coll Cardiol.* 2004;44(6):1200–1209.
3. Koreny M, et al. Arterial puncture closing devices compared with standard manual compression after cardiac catheterization: systematic review and meta-analysis. *JAMA.* 2004;291(3):350–357.
4. Applegate RJ, et al. Vascular complications with newer generations of angioseal vascular closure devices. *J Interv Cardiol.* 2006;19(1):67–74.
5. Dauerman HL, Applegate RJ, Cohen DJ. Vascular closure devices: the second decade. *J Am Coll Cardiol.* 2007;50(17):1617–1626.
6. Schulz-Schupke S, et al. Comparison of vascular closure devices vs manual compression after femoral artery puncture: the ISAR-CLOSURE randomized clinical trial. *JAMA.* 2014;312(19):1981–1987.
7. Robertson L, et al. Vascular closure devices for femoral arterial puncture site haemostasis. *Cochrane Database Syst Rev.* 2016;3:CD009541.

8. Cox T, et al. Systematic review of randomized controlled trials comparing manual compression to vascular closure devices for diagnostic and therapeutic arterial procedures. *Surg Technol Int.* 2015;27:32–44.
9. Ortiz D, et al. Access site complications after peripheral vascular interventions: incidence, predictors, and outcomes. *Circ Cardiovasc Interv.* 2014; 7(6):821–828.
10. Seto AH, et al. Real-time ultrasound guidance facilitates femoral arterial access and reduces vascular complications: FAUST (Femoral Arterial Access With Ultrasound Trial). *JACC Cardiovasc Interv.* 2010;3(7): 751–758.
11. Krishnasamy VP, et al. Vascular closure devices: Technical tips, complications, and management. *Tech Vasc Interv Radiol.* 2015;18(2):100–112.
12. Hadziomerovic A, Jetty P, Gupta A. Angioseal-assisted closure of Iatrogenic refractory femoral arterial pseudoaneurysm: A novel technique. *JACC Cardiovasc Interv.* 2016;9(6):e55–57.

4

General Complications of EVAR

Tracy J. Cheun, MD, Lalithapriya Jayakumar, MD and Mark G. Davies, MD, PhD, MBA

Endovascular aortic aneurysm repair (EVAR) was first performed in 1987[1]; however, a more popularized adaptation was introduced in the early 1990s.[2] Since then, EVAR's popularity and methods have expanded with a constantly evolving and growing list of techniques, devices, and indications. Several large-scale trials have proven the early morbidity and mortality benefit of EVAR over open infrarenal aortic aneurysm repair (OAR) in a variety of patient populations; however, trials with earlier device models have demonstrated a possible expiration date to this benefit and a higher rate of graft complications and need for reinterventions with EVAR compared with OAR, with an estimated complication rate in most series of approximately 30% and a 5-year reintervention rate of 20% to 30%.[3,4] While the Dutch Randomized Endovascular Aneurysm Management (DREAM) trial 2017 update noted a 38.8% reintervention rate for EVAR compared with 21.1% for OAR at 12 years, it found no significant survival difference (38.5% EVAR versus 42.2% OAR).[5] This provides further corroboration of EVAR's safety but critiques its durability and reemphasizes the potential for improvement.

As with any other procedure, a critical factor to minimize complications, both peri- and postoperatively, is the preoperative evaluation and preparation. The Society for Vascular Surgery (SVS) published reporting standards for EVAR,[6] outlining definitions of success when performing an EVAR (Table 4.1). Preoperative risk stratification and medical optimization prior to implantation are as critical as technical preparations with imaging studies and device selection for the overall success of the procedure with minimal complications. A thorough and accurate understanding of a patient's preoperative status and mitigation of physiological risk is of critical importance in safe peri- and postoperative care. However, all untoward outcomes cannot be avoided. This chapter aims to describe the general complications of EVAR and practices to prevent, recognize, and manage them as they arise.

EVAR General Complication Classes

- Cardiovascular
- Pulmonary
- Renal
- Thromboembolic
- Ischemia
- Sedation
- Radiation
- Postimplantation syndrome
- Infection

PREDICTING COMPLICATION

Most reinterventions after EVAR are performed with the overall goal of prevention of aneurysm expansion and rupture. Given that there is approximately a 1% per year risk of rupture across series after EVAR with most of these being fatal, lifelong surveillance is recommended and remains a major downside of EVAR compared with open repair.[7] A systematic review identified predictors of reintervention after EVAR to attempt to tailor surveillance schedules to risk-stratified individuals.[3] Although no conclusive amendments to surveillance were devised, common high-risk characteristics were identified. Across studies, the most common and the strongest predictors of reintervention remain morphologic characteristics, such as preoperative abdominal aortic aneurysm (AAA) size greater than 65 mm, common iliac artery size greater than 20 mm, tortuous diseased iliac arteries, complex aneurysm neck anatomy (increased diameter, decreased length, increased angulation), and non-adherence to the instructions for use.[3]

The SVS published a complex Anatomic Severity Grading score for predicting various aortic complications, factoring in a multitude of morphologic characteristics such as aortic neck diameter, length, and angulation; iliac vessel tortuosity, calcification, and diameter; presence and number of branch vessels; as well as several other factors. To date, there are several such risk prediction tools of reintervention risk after

TABLE 4.1 SVS definitions for EVAR reporting standards.

Clear definitions of EVAR success are equally important to reporting successes and failures.[6]

Technical success (first 24 hours)	Successful device introduction and deployment
	Adequate proximal and distal fixation
	Access from remote site without artificial conduit
	Absence of rupture, death, or conversion to open surgery
	Absence of Type I or III endoleak
	Graft patency without kinks, twists, or occlusions
Clinical success (initial = 0–30 days) (early = 30 days to 6 months) (mid = 6 months to 5 years) (late ≥5 years)	Technical success
	Absence of aneurysm expansion (≥5 mm diameter or ≥5% volume)
	Absence of graft migration (≥10 mm proximal edge)
	Absence of graft dilation (≥20% diameter)
	Absence of graft infection
	Absence of failure of graft integrity
Primary success	Success by above terms without need for additional intervention
Primary assisted success	Success with additional unplanned endovascular intervention
Secondary success	Success with additional unplanned surgical intervention

EVAR. The St George's Vascular Institute (SGVI) risk score (Fig. 4.1), which has performed well in external validation studies, dichotomizes patients into high- and low-risk groups for reintervention risk based on two parameters: maximum aortic diameter and common iliac artery diameter.[8] The DREAM Study Group performed a retrospective validation study of the SGVI score[9] and found that it reliably predicts a 5-year reintervention risk between high- and low-risk groups (hazard ratio = 4.06). The implications of such scoring tools lie in the potential to customize postoperative patient care and graft surveillance; however, there remains a need for further prospective studies and external multicenter validation to validate their widespread introduction and to affect changes to management guidelines.

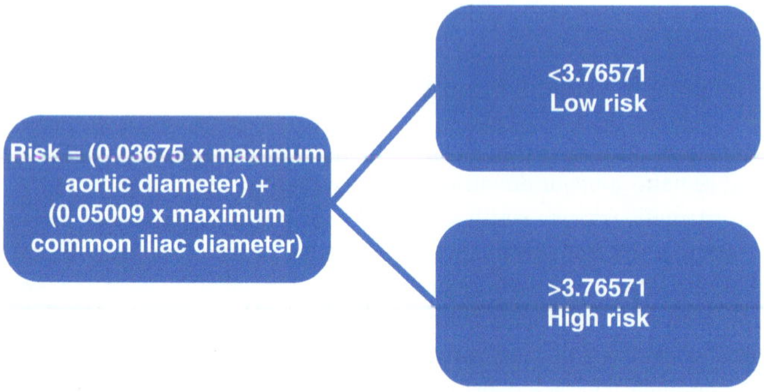

Fig. 4.1 St. George's Vascular Institute Score. This scoring index dichotomizes patients into low- and high-risk groups with regard to post-EVAR aortic complications.

(Data from Karthikesalingam A, Holt P, Vidal-Diez A, et al. Predicting aortic complications after endovascular aneurysm repair. *Br J Surg.* 2013;1302–1311.)

SYSTEMIC COMPLICATIONS

EVAR patients can be elderly and frail with multiple comorbidities and have a high incidence of cardiac and cerebrovascular disease, both known and occult. As a result, preoperative risk stratification is paramount to ensure safe care. Chaikof et al. published a medical comorbidity grading system (Table 4.2) based on the systemic complications of EVAR published by the SVS in 2002, dividing and weighing risk based on cardiac, pulmonary, and renal factors, which generates a global assessment of a patient's clinical risk.[10] Morbidity and mortality are also predicted by frailty, defined loosely as a diminution of physiologic reserve.[11] The Modified Frailty Index (mFI), for example, has been used to demonstrate this association between frailty and morbidity and mortality after EVAR. A study of 17,668 patients in the National Surgical Quality Improvement Program (NSQIP) database who underwent elective EVAR demonstrated a reliable and direct association, with increasing morbidity and mortality with each point increase in the mFI.[12]

TABLE 4.2 SVS medical comorbidity grading system.

The weighted scores are summed and divided by 3 to generate a score on a 3-point scale that reflects the patient's global systemic complication risk.[6]

Components		Pts	Characteristics
Major	Cardiac (weight × 4)	0	Asymptomatic Normal EKG
		1	Asymptomatic or Miocardial Infarction (MI) MI >6 months ago or occult MI on EKG or fixed defect on reperfusion scan
		2	Stable angina or significant reversible defect on reperfusion scan or significant silent ischemia on Holter monitor or EF 25% to 45% or controlled ectopy or asymptomatic dysrhythmia or compensated CHF
		3	Unstable angina or symptomatic or poorly controlled ectopy or dysrhythmia or poorly compensated CHF or EF <25% or MI <6 months ago
	Pulmonary (weight × 2)	0	Asymptomatic and normal chest x-ray and PFT within 20% of predicted
		1	Asymptomatic or mild exertional dyspnea and mild chronic parenchymal changes on chest x-ray and PFT 65% to 80% of predicted
		2	Between 1 and 3
		3	Vital capacity <1.85 L or FEV_1 <1.2 L or <35% of predicted or maximal voluntary ventilation <50% of predicted or PCO_2 >45 mmHg or supplemental oxygen use or pulmonary hypertension
	Renal (weight × 2)	0	No known renal disease and normal serum creatinine
		1	Moderately elevated serum creatinine but <2.2 mg/dL
		2	Serum creatinine 2.5 mg/dL to 5.9 mg/dL
		3	Serum creatinine >6 mg/dL or hemodialysis or history of kidney transplant
Minor	Hypertension (weight × 1)	0	None
		1	Controlled with single drug
		2	Controlled with two drugs
		3	Uncontrolled or requires >2 drugs
	Age (weight × 1)	0	<55 years
		1	55–69 years
		2	70–79 years
		3	>80 years

Cardiovascular Complications

Cardiac complications remain the most common cause of post-EVAR mortality. According to a 2017 study of 24,813 patients in the NSQIP Participant Use Data Files who underwent EVAR between 2005 and 2013, the overall 30-day mortality for EVAR was 1.4% and the incidence of postoperative myocardial infarction (MI) or cardiac arrest was 1.4%.[13] These events increased to 8.5% and 4.3%, respectively, among patients with three comorbidities from the surgical risk factor inclusion criteria list (Box 4.1).

Preoperative cardiopulmonary evaluation (Fig. 4.2) begins with a detailed history of prior cardiac events and interventions as well as the existence of coronary artery disease equivalents and active disease. All patients should have routine blood work, a chest radiograph, and an electrocardiogram as indicated. Further cardiac workup is dictated by their risk stratification. Patients with acceptable exercise tolerance and those classified as low risk by the Vascular Study Group of New England Cardiac Risk Index[14] do not require further cardiac testing, whereas patients with low or unknown exercise tolerance and a "high risk" classification merit further workup.[15] Patients with new cardiac murmurs and/or signs or symptoms concerning unrecognized heart failure should have a preoperative echocardiogram and a stress test prior to elective EVAR to address potential valvular disease and/or heart failure and reduce the risk of perioperative adverse cardiac events. Medical management to optimize the patient is recommended prior to intervention. Patients with stable cardiac disease have not been shown to receive any mortality benefit from coronary revascularization unless it was planned prior to the decision to pursue aneurysm repair.

Cardioprudent medications such as beta blockers, statins, and antiplatelet agents should be evaluated and optimized appropriately, preferably one month prior to surgery. The beneficial effects of statins, which are derived from both serum cholesterol-lowering and pleiotropic effects, have been shown in multiple prospective randomized studies to reduce perioperative cardiac mortality significantly.[16] Beta blockade should not be discontinued or initiated abruptly prior to surgery. However, in high-cardiac-risk individuals, initiation of beta blockade a week to a month prior to surgery can confer a survival benefit.[17]

Concern regarding bleeding risk and other complications with the continued use of antiplatelet agents or other anticoagulants has been evaluated in several studies. One such study of 407 patients on chronic antiplatelet or anticoagulation therapy who underwent EVAR found no significant difference in the rate of endoleaks or aneurysmal sac expansion compared with patients not on therapy over a median follow-up period of 18 months.[18] Antiplatelet agents can be safely continued through the perioperative period for EVAR. Chronic anticoagulation should be evaluated on a case-by-case basis to determine whether cessation or a heparin bridge is appropriate depending on indication for therapy and individual bleeding risk.

BOX 4.1 High-risk comorbidities. These inclusion criteria for a 2017 NSQIP study, adapted from the Endovascular Aneurysm Repair Trial 2, were noted to be associated with increasing complication rates.[13]

MI within 6 months
Any history of cardiac intervention
Angina within 30 days
CHF within 30 days
History of COPD within 30 days
Cr >2.26 mg/dL
Hemodialysis within 2 weeks

Pulmonary Complications

Tobacco use and variants of chronic obstructive pulmonary disease (COPD) can be intimately related to aneurysm development. Many EVAR patients may have underlying pulmonary disease, which can be diagnosed or undiagnosed at the time of presentation. According to an analysis of the NSQIP database, 30% of EVAR patients are active smokers at the time of intervention.[13] With the decreased use of general anesthesia with EVAR compared with OAR, the incidence of respiratory

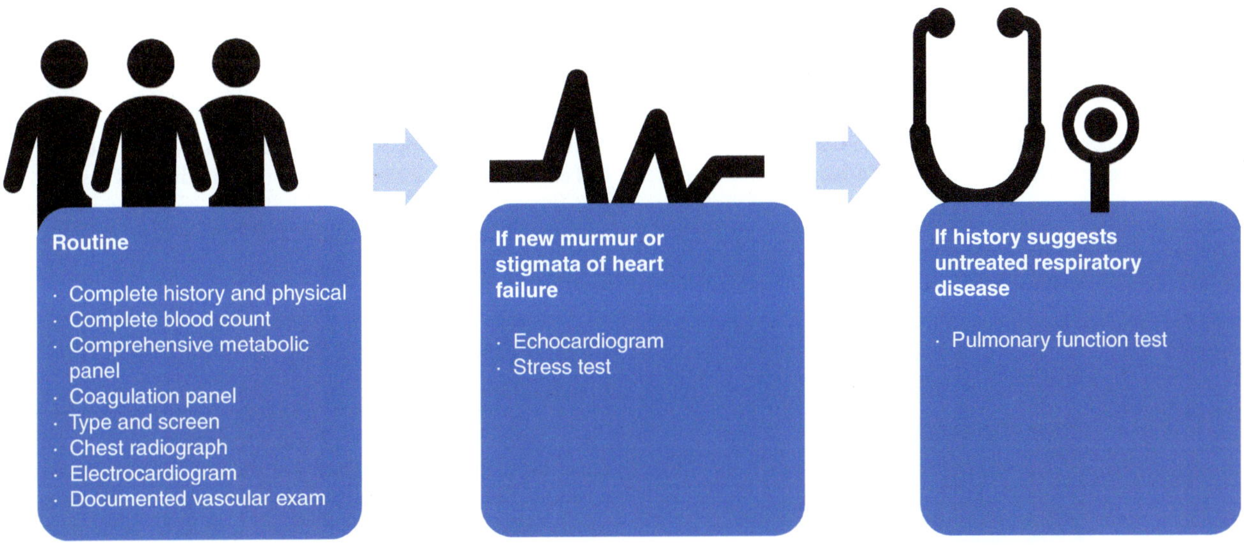

Fig. 4.2 Preoperative Workup. The preoperative cardiac workup for EVAR differs based on history and risk factors.

complications is lower, but continues to be a significant source of morbidity and the second most common cause of mortality after EVAR.[19] The incidence of post-EVAR pneumonia is 1.3%, unplanned reintubation 1.5%, and prolonged ventilator dependence 1.2%.[13]

Severe COPD has been spirometrically defined as FEV_1 to FVC ratio of less than 0.7 or FEV_1 less than 30% of predicted.[20] Severe COPD, decreased FEV_1 (1.9 L among nonsurvivors versus 2.3 L among survivors), and decreased FVC (3.0 L among nonsurvivors versus 3.4 L among survivors) have been independently associated with significantly lower 5-year survival after EVAR. Therefore, it is crucial to characterize and to optimize respiratory status preoperatively prior to intervention.[21] Despite this, pulmonary function assessment prior to EVAR is often overlooked. A prospective observational study of 200 EVAR patients found when all patients underwent preoperative pulmonary function tests (PFTs), 57% of patients were found to have previously undiagnosed and untreated respiratory disease.[22]

Active smokers should quit smoking at least 2 to 4 weeks prior to intervention to exceed the postcessation window of hypersecretion and impaired ciliary clearance (Fig. 4.3). A risk index for pulmonary complications, such as the ARISCAT risk index, can stratify patients by risk to determine who may require further preoperative testing.[23] Given the association between poor pulmonary function and post-EVAR mortality, any patient with history or physical examination for respiratory disease should undergo preoperative PFTs and medical optimization of pulmonary function.

Renal Complications

Renal dysfunction following EVAR has a wide range of reported incidences depending on the definition of postoperative renal dysfunction used. A recent systematic review of post-EVAR renal dysfunction estimated a risk of clinically relevant renal dysfunction at one year to be 18%.[24] This injury is attributed to a combination of contrast-induced nephropathy from intraoperative contrast usage, surveillance imaging, renal infarction secondary to suprarenal renal fixation or microembolic disease from juxtarenal device manipulation, and ischemia-reperfusion injury. Moreover, this injury has potential life-long implications. A study of 212 consecutive EVAR patients identified a significantly increased rate of chronic kidney disease in EVAR patients compared with risk-controlled nonoperated aneurysm patients (23.5% versus 6.7%), and postprocedural acute kidney injury (AKI) was a significant risk factor for CKD.[25]

Furthermore, postoperative AKI has been directly associated with increased incidence of cardiovascular events and all-cause mortality. A study of 947 patients undergoing EVAR followed over a period of 33 months postprocedurally found that those who developed AKI had a higher risk of mortality (32.1% versus 1.7%) than those who did not develop AKI. Pre-existing renal disease was the most significant risk factor for post-EVAR AKI.[26] These studies identified other variables such as longer operative time, larger volume of contrast used, preoperative ACE inhibitor use, decreased preoperative cardiovascular reserve, and advanced age as prominent risk factors for perioperative kidney injury.

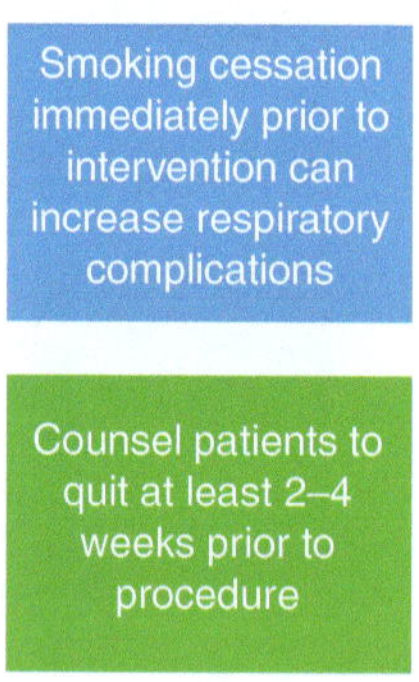

Fig. 4.3 Smoking cessation recommendations.

Pre- and intraoperative intravenous hydration may mitigate contrast-induced nephropathy (CIN), although results of studies regarding its efficacy are conflicting. Risk of CIN can also be decreased through the utilization of carbon dioxide as the contrast medium whenever feasible. One series achieved an 85% technical success rate for EVAR solely using carbon dioxide angiography, with only one case requiring reversion to iodinated contrast because of inadequate image quality.[27] The patients with endoleaks were able to be diagnosed using carbon dioxide angiography and treated using very small volumes of iodinated contrast material. The risk of CIN can also be avoided through the increasing use of contrast-enhanced ultrasound (CEUS) for graft surveillance, which carries no additional risk of renal dysfunction as opposed to serial Computer Tomographic Angiography (CTA) examinations.[28]

The association between suprarenal fixation and postoperative renal dysfunction has not yet been clearly elucidated in well-powered, long-term, controlled studies. Suprarenal fixation, while shown to decrease the incidence of EVAR graft migration, may be a nidus for thrombus with partial or complete occlusion of a renal artery over time. A study of 2574 EVAR patients found that suprarenal fixation was associated with a significantly higher incidence of serum creatinine increase of at least 0.5 mg/dL (3.7% versus 2%) and twice the likelihood of clinical renal deterioration.[29] However, this study, as with the majority of other similar reports, failed to account completely for patient and graft selection bias, as patients for whom suprarenal fixation was utilized tended to have more severe juxtarenal disease at the time of intervention.

Another important consideration is the presence of an accessory renal artery (ARA), which can have a prevalence of up to one-third of the population.[30] A clinically relevant ARA originates inferior to the main renal artery, supplies one-third of the renal parenchyma, and has a diameter greater than 4 mm.[31] Exclusion of a clinically relevant ARA can lead to renal infarction with or without a decrease in glomerular filtration rate (GFR). A study of 34 patients with ARA who underwent EVAR compared with 102 matched patients without ARA found a significantly higher incidence of depressed GFR in the ARA group (decrease of 10.7 versus 1.2 mL/min/1.73 m^2). This study demonstrated that the presence of ARA is a clinically significant anatomic variant that merits attention in the preoperative workup with potentially serious implications if overlooked.[32] Furthermore, there are techniques described to preserve clinically relevant ARA such as parallel graft placement during the EVAR implantation. In a small series of nine infrarenal EVARs that had chimney grafts placed in clinically relevant ARAs, over a mean follow-up of 13 months, eight of the nine patients had either no change or an improvement in their CKD stage.[31] Given that short- and long-term renal decline is associated with increased morbidity and mortality, preservation of renal parenchyma and function should be considered in regard to clinically relevant ARA.

DEEP VEIN THROMBOSIS AND PULMONARY EMBOLISM

The incidence of acute deep vein thrombosis (DVT) after EVAR according to the NSQIP database is 0.5%, with similar rates across multiple large series.[13,33,34] There exists some concern that percutaneous EVAR (PEVAR) with suture-mediated "pre-close" technique may precipitate development of a DVT. A series of 52 PEVAR patients retrospectively analyzed demonstrated a 4% incidence of proximal lower extremity DVT, which is comparable to that of other vascular procedures including open aneurysm repair.[35] Pulmonary embolism after EVAR is an even less common complication, reported at 0.2% in the NSQIP database; however, any provider caring for a patient with an AAA must be aware of the heightened risk of venous thromboembolic disease among aortic aneurysm patients. A cohort study of the National Health Research Institutes database in Taiwan noted that, after matching age, prothrombotic comorbidity, and length of hospitalization, untreated patients with AAA had a 1.89-fold higher risk of DVT and/or PE compared with non-AAA patients.[36] Therefore, while postoperative EVAR patients do not warrant heightened DVT or PE testing unless otherwise clinically indicated, clinical suspicion should be maintained given their higher baseline risk.

ISCHEMIC COMPLICATIONS

The main mechanisms of ischemia are cholesterol or thrombus embolization, thrombosis, and inadvertent vessel coverage, most commonly affecting the lower extremities, pelvis, and kidneys. However, atheromatous debris can embolize to every conceivable vascular bed. In a study of a series of 311 infrarenal EVAR patients, the total ischemic complication rate was 9%, with 6.8% lower extremity ischemia, 2.3% pelvis ischemia, and 0.6% spinal cord ischemia.[37] The presentation naturally depends on the location of ischemia. Skin manifestations may occur in the form of petechiae, cyanosis, livedo reticularis, or frank necrosis.

Spinal Cord

Spinal cord ischemia resulting in paraparesis or paraplegia after infrarenal EVAR is an extremely rare complication and one that is not commonly reported in studies. In an analysis of the EUROSTAR database, the incidence of spinal cord ischemia was 0.2%.[38] While a rare complication, this highlights the importance of understanding the patient's anatomy and vascular supply to the spinal cord prior to intervention, which should be reviewed prior to graft deployment.

EVAR patients presenting with paraparesis or paralysis require expeditious workup with an immediate CT of the abdomen and pelvis to evaluate for hematoma compressing the cord followed by an MRI to confirm spinal cord infarction if the graft is MR-compatible. Neurosurgical consultation for possible lumbar drain placement should be made early.

Lower Extremity

Ischemia of the lower extremities can be a result of embolism as well as thrombotic occlusion. The incidence of leg ischemia during EVAR is approximately 7%.[37] Delineation of the vascular status of the lower extremity preoperatively and careful perioperative monitoring of the vascular exam are paramount to awareness of ischemic time and the possibility of compartment syndrome and consequent need for decompressive fasciotomy. The use of large-caliber sheaths can cause occlusive ischemic insult. Therefore, the largest sheath should be removed first in order to evaluate for ischemia while maintaining access in the event that a diagnostic angiogram is indicated. In other cases, patients may present days to weeks postoperatively with claudication, rest pain, or even frank gangrene. Management of lower extremity ischemia takes many different forms depending on the etiology and the presentation: catheter-directed thrombolysis, angioplasty and stenting, embolectomy, endarterectomy with or without patch angioplasty, bypass grafting, and major amputation.

Colon

Intestinal ischemia has a reported incidence of 1.5% to 3% after EVAR.[39] While uncommon, vigilant perioperative monitoring for this potentially devastating complication is of utmost importance. The prevalence of mesenteric atherosclerosis, often occult, has been found on autopsy studies to be in the range of 6% to 10%. While intestinal perfusion can be maintained through various anastomoses between the celiac (CA), superior mesenteric (SMA), and inferior mesenteric arteries (IMA), if one vessel is chronically occluded and a widely patent IMA is excluded by stent graft deployment, the single remaining visceral branch may provide inadequate perfusion. Alternatively, atheroembolism to any of the visceral branch vessels can cause similar hypoperfusion injuries.

The effect of hypogastric artery interruption has been shown in some series to be associated with a significantly increased number of pelvic complications, but in others bilateral embolization has not been shown to be associated with any serious ischemic complications. A small retrospective study of 16 patients who underwent preoperative hypogastric artery occlusion found no association with serious pelvic complications, including bowel ischemia.[40] The only complications noted were buttock claudication and sexual dysfunction. Ultee et al., however, noted in a series of 4675 EVAR patients that unilateral hypogastric artery coverage yielded a 1:7 odds ratio of bowel ischemia.[41]

Risk factors for bowel ischemia are difficult to define cleanly given that it shares many factors with the frequent comorbidities of AAA patients, such as smoking, dysrhythmia, and heart failure. Moghadamyeghaneh et al. conducted a retrospective study of 3082 EVAR patients who developed postoperative mesenteric ischemia and determined a number of risk-adjusted factors associated with postoperative mortality (Table 4.3).[39] Ruptured aneurysm and transfusion requirement were the strongest predictors of post-EVAR bowel ischemia, theorized to be caused by the interruption of perfusion through the IMA in these scenarios. Patients who developed bowel ischemia had a fourfold increased risk of postoperative mortality, further underscoring the gravity of this complication.[39]

Bowel ischemia can present with a slow insidious course or an abrupt onset of abdominal pain. The classic presentation of abdominal pain out of proportion to the examination, as well as postprandial pain, fever, tachycardia, leukocytosis, or lactic acidosis in addition to a history of an EVAR, should raise the suspicion of possible bowel ischemia.

Preoperative and intraoperative imaging should be scrutinized before and during EVAR for patency of the CA and SMA, with recanalization and/or stenting as indicated. In the case of a patient presenting with post-EVAR bowel ischemia, recanalization and stenting may be possible. However, if endovascular salvage is unsuccessful, open mesenteric bypass may be indicated.

SEDATION COMPLICATIONS

The main advantage of EVAR over open aneurysm repair is its overall minimally invasive nature, which confers upon EVAR a lesser

TABLE 4.3 Risk-adjusted factors associated with post-EVAR ischemic colitis.[39]

Factor	Adjusted odds ratio
Emergency admission	3.2
Intra- or postoperative transfusion	2.06
Ruptured aneurysm	4.07
Renal failure requiring hemodialysis	3.86
Proximal aneurysm extension	2.19
Diabetes	1.87
Female gender	1.75

inflammatory response, reduced cardiac stress, and decreased hemodynamic fluctuations. It is also advantageous in that it allows the use of locoregional anesthesia, when appropriate, and avoidance of the various risks that arise with general anesthesia.

The most common anesthetic technique utilized for EVAR in the United States is a combination of local anesthesia with monitored anesthesia care (MAC). The choice of anesthetic technique (general versus neuroaxial versus local/MAC) has not been shown in large-scale studies to be associated with differing mortality risk. However, locoregional anesthesia has been associated in multiple studies with decreased operative time, length of stay, rate of postoperative intensive care unit admission, and incidence of adverse cardiac, pulmonary, and renal events. In a retrospective study of 302 EVAR patients, those who underwent general anesthesia had a 30-day cardiac event rate of 13.3% versus 4.7% among those who underwent locoregional anesthesia.[15] In this same series, no pulmonary complications were noted in the locoregional anesthesia group compared with 2.9% in the general anesthesia group. A systematic review and meta-analysis of similar studies corroborated these findings of locoregional anesthesia's association with decreased operative time, length of stay, and postoperative complications.[19] However, these results are heavily influenced by selection bias, and as such the general conclusion is that comorbidity and challenging morphology are more likely to be the causal agents in the outcome differences rather than the choice of anesthesia. Therefore, anesthetic technique should be tailored to each patient based on comorbidity and operative plan after a discussion between surgeon and anesthesiologist.

RADIATION COMPLICATIONS

EVAR exposes both patients and staff to a significant amount of ionizing radiation, the effects of which can be divided into two categories: deterministic and stochastic effects. Deterministic effects are those dose-dependent effects such as cataracts, erythema, hair loss, desquamation, and skin necrosis. These were known to begin at a threshold dose of 2 Gy, with erythema typically presenting early within 24–48 hours of exposure while necrosis typically presents days or weeks after exposure. The International Commission on Radiological Protection recently lowered the safe occupational threshold exposure for prevention of radiation-induced cataracts (Fig. 4.4).[42] Stochastic effects, by contrast, have no known threshold dose and generally refer to long-term side effects, primarily to an elevated lifetime risk of malignancy. The mean effective dose for a straightforward bifurcated infrarenal EVAR is reported around 20 mSv. Approximately 100 mSv of exposure over 2 years is associated with a 2.7% lifetime increase in leukemia and solid tumor malignancy in patients with a life expectancy greater than 15 years.[43]

There are several risk factors for radiation-induced injury (Box 4.2); however, all patients, regardless of risk profile, should be exposed to the least amount of radiation necessary for a procedure, counseled on this risk, and mindfully monitored for signs of injury in the hours to months following EVAR. Careful inspection of postoperative patients, with the knowledge that radiation-induced burns typically appear on the patient's posterior aspect, is key to early detection.

Several techniques can be used to minimize radiation exposure and risk of injury. Exposure can be reduced by providing proper lead shields and eye protection as well as minimizing operative and fluoroscopy times. Inadvertent engagement of the foot pedal can be responsible for a significant additional radiation burden. Utilization of pulse mode in a low or half-dose setting, as much as possible, as opposed to continuous mode, yields a significant dose reduction without compromise of image quality. Limiting the use of digital subtraction angiography, which utilizes a substantially higher quantity of radiation, and instead using digitally stored fluoroscopy loops can also significantly reduce exposure. Collimation reduces the field of view and proportionately reduces the degree of scatter and area of unnecessarily exposed tissue. Operator-controlled imaging has been reported to be associated with a 30% dose reduction compared with radiographer-controlled imaging secondary to a decrease in erroneous exposures as a result of miscommunication. Equipment with image fusion technology has been shown to reduce exposure by utilizing a digitally produced 3-dimensional "road-map" from the preoperative CT angiography that obviates the need for a diagnostic run at the start of the procedure.[44]

Minimizing radiation exposure during the index procedure is important; however, given that more than 90% of aneurysm-related imaging in a patient's lifetime is composed of surveillance CT scans, the manner of surveillance has been rightfully under scrutiny.[45] A surveillance CT schedule of scans at 0, 1, and 12 months postoperatively, then annually thereafter (with an additional scan at month 6 if the month 1 scan was abnormal), has been standard after EVAR for detection of endoleaks, graft migration, fractures, stenosis, and enlarging aneurysm sac.[46] However, multiple prospective studies have demonstrated that contrast enhanced ultrasound (CEUS) in post-EVAR surveillance has excellent diagnostic performance without the radiation exposure, renal impairment, and higher cost of monitoring with CT angiography.[28] The use of CEUS is limited by its operator-dependent

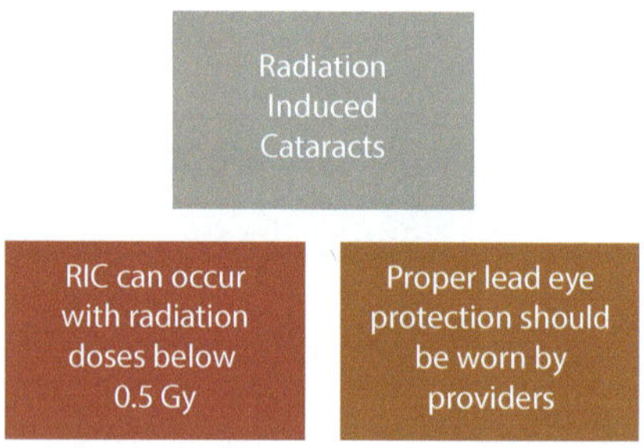

Fig. 4.4 Radiation-induced cataracts.

(Data from Rehani M, Ciraj-Bjelac O, Vano E, et al. Radiological protection in fluoroscopically guided procedures performed outside the imaging department. *Annals of the ICRP* 2010;40(6).)

BOX 4.2 Risk factors for radiation-induced injury. Knowledge of risk factors and proper risk mitigation is essential for minimizing injury secondary to ionizing radiation exposure during EVAR.[44]

Diabetes
Obesity (overlapping skin folds)
Hyperthyroidism
Malnourishment
Active tobacco smoking
Mutations of impaired DNA stability or repair (e.g., ataxia-telangiectasia)
Significant history of radiation exposure (cumulative lifetime effect)

nature; therefore, it can be reliably used only at vascular centers and institutions with adequately trained and experienced vascular laboratory technologists.

POST-IMPLANTATION SYNDROME

Post implantation syndrome (PIS) is a common phenomenon after EVAR, with a reported incidence of 34% to 39% across multiple series,[47] yet it remains a poorly characterized entity. There is no consensus on a definition of or treatment for PIS; however, generally it is marked by fever, elevated white blood cell count, an increase in inflammatory markers (such as C-reactive protein and interleukin 6), and normal procalcitonin without an identified source of infection. It is thought that the graft material and systemic response to new burden of thrombus within the excluded aneurysm sac may elicit this generally benign inflammatory response. Its occurrence can be difficult to distinguish from systemic infection and it can lead to prolonged hospital stays and costly further imaging and interventions. In addition, PIS was found to be associated with an increase in the incidence of major adverse cardiovascular events over a one-year followup period.[48]

Management of PIS consists of clinical evaluation to rule out infection. There is no established treatment described or indicated; however, in practice the use of a short course of nonsteroidal antiinflammatory drugs (NSAIDs) is most common to reduce the convalescent period. The use of systemic corticosteroids has also been described. One randomized controlled trial comparing preoperative methylprednisolone administration with placebo in EVAR patients demonstrated a reduced postoperative systemic inflammatory response syndrome and reduced plasma inflammatory markers; however, 30-day morbidity was comparable.[49]

WOUND INFECTION

Percutaneous access with a closure device, compared with open femoral access, is associated with shorter operating time and hospital length of stay as well as decreased incidence of postoperative wound complications according to multiple retrospective studies.[50,51] The PEVAR Trial, a multicenter, randomized, controlled trial of PEVAR versus open femoral artery access, found PEVAR to be noninferior in terms of safety and technical success. It also found PEVAR to be associated with shorter operative time and decreased blood loss.[52] This is particularly important among the increasing number of obese (body mass index [BMI] greater than 30 kg/m^2) and morbidly obese (BMI greater than 40 kg/m^2) patients undergoing aneurysm repair. This population typically has higher incidence of wound infection and dehiscence as well as prolonged convalescence following surgery given the extra challenge to hygiene and mobility their habitus poses. A study of the NSQIP database comparing outcomes of aneurysm repair between obese and nonobese patients found that obesity of any class was predictive of wound complications in EVAR patients (odds ratio = 3:1). While the incidence of other typical risk factors for wound complications such as COPD, steroid use, and diabetes, steadily increases with BMI in this cohort, multivariate logistic regression confirmed that obesity is an independent risk factor for wound complications.[51]

The benefit of EVAR over traditional open repair continues to evolve and expand; however, it comes at the expense of increased complications and need for reinterventions. Diligent preoperative workup, intraoperative preparation for anticipated complications, and postoperative vigilance for expected complications, as well as constant readiness for conversion to open repair as needed, are crucial to safe delivery of endovascular aneurysm repair.

Take-home points

- The risk of general systemic complications from EVAR is directly proportional to the patient's preoperative comorbidities and risk factors.
- The preoperative evaluation and risk stratification is paramount to minimization of risk.
- Cardiovascular and pulmonary complication risk can be mitigated with appropriate preoperative testing and medical optimization.
- All active tobacco users should be strongly advised to quit at least 2 to 4 weeks prior to EVAR.
- Renal injury secondary to iodinated contrast use can be mitigated by judicious pre- and intraoperative intravenous hydration.
- Case-by-case inclusion of clinically relevant accessory renal arteries should be considered to prevent renal ischemia or infarction.
- A high index of suspicion must be maintained for ischemia of the limbs, spinal cord, and colon.
- In appropriate patients, neuraxial anesthesia should be considered to reduce the risk of the systemic complications of general anesthesia.
- Techniques and practices to reduce the risk and severity of radiation-induced injury to both patient and operator include the use of appropriate shields and dose reduction techniques.

REFERENCES

1. Volodos N, Karpovich I, Troyan V, et al. Clinical experience of the use of self-fixing synthetic prosthesis for remote endoprosthetics of the thoracic and the abdominal aorta and iliac arteries through the femoral artery and as intraoperative endoprosthesis for aorta reconstruction. *Vasa Suppl.* 1991;33:93–95.
2. Parodi J, Palmaz J, Barone H. Transfermoral intraluminal graft implantation for abdominal aortic aneurysms. *Ann Vasc Surg.* 1991;5:491–499.
3. Patel S, Allen C, Grima M, et al. A systematic review of predictors of reintervention after EVAR: guidance for risk-stratified surveillance. *Vasc Endovascular Surg.* 2017;51(6):417–428.
4. de Bruin J, Baas A, Buth J, et al. Long-term outcome of open or endovascular repair of abdominal aortic aneurysm. *N Engl J Med.* 2010;362:1881–1889.
5. van Schaik T, Yeung K, Verhagen H, et al. Long-term survival and secondary procedures after open or endovascular repair of abdominal aortic aneurysms. *J Vasc Surg.* 2017;66(5):1379–1389.
6. Chaikof E, Blankensteijn J, Harris P, et al. Reporting standards for endovascular aortic aneurysm repair. *J Vasc Surg.* 2002;35(5):1048–1060.
7. Franks S, Sutton A, Brown M, Sayers R. Systematic review and meta-analysis of 12 years of endovascular abdominal aortic aneurysm repair. *Eur J Vasc Endovascular Surg.* 2007;33:154–171.
8. Karthikesalingam A, Holt P, Vidal-Diez A, et al. Predicting aortic complications after endovascular aneurysm repair. *Br J Surg.* 2013;1302–1311.
9. de Bruin J, Karthikesalingam A, Holt P, et al. Predicting reinterventions after open and endovascular aneurysm repair using the St George's Vascular Institute score. *J Vasc Surg.* 2016;63(6):1428–1433. e1.
10. Chaikof E, Fillinger M, Matsumura J, et al. Identifying and grading factors that modify the outcome of endovascular aortic aneurysm repair. *J Vasc Surg.* 2002;1061–1066.
11. Fried L, Tangen C, Walston J, et al. Frailty in older adults: evidence for a phenotype. *J Gerontol.* 2001;56(3):146–157.
12. Arya S, Kim S, Duwayri Y, et al. Frailty increases the risk of 30-day mortality, morbidity, and failure to rescue after elective abdominal aortic aneurysm repair independent of age and comorbidities. *J Vasc Surg.* 2015;61:324–331.
13. Adkar S, Turner M, Leraas H, et al. Low mortality rates after endovascular aortic repair expand use to high-risk patients. *J Vasc Surg.* 2017;1–9.

14. Bertges D, Neal D, Schanzer A, et al. The Vascular Quality Initiative Cardiac Risk Index for prediction of myocardial infarction after vascular surgery. *J Vasc Surg.* 2016;64(5):1411–1421.
15. Bakker E, van de Luijtgaarden K, van Lier F, et al. General anaesthesia is associated with adverse cardiac outcome after endovascular aneurysm repair. *Eur J Vasc Endovascular Surg.* 2012;(44)121–125.
16. Durazzo A, Machado F, Ikeoka D, et al. Reduction in cardiovascular events after vascular surgery with atorvastatin: a randomized trial. *J Vasc Surg.* 2004;39:967–976.
17. Auerbach A, Goldman L. Beta-blockers and reduction of cardiac events in noncardiac surgery: clinical applications. *J Am Med Assoc.* 2002;287(11): 1445–1447.
18. Wild J, Dattani N, Stather P, et al. Effect of anticoagulation and antiplatelet therapy on incidence of endoleaks and sac size expansions after endovascular aneurysm repair. *Ann Vasc Surg.* 2014;28(3):554–559.
19. Karthikesalingam A, Thrumurthy S, Young E, et al. Locoregional anesthesia for endovascular aneurysm repair. *J Vasc Surg.* 2012;56(2):510–519.
20. Pauwels R, Buist S, Calverley P, et al. Global strategy for the diagnosis, management, and prevention of chronic obstructive pulmonary disease. *Am J Respir Crit Care Med.* 2001;163:1256–2001.
21. Ohrlander T, Dencker M, Acosta S. Preoperative spirometry results as a determinant for long-term mortality after EVAR for AAA. *Eur J Vasc Endovascular Surg.* 2012;43:43–47.
22. Dawson J, Vig S, Choke E, et al. Medical optimisation can reduce morbidity and mortality associated with elective aortic aneurysm repair. *Eur J Vasc Endovascular Surg.* 2007;33:100–104.
23. Canet J, Gallart L, Gomar C, et al. Prediction of postoperative pulmonary complications in a population-based surgical cohort. *Anesthesiology.* 2010;113(6):1338–1350.
24. Karthikesalingam A, Bahia S, Patel S, et al. A systematic review and meta-analysis indicates underreporting of renal dysfunction following endovascular aneurysm repair. *Kidney Int.* 2015;87:442–451.
25. van Eps RG, Nemeth B, Mairuhu RT, et al. Determinants of acute kidney injury and renal function decline after endovascular abdominal aortic aneurysm repair. *Eur J Vasc Endovascular Surg.* December 1, 2017;54 (6):712–720. Retrieved from https://doi.org/10.1016/j.ejvs.2017.09.011.
26. Saratzis A, Melas N, Mahmood A, Sarafidis P. Incidence of acute kidney injury (AKI) after endovascular abdominal aortic aneurysm repair (EVAR) and impact on outcome. *Eur J Vasc Endovascular Surg.* 2015;49(5):534–540.
27. de Angelis C, Sardanelli F, Perego M, et al. Carbon dioxide angiography as an option for endovascular abdominal aortic aneurysm repair in patients with chronic kidney disease. *Int J Cardiovasc Imaging.* 2017; 33(11):1655–1662.
28. Partovi S, Kaspar M, Aschwanden M, et al. Contrast-enhanced ultrasound after endovascular aortic repair—current status and future perspectives. *Cardiovasc Diagn Ther.* 2015;5(6):454–463.
29. Zettervall S, Deery S, Soden P, et al. Renal complications after EVAR with suprarenal versus infrarenal fixation among all users and routine users. *Eur J Vasc Endovascular Surg.* 2017;54(3):287–293.
30. Urban B, Ratner L, Fishman E. Three-dimensional volume-rendered CT angiography of the renal arteries and veins: normal anatomy, variants, and clinical applications. *Radiographics.* 2001;21(2):373–386.
31. Abu Bakr N, Torsello G, Pitoulias G, et al. Preservation of clinically relevant accessory renal arteries in infrarenal AAA patients with adequate proximal landing zones undergoing EVAR. *J Endovascular Ther.* 2016;23 (2):314–320.
32. Sadeghi-Azandaryani M, Zimmermann H, Korten I, et al. Altered renal functions in patients with occlusion of an accessory renal artery after endovascular stenting of an infrarenal aneurysm. *J Vasc Surg.* 2017;65:635–642.
33. Eagleton M, Grigoryants V, Peterson D, et al. Endovascular treatment of abdominal aortic aneurysm is associated with a low incidence of deep vein thrombosis. *J Vasc Surg.* 2002;36:912–916.
34. Ramanan B, Gupta P, Sundaram A, et al. In-hospital and postdischarge venous thromboembolism after vascular surgery. *J Vasc Surg.* 2013;57:1589–1596.
35. Morgan C, Herm-Barabasz R, Rodriguez H, et al. Incidence of acute lower extremity venous thrombosis after percutaneous endovascular aneurysm repair. *J Vasc Surg.* 2015;62(2):351–354.
36. Lee FY, Chen WK, Chiu CH, Lin CL, Kao CH, Chen CH, et al. Increased risk of deep vein thrombosis and pulmonary thromboembolism in patients with aortic aneurysms: A nationwide cohort study. *PloS one.* June 7, 2017;12(6):e0178587. Accessed November 2, 2017. http://journals.plos.org/plosone/article?id=10.1371/journal.pone.0178587.
37. Maldonado T, Rockman C, Riles E, et al. Ischemic complications after endovascular abdominal aortic aneurysm repair. *J Vasc Surg.* 2004; 40(4):703–710.
38. Berg P, Kaufmann D, van Marrewijk C, Buth J. Spinal cord ischemia after stent-graft treatment for infra-renal abdominal aortic aneurysms. Analysis of the EUROSTAR database. *Eur J Endovascular Surg.* 2001;22:342–347.
39. Moghadamyeghaneh Z, Sgroi M, Chen S, et al. Risk factors and outcomes of postoperative ischemic colitis in contemporary open and endovascular abdominal aortic aneurysm repair. *J Vasc Surg.* 2016;63:866–872.
40. Engelke C, Elford J, Morgan RA, Belli AM. Internal iliac artery embolization with bilateral occlusion before endovascular aortoiliac aneurysm repair—clinical outcome of simultaneous and sequential intervention. *Journal of vascular and interventional radiology.* July 1, 2002;13(7):667–76.
41. Ultee K, Zettervall S, Soden P, et al. Incidence of and risk factors for bowel ischemia after abdominal aortic aneurysm repair. *J Vasc Surg.* 2016;64:1384–1391.
42. Rehani M, Ciraj-Bjelac O, Vano E, et al. ICRP, 2010. Radiological protection in fluoroscopically guided procedures performed outside the imaging department. *Ann ICRP.* 2010;40(6).
43. Zoli S, Trabattoni P, Dainese L, et al. Cumulative radiation exposure during thoracic endovascular aneurysm repair and subsequent follow-up. *Eur J Cardiothorac Surg.* 2012;42(2):254–259.
44. Hertault A, Maurel B, Midulla M, et al. Editor's choice—minimizing radiation exposure during endovascular procedures: basic knowledge, literature review, and reporting standards. *Eur J Vasc Endovascular Surg.* 2015;50(1):21–36.
45. White H, Macdonald S. Estimating risk associated with radiation exposure during follow-up after endovascular aortic repair (EVAR). *J Cardiovasc Surg.* 2010;51:95–104.
46. Chaikof E, Brewster D, Dalman R, et al. SVS practice guidelines for the care of patients with an abdominal aortic aneurysm. *J Vasc Surg.* 2009; 50(4):880–896.
47. Arnaoutoglou E, Kouvelos G, Papa N, et al. Prospective evaluation of postimplantation syndrome evolution on patient outcomes after endovascular aneurysm repair for abdominal aortic aneurysm. *J Vasc Surg.* 2016;63(5):1248–1255.
48. Sartipy F, Lindstrom D, Gillgren P, Ternhag A. The impact of stent graft material on the inflammatory response after EVAR. *Vasc Endovascular Surg.* 2015;49(3–4):79–83.
49. de la Motte L, Kehlet H, Vogt K, Nielsen CH, et al. Preoperative methylprednisolone enhances recovery after endovascular aortic repair: a randomized, double-blind, placebo-controlled clinical trial. *Annals of Surgery.* September 1, 2014;260(3):540–549.
50. Chin J, Skrip L, Sumpio B, et al. Percutaneous endovascular aneurysm repair in morbidly obese patients. *J Vasc Surg.* 2017;65(3):643–650.e1.
51. Johnson O, Sidawy A, Scanlon J, et al. Impact of obesity on outcomes after open surgical and endovascular abdominal aortic aneurysm repair. *J Am Coll Surg.* 2010;210:166–177.
52. Nelson P, Kracjer Z, Kansal N, et al. A multicenter, randomized, controlled trial of totally percutaneous access versus open femoral exposure for endovascular aortic aneurysm repair (the PEVAR trial). *J Vasc Surg.* 2014;59:1181–1194.

FURTHER READING

Alric P, Hinchliffe R, MacsSweeney S, et al. The Zenith aortic stent-graft: a 5-year single-center experience. *J Endovascular Ther.* 2002;9:719–728.

Bhama J, Lin P, Voloyiannis T, et al. Delayed neurologic deficit after endovascular abdominal aortic aneurysm repair. *J Vasc Surg.* 2003;37(3):690–692.

Candell L, Tucker L, Goodney P, et al. Early and delayed rupture after endovascular abdominal aortic aneurysm repair in a 10-year multicenter registry. *J Vasc Surg.* 2014;60:1146–1153.

Fowkes F, Anandan C, Lee A, et al. Reduced lung function in patients with abdominal aortic aneurysm is associated with activation of inflammation and hemostasis, not smoking or cardiovascular disease. *J Vasc Surg.* 2006;43(3):474–480.

Ilyas S, Shaida N, Thakor A, et al. Endovascular aneurysm repair follow-up imaging: the assessment and treatment of common postoperative complications. *Clin Radiol.* 2015;70(2):183–196.

Mahlmann A, Weiss N. Anesthesia management during aortic surgery: preoperative patient assessment. *Best Pract Res Clin Anaesthesiol.* 2016;30(3): 249–255.

Patel R, Sweeting M, Powell J, Greenhalgh R. Endovascular versus open repair of abdominal aortic aneurysm in 15-years' follow-up of the UK endovascular aneurysm repair trial 1 (EVAR trial 1): a randomised controlled trial. *Lancet.* 2016;388:2366–2374.

Reid J, Mole D, Johnston L, Lee B. Delayed paraplegia after endovascular repair of abdominal aortic aneurysm. *J Vasc Surg.* 2003;37(6):1322–1323.

Rockman C, Riles T, Landis R. Lower extremity paraparesis or paraplegia subsequent to endovascular management of abdominal aortic aneurysms. *J Vasc Surg.* 2001;33:178–180.

Sailer A, Nelemans P, van Berlo C, et al. Endovascular treatment of complex aortic aneurysms: prevalence of acute kidney injury and effect on long-term renal function. *Eur Radiol.* 2016;26:1613–1619.

Su Z, Pan T, Lian W, et al. Celiac artery stenting in the treatment of intestinal ischemia due to the sacrifice of the dominant inferior mesenteric artery during endovascular aortic repair. *Vasc Endovascular Surg.* 2016;50 (6):446–450.

Thurley P, Glasby M, Pollock J, et al. Endovascular management of delayed complete graft thrombosis after endovascular aneurysm repair. *Cardiovasc Intervent Radiol.* 2009;33(4):840–843.

Tunick P, Nayar A, Goodkin G, et al. Effect of treatment on the incidence of stroke and other emboli in 519 patients with severe thoracic aortic plaque. *Am J Cardiol.* 2002;90(12):1320–1325.

Verzini F, Romano L, Parlani G, et al. Fourteen-year outcomes of abdominal aortic endovascular repair with the Zenith stent graft. *J Vasc Surg.* 2017; 65(2):318–329.

Wang G, Zhai S, Li T, et al. Limb graft occlusion following endovascular aortic repair: incidence, causes, treatment and prevention in a study cohort. *Exp Ther Med.* 2017;14(2):1763–1768.

5

Gore Excluder

Clayton J. Brinster, MD, FACS and Ross Milner, MD, FACS

INTRODUCTION

Endovascular aortic repair (EVAR) has become the standard of care in the treatment of infrarenal abdominal aortic aneurysm (AAA), with low perioperative morbidity and mortality and comparable long-term outcomes to open surgical repair.[1,2] Successful EVAR requires meticulous intraoperative execution and careful consideration of a variety of anatomic factors during preoperative planning. Of these anatomic features, perhaps the most important are the characteristics of the infrarenal aortic neck. Hostile proximal neck anatomy, in the form of severe angulation, copious thrombus or calcification, or short overall length, is associated with worse short- and long-term outcome after EVAR.[2,3] In order to improve these outcomes, continuous technological innovation in EVAR has focused on broadening the anatomic applicability of currently available devices and improving endograft performance in the infrarenal neck. These advances and a steadily increasing comfort level with EVAR among vascular specialists have led to an increasing number of aortic stent grafts placed over the past 10 years, with a significant percentage placed outside device specific indications for use (IFU). Given this trend of EVAR application in cases with challenging anatomy, the use of a repositionable stent graft offers several potential advantages, including increased deployment accuracy, potentially reduced procedure and fluoroscopy time, and a potential cost reduction by reduced need for aortic cuffs following inaccurate initial deployment or to treat proximal endoleak. With these potential advantages novel complications also emerge, specific to intraoperative repositioning of the device. This chapter will examine the unique attributes and potential complications of the only commercially available, repositionable device for EVAR, the Gore Excluder with its C3 delivery system (W.L. Gore & Associates, Flagstaff, AZ).

EVOLUTION OF THE GORE EXCLUDER AAA ENDOPROSTHESIS

Since the introduction of EVAR, technological innovation has focused on increased anatomic applicability of respective stent grafts and on improved short- and long-term outcomes following aortic repair. The Gore Excluder, now in its third iteration, has been implanted in over 300,000 patients and has undergone several design modifications and improvements since its initial FDA approval in 1997. The first major improvement, in 2004, was the modification of the original ePTFE (expanded polytetrafluoroethylene) microstructure, reducing porosity and subsequent fluid transmigration.[4] The newer, low permeability Excluder was shown not only to reduce the incidence of sac enlargement and associated endotension, but also to promote early aneurysm sack shrinkage.[4,5] Although known for its inherent overall flexibility and performance in challenging iliac anatomy, accurate proximal deployment of the Excluder still remained a concern among clinicians.

A critical second modification to the Excluder was the complete redesign of the traditional "rip-cord" mechanism or sim-pull technology of proximal graft deployment, which was occasionally imprecise in the setting of severe proximal neck angulation, to a repositionable deployment system.[6,7] The modified C3 delivery system allows the operator to reconstrain the proximal aspect of the stent graft twice and reposition the device before final deployment. This novel feature means the graft can be repositioned when the proximal aspect of the main body graft fabric lands either too far proximally or too far distally with respect to the lower renal artery. The proximal aspect of the stent graft is constrained to approximately 30% of its full diameter, withdrawing the proximal anchors away from the aortic wall and allowing proximal or distal adjustment. In addition, when contralateral gate catheterization is challenging, the proximal aspect of the stent graft can be reconstrained and the graft rotated to allow a more favorable orientation.

EXCLUDER WITH C3 DELIVERY SYSTEM DEPLOYMENT

Deployment of the Excluder with C3 delivery system occurs with three sequential steps: (1) opening of the main body and contralateral gate; (2) removal of the constraining wire and loop; and (3) deployment of the ipsilateral limb.

Step 1

First, to initiate the deployment sequence after the usual maneuvers to establish access and perform diagnostic aortography are accomplished, the outer white deployment knob is rotated 90 degrees counter-clockwise, then slowly and steadily pulled (Fig. 5.1). This maneuver will deploy the main body of the endograft and spring the contralateral gate. If the proximal position of the stent graft is acceptable, the procedure continues with cannulation of the contralateral gate. If the endograft requires adjustment to maximize proximal seal, the main body can be reconstrained and the endograft moved cephalad or caudad for ideal positioning. In order to reposition, the gray dial is rotated clockwise to reconstrain the proximal end, until the handle stops turning, moving the black nut toward the trailing end of the catheter handle, as seen through the transparent aspect of the manifold. While the main body of the endograft is reconstrained, the entire device can be manipulated proximally or distally to improve the position of the proximal landing zone, or along its rotational axis to improve the position of the contralateral gate. When the desired position of the proximal graft and gate is achieved, redeployment of the main body is accomplished by turning the same gray dial counterclockwise as far as possible. The black nut will be seen to move proximally. Fig. 5.2 displays these constrainment maneuvers and corresponding graft behavior (Boxes 5.1 and 5.2).

Step 2

After the main body and contralateral gate are optimally positioned and proximal position is verified, the graft is released from the constraining wire and loop by pulling back and holding in place the red safety lock. The entire transparent knob is then rotated 90 degrees counterclockwise and pulled completely out of the catheter handle (Fig. 5.3).

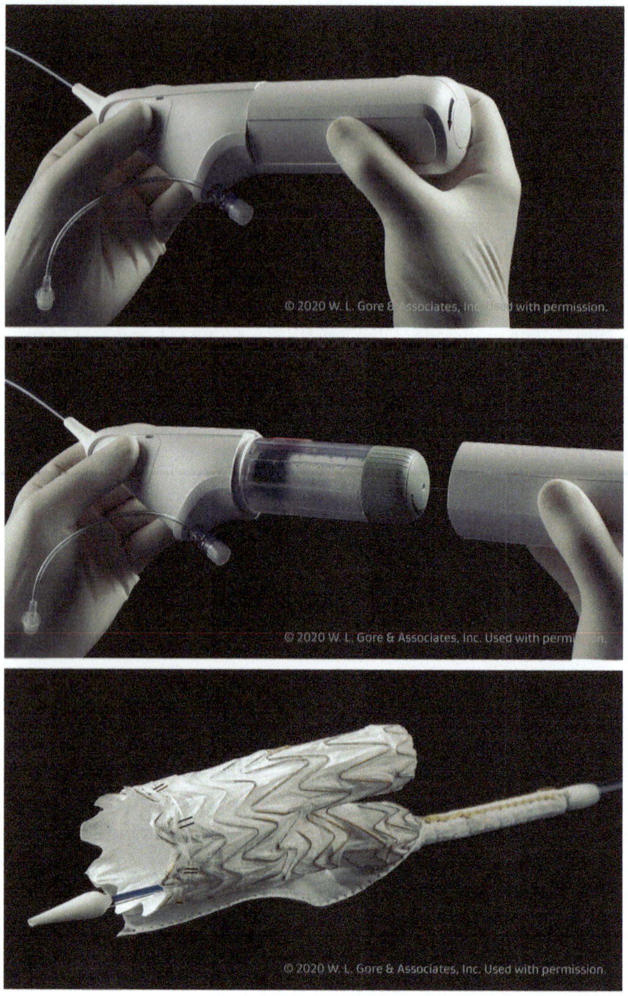

Fig. 5.1 Excluder Deployment. Deployment of the main body and release of the contralateral gate are achieved as the outer white deployment knob is rotated 90 degrees in counterclockwise direction, then slowly and steadily pulled.

(Images provided by W.L. Gore and Associates, Flagstaff, Arizona.)

Step 3

Ipsilateral limb deployment is completed by loosening the gray deployment knob, then pulling it straight out of the catheter handle using a slow, steady motion (Fig. 5.3). The contralateral limb can then be placed to complete the procedure.

CRITICAL TECHNICAL CONSIDERATIONS, POTENTIAL PITFALLS, TROUBLESHOOTING

The C3 deployment system offers a number of options for repositioning and readjustment of both the proximal main body and the contralateral gate of the main body Excluder device, which are useful in a variety of clinical scenarios.[8] The ability to deploy, recapture, and reposition the proximal aspect of the endograft relative to the lower renal artery is advantageous for both the inexperienced operator in cases with routine anatomy and for the experienced operator in cases that feature hostile proximal neck anatomy. Recapturing the proximal aspect of the main body for rotational adjustment of the endograft along its longitudinal axis also allows for reorientation of the contralateral gate to a more favorable position to facilitate cannulation.

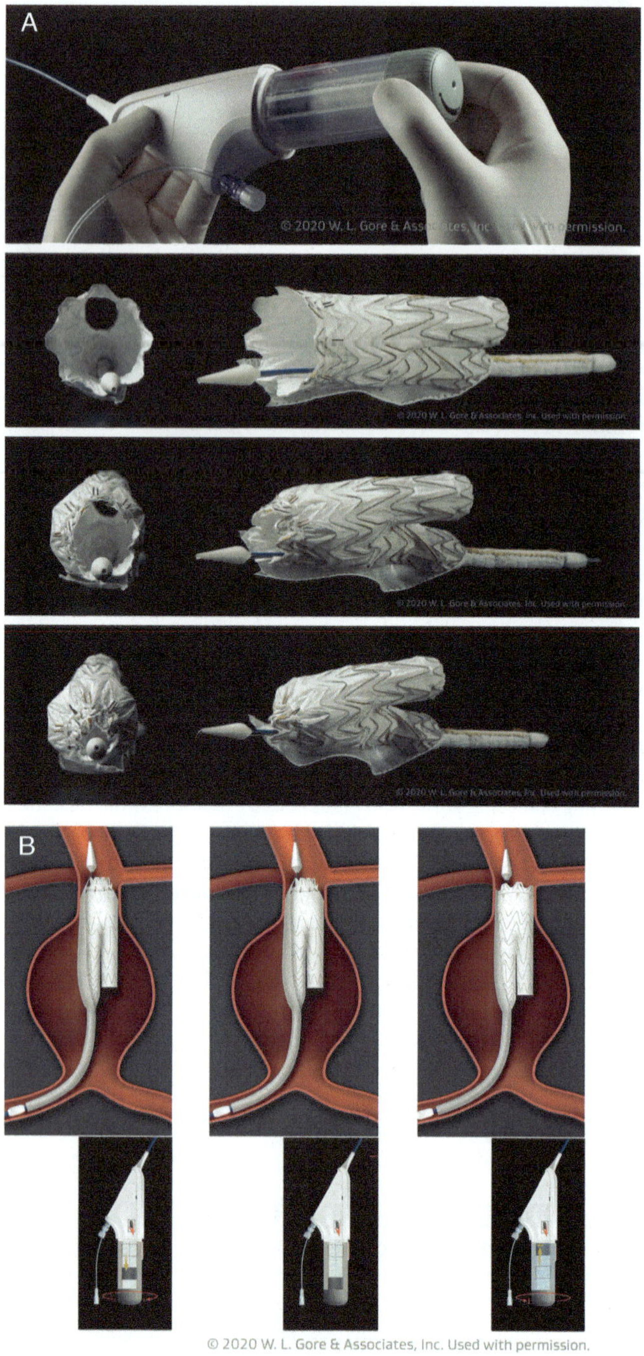

Fig. 5.2 Excluder Reconstrainment and Repositioning. The C3 delivery system allows the main body to be reconstrained (A) with clockwise rotation of the gray dial *(yellow arrow)* and redeployed after repositioning (B) with counterclockwise rotation of the gray dial *(red arrows)*.

(Images provided by W.L. Gore & Associates, Flagstaff, Arizona.)

Several critical technical points should be considered by the operator when repositioning is undertaken:

- The endoprosthesis should not be constrained and reopened more than two times during a procedure, because device or catheter damage may occur.
- Repositioning should not be performed with the endoprosthesis while the trunk is at its maximum diameter. Vessel damage or device misplacement may result.

- The endoprosthesis should be repositioned only when fully constrained.

The IFU for the Excluder recommends a maximum of two reconstrain/reposition maneuvers, and there are fundamental risks involved with excessive repositioning (Box 5.3). Reconstraining the stent graft with subsequent upward force applied to move the endograft proximally can be difficult in severely angulated, heavily calcified, short, narrow, or otherwise hostile necks. The increased friction generated with cranial force on the delivery system in these anatomic conformations can limit trackability during reorientation or, with excessive force, potentially result in aortic dissection or rupture. With this type of challenging proximal anatomy, Verhoeven and colleagues[8] in reviewing the 1-year experience of C3 Excluder in the GREAT (Global Registry for Endovascular Aortic Treatment) recommend aggressive deployment of the stent graft at the level of the renal arteries or even a few millimeters higher, with the option to withdraw the endograft to a slightly lower position if needed.

When challenging aortic or iliac anatomy is encountered, the endograft main body may not advance to optimal position in the aortic neck. If excessive resistance is noted during attempts to advance the endograft to the desired position, the main body should be deployed in lower than normal position following the standard deployment sequence described. An aortic cuff, which is typically easier to track and push in the setting of challenging anatomy because of its shorter length, should be advanced and deployed in the desired infrarenal position. A minimum overlap of approximately 3 cm between the cuff and main body endograft is preferred to prevent component separation and consequent type III endoleak because the aorta remodels over time. In addition, before deployment of the main body in lower-than-desired anatomic position, the operator must ensure that there is adequate infrarenal aortic length to allow the contralateral gate to open for cannulation. If a proximal extension cuff is unavailable, a possible alternative approach would involve establishment

BOX 5.1 Warning

Do not rotate the device delivery catheter while the endoprosthesis is inside the introducer sheath. Catheter breakage or premature deployment may occur.

BOX 5.2 Warning

Do not continue advancing any portion of the delivery system if resistance is felt during advancement of the guidewire, sheath, or catheter. Arterial or catheter damage may occur. Instead, stop and assess the cause of resistance.

BOX 5.3 Warning

Do not rotate the trunk delivery catheter beyond 360 degrees to avoid delivery system kinking, structural damage, or premature deployment.

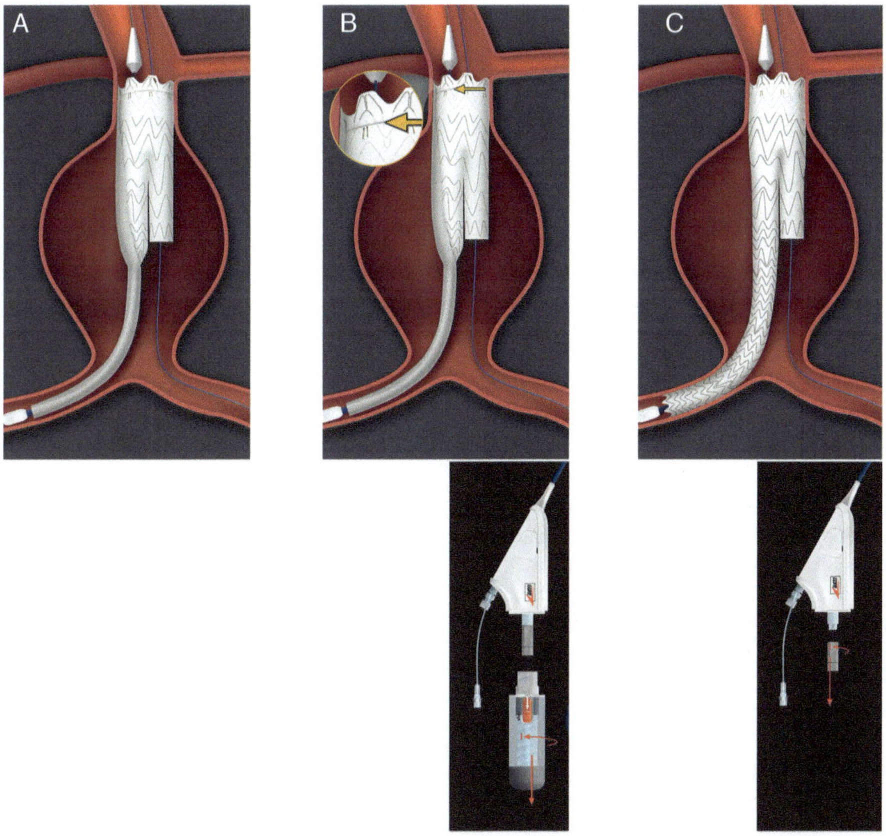

Fig. 5.3 Excluder Final Main Body and Ipsilateral Limb Deployment. After repositioning (if desired) is complete, the contralateral gate is cannulated (A). The graft is released from the constraining wire *(yellow arrow)* and loop by pulling back and holding in place the red safety lock, rotating the transparent handle 90 degrees counterclockwise *(red arrows)*, then removing it (B). Ipsilateral limb deployment is completed by loosening the gray deployment knob, then pulling it straight out of the catheter handle with a slow, steady motion *(red arrows)* (C).

(Images provided by W.L. Gore and Associates, Flagstaff, Arizona.)

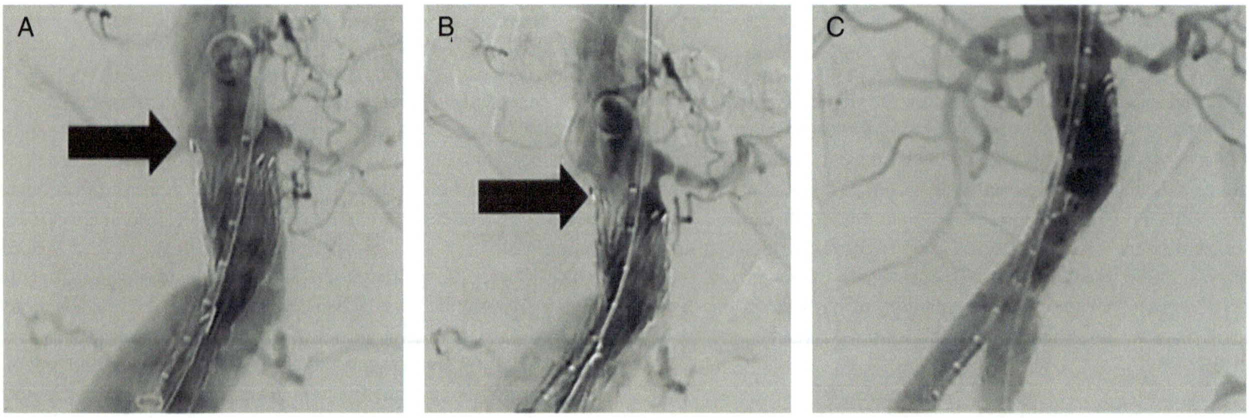

Fig. 5.4 Reconstrainment and Repositioning of the Excluder to Preserve Renal Artery Patency. (A) Right renal artery covered by the proximal fabric of the Excluder during initial deployment (**arrow**). (B) The proximal graft was reconstrained and repositioned distally (**arrow**). (C) Completion angiogram demonstrating a patent right renal artery and no evidence of an endoleak.

BOX 5.4 Warning

Do not attempt to reposition the endoprosthesis after complete deployment of the device. Arterial damage or device misplacement may result.

of brachial access, snaring the stiff wire from the brachial access sheath and creating a "rail" over which the main body is then advanced. Note: this technique should be attempted by experienced operators only, because potentially catastrophic aortic disruption can occur with excessive force.

Additional hazards may be encountered while reconstraining and repositioning the stent graft system along its longitudinal axis. Specifically, excessive rotation may cause ipsilateral limb twisting and kinking. When reorientation of the graft has been preformed to facilitate contralateral gate access, deployment of the ipsilateral limb in sequence should be performed slowly under continued magnification fluoroscopy. This gradual maneuver allows the ipsilateral limb to be untwisted, or "derotated," if necessary before deployment is completed.

Manipulation of the stent graft during the final step, deployment of the ipsilateral limb, may also result in technical complication. Excessive upward device displacement to avoid encroachment upon the hypogastric artery during ipsilateral limb deployment can result in upward migration of the entire stent graft system, partially or totally covering a renal artery in the process.[9] Vigilant observation of the proximal graft fabric position is required if this maneuver is undertaken. Katsargyris and colleagues recommend an adjunctive technical approach if the risk of proximal endograft migration is high during repositioning, and preservation of the hypogastric artery is essential. An inflated coda balloon can be introduced via the contralateral side and inflated in the main body of the stent graft, thereby fixing the system in place while the distal aspect of the ipsilateral limb is adjusted to a more proximal position.[9] If partial or complete renal artery coverage is suspected, urgent endovascular salvage with renal artery stenting should be attempted. Fig. 5.4 demonstrates coverage of a renal artery during initial main body deployment, followed by distal repositioning to restore flow to the renal artery and maintain proximal seal (Box 5.4).

Alternatively, the graft may be gently retracted by either inflating a coda balloon in the main body and gently attempting caudal adjustment, or positioning a stiff wire "up and over" the flow divider, snaring the wire via the contralateral access sheath, and pulling the graft caudally. Note: movement of the endograft main body in caudal fashion after deployment and engagement of the active fixation barbs may result in intimal trauma, aortic dissection, or aortic rupture and should be attempted only by experienced operators.

EXCLUDER WITH C3 DELIVERY SYSTEM FAILURE MODES

Operators should be familiar with several bailout techniques available with the Excluder in the event of a graft deployment malfunction. If counterclockwise rotation of the gray constraining dial does not reopen the proximal aspect of the graft after recapture and repositioning, the following maneuvers should be performed in sequence: (1) verify the position of the proximal fabric of the endograft relative to the lower renal artery; (2) manually stabilize the delivery system at the introducer sheath and likewise stabilize the sheath relative to the patient to prevent graft migration; (3) disengage the constraining mechanism by sliding the red safety lock back while rotating the entire transparent knob 90 degrees counterclockwise; and, finally, (4) remove the constraining mechanism by pulling the transparent knob straight out from the catheter handle (Fig. 5.5). These four maneuvers will allow the release and removal of the endograft constraining mechanism and reopen the proximal aspect of the main body (Box 5.5).

If the stent graft does not deploy when standard maneuvers are performed, the Excluder manifold features a failure mode "deployment line access hatch" that can be readily accessed (Fig. 5.6). If removal of the white outer deployment knob does not initiate the deployment of the proximal main body, the access hatch should be opened manually. The first deployment line, labeled "1", should be grasped and pulled with a surgical instrument and the line fully removed in a steady, continuous motion. Removal of this line will deploy the main body and spring the contralateral gate (Box 5.6).

Additionally, if rotation of the transparent knob does not initiate removal of the constraining mechanism, the silver lock pin line, labeled "2," should be cut, grasped with a clamp and removed in a slow, steady motion. The gray constraining loop line, labeled "3," should then be withdrawn in a similar fashion. Removal of the lock pin line and the constraining loop line will release the endograft from the constraining mechanism. Finally, if the removal of the gray deployment knob does not initiate deployment of the ipsilateral limb, the second deployment line, labeled "4," should be grasped and slowly removed to deploy the limb (Box 5.7).

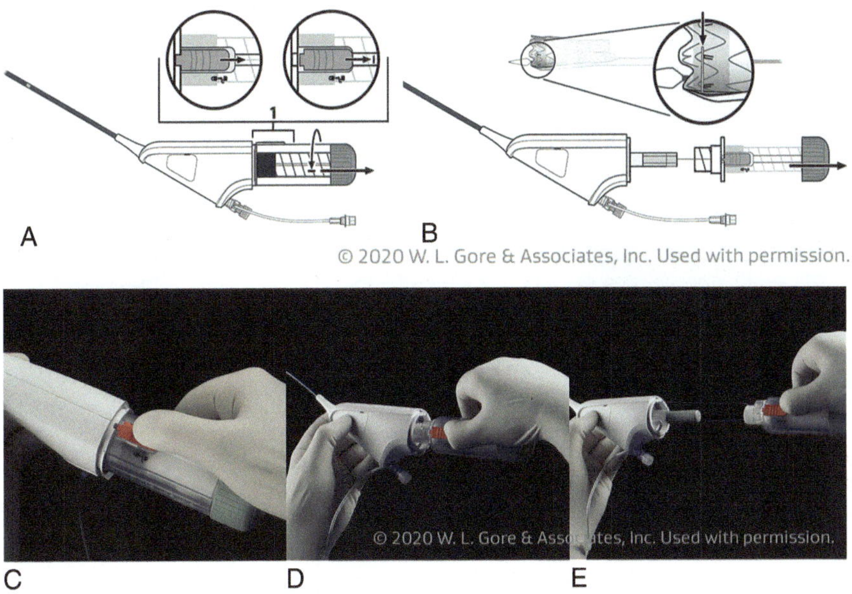

Fig. 5.5 **Bailout Manuevers–Release and Removal of Endograph Constraining Mechanism.** (A) Disengage the constraining mechanism by sliding the red safety lock back while rotating the entire transparent knob 90 degrees counterclockwise *(arrows)* and (B) remove the constraining mechanism by pulling the transparent knob straight out from the catheter handle *(arrows)*. (C, D, E) Bailout maneuvers in sequence.
(Images provided by W.L. Gore and Associates, Flagstaff, Arizona.)

BOX 5.5 Warning

Do not attempt to withdraw any undeployed endoprosthesis through the 12 Fr, 18 Fr, or 20 Fr introducer sheath. Instead, the sheath and catheter must be removed together.

BOX 5.6 Warning

Do not cut the first deployment line (labeled "2") Patient injury, catheter damage, or device damage may occur.

BOX 5.7 Warning

The constraining mechanism cannot be removed unless the proximal end of the trunk device is fully opened. Prior to removing the constraining mechanism, check that the gray constraining dial is rotated counterclockwise until it stops. Attempting to remove the constraining mechanism while the main body is constrained may result in catastrophic injury or structural damage to the stent graft.

CLINICAL APPLICATION OF THE EXCLUDER WITH C3 DELIVERY SYSTEM

Data from comprehensive registries and robust clinical series have demonstrated excellent performance of the C3 Excluder, with low morbidity and mortality and superb rates of technical success.[8,10] The incorporation of the C3 delivery system was intended to broaden the applicability of the Excluder, especially in the challenging infrarenal aortic neck. While the unique ability to reconstrain and reposition the endograft to achieve better seal in these situations can increase the likelihood of successful EVAR in experienced hands, it could also encourage operators to perform cases outside the Excluder IFU. It should be noted that the IFU for the Excluder were not changed with the incorporation of the C3 delivery system, however, and a conservative approach should be undertaken when considering use of this endograft in all types of challenging anatomic scenarios.

Accumulated evidence suggests that better outcomes are achieved when EVAR is performed within device-specific IFU.[11] Morasch and colleagues have noted that, historically, major adverse events following EVAR performed outside IFU may not be related to initial endograft positioning (the major variable the C3 system was designed to improve).[12] Verhoeven et al., when reviewing 400 C3 Excluder cases for the GREAT registry, noted that 17% of patients were treated outside the IFU with no difference in device delivery, positioning, or deployment.[8] Two early Type Ia endoleaks requiring intervention did occur in this group, however, leading the authors to conclude that the C3 Excluder should not be advocated to treat hostile necks outside the IFU, especially if other treatment options are available. Unless more comprehensive data emerge to suggest otherwise, it should not be assumed, therefore, that use of the C3 Excluder will improve outcomes in cases outside the IFU.

CONCLUSION

Although EVAR has gained wide acceptance in the treatment of AAA and the comfort level with a variety of devices has increased among vascular specialists worldwide, the individual operator should be prepared for potential intraoperative complications. When significant issues arise during the deployment process, the alternative techniques described in this chapter should be performed slowly and deliberately, and, in most cases, with magnification fluoroscopy. Experienced operators and Gore Excluder representatives should be called for assistance. Significant resistance with any maneuver during deployment should signal to the operator that something is wrong, and excessively applied force at any time can lead to catastrophic arterial injury. Meticulous attention to detail during preoperative planning and intraoperative deployment is essential to achieve good outcomes with any endovascular procedure. Finally, while the unique attributes of the C3 deployment

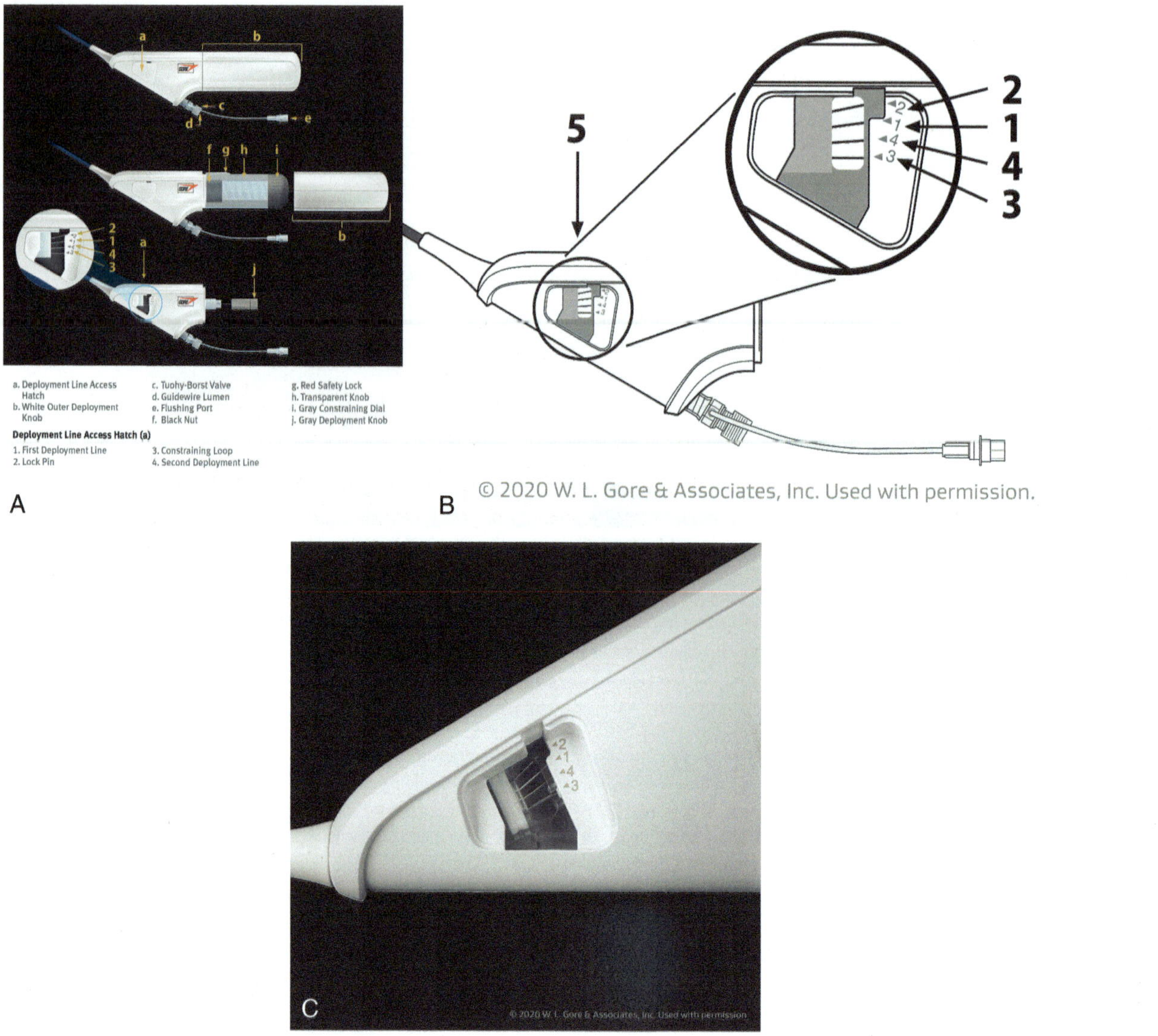

Fig. 5.6 (A) Excluder with C3 delivery system, (B) bailout deployment line access hatch, and (C) access hatch as appears with device. (Images provided by W.L. Gore and Associates, Flagstaff, Arizona.)

system may allow utilization of the Excluder with hostile neck anatomy, only the most experienced operators should attempt these cases.

REFERENCES

1 De Bruin J, Baas AF, Buth J, et al. Long-term outcome of open or endovascular repair of abdominal aortic aneurysm. *N Engl J Med.* 2010;362:1881–1889.

2 Jackson RS, Chang DC, Freischlag JA. Comparison of long-term survival after open vs endovascular repair of intact abdominal aortic aneurysm among Medicare beneficiaries. *JAMA.* 2012;307:1621–1628.

3 AbuRahma AF, Campbell J, Stone PA, et al. The correlation of aortic neck length to early and late outcomes in endovascular aneurysm repair patients. *J Vasc Surg.* 2009;50:738–748.

4 Fillinger M. Three-dimensional analysis of enlarging aneurysms after endovascular abdominal aortic aneurysm repair in the Gore Excluder pivotal clinical trial. *J Vasc Surg.* 2006;43:888–895.

5 Haider SE, Najjar SF, Cho JS, et al. Sac behavior after aneurysm treatment with the Gore Excluder low-permeability aortic endoprosthesis: 12-month comparison to the original Excluder device. *J Vasc Surg.* 2006;44:694–700.

6 Tanski W, 3rd, Fillinger M. Outcomes of original and low-permeability Gore Excluder endoprosthesis for endovascular abdominal aortic aneurysm repair. *J Vasc Surg.* 2007;45:243–249.

7 Verhoeven EL, Oikonomou K. Mohner, et al. First experience with the new repositionable C3 excluder stent-graft. *J Cardiovasc Surg.* 2011;52:637–642.

8 Verhoeven EL, Katsargyris A, Bachoo P, et al. GREAT European C3 module investigators. Real-world performance of the new C3 Gore Excluder stent-graft: 1-year results from the European C3 module of the Global Registry for Endovascular Aortic Treatment (GREAT). *Eur J Vasc Endovasc Surg.* 2014;48:131–137.

9 Katsargyris A, Oikonomou K, Bracale UM, et al. Unexpected complication with the new C3 Excluder: cause and treatment. *Cardiovasc Intervent Radiol.* 2013;36:536–539.

10 Poublon CG, Holewijn S, van Sterkenburg SMM, et al. Long-term outcome of the GORE EXCLUDER AAA endoprosthesis for treatment of infrarenal aortic aneurysms. *J Vasc Interv Radiol.* 2017;28(5):637–644.

11 Schanzer A, Greenberg RK, Hevelone N, et al. Predictors of abdominal aortic aneurysm sac enlargement after endovascular repair. *Circulation.* 2011;123(24):2848–2855.

12 Lee CJ, Keldahl ML, Morasch MD. Gore Excluder device with the C3 delivery system for management of abdominal aortic aneurysm. *Open Access Surg.* 2012;5:15–21.

6

Complications of the Medtronic Endurant Stent Graft

Michael Shih, MD, Jason Chang, MD and Robert Rhee, MD

BACKGROUND OF THE MEDTRONIC ENDURANT STENT GRAFT DEVICE

The Endurant stent graft system is an evolution of previous abdominal stent graft systems to meet the challenges of hostile abdominal aortic aneurysm anatomy. After gaining CE marking in Europe in 2008 and FDA approval in 2010, it has become one of the preeminent endograft systems in the world. It consists of a high-density multifilament polyester graft with low porosity, externally supported by a nitinol stent structure (Fig. 6.1).

Proximally, there is a suprarenal fixation system consisting of a nitinol stent with anchoring pins. Next is a series of nitinol stents constructed into a low amplitude sinusoidal M-shape, which allows more flexibility, conformability, and improved seal in short and angulated proximal aneurysm necks. The reduction of columnar strength also contributes to the flexibility of the stent graft. The Endurant II improved upon the previous iteration by extending the hydrophilic coating, loading the 28 mm graft into the smaller 18 French delivery system, introducing more contralateral limb lengths, and increasing the radiopacity of the markers for better visualization. Recently, the Endurant IIs (EIIs) was added to the armamentarium. The EIIs is a 3-piece system with standardized limbs, which allows more options with a smaller range of components and streamlines sizing and inventory.

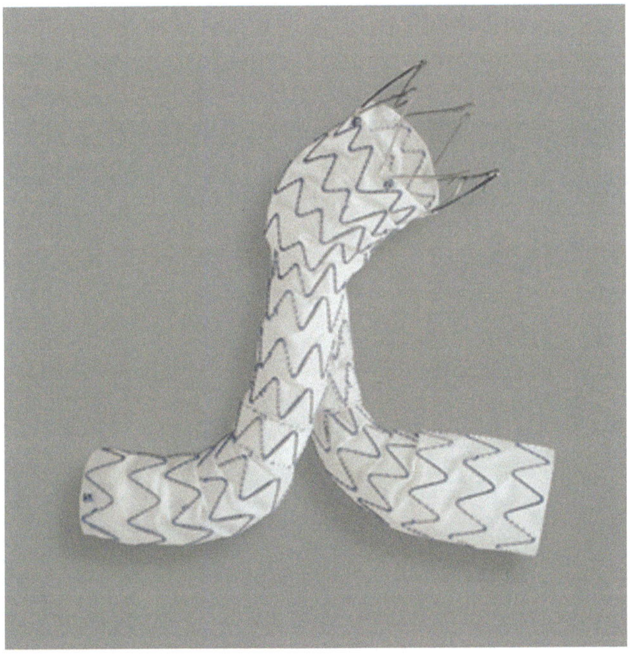

Fig. 6.1 Endurant II Abdominal Aortic Endograft System. Modular stent graft system consisting of a polyester graft with externally supported nitinol stents, and a suprarenal fixation stent with anchoring pins.

The Endurant II and EIIs stent graft systems are indicated in treatment of aneurysms with a proximal neck ranging from 19 mm to 32 mm in diameter, length greater than or equal to 10 mm, and infrarenal neck angulation less than or equal to 60 degrees. The Endurant delivery system provides a stepwise, gradual deployment for utmost precision. The tip capture mechanism allows for fine adjustments until the very last moment before release of the suprarenal fixation pins. Combined with its low profile, hydrophilic delivery sheath, the Endurant system has been developed to become an industry standard.

The evolution of the Endurant endograft has not been without its growing pains. Minor, early design flaws and physician inexperience have occasionally resulted in suboptimal deployment, inadvertent occlusion of inflow or outflow vessels, additional procedures, and occasional conversion to an open repair. Some of these difficulties have been eliminated or reduced by improvements in design. For example, the graft fabric was changed to reduce the incidence of Type IV endoleaks (Fig. 6.2), and a minor geometry change to the spindle component of the tip capture mechanism was made right after commercial launch in the United States. However, occasional complications still arise. These issues will be addressed in the following sections, along with some tips in managing these challenging situations.

ENDURANT SPECIFIC COMPLICATIONS

Deployment and Tip Capture

There are very few known issues with the Endurant device that do not apply to all endografts used to treat abdominal aortic aneurysms. One potential area that was identified early after its full clinical release is with the deployment mechanism of the endograft. Once position of the graft is satisfactory, deployment consists of rotating the backend thumb wheel, which advances the constraining tip to release the suprarenal stent and anchor pins (Figs. 6.3 and 6.4). The potential malfunction of this mechanism is addressed within the Medtronic (Minneapolis, Minnesota) Endurant II/IIs Instructions for Use (IFU). In the section labeled "Bail-Out Techniques" the company outlines its recommendations in cases of delivery system failure.[1]

The first situation is if there is partial deployment as a result of graft cover severance. In this incidence, the screw gear handle can be disassembled. This allows for manual retraction of the graft cover, salvaging a potentially devastating complication of a retained, partially deployed endograft. Hemostats can be inserted into the screw gear handle disassembly ports to disengage the front grip from the screw gear. After the front grip is removed, the screw gear can be separated in half to reveal the graft cover, which can then be manually retracted with a clamp.

Another rare situation that may be encountered is if the captured proximal tip of the suprarenal stent cannot be deployed. If the

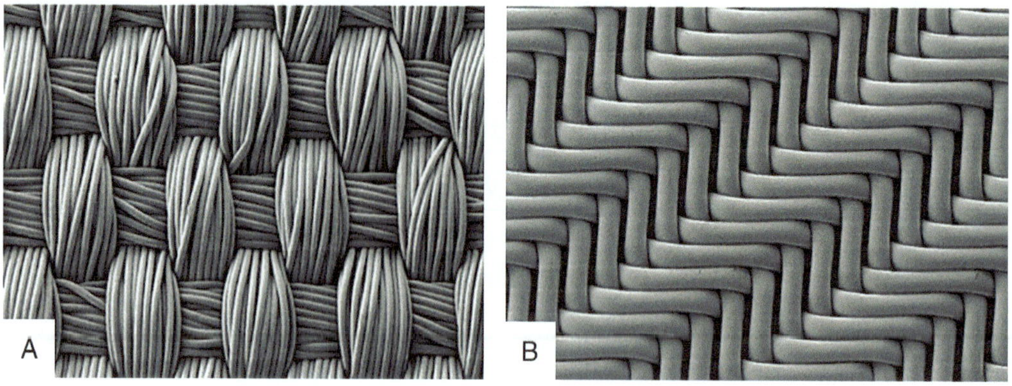

Fig. 6.2 Magnified View of Stent Graft Fabric. Comparison of (A) the Medtronic Endurant multifilament polyester fabric and (B) the older Medtronic Talent monofilament fabric.

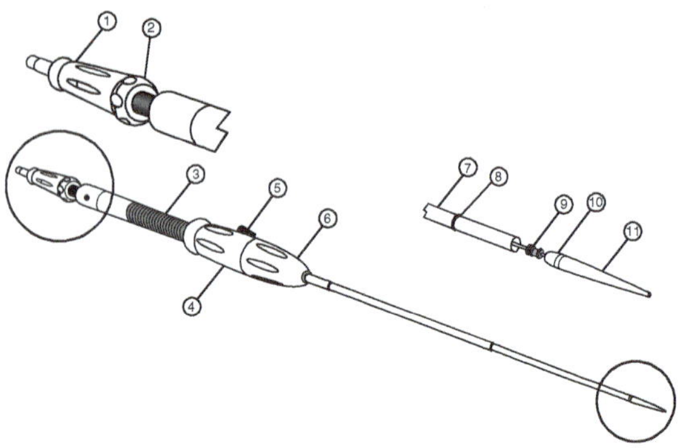

1. Rear Handle
2. Back-End Wheel
3. Screw Gear
4. External Slider
5. Trigger
6. Front Grip
7. Graft Cover
8. Markerband
9. Spindle
10. Sleeve
11. Tapered Tip

Fig. 6.3 Schematic of Endurant II Delivery System. Taken from the Endurant II/IIs Instructions for Use.
(Reproduced with permission of Medtronic.)

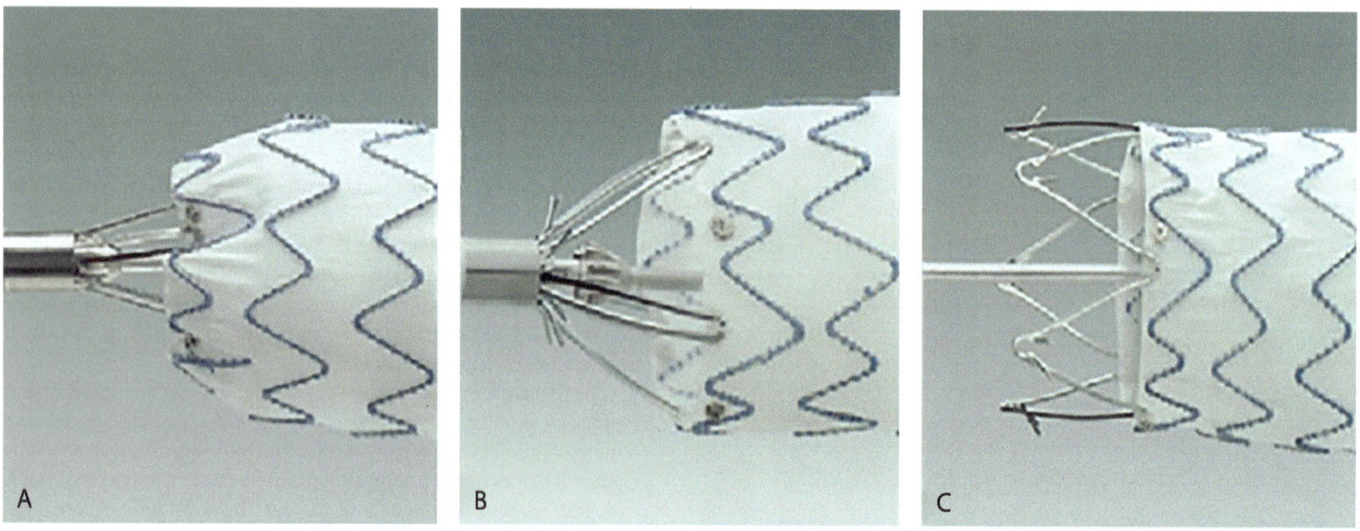

Fig. 6.4 Endurant II Proximal Neck Deployment. (A) The suprarenal stent restrained in the delivery tip; (B) the suprarenal stent partially deployed with visualization of the anchor pins; (C) the suprarenal stent fully deployed.
(Reproduced with permission of Medtronic.)

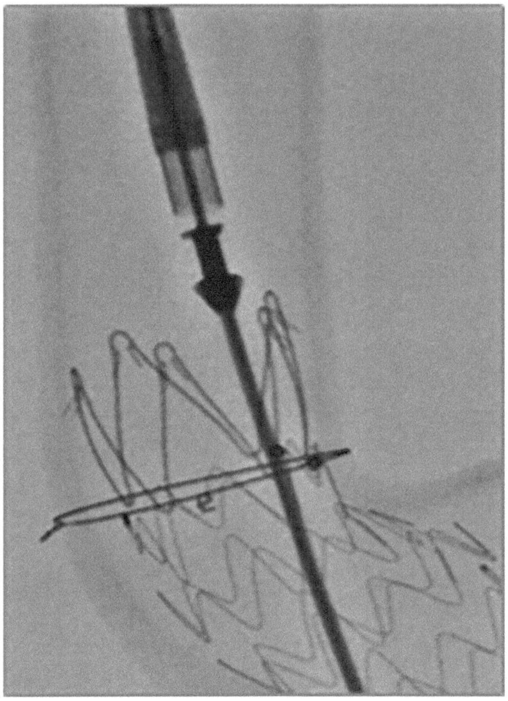

Fig. 6.5 **Delivery Tip and Proximal Stent Graft.** Fluoroscopic view of an Endurant endograft in a model with the delivery tip and spindle near the suprarenal stent.

back-end wheel still works, a ballooning technique is described that may allow continued deployment of the endoprosthesis. To accomplish this, a compliant balloon is placed within the main body and inflated to profile. The balloon catheter is used to stabilize the stent graft position, while the tip capture deployment can be carried out per the IFU, followed by delivery system removal. However, if the deployment of the suprarenal stent fails because of a failure of the back-end wheel, the back-end handle can be disassembled to attempt manual disengagement. This involves inserting a hemostat into the rear handle disassembly port, allowing retraction of the handle from the delivery system. The spindle and tapered tip can then be manually advanced/withdrawn by pushing and pulling the exposed tabs of the back-end T-tube. In this situation, backward tension must be maintained on the tabs during system removal to keep the tapered tip recaptured over the spindle. The entire delivery system can then be removed from the patient as usual.

Lastly, the manufacturer discusses a snare technique if the deployment of the suprarenal stent is unable to be completed even after disassembling the back-end handle. A snare is introduced from a brachial or axillary access. Under fluoroscopy, the delivery tip is snared. The snare is then pulled back while stabilizing the distal delivery system from the femoral access. This should facilitate separation of the tip and sleeve from the suprarenal stent, allowing for full deployment. The remainder of the steps for removing the system follows those outlined earlier.

Tip Retrieval

Another step that can be an issue with the Endurant stent graft is with retrieving the tapered tip, sleeve, and spindle after graft deployment[2,3] (Fig. 6.5). This is relevant particularly in situations of highly tortuous vessels and severely angulated necks. After deployment, the delivery tip must be withdrawn from the aorta, through the stent graft, and out of the femoral access site. There are multiple areas where this can catch during its extraction. Excessive force can lead to migration of the endoprosthesis or injury to the vessels. After identifying this issue with earlier iterations of the device, Medtronic adjusted the design to include a reverse taper on the spindle to streamline the profile. This has greatly reduced the occurrence of this complication with the Endurant II and EIIs endografts.

During deployment, it is critical to adhere to the IFU, which includes specific maneuvers designed to ensure smooth retrieval of the tapered tip and spindle beyond the suprarenal stents. Specifically, one must confirm that the spindle has fully separated from the suprarenal stent by gently torquing the device and advancing it approximately 3 cm; then, recapture the spindle in the sleeve of the tip under fluoroscopy. If the spindle catches on the suprarenal stent, advance with gentle rotation until the spindle slips past the suprarenal stent and restart the capture process. When withdrawing the captured spindle and tip past the stent graft, again apply a gentle rotation until the delivery system is within the fabric portion of the graft.

Beyond the suprarenal stent, there are other locations where the delivery system may have potential difficulty maneuvering, especially in severely angulated necks or tortuous iliac arteries. Georgiadis et al. nicely summarize several different scenarios where the delivery system could get caught, as well as some tips for recovery.[4] Note that while these techniques were described with the Endurant graft in mind, these can be applied to any graft where there is difficulty removing the delivery catheter at the given locations.

The first scenario is if the tip sleeve is caught within the suprarenal bare-stent anchoring pins. The flexibility of the delivery system will displace the shaft off the centerline, and at times hug the aortic wall if there is severe angulation. This can cause one side of the tip sleeve to catch on one of the suprarenal stents. The following techniques can be utilized to remove the delivery system.

The first step is to remove the stiff guidewire from inside the delivery system, which allows the graft to better conform to the natural aortic anatomy. This causes the delivery system to follow a more curved path, thus avoiding catching at the level of the anchoring pins. Similar to standard withdrawal, gently torquing the delivery system past the suprarenal stents reduces the likelihood of it snagging. Deployment of the contralateral limb should precede delivery system withdrawal to ensure proper positioning and to stabilize the main body.

In contrast, where the delivery system was encouraged to follow the curve of the aorta, an attempt can be made to straighten the aorta and alter the path that the system follows during its retraction. After deployment of the contralateral docking limb, a stiff wire and large introducer sheath can be advanced to beyond the level of the suprarenal stent, straightening the aorta. A wire can also be snared from a brachial access to create a rail from the femoral artery to straighten the aortic neck further to allow passage of the tip.

Another reasonable option would be to partially inflate a molding balloon (e.g. Reliant) at the level of the pins as the delivery system is withdrawn (Fig. 6.6A,B). This technique alters the trajectory, using the balloon as a bumper to deflect the tip as it slides past the suprarenal stents.

The last option utilizes a snare device that is introduced through a left brachial artery access. The top cap and spindle are captured via the snare and held on slight tension, while the delivery system is simultaneously retracted with slow rotational movements, thus keeping the tip away from the edges of the stent graft (Fig. 6.6C).

The next theoretical place for the delivery system to catch is at the flow divider. A molding balloon can again be used. After deployment of the contralateral limb, a compliant balloon can be inserted and positioned to straddle the flow divider. The balloon is inflated to guide the

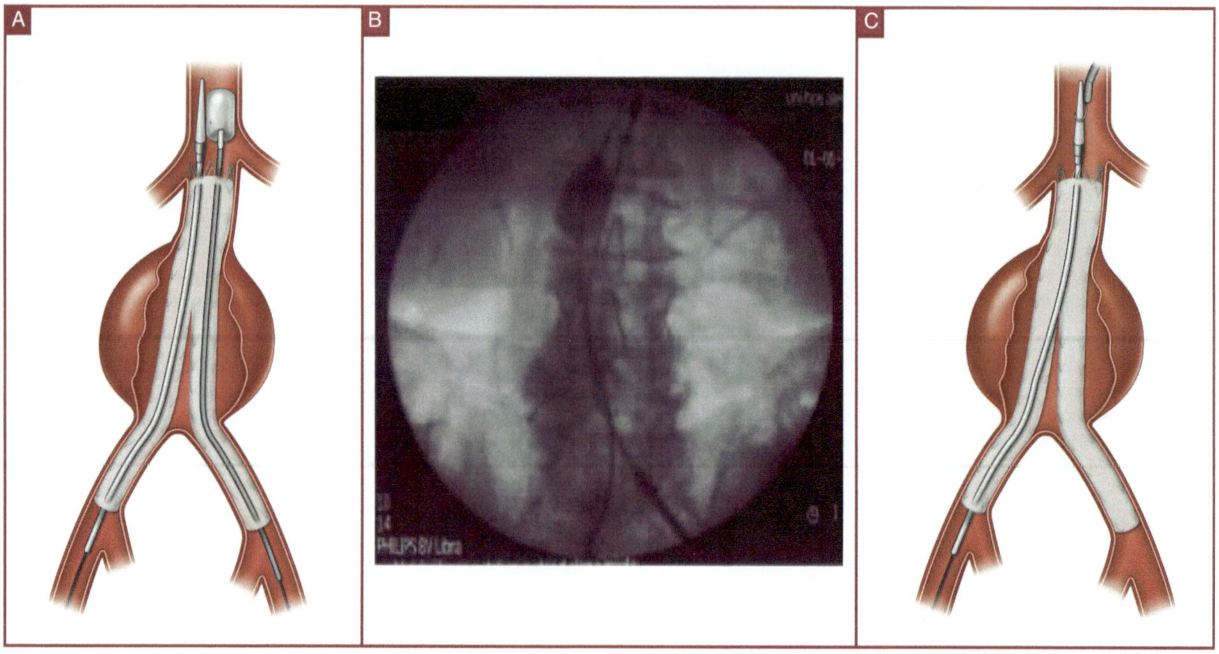

Fig. 6.6 Maneuver: Delivery Tip Catches at Suprarenal Stent. Inflation of a molding balloon at the level of the suprarenal stent to deflect the tip during withdrawal of the delivery system (A). Fluoroscopic view of the maneuver described in (A and B). Use of a snare device to capture the tip, straightening it as it passes by the fixation pins (C).

(Georgiadis G, Antoniou G, Trellopoulos G, et al. Troubleshooting techniques for the Endurant device in endovascular aortic aneurysm repair. *Cardiovasc J Afr.* 2014;25(5):239–243.)

delivery system away from the flow divider towards the centerline of the ipsilateral limb as it is slowly retracted (Fig. 6.7).

In cases where the iliac arteries are very tortuous, there is the possibility of the delivery tip being caught in the ipsilateral limb. Changing the stiffness of the wire may change the configuration enough to allow easy withdrawal. Otherwise, two molding balloons can be used to stabilize the endograft, one at the level of the suprarenal stent and one at the contralateral limb near the flow divider (Fig. 6.8). The delivery system is simultaneously retracted downward while the balloons are inflated. It may be most efficacious if the proximal balloon is inserted from a brachial approach.

The delivery system can also catch at the external iliac artery, especially in stenotic or tortuous iliac arteries. In this situation, angioplasty of the external iliac artery may be all that is needed to create enough space to pass the device. Ideally, this would be recognized on preoperative imaging and the angioplasty performed prior to device introduction. However, if it is not recognized until after the endograft is inserted, the delivery system sheath can be directly punctured with a single wall needle (Fig. 6.9). A wire and 6-French sheath can be inserted into the delivery system. An angioplasty of the external iliac artery can then be performed, followed by removal of the entire system.

Limb Occlusions

While not exclusive to the Endurant graft, limb occlusion has been found to occur at a slightly higher rate than expected.[5] This may have been because the Endurant was the first of the low profile systems, and therefore, many of the patients treated had smaller and more diseased iliac arteries to begin with. Reports in the literature describe limb occlusion rates ranging from 2.7% to 5.6%.[2,6–9] When deployed according to the IFU, the Endurant US Pivotal Trial Investigators found a limb occlusion rate of 3%, which was unexpected given the improved flexibility in the graft. This compares with the 1%–3% range seen for other devices of its generation[10], albeit at the higher end.

Mannetje et al. found a higher incidence of limb occlusion with the Endurant stent graft compared with the older generation Talent endograft (Medtronic).[11] They reported a limb occlusion rate of 5.6% versus 0%, with an additional 4.8% of patients in the Endurant group having an iliac stenosis.

In real-world scenarios, where application of the device outside the IFU is seen, the Endurant graft compares favorably.[12] The Endurant Stent Graft Natural Selection Global Postmarket Registry (ENGAGE) is a large, prospective, consecutive, international patient registry that collected data on over 1200 patients from 79 high-volume centers across 30 countries between 2009 and 2011. Data included patients who were treated within the IFU and those outside of it. Stokmans et al. demonstrated an occlusion rate of 2% at 1 year.[3] However, they also reported that an additional 1.7% of patients had kinks in the stent graft, and a further 1.4% of patients had stenosis, indicating that 5.1% of patients treated with the Endurant graft had a limb occlusion or were at risk of one developing. Continued analysis of the registry demonstrated an occlusion rate of 3.4% at 2 years.[10]

It is unclear whether the graft itself has led to the higher incidence of limb occlusions seen with the Endurant when compared with the older Talent graft. The Endurant was designed to be more pliable and have limbs that are more conformable compared with the Talent, which was prone to kinking as a result of a supportive wire in the limbs. This may have allowed increased compression of the graft, especially in tortuous or stenotic vessels. Alternatively, the improved flexibility and profile of the device may have had the paradoxical effect of increasing its use in cases with challenging anatomy, thus increasing the risk of occlusive complications.

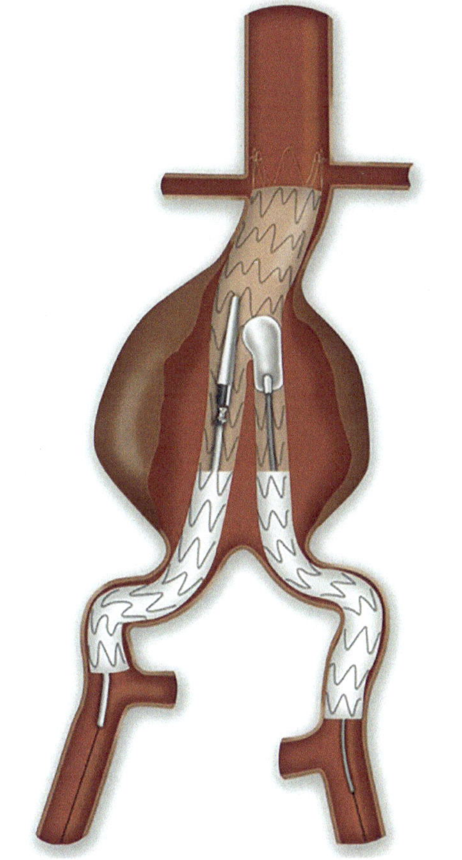

Fig. 6.7 Maneuver: Delivery Tip Catches at Flow Divider. Inflation of a balloon at the flow divider pushes the delivery system to the ipsilateral side.

(Georgiadis G, Antoniou G, Trellopoulos G, et al. Troubleshooting techniques for the Endurant device in endovascular aortic aneurysm repair. *Cardiovasc J Afr.* 2014;25(5):239–243.)

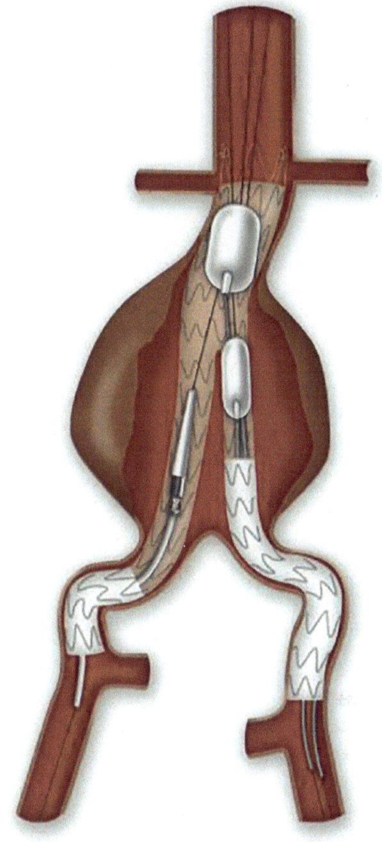

Fig. 6.8 Maneuver: Delivery Tip Catches in Ipsilateral Limb. Using two balloons to stabilize the endograft and maintain its position while simultaneously placing downward traction on the delivery system.

(Georgiadis G, Antoniou G, Trellopoulos G, et al. Troubleshooting techniques for the Endurant device in endovascular aortic aneurysm repair. *Cardiovasc J Afr.* 2014;25(5):239–243.)

Multiple groups have examined the risk factors that may predispose to limb occlusion. Based on the ENGAGE registry, Faure et al. found that the strongest independent predictors of limb occlusion were distal landing zone in the external iliac artery, external iliac artery diameter ≤10mm, maximum aneurysm diameter <59 mm, needing corrective action for an endoleak, and kinking of the graft.[10] They then created a decision tree that divided patients into high risk and low risk for limb occlusion to help direct the physician toward adjunctive measures or adjustment of follow-up protocol, or toward alternative approaches such as an aorto-uni-iliac device with a femoral–femoral bypass.

Avoiding situations that predispose to graft occlusion is of paramount importance. Building the limbs through any tortuous segments of the iliac arteries, as opposed to landing at a bend, can avoid the kink or flow disruption caused by the end of the graft (Fig. 6.9). Other recommendations include treating any stenotic lesions to prevent future iliac limb occlusion, and to avoid excessive oversizing of the distal limbs.

Once a graft is deployed, additional maneuvers to help detect patients at risk of occlusion include two directional angiography or cone beam CT, angiography after removal of the stiff guidewires, measuring iliac/femoral pressures, and the use of intravascular ultrasound or Duplex ultrasound. Additionally, if a limb is deemed at risk, the use of less compliant balloons, kissing balloons, or additional stent components for reinforcement should be considered. Closer follow-up of patients who have higher-risk anatomy or who underwent additional maneuvers may be prudent.

The newer EIIs stent graft is a three-piece system with a short bifurcated main body and bilateral docking limbs. This design has the potential advantage of having the modular connection between the limbs and the bifurcated main body located proximal to the often smaller distal aorta. The two limbs also have equal radial force in the overlap areas. The proximal overlap location and equal radial force between the limbs ensure full limb diameter expansion. This might reduce the potential for limb occlusions and long-term data might show the EIIs to be superior to the Endurant/Endurant II in terms of limb occlusion. Troisi et al. reported no limb occlusions at 1 year in a series of 79 EIIs implants.[13]

CONCLUSION

No aortic endograft system is without some inherent risk. Knowing the potential areas where trouble might be encountered for each particular graft allows for improved preoperative planning. With careful planning and attention to detail, the incidence of any major adverse events has remained acceptably low with the Endurant system. Future iterations of this graft will surely address some of these issues and will continue to improve function and safety from generation to generation.

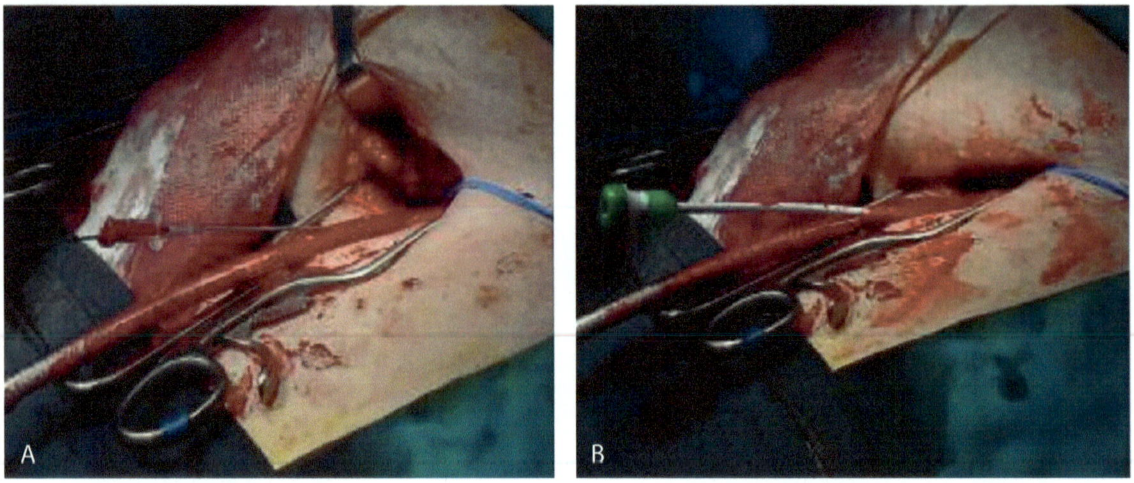

Fig. 6.9 Maneuver: Delivery Tip Catches at Stenosis in External Iliac Artery. The delivery system can be directly accessed with a needle (A). A sheath can then be inserted into the device and angioplasty can be performed through the sheath (B).

(Georgiadis G, Antoniou G, Trellopoulos G, et al. Troubleshooting techniques for the Endurant device in endovascular aortic aneurysm repair. *Cardiovasc J Afr.* 2014;25(5):239–243.)

TIP BOX 6.1

- Careful preprocedural planning is of utmost importance to predict and prevent potential complications.
- The Endurant II/IIs Instructions for Use should be referred to in cases where the mechanical thumb wheel fails to disengage the graft from the delivery catheter.
- Creative solutions may be needed to manipulate the delivery tip in cases where it becomes caught within the graft or native vessels.
- Different combinations of balloons and wires may be used to try to change the configuration of the vessels and graft to allow removal of the delivery tip.

WARNING BOX

- Strict adherence to the manufacturer's Instructions for Use will help minimize the chance of an adverse event with the endograft.
- Severe angulation at the aortic neck or tortuosity of the iliac arteries should heighten awareness of the possibility of difficulty with retrieval of the delivery system.
- Small, tortuous iliac vessels can also predispose to limb occlusion and should be considered in the planning stages of the repair.

REFERENCES

1. Medtronic. Endurant II Endurant IIs Stent Graft System: Instructions for Use. https://www.medtronic.com/us-en/healthcare-professionals/products/cardiovascular/aortic-stent-grafts/endurantii.html; 2019.
2. Rowed EV, Tersely G, de Vries JP, et al. Final results of the prospective European trial of the Endurant stent graft for endovascular abdominal aortic aneurysm repair. *Eur J Vasc Endovasc Surg.* 2011;42:489–497.
3. Stokmans RA, Teijink JAW, Forbes TL, et al. Early results from the ENGAGE Registry: real-world performance of the Endurant stent graft for endovascular AAA repair in 1262 patients. *Eur J Vasc Endovasc Surg.* 2012;44:369–375.
4. Georgiadis GS, Antoniou GA, Trellopoulos G, et al. Troubleshooting techniques for the Endurant™ device in endovascular aortic aneurysm repair. *Cardiovasc J Afr.* 2014;25:239–243.
5. Makaroun MS, Tuchek M, Massop D, et al. One year outcomes of the United States regulatory trial of the Endurant Stent Graft System. *J Vasc Surg.* 2011;54:601–608.
6. van Keulen JW, de Vries JP, Dekker H, et al. One-year multicenter results of 100 abdominal aortic aneurysm patients treated with the Endurant stent graft. *J Vasc Surg.* 2011;54:609–615.
7. van Zeggeren L, Bastos Gonçalves F, van Herwaarden JA, et al. Incidence and treatment results of Endurant endograft occlusion. *J Vasc Surg.* 2013;57:1246–1254.
8. Singh MJ, Fairman R, Anain P, et al. Final results of the Endurant Stent Graft System in the United States regulatory trial. *J Vasc Surg.* 2016;64:55–62.
9. Bisdas T, Weiss K, Eisenack M, et al. Durability of the Endurant stent graft in patients undergoing endovascular abdominal aortic aneurysm repair. *J Vasc Surg.* 2014;60:1125–1131.
10. Faure EM, Becquemin JP, Cochennec F. on behalf of ENGAGE collaborators. Predictive factors for limb occlusions after endovascular aneurysm repair. *J Vasc Surg.* 2015;61:1138–1145.
11. Mannetje YW, Cuypers PWM, Saleem BR, et al. Comparison of midterm results for the Talent and Endurant stent graft. *J Vasc Surg.* 2017;66:735–742.
12. Pecoraro F, Corte G, Dinoto E, et al. Clinical outcomes of Endurant II stent-graft for infrarenal aortic aneurysm repair: comparison of on-label versus off-label use. *Diagn Interv Radiol.* 2016;22:450–454.
13. Troisi N, Pitoulias G, Michelagnoli S, et al. Preliminary experience with the Endurant II short form stent-graft system. *J Cardiovasc Surg.* 2019;60(3):364–368. DOI: 10.23736/S0021-9509.17.09862-7 Epub ahead of print.

7

Endologix Ovation

Sikandar Z. Khan, MD and Richard Curl, MD

The Ovation abdominal stent graft system is a unique polymer-based trimodular endoprosthesis that has demonstrated safety and effectiveness in treatment of abdominal aortic aneurysms, especially in patients with challenging neck anatomy and narrow iliac vessels[1] (Fig. 7.1). The stent graft is made of a 32 mm long nitinol suprarenal stent, with radiopaque (RO) markers near the proximal edge of the graft. The main stent graft body is made up of low-permeability PTFE (polytetrafluoroethylene) and lacks a metallic frame. There are two O-rings proximally with polymer channels and smaller rings along the main body and limbs, providing support to the stent graft. By replacing the metallic stent with polymer channels, the stent graft profile is reduced and is deliverable through 14 or 15 French sheaths. While other aortic stent grafts achieve fixation and sealing with an outward radial force of a self-expanding nitinol stent, the Ovation stent graft uncouples fixation and sealing (Fig. 7.2). Fixation is achieved by the nitinol suprarenal stent and sealing is achieved by filling the graft's proximal most conformable O-ring with a polymer during graft deployment (Fig. 7.2). The sealing rings conform to vessel wall and create a circumferential seal without exerting a chronic radial force. Lack of radial force removes pressure from the neck and is thought to prevent neck dilatation, migration and type IA endoleaks. The rings inflate gradually, allowing them to conform to neck irregularities such as thrombus and calcifications. The polymer fills the stent graft bottom-to-top and then the contralateral limb. The polymer filling is diverted away from the sealing ring when it comes across an aortic wall irregularity, and excess inflation is diverted inwards into the aortic lumen, avoiding any significant stress on the aortic wall.

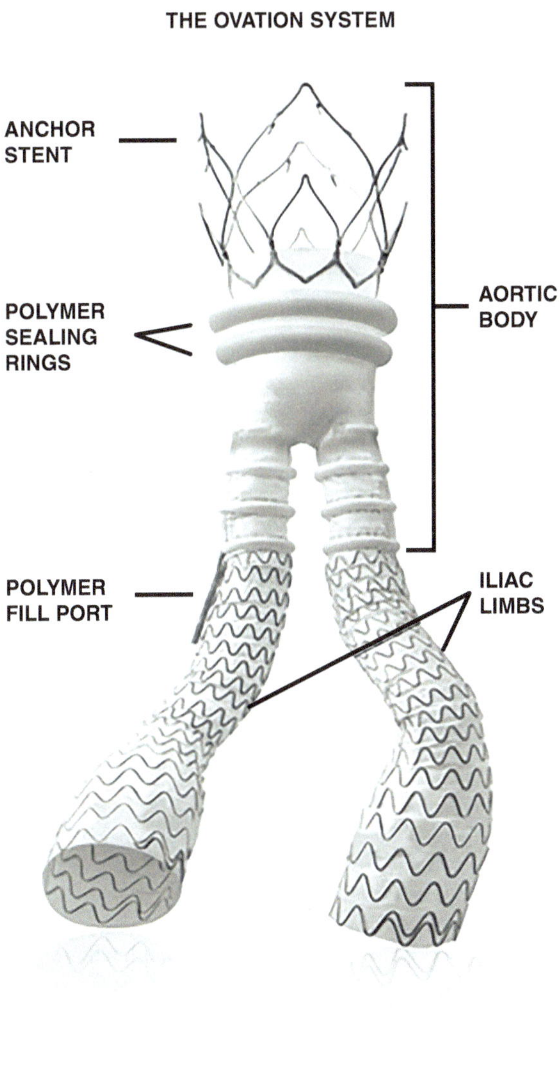

Fig. 7.1 The Ovation Stent Main Body and Iliac Limbs. The figure shows the suprarenal stent, sealing O-rings, and polymer rings along the main body limbs. The main body is made up of PTFE and lacks a metallic frame. Image provided courtesy of Endologix, Inc.

DEPLOYMENT

After delivery of the stent graft, it is unsheathed and the proximal nitinol stent is deployed in two stages with the RO markers ensuring proper positioning of the graft (Fig. 7.3B). After the release of the first knob, the mid-crown is deployed. The stent graft can still be repositioned at this time. It is prudent to start deployment higher than the intended final position, since it is easier to pull the stent graft down than to push it up. After the second knob is released, the suprarenal stent is completely deployed, anchoring the stent graft. The polymer is mixed in the two syringes of the polymer kit and infused using the autoinjector (Fig. 7.3A). The polymer begins to fill the stent graft, inflating the sealing ring against the aortic wall. The autoinjector exerts a constant pressure against the aortic wall allowing the seal to conform to the aortic wall. Holding the stent delivery system or applying forward pressure on it is not recommended. The stiff wire is withdrawn into the body of the graft to facilitate conformance of the stent to native aortic anatomy, especially when acute angulation is present. The deployment of the main body is completed by turning the third knob to disconnect the filling tube from the stent graft.

INSTRUCTIONS FOR USE (IFU)

According to the IFU, the anatomic criteria for the use of the Ovation stent graft include proximal aortic diameter between 16 and 30 mm at 13 mm below the inferior most renal artery, with an aortic angle of $\leq$60 degrees if proximal neck is $\geq$10 mm and $\leq$45 degrees if proximal neck is $<$10 mm. There should be at least 10 mm iliac landing zone with

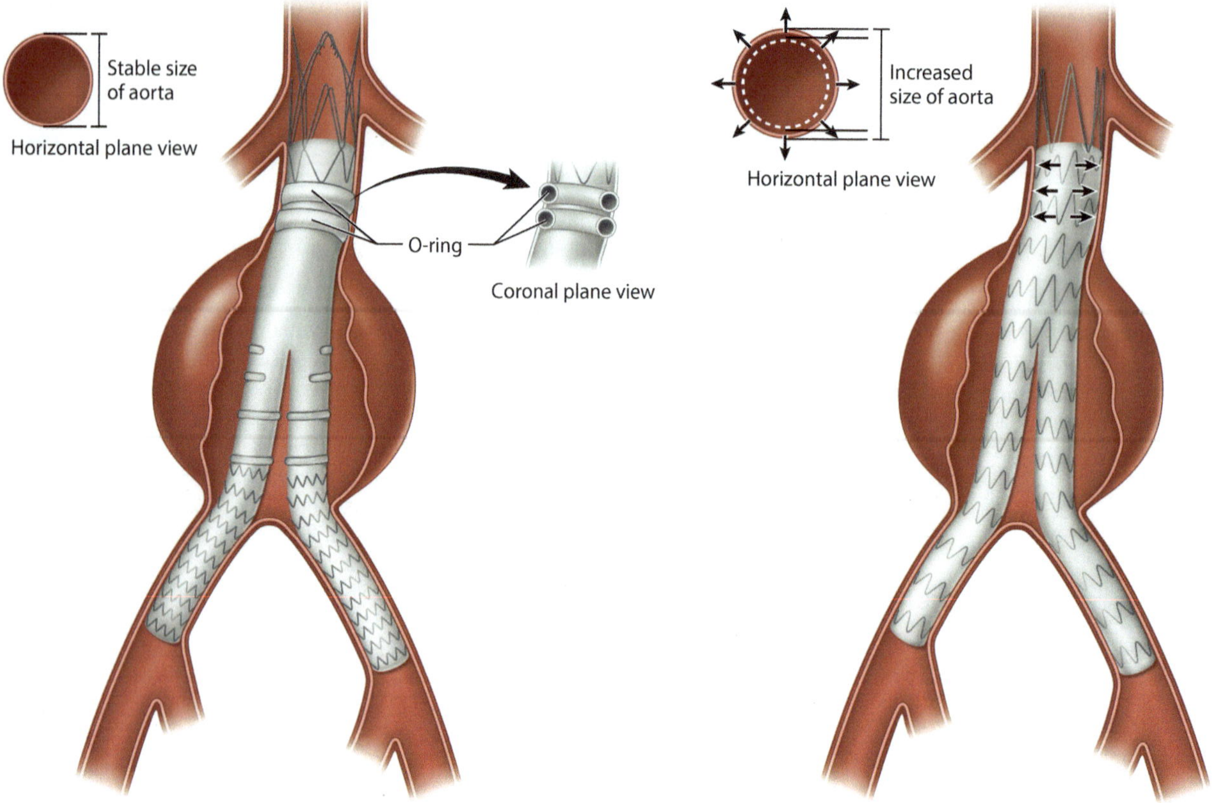

Fig. 7.2 The Ovation stent has a unique sealing mechanism consisting of polymer-filled sealing rings that exert minimal radial force, unlike other aortic stent grafts. Image provided courtesy of Endologix, Inc.

diameters between 8 and 20 mm. Patients with known allergy to the device materials (including PTFE, polyethylene glycol (PEG)-based polymers, fluorinated ethylene propylene [FEP] or nitinol) should not be treated with the Ovation stent graft.

POLYMER-RELATED COMPLICATIONS

As mentioned above, the Ovation stent graft is contraindicated in patients who are allergic to device materials including PTFE, PEG, or nitinol. There have been reports of inadvertent leakage of polymer into the systemic circulation with resulting allergic reactions including anaphylaxis.[2,3] In the majority of cases, the exact cause of the leakage was not identified and was attributed to defects in the polymer kit system.[2–4]

Polymer-related complications

- Polymer should be injected using the autoinjector only
- DO NOT detach delivery system prematurely unless there has been an allergic reaction
- If there is leakage, detach autoinjector and polymer syringe immediately
- In case of allergic reaction/anaphylaxis, use antihistamines, steroids, vasopressors, and airway protection as necessary

To prevent polymer-related complications, the IFU should be followed when deploying the stent. The following steps and key points should be considered to prevent polymer-related issues:

- After deployment of the suprarenal stent, the delivery system should not be pulled as it may cause inadvertent detachment of the polymer fill connecter from the main body leading to leakage of the polymer into the blood.
- The delivery system should not be detached prematurely (time to polymerize is 20 minutes for the TriVascular Fill Polymer Kit or 14 minutes for the CustomSeal Kit) to prevent leakage of the polymer.
- The patient's body temperature should also be considered. The polymer is designed to cure at core body temperature of 37°C and might take longer at lower temperatures. If the core body temperature is lower than 35°C, it may require at least one additional minute per degree below 35°C prior to disconnection.
- If there is an error in mixing or transferring the polymer or delay in infusing after mixing (3 or more minutes after mixing if using the TriVascular Fill Polymer Kit or injection has been delayed 2 or more minutes using the CustomSeal Kit), the polymer should be discarded and a new kit opened.
- The polymer should be infused using the autoinjector only; hand injections can damage the stent causing delamination of the polymer channels.
- The filling of the polymer should be initially observed under fluoroscopy. Lack of filling of the polymer channels or rapid emptying of the syringe may indicate that the polymer is not being infused into the stent and may be leaking into the blood.

If there is suspicion or evidence of leakage, the autoinjector and the polymer fill syringe should be immediately detached from the delivery system to ensure patient safety.

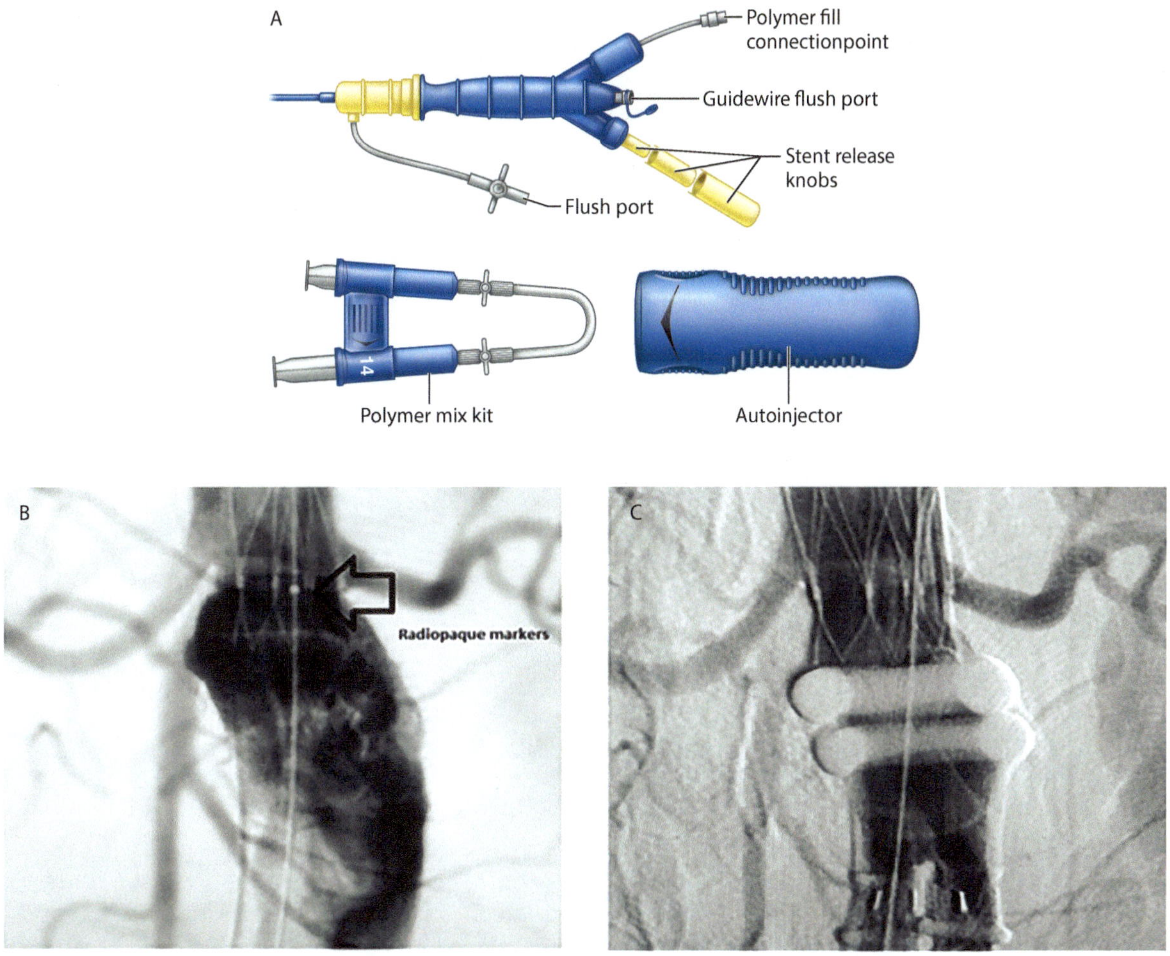

Fig. 7.3 (A) Ovation deployment system. (B, C) Positioning of the stent using the RO markers, deployment and sealing with inflated polymer rings. Image provided courtesy of Endologix, Inc.

In case of allergic reactions, standard treatment (antihistamines, steroids, vasopressors, airway protection) should be administered.

TYPE IA ENDOLEAK

Type IA can result from incomplete or lack of filling of the sealing rings or secondary to in-folding of the sealing ring. The IFU and the key points described in the previous section should be followed to prevent and minimize the chances of a type IA endoleak.

INCOMPLETE FILLING OF CHAMBERS

In case of incomplete or no filling of the sealing ring, proximal seal can be achieved by deployment of a Palmaz stent (Cordis, Miami Lakes, Florida).

- The Palmaz stent can be mounted on a compliant or non-compliant balloon, which is sized to match the native aorta. We routinely use the Z-Med balloon (B. Braun Medical Inc, Bethlehem, Pennsylvania) to deploy the Palmaz stent.
- The main body as well as the bilateral iliac limbs are completely deployed.
- A sheath is advanced to the level of the sealing rings, protecting the Palmaz stent as it is delivered to the desired deployment area, to prevent dislodgement of the stent during transit.
- The proximal edge of the Palmaz is then aligned with the RO markers of the Ovation stent.
- Before deployment of the Palmaz, all wires and catheters should be withdrawn to avoid entrapment behind the stent and the sheath pulled back to just below the stent.

IN-FLOW STENOSIS/SEALING RING IN-FOLDING

The sealing rings inflate slowly and any excess inflation is directed inward into the aortic lumen to limit stress on the aortic neck. This can lead to circumferential aortic lumen narrowing, especially in patients with heavily calcified, irregular neck (Fig. 7.4). While this can lead to up to 60% in-flow stenosis, there is no evidence that this is hemodynamically significant.[5,6] In-folding can be prevented by avoiding excessive oversizing. The O-rings are designed to inflate to a specific diameter and if cramped within a small aortic neck, the rings will expand inward when outward expansion is limited by the aortic wall. While other stent grafts rely on oversizing and outward radial force for seal, the Ovation stent graft, with its unique sealing mechanism, does not need to be unduly oversized. The manufacturer-recommended sizing incorporates adequate oversizing for different aortic diameters and should be followed. In case of excessive stenosis or in-folding, the following steps can be taken:

- A compliant or non-compliant balloon can be inflated 14–25 minutes after polymer mix for Custom Seal and 20–40 minutes

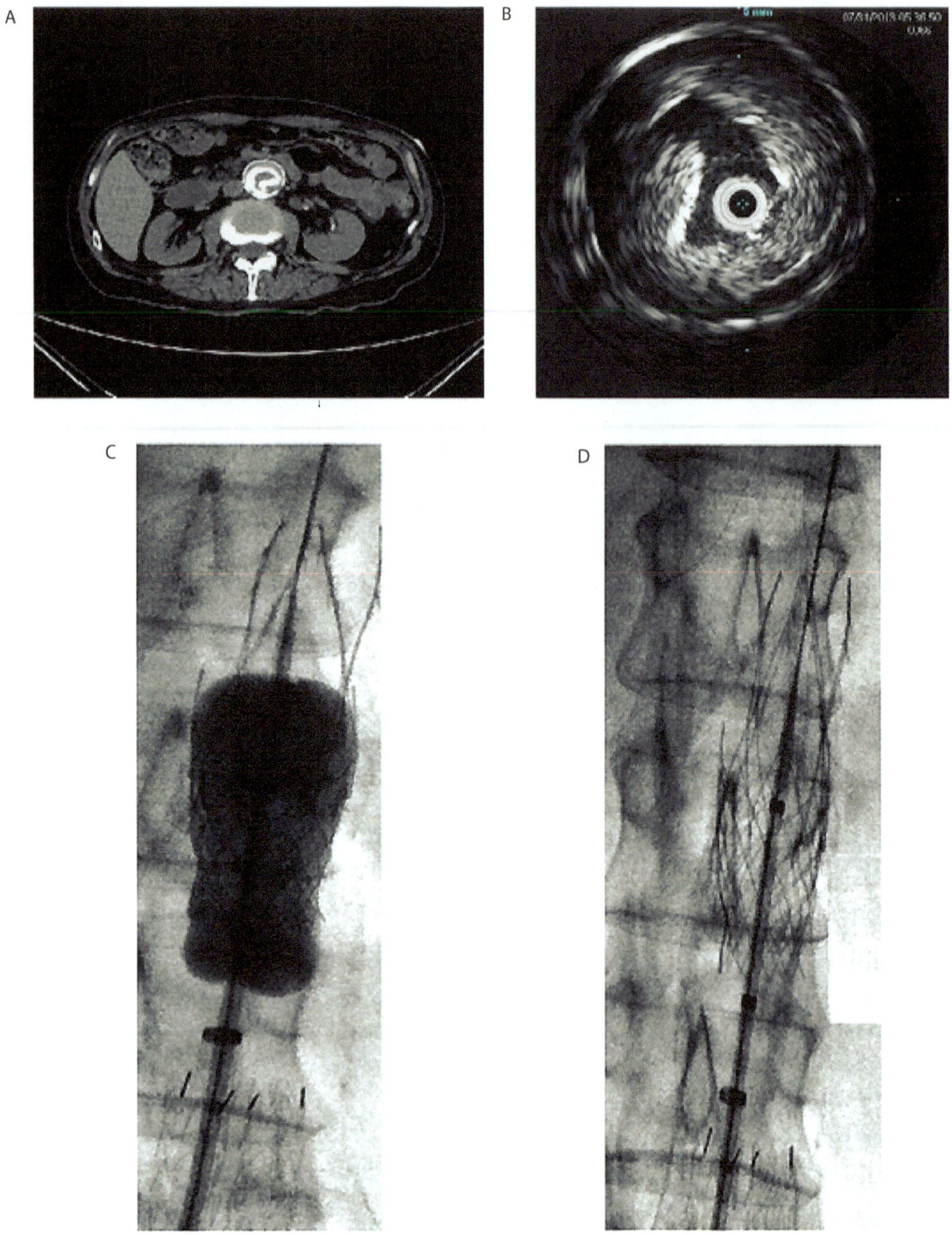

Fig. 7.4 CT scan (A) and intravascular ultrasound (B) showing in-folding of the sealing rings. This was treated with placement of a Palmaz stent (C, D).

for the Ovation Polymer. The balloon is centered over the middle of the sealing rings and inflated to conform to the rings or resolve any in-folding.

- If stenosis/in-folding persists, it can be treated by placement of a Palmaz stent as described earlier (Fig. 7.4).

A type IA endoleak may be present even after complete and appropriate filling of the sealing rings and without any in-folding. There are a few options to achieve seal.

- A compliant or non-compliant balloon, sized to match the native aorta, should be inflated 14–25 minutes after polymer mix for Custom Seal and 20–40 minutes for the Ovation Polymer. The balloon is centered over the middle of the sealing rings and inflated for 30 seconds.
- A Palmaz stent can be used to achieve seal as described earlier.
- A third option is coil embolization or embolic agents.

TWO LIMBS IN ONE GATE

There have been several reported cases of inadvertent cannulation of the ipsilateral gate and deployment of an iliac limb from the ipsilateral

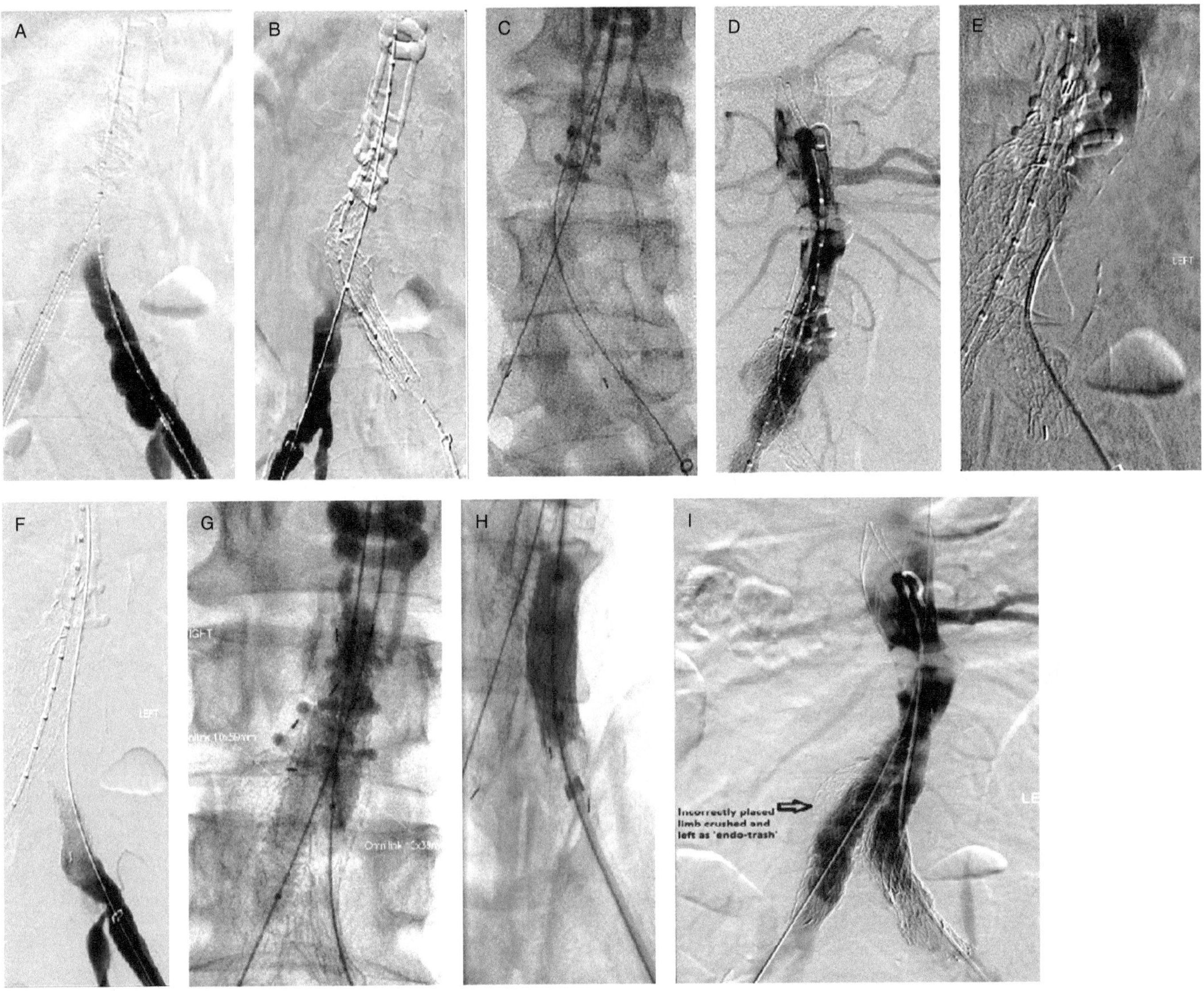

Fig. 7.5 Inadvertent placement of two iliac limbs in the ipsilateral gate, (A) cannulation of the ipsilateral gate from the contralateral iliac artery followed by (B) cannulation of the ipsilateral gate from the ipsilateral iliac resulting in two iliac limbs in the ipsilateral gate (C, D). Gain access to the contralateral iliac gate from the contralateral iliac artery (E) followed by correct contralateral limb deployment (F) and crushing of the incorrectly placed limb by inflating a balloon in the ipsilateral gate (G) and in the iliac artery (H). This should exclude the aneurysm with intact flow into both iliac arteries; the misplaced limb is left as "endo-trash" (I).

gate to the contralateral iliac artery (Fig. 7.5A,B).[7] Both iliac gates are essentially identical in appearance and length, particularly after the stiff wire has been withdrawn from the graft during polymer infusion, making it more likely that such a mistake could occur during cannulation. Of note, in the next generation Alto device the contralateral gate will be longer than the ipsilateral gate, thus facilitating correct identification of the limbs. The error is generally recognized once attempts are made to re-advance the wire through the ipsilateral gate, discovering that it is blocked by the contralateral iliac limb. Techniques to minimize the chance of this error include:

- Adjust the C-arm angle to maximize separation and improve identification of the iliac gates.
- Consider leaving the floppy portion of the stiff wire in the ipsilateral iliac gate during polymer fill, to help distinguish it from the contralateral gate.
- Cannulation of the contralateral gate can also be confirmed with angiography by injecting contrast into the contralateral gate through a sheath or catheter.
- Consider inflating a balloon with in the contralateral gate and rocking it. The contralateral gate will move with the balloon, in contrast to the ipsilateral gate, which is still attached to the delivery system.
- Use the Ovation iX integrated cross-over lumen for contralateral gate access.

If the error has been recognized before the second limb is deployed (Fig. 7.5B), the following solution is possible:

- Leave the misplaced limb in place.
- After de-mating, attempt to cannulate the contralateral gate from the ipsilateral side, either directly, or with Ovation iX, by snaring a wire advanced through the cross-over lumen.

- If successful, a limb can then be placed from the contralateral gate to the ipsilateral side, thus reversing ipsilateral and contralateral orientation.

But if the error is not recognized early and two limbs are deployed in the ipsilateral gate (Fig. 7.5C,D), the following technical fix has been used (Fig. 7.5E–I). It may be prudent to confirm proximal seal and balloon, if necessary, through the misplaced limb before proceeding:

- After de-mating of the polymer injection system, gain wire access from the contralateral side into the aneurysm (Fig. 7.5E), followed by balloon crushing of the iliac end of the limb and placement of a sheath, allowing cannulation of the correct contralateral gate and placement of a new contralateral limb (Fig. 7.5F), again employing necessary ballooning (Fig. 7.5G,H) and stenting if needed to ensure full expansion of the correct contralateral limb.
- Maintain wire access on the ipsilateral side through the correct ipsilateral iliac limb, and inflate an 8- to 10-mm high-pressure balloon in the gate to crush the inadvertently placed limb (Fig. 7.5G). If needed, a balloon expandable stent can be used to ensure full expansion of the correct ipsilateral limb.

DIFFICULT RETRIEVAL OF THE NOSE CONE

Another complication that has been reported is the nose cone getting caught on the suprarenal stent during withdrawal. This has the potential to cause dislodgement of the graft if not recognized.

- Always withdraw the nose cone under direct fluoroscopic visualization.
- If the nose cone becomes caught, avoid downward pulling, use upward pressure or twisting of the inner core to free the nose cone and buttress the graft by putting forward pressure on the sheath to prevent downward dislodgement of the graft.
- Remove stiff wire to alleviate possible wire bias forcing the nose cone to the side.
- Insert a large balloon from contralateral side and inflate next to the nose cone to push it away from crown.
- External manipulation of the aorta by pressing on the abdomen can also sometimes push the nose cone away from the aortic wall.

Difficult retrieval of the nose cone

- Withdraw nose cone under fluoroscopy
- Use forward pressure and twist the inner core to free the nose cone if it tethers to the suprarenal stents
- Use balloon inflation to separate the nose cone from the suprarenal stent if necessary

DISTORTION/CRUSHING OF THE LIMBS

Limb crush/distortion

- Gain wire access across the limb by using the cross-over lumen or brachial access
- Restore patency by balloon angioplasty or stent placement
- If limb remains crushed, convert to aorto-uni-iliac and femoral–femoral bypass

The Ovation main body platform, particularly the contralateral iliac gate, because of a lack of structural form or rigidity prior to infusion of the polymer, is vulnerable to being crushed against the wall of the aneurysm. This can lead to the inability to infuse polymer, as discussed earlier, and also the inability to cannulate. As with most potential complications, prevention is of primary importance:

- Careful analysis of the aneurysm, with identification of potential areas where there may be limited room for the iliac gates, may allow positioning of the device in such a way as to diminish the risk of this occurring.
- Problems with the gates will most likely become apparent at the time of polymer filling, with distortion of the gates and incomplete filling of the polymer rings.

Incomplete filling of rings, persistent Type IA endoleak, or inflow stenosis

- Consider using a Palmaz stent

If significant distortion of the gate is present, the following approach is recommended:

- An initial attempt at gate cannulation may be attempted, but is unlikely to be successful.
- Access to the gate may then be attempted by snaring a wire advanced either through the cross-over lumen with Ovation iX, directed over the bifurcation by a catheter, or advanced from brachial access.

Wrong gate cannulation

Prevent by

- Adjusting C-arm angle to separate and identify the limbs
- Confirm cannulation of the contralateral gate with angiography or inflating a balloon within the gate

If error is recognized after cannulation of the ipsilateral gate and before the second limb is deployed

- Cannulate contralateral gate from the ipsilateral side, thus reversing ipsilateral and contralateral orientation

Two limbs in one gate

- Gain wire access to the contralateral gate from the contralateral iliac
- Deploy a third iliac limb from the contralateral gate into the contralateral iliac
- Endo-trash the inadvertently placed limb and maintain patency of the correctly placed limbs by balloon angioplasty and/or stent placement (see text for details)

- Once wire access to the gate has been achieved, then patency can be restored by balloon angioplasty, followed by limb extension placement, and the additional use of a self-expanding or balloon expandable stent, if needed.
- As a last resort, conversion to an aorto-uni-iliac graft and a femoral–femoral bypass may be required. Aorto-uni-iliac conversion can be achieved by occlusion of the contralateral gate with coils or an Amplatzer plug.

REFERENCES

1. Mehta M, Valdés FE, Nolte T, et al. One-year outcomes from an international study of the Ovation Abdominal Stent Graft System for endovascular aneurysm repair. *J Vasc Surg*. 2014;59(1):65–73.
2. Siani A, Accrocca F, De Vivo G, Mounayergi F, Siani LM, Antonelli R. Anaphylactic reaction during implantation of ovation abdominal stent graft in patients with abdominal aortic Aneurysm. *Ann Vasc Surg*. 2017;39:289.
3. Sfyroeras GS, Moulakakis KG, Antonopoulos CN, et al. Anaphylactic reaction during implantation of the Ovation Stent-Graft System in a patient with abdominal aortic aneurysm. *J Endovasc Ther*. 2015;22:620–622.
4. Georgakarakos E, Ioannou CV, Georgiadis GS, et al. The ovation abdominal stent graft for the treatment of abdominal aortic aneurysms: current evidence and future perspectives. *Expert Rev Med Devices*. 2016;13(3): 253–262.
5. Ioannou CV, Kontopodis N, Metaxa E, et al. Graft inflow stenosis induced by the inflatable ring fixation mechanism of the Ovation Stent-Graft system: hemodynamic and clinical implications. *J Endovasc Ther*. 2014; 21(6):829–838.
6. Georgakarakos E, Argyriou C, Georgiadis GS, Lazarides MK. Pulse wave analysis after treatment of abdominal aortic aneurysms with the ovation device. *Ann Vasc Surg*. 2017;40:146–153.
7. Georgakarakos E, Ioannou CV, Kontopodis N, Tsetis D. A case of difficult catheterization of the contralateral limb of the Ovation Abdominal Stent Graft System in challenging aortoiliac anatomy, facilitated through the brachial access: a word of caution. *Ann Vasc Surg*. 2015;29(2):392–396.

8

Endologix AFX

Sikandar Z. Khan, MD, Nicolas J. Mouawad, MD, MPH, MBA, FSVS, FACS, FRCS, RPVI and Richard Curl, MD

The original Endologix endovascular graft is currently called AFX, mainly to distinguish it from the other Endologix products, Ovation and Nellix (Endologix, Irvine, California). The AFX2 is the third-generation endovascular system after the earlier Powerlink and AFX stent grafts. The AFX is a unibody, bifurcated system consisting of a self-expanding cobalt-chromium alloy stent attached to a fabric cover (Fig. 8.1). The fabric is a proprietary form of polytetrafluoroethylene (PTFE), an ultra-high-density, multi-layered material referred to as Duraply, which is conformable and tear resistant. There are some unique characteristics of the AFX, differentiating it from other stent graft systems. First, AFX is the only stent graft that sits on the aortic bifurcation to provide anatomic fixation thus maintaining the native bifurcation. Second, the PTFE fabric is externally mounted and attached only to the proximal and distal ends of the stent. This allows the fabric to move independently from the stent conforming to varied shapes of the aortic neck and bifurcation achieving an ActiveSeal (Fig. 8.2).[1,2] The VELA proximal extension comes in two configurations, with and without suprarenal bare-metal stent, and achieves seal at the aortic neck (Fig. 8.1). The iliac limb extensions come in straight, tapered, flared, and stepped configurations to treat different iliac anatomies (Fig. 8.1).

DEPLOYMENT

The AFX2 system is delivered through a 17-French AFX Introducer sheath and a 7-French contralateral sheath. The three types of stent grafts delivered through the introducer sheath include the bifurcated main body stent graft, VELA extension, and iliac limb extensions. The AFX2 system incorporates a 0.035 contralateral wire that is fed through the ipsilateral sheath along with the main body and snared from the contralateral side (Fig. 8.3). The wire is withdrawn from the contralateral sheath and the stent graft main body is delivered through the sheath over a stiff wire, ensuring that the contralateral wire is not wrapped around the inner core of the delivery system. After confirming proper alignment, the stent graft is pulled down to seat it on the aortic bifurcation, guiding each limb into its respective iliac artery (Fig. 8.3). The main body, contralateral limb, and the ipsilateral limb are then sequentially deployed. The AFX main body delivery system is removed and can be followed by the VELA extension or iliac limb extensions as necessary. This novel fixation technique prevents distal migration of the graft beyond the bifurcation and allows for easy up-and-over access across the bifurcation from one femoral access to the contralateral leg. This unique design has prompted the use of the AFX main body in the treatment of aortoiliac occlusive disease, which is currently an off-label use and will not be considered further in this chapter.

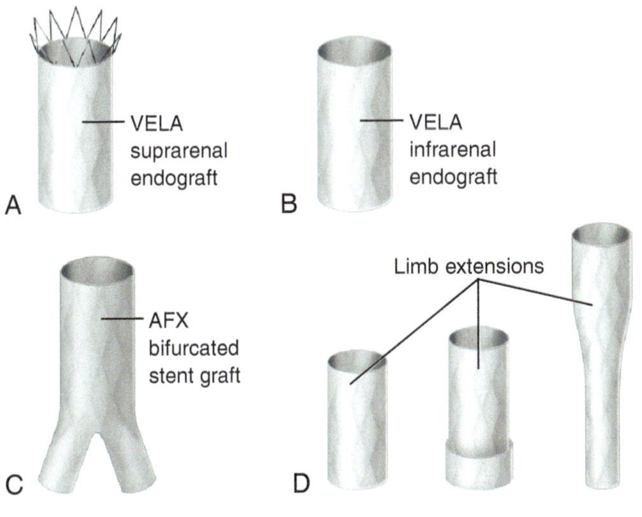

Fig. 8.1 (A) VELA proximal extension with suprarenal bare-metal stent, (B) VELA proximal extension without suprarenal bare-metal stent, (C) bifurcated main body, (D) iliac limb extensions.

(From Endologix, Irvine, California.)

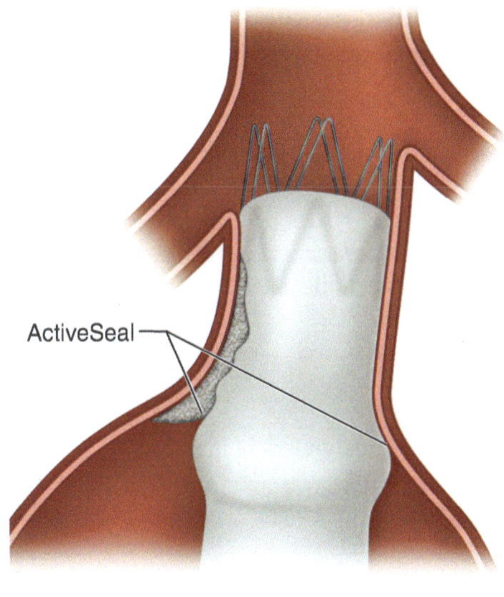

Fig. 8.2 ActiveSeal Technology. PTFE is attached to the proximal and distal ends only allowing it to move independently and conform to the aortic wall.

(From Endologix, Irvine, California.)

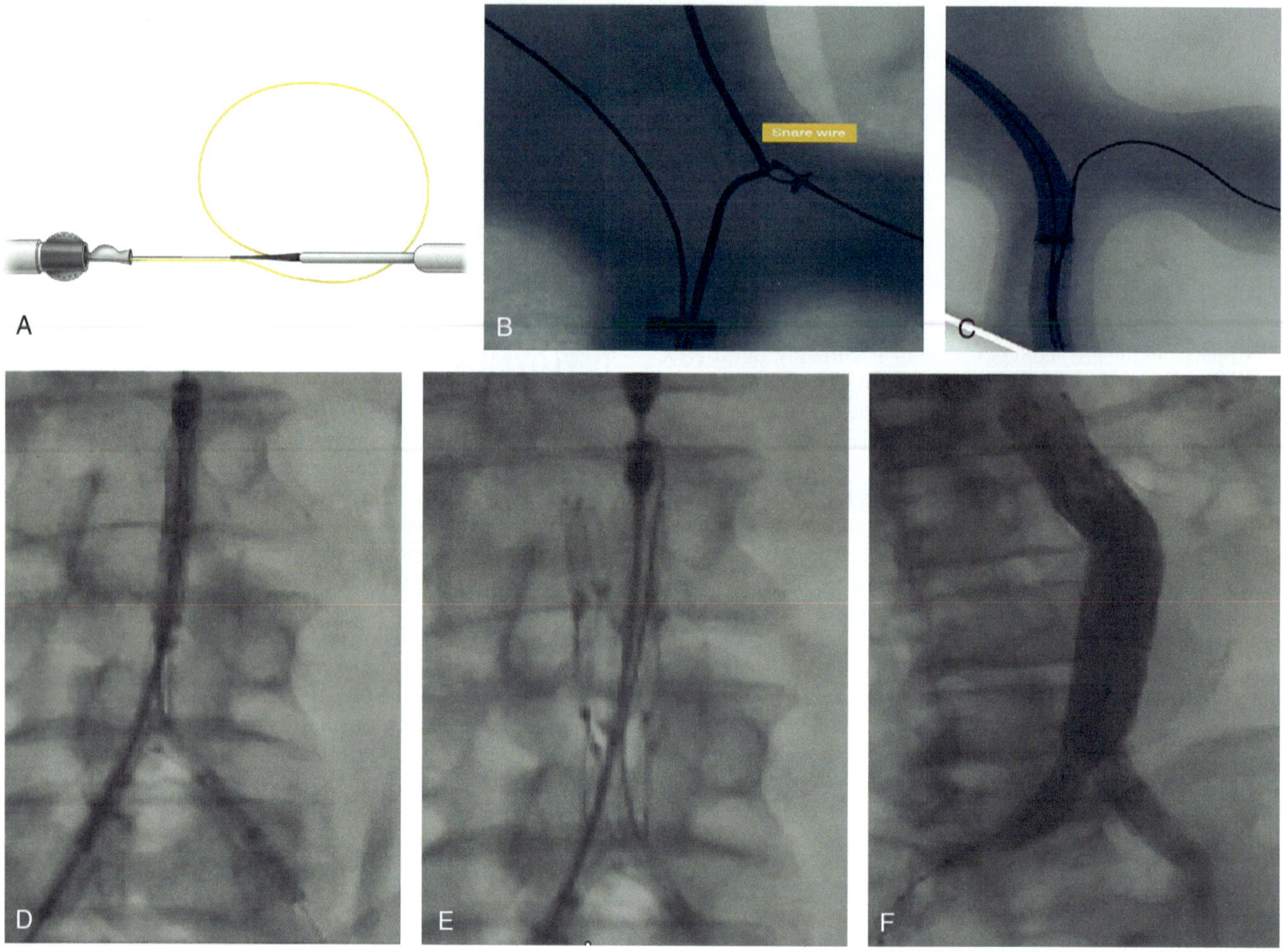

Fig. 8.3 Deployment. (A) Passing the contralateral wire through the ipsilateral delivery sheath; (B) snaring of contralateral wire from the contralateral side; (C) contralateral wire should be on the medial side of the main body stent graft; (D) pre-deployment stent graft with iliac limbs lined with respective iliac arteries; (E) deployment of bifurcated main body and seating on the aortic bifurcation; (F) angiography after deployment of the proximal VELA extension.

(A–C from Endologix, Irvine, California.)

INSTRUCTIONS FOR USE (IFU)

The AFX stent graft system is indicated for patients with suitable abdominal aortic aneurysm morphology including:

1. Adequate access vessels (diameter ≥6.5 mm) compatible with the AFX delivery system.
2. Non-aneurysmal aortic neck between the renal arteries and the aneurysm:
   a. ≥15 mm length
   b. diameter of ≥18 mm and ≤32 mm
   c. neck angle of ≤60 degrees
3. Aortic length ≥1.0 cm longer than the body portion of the chosen bifurcated model.
4. Common iliac artery distal fixation site:
   a. distal fixation length of ≥15 mm
   b. diameter of ≥10 mm and ≤23 mm
   c. iliac angle of ≤90 degrees to the aortic bifurcation
5. Extension stent grafts must have the ability to overlap the bifurcated stent graft by at least 30 to 40 mm proximally and at least 15 to 20 mm distally.
6. At least one hypogastric artery is preserved.

Patients with known allergy to the device materials or any condition that could result in graft infection should not be treated with the AFX stent graft system.

Like all stent grafts, the AFX device is subject to some of the same generic complications common to all devices. However, it is also subject to some unique problems, which will be discussed in this chapter.

WIRE WRAP

As discussed earlier, deployment of the stent graft main body requires snaring of the contralateral wire from the contralateral femoral side (Fig. 8.3). This is done prior to advancing the stent graft main body through the sheath. Wire wrap can occur if the contralateral wire takes a spiral path around the ipsilateral wire as it is advanced through the sheath. This is an extremely common event and correction of wire wrap is a routine part of AFX deployment. Nonetheless, failure to recognize and correct this can lead to problems with and even failure to successfully seat the graft on the aortic bifurcation. Steps to prevent or to minimize wire wrap include:

- Insert the contralateral wire on the medial side of the sheath, medial to the ipsilateral wire.

- Once the contralateral wire emerges from the end of the sheath, attempt to snare it on the medial side of the ipsilateral wire (Fig. 8.3B,C).
- Once the wire is snared and brought out of the contralateral groin, the main body is advanced through the sheath, keeping tension on the contralateral wire. During this time, care must be taken to recognize and treat wire wrap.
- The main body and its relation to the contralateral wire is carefully observed under magnified fluoroscopy as the device is advanced beyond the sheath. The wire should be on the medial side of the stent graft (Fig. 8.3C).
- Confirm the proper orientation of the contralateral limb marker on the medial side of the sheath.
- If the wire appears lateral to the main body or it appears to be crossing over the device from medial to lateral, then a wire wrap must be assumed.

Wire wrap

- Ensure that contralateral wire and limb are on the medial side of the sheath
- Maintain tension on the contralateral wire as the main body is advanced
- If wire wrap is identified, rotate the sheath and device as a unit in a clockwise or counterclockwise direction under fluoroscopy to unwrap

Once wire wrap is diagnosed, it must be treated appropriately. It is usually difficult to ascertain the direction in which the wire is wrapped, so correction must be done with careful fluoroscopic monitoring:

- Rotate the sheath and device as a unit, in either a clockwise or counterclockwise direction, while maintaining some tension on the contralateral wire.
- If the wire orientation to the device appears to be correcting, and the contralateral wire feels like it is being "reeled out", continue rotating until the wrap is completely corrected. Both the wire at the top of the sheath and the contralateral limb marker should be on the medial side.
- If the wire orientation is not correcting, or the wire feels like it is being "reeled in", then the direction of rotation should be reversed and continued until the wrap is corrected.

Once wire wrap is corrected, the main body can be advanced and seated on the aortic bifurcation by guiding the limbs into their respective iliac arteries (Fig. 8.3D,E). Rarely, the wire wrap is discovered after the main body is out of the sheath. This must be corrected before the device can be seated on the bifurcation. The same technique as described earlier is used, with careful rotation of the device while maintaining mild tension on the contralateral wire. While this usually results in successful deployment, it should be noted that rotation of the unconstrained device in the aortic sac increases the risk of embolization due to dislodgment of mural thrombus.

PLACEMENT OF COMPONENTS BEHIND STENT STRUTS

As noted earlier, a unique feature of the Endologix AFX device and its previous versions is that the covering fabric is attached to the stent only at the proximal and distal ends. This allows a guide wire to pass between the stent strut and the fabric. While this is usually not an issue with routine use of the graft, it can lead to potential problems when wire access is inadvertently lost during deployment, or when secondary procedures are required, necessitating wire replacement through the device. It should be noted that inadvertent routing of low-profile catheters, balloons or sheaths behind the stent struts rarely cause complications. However, attempts to advance large diameter sheaths or limb extensions behind the stent can lead to disruption of the device or limb occlusion. Efforts to avoid wire placement behind a stent strut include:

- Use a pigtail or similar reverse curve catheter to advance through the device, because it is less likely to find its way behind a stent strut (Fig. 8.4A).
- Once wire access is achieved, examine the wire at 90-degree angles to ensure it is centrally located in the device.
- Advance an angioplasty balloon (8–12 mm) over the wire and then retract the inflated balloon under fluoroscopy, watching for any areas of hang up or distortion as it is pulled through (Fig. 8.4B–E).
- Intravascular ultrasound (IVUS) can be also be used to confirm the central location of the wire. During IVUS, stent struts can appear to be crossing into the lumen. This may be caused by angulation or fracture (Fig. 8.4F).
- If there is any question about the location of the wire, remove it, and try again to advance it.

Ensuring wire is not behind stent struts

- Use pigtail catheter to advance through the stent graft
- Inflate and drag an 8–12 mm balloon under fluoroscopy and look for any areas of hang up or distortion
- Use multiple angles to ensure central location of the wire
- IVUS can be used to confirm central location of the wire

The consequences and treatment of a component being inadvertently deployed behind a strut depend on the nature and location of the component. An example would be an iliac limb extension placed behind a stent strut in the main body, which can lead to occlusion of the limb. Attempts to open the trapped end of the limb with forceful balloon angioplasty behind the strut may result in disruption of the main body. Options to treat this complication would be:

- Gain wire access outside the extension in the iliac artery, crush the misplaced extension with a balloon, and place a parallel limb.
- Femoral–femoral bypass to restore perfusion to the leg if endovascular options fail.

TYPE III ENDOLEAK AND COMPONENT SEPARATION

An increased incidence of Type III endoleak has been reported with the Endologix Powerlink and AFX stent grafts.[3–5] Type III endoleaks are subdivided into stent graft component separation (Type IIIa) and a tear in the fabric (Type IIIb) (Figs. 8.5 and 8.6). The distinction is important with regard to the AFX stent graft system and the mechanism of repair. Type IIIa endoleak risk factors include:

- inadequate overlap between the bifurcated main body and the proximal or distal extensions during the index operation;
- lateral movement of the stent grafts in tortuous or large aortas leading to a reduction of overlap;
- deployment of an excessively oversized proximal extension into the bifurcated unibody device.

It has also been hypothesized that a reverse windsock effect, with the fabric billowing on the proximal aortic extension, may increase the distraction forces on the proximal extension and the bifurcated main body leading to separation.[4]

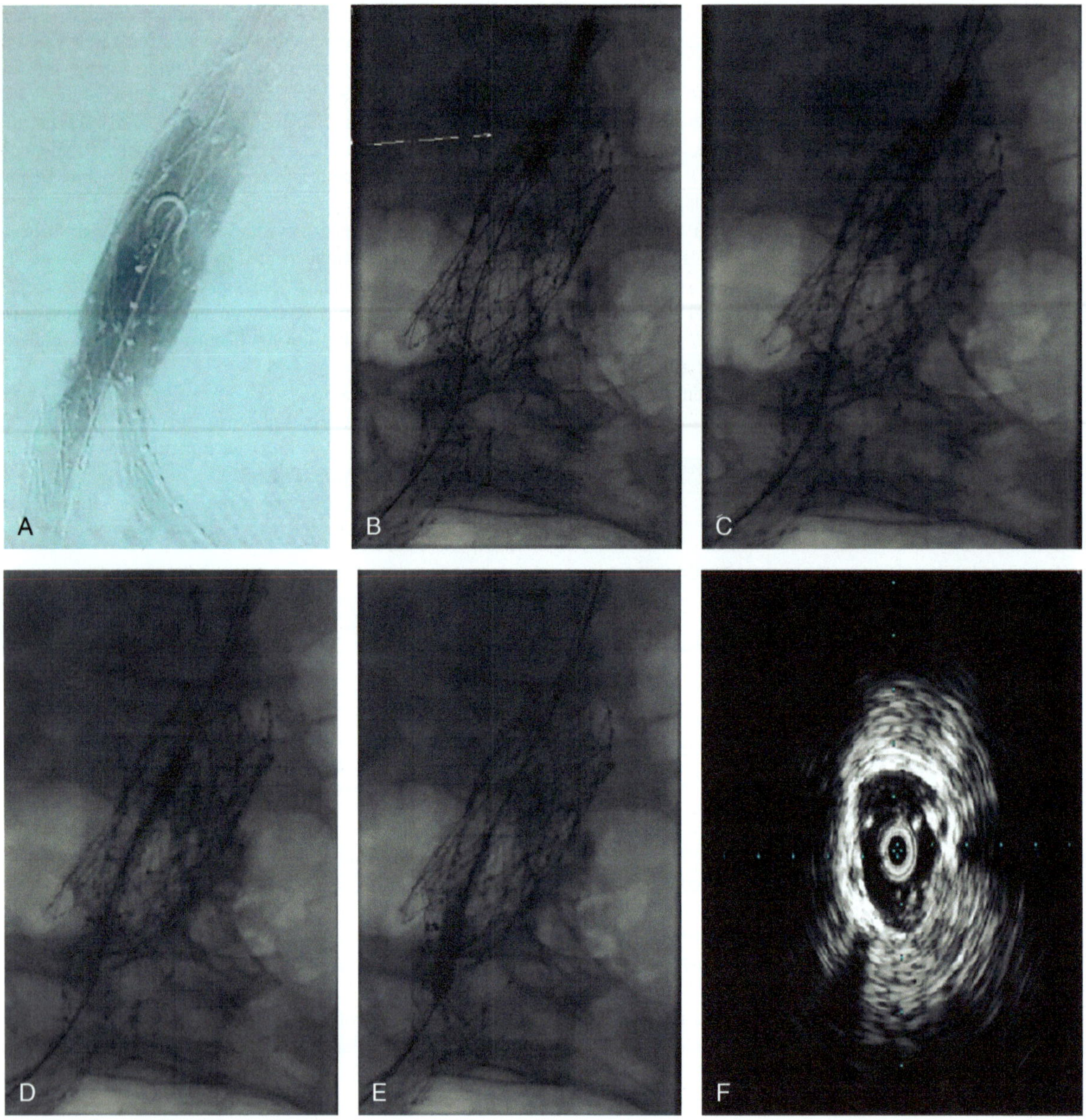

Fig. 8.4 Steps to Avoid Wire Placement Behind a Stent Strut. (A) Advance a reverse curve catheter through the device as it is less likely to find its way behind a strut; (B–E) retract an inflated balloon under fluoroscopy, watching for any areas of hang up or distortion as it is pulled through; (F) use IVUS to confirm central location of the wire.

Preventing Type IIIa endoleak/component separation

- Maximize overlap between stent graft components
- Use additional overlapping stent grafts in angulated aortic neck, tortuous aorta, long renal to bifurcation length, and large aneurysm diameter (>70 mm)
- Avoid excessive oversizing of the proximal extension relative to the main body

Repair of Type IIIa endoleak/component separation

- Obtain wire access across the separated components, ensuring that the wire is not behind the struts
- Deploy bridging stent graft with adequate overlap

To decrease the risk of component separation, the following recommendations have been made by the manufacturer[5]:

- maximize component overlap (OL): OL must be greater than the aneurysm radius (AR) + 20 mm ($OL \geq AR + 20$ mm);
- avoid excessive oversizing of the proximal extension relative to the main body;
- use another overlapping stent graft in patients with an angulated aortic neck, tortuous aorta, long renal to bifurcation length, and large aneurysm diameter (>70 mm).

Patients with type III endoleak can present with aortic sac enlargement and aortic rupture. In cases with complete separation of the stent graft components, patients can also present with symptoms of distal ischemia if there is obstruction of flow. Endovascular repair of a Type IIIa endoleak can usually be achieved by bridging the two separated components with a new stent graft of appropriate size (Fig. 8.6).

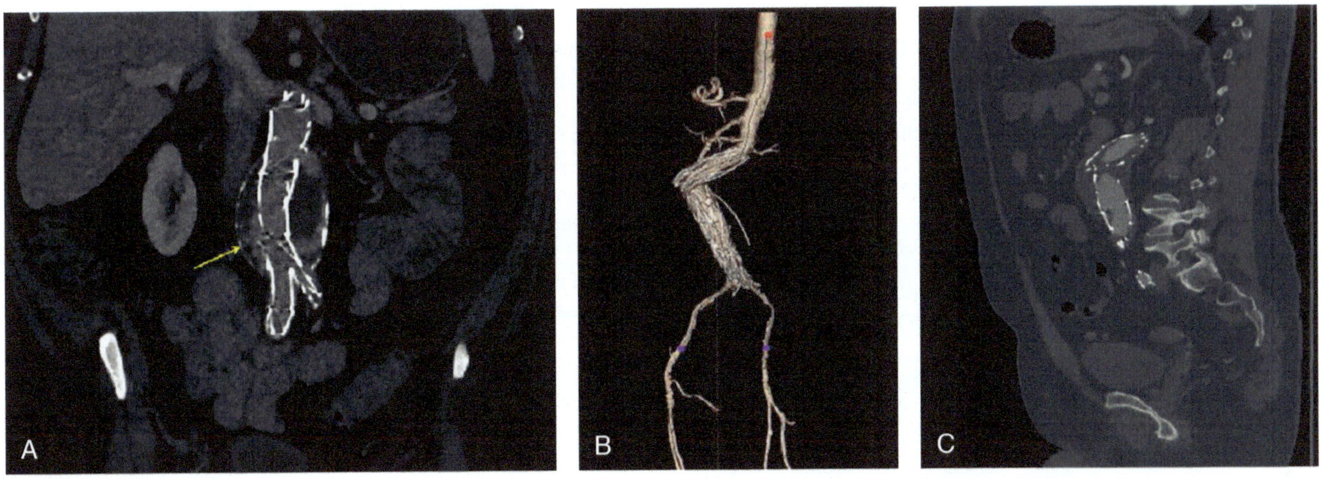

Fig. 8.5 Type III Endoleaks. (A) Type IIIb endoleak caused by disruption of fabric *(arrow)*. (B, C) Type IIIa endoleak caused by separation of proximal extension and main body.

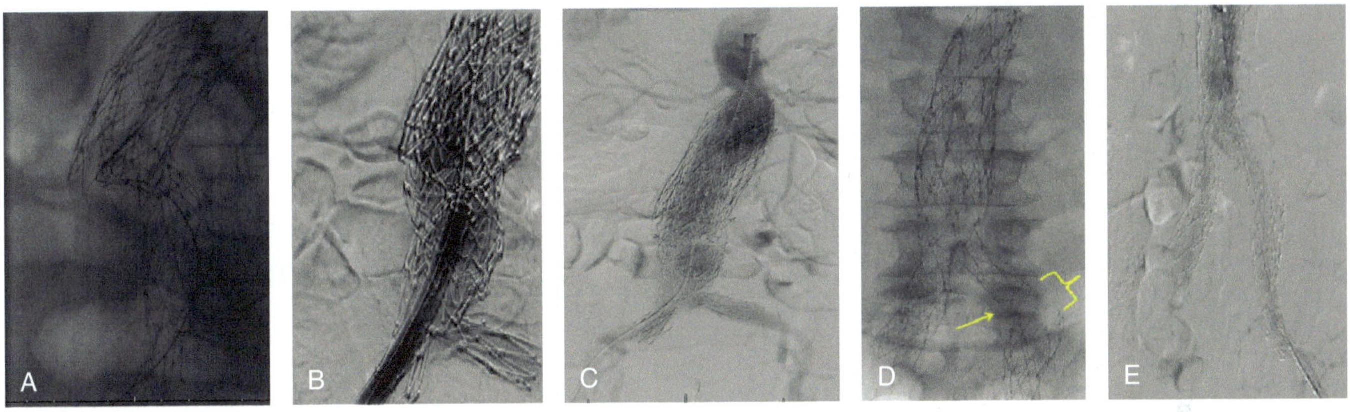

Fig. 8.6 Repair of Type IIIa Endoleaks. (A) Type IIIa endoleak caused by separation of proximal extension and main body. (B, C) Repair with stent graft bridging and deployment of Palmaz stent. (D) Type IIIa endoleak caused by separation of main body and iliac extension (arrow and bracket). (E) Repair with stent graft placement.

Technical challenges during repair are proportional to the degree of separation, angulation, and distortion of the stent graft components.

- Get wire access across the separated components, ensuring that the wire is not behind the struts as discussed in detail earlier.
- Wire access can usually be obtained retrograde, however, in cases with severe distortion of the bifurcated main body, antegrade access from brachial or axillary access with subsequent snaring maybe necessary.
- Confirm wire position by inflating and dragging an 8–12 mm balloon under fluoroscopy.
- Advance the delivery sheath, ideally to the level of deployment, under fluoroscopy to ensure it does not catch the stent graft.
- In case of severe angulation and separation, delivery of sheath and the stent graft may be difficult. This can be facilitated by having a stiff wire across the separated stents in a "body floss" fashion (combined femoral and brachial/axillary access), which provides a stable "rail" to work with.
- Although any stent graft of appropriate diameter and length can be used to bridge the separated main body and proximal extension, stent grafts with good radial force should be used in cases of severe angulation, separation, and distortion of the original components to ensure straightening and adequate lumen size. In certain cases, deployment of a Palmaz stent (Cordis, Miami Lakes, FL, USA) inside the stent graft may be necessary to achieve the desired radial force.
- If the anatomy allows, it can also be treated by placement of a new bimodular aortic stent graft (Fig. 8.7).
- Open conversion with complete or partial stent graft excision is also an option in low-risk patients.

Type IIIb endoleaks have been noted to occur in the AFX stent graft usually at the saddle that sits on the native aortic bifurcation. Factors that can lead to fabric damage include inappropriate guidewire and catheter manipulation or excessive balloon angioplasty within the stent graft, lateral movement with changes in stent graft stability, and deployment in severe calcific vessels. In October 2014, Endologix announced a change in their PTFE design from Strata to a new ultra-high-density, multi-layered material referred to as Duraply. Duraply has increased strength compared with the earlier fabric versions with an unchanged conformability and biocompatibility profile. Since the introduction of these changes, the rate of Type III endoleaks has decreased.

As a result of difficulty in identifying the exact location of the tear, complete relining of the endograft is recommended to exclude the endoleak. This can be done using other commercially available stent graft systems depending on the aortic anatomy (Fig. 8.7). Open conversion with complete or partial stent graft excision remains an option.

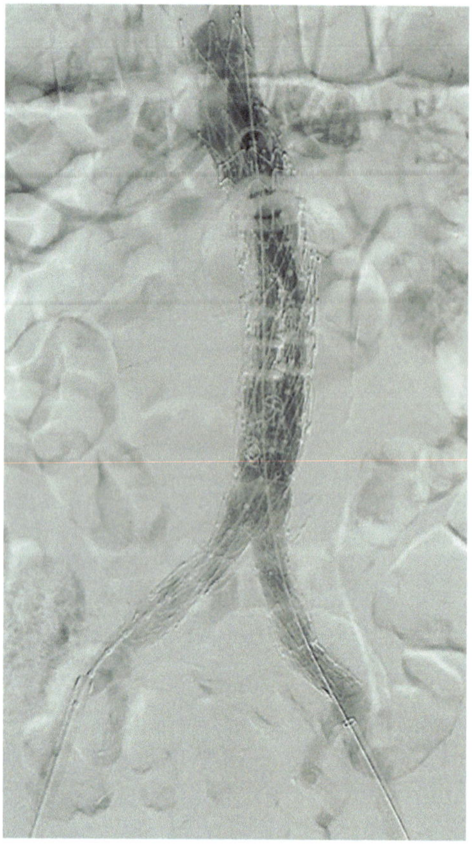

Fig. 8.7 Deployment of an Ovation stent graft system in a patient with a previous AFX with aortic sac enlargement and unidentifiable endoleak.

DIFFICULT RETRIEVAL OF THE NOSE CONE

Another issue that may be encountered is resistance as the nose cone and inner core are withdrawn after deployment of the bifurcated main body. This has the potential to cause distortion and dislodgment of the graft if not recognized.

- Always withdraw the nose cone under direct fluoroscopic visualization.
- If it becomes caught, rotate the inner core 90 degrees to reposition the wing on the delivery system, and proceed with withdrawal.
- Withdraw the stiff wire to alleviate possible wire bias forcing the nose cone to the side.
- Insert a large balloon from the contralateral side and inflate next to the nose cone to push it away from the stent graft.
- External manipulation of the aorta by pressing on the abdomen can also sometimes push the nose cone away from the aortic wall.

Difficult retrieval of the nose cone

- Withdraw nose cone under fluoroscopy
- Rotate the inner core 90 degrees to reposition the wing on the delivery system if it appears to be catching the stent graft
- Use balloon inflation to separate the nose cone from the stent if necessary

MALFUNCTION OF THE CONTRALATERAL WIRE

The 0.035 contralateral wire is attached to a wire lock near the nose cone, which is released by threading a pigtail catheter over the wire, holding the catheter against the wire lock and pulling the wire to release it (Fig. 8.8). This is a unique feature of the AFX2 system, designed to reduce the number and complexity of deployment steps.

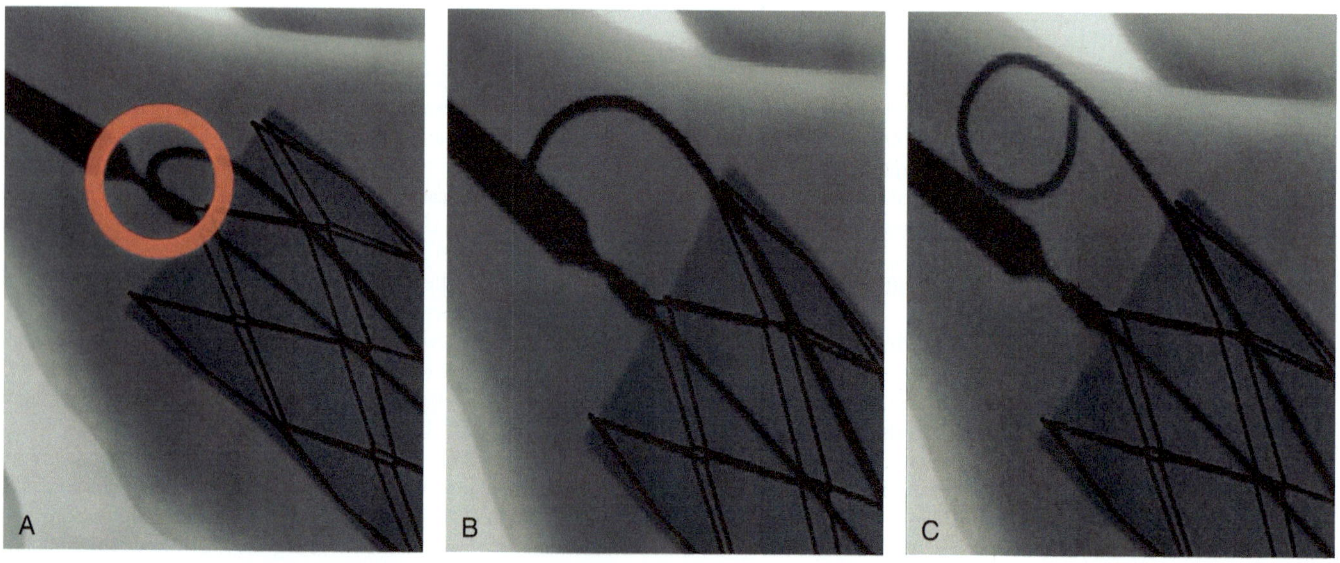

Fig. 8.8 Release of Contralateral Wire. (A) Pass a pigtail catheter over the contralateral wire; (B) hold the catheter against the wire lock to form a loop; (C) pull on the wire to release it and keep catheter to maintain access.
(From Endologix, Irvine, California.)

Sometimes, the wire lock deploys prematurely before the catheter is threaded through the contralateral limb. When this happens, the contralateral limb should be completely deployed by pulling on the yellow wire cover and completely removing it. The deployed limb is then cannulated using standard technique to maintain contralateral access.

In rare cases, the contralateral wire fails to release from the wire lock. The following steps should be taken:

- The pigtail catheter is withdrawn to the level of the aortic bifurcation.
- The inner core is pulled down while simultaneously pulling on the contralateral wire so that the wire lock is positioned just above the aortic bifurcation.
- The delivery sheath and inner core are retracted to deploy the ipsilateral limb.
- The inner core is retracted all the way into the sheath with the contralateral wire still attached until a stop is felt.
- Detach the delivery system from the introducer sheath and disconnect the wire from the locking mechanism.

DIFFICULTY IN DELIVERING THE PROXIMAL EXTENSION

The VELA extension is delivered after deployment of the bifurcated main body. Sometimes the extension is tethered to the main body and advancing the VELA extension may lead to malpositioning of the main body. To avoid this, the following steps should be taken:

- Always advance the VELA extension delivery system under direct fluoroscopy;
- Anchor the main body by inflating an appropriately sized balloon from the contralateral side in the contralateral iliac limb.

MALFUNCTION OF THE CONTROL CORD

The main body is deployed by pulling on the control cord, which pulls the body cover off the stent graft. If the control cord does not work, the following steps should be taken:

- Do not cut the control cord handle.
- Hold the introducer sheath and retract the inner core slowly through the main body under fluoroscopic guidance. This will lead to deployment of the stent graft as the inner core breaks up the sutures.

REFERENCES

1. Welborn MB, McDaniel HB, Johnson RC, et al. Clinical outcome of an extended proximal seal zone with the AFX endovascular aortic aneurysm system. *J Vasc Surg*. 2014 Oct;60(4):876–883.
2. Diethrich EB. Novel sealing concept in the Endologix AFX unibody stent-graft. *J Cardiovasc Surg (Torino)*. 2014;55(1):93–102.
3. Skibba AA, Evans JR, Greenfield DT, et al. Management of late main body aortic endograft component uncoupling and type IIIa endoleak encountered with the Endologix Powerlink and AFX platforms. *J Vasc Surg*. 2015;62(4):868–875.
4. Lemmon GW, Motaganahalli RL, Chang T, et al. Failure mode analysis of the Endologix endograft. *J Vasc Surg*. 2016;64(3):571–576.
5. [ENDOLOGIX UPDATE 2015] https://endologix.com/wp-content/uploads/2016/12/12-30-Physician-Letter-AFX-TIII-Endoleak-FINAL.pdf

9

Graft-Specific Issues for EVAR: The Aorfix Endograft

Hanaa Dakour Aridi, MD, Sophie Wang, MD and Mahmoud B. Malas, MD, MHS, RPVI, FACS

INTRODUCTION

Anatomical characteristics of infrarenal abdominal aortic aneurysms (AAA) are the most critical factors for successful endovascular repair (EVAR).[1] The long-term durability of EVAR is highly dependent on the integrity of the proximal fixation site.[2] Severe proximal aortic neck angulation (i.e., ≥60 degree angulation between the infrarenal aortic neck and the longitudinal axis of the aneurysm) and iliac angulation/tortuosity make it difficult to introduce the delivery system and deploy the Stent-Graft which tends to kink when encountering severe proximal neck angulation or compound curvatures of the iliac arteries. High proximal aortic neck angulation increases EVAR complexity and is associated with several postoperative complications including persistent Type Ia Endoleak, graft migration, aneurysm sac expansion with late rupture, and requirement for remedial procedures or delayed open conversion.[1−5] Severe iliac artery tortuosity increases the risk of iliac limb occlusion and Type Ib endoleak.[1]

Patients with these unfavorable anatomical features comprise a large proportion of those who eventually receive EVAR.[6] Initial landmark clinical trials excluded up to 20% of patients with an infrarenal aortic neck angle >60 degrees from receiving EVAR since they did not meet the anatomic restrictions in the instructions for use (IFU) for the endografts available at the time of these trials.[7] Newer generation devices have attempted to accommodate a wider range of aortoiliac anatomies.[7,8] The Lombard Aorfix endograft (Lombard Medical Inc., Oxfordshire, United Kingdom) is a highly conformable nitinol/polyester device designed for transrenal fixation and accommodates highly angulated aortic necks of up to 90 degrees. Aorfix has been on the European market since late 2004 and was approved by the US Food and Drug Administration (FDA) in 2013 after initial early results of the Prospective Aneurysm Trial: High Angle Aorfix Bifurcated Stent-Graft (PYTHAGORAS) trial showed that outcomes associated with the use of the Aorfix were comparable to those of other endografts used in normal anatomy.[7,9] The use of the Aorfix increased the number of patients eligible for EVAR, who were previously excluded from this type of treatment.

The Aorfix endograft remains the only on-label alternative to open repair for patients with highly angulated aortic necks.[9] The device uses the ring stent concept and is designed to be flexible and conformable to the vessel, resistant to kinking and twisting, and able to shorten without kinking (Fig. 9.1). These features make it particularly suitable when proximal and/or distal landing zones are considerably angulated, especially in larger aneurysms with elongated aorta and iliac arteries. When implanted, the Stent-Graft rings are reformed to have a saddle or "fish-mouth" shape hugging the renal artery orifice and allowing the endograft to be placed pararenally. The fish-mouth troughs are aligned with the renal arteries juxtarenally and the fish-mouth peak extends suprarenally. This provides optimum seal positioning, which might reduce endoleak risk[1,10−12] (Fig. 9.2). The Stent-Graft can also be used in patients with standard anatomy, which helps increase operator familiarity with the device.[13] On certain occasions, namely in patients with tortuous iliac vessels and wide proximal aneurysm necks, main bodies made by other manufacturers in conjunction with the Aorfix iliac limbs have been used[10] (Box 9.1).

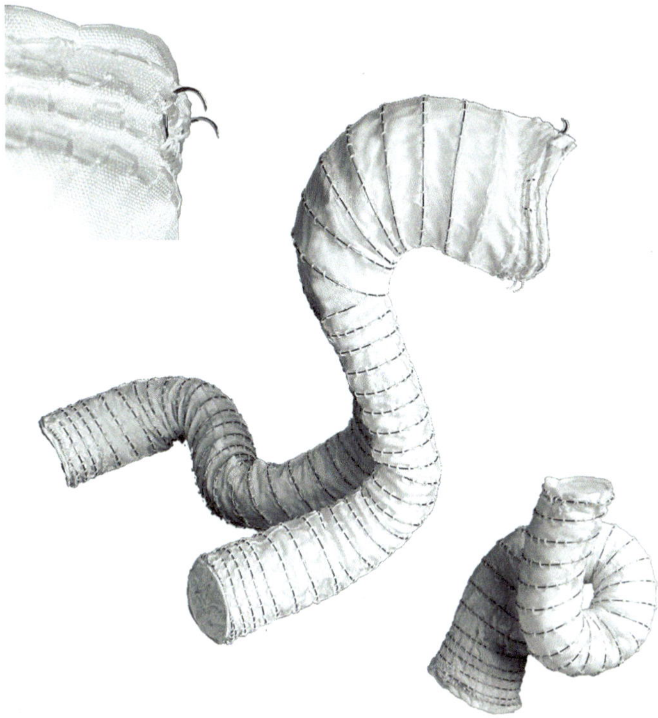

Fig. 9.1 The Aorfix endograft (Lombard Medical Inc., California). Notice the double hooks or barbs at the proximal end of the graft within an 8-mm primary sealing ring, which enhance transrenal fixation.

EVAR AND DEVICE-SPECIFIC COMPLICATIONS

Technical Failure

The first intraoperative difficulty that may be encountered with the Aorfix Stent-Graft is the introduction of the delivery system through the angulated neck. This problem can be solved by applying gentle external compression on the abdomen to the aneurysm via a simple hand maneuver. An additional option would be adding a stiff buddy wire to straighten the anatomy. In cases where there is difficulty in cannulating the contralateral limb, the bifurcated graft can be converted to an aorto-uni-iliac (AUI) stent graft.[13]

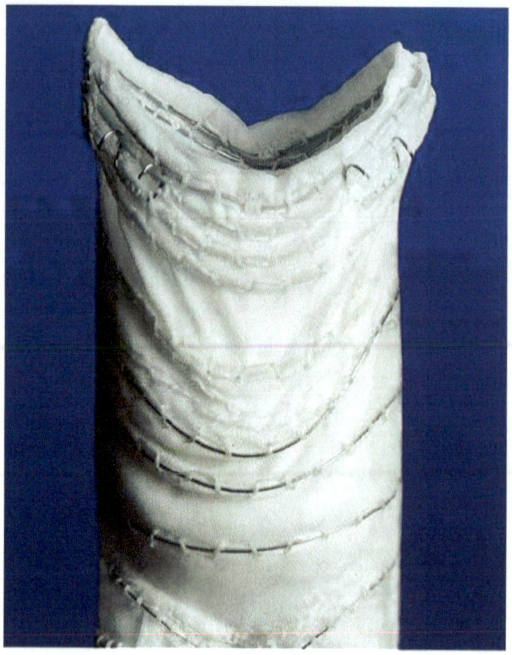

Fig. 9.2 Lateral view of a 24-mm Stent-Graft once deployed, showing the fish-mouth shape.

(Lombard Medical Inc., California. Instructions for use of the Aorfix AAA Flexible Stent-Graft System and Aorfix Plus AAA Flexible Stent-Graft System. Available at: https://www.accessdata.fda.gov/cdrh_docs/pdf11/P110032C.pdf.)

BOX 9.1

Care needs to be taken when sizing the proximal fish-mouth section of the graft, as gross oversizing may cause luminal distortion. An oversizing between 10% and 30% proximally in the aortic neck and 1–2 mm in the iliac component is recommended. However, it is important to note that the outside diameter of Aorfix stent grafts is 1 mm larger than the label diameter which refers to the lumen of the graft. Oversizing is calculated from this outside diameter. Moreover, some familiarity with the orientation of the proximal fish-mouth configuration of the graft is essential for a successful deployment. Once this process is mastered, the subsequent steps can be implemented with minimal difficulty.[10]

In the PYTHAGORAS trial, graft deployment was unsuccessful in eight patients out of 218 patients because of iliofemoral access issues.[12] In one case, no attempt was made to insert the endograft after failure to introduce appropriate dilators.[12] However, in all other cases, various degrees of difficulty were encountered that resulted in failure to gain adequate access to deploy the graft (Box 9.2). Notably, the low profile Intelliflex delivery system for Aorfix is not available in the United States, and PYTHAGORAS and other US experience is currently limited to early versions of the deployment device which featured a larger profile and different delivery mechanism.

BOX 9.2 Tips to avoid technical failure

- Careful preoperative imaging with thin-slice computed tomography angiography (CTA) and 3D reconstruction are very valuable in determining adequate access vessels and the appropriate side for introduction of the endograft. This is helpful in preventing technical failure at this stage. In patients with highly tortuous aortic neck and iliac arteries, meticulous assessment of anatomy prior to the procedure in all three CTA planes can help choose the side with the least angulation for the introduction of the main graft delivery system. For example, in the case of severe neck angulation seen in the coronal plane toward the right, introduction from the contralateral left side will facilitate the passage at the top of the bend and allow for C-shape curve on the delivery system. The use of a super stiff guide wire, such as the Lundequist (Cook Inc., Bloomington, Indiana), is also invaluable.
- For cases with small iliac diameters, extending the groin incision or a retroperitoneal exposure with placement of a conduit might be required as with any other endografts.
- Do not use excessive force to advance or withdraw the delivery device when resistance is encountered.
- If the delivery device kinks during insertion, do not attempt to deploy the Stent-Graft component; remove the device and replace it with a new one.[13]

Endoleaks

Type I Endoleak

Intraoperative proximal endoleak in the interventional suite is not a rare event in cases with hostile infrarenal necks.[15] Their occurrence is highly associated with the learning curve for the Aorfix endograft.[15] In preliminary single-institutional experiences with the Aorfix Stent-Graft, intraoperative Type I endoleaks were detected in 5% to 24.1% of patients.[1,14] In one patient, the Stent-Graft was positioned too low beneath the lowermost renal artery and was treated successfully using proximal extension. In another patient, the Type I endoleak persisted despite positioning the proximal extender at the renal arteries and was left untreated because no Palmaz stent was available at the time and conversion to open repair could not be attempted because of the poor general condition of the patient.[14] In two other patients, simple dilation with an aortic balloon was performed. However, it failed in one patient and a giant P4014 Palmaz stent (Cordis, Miami, Florida) was successfully deployed.[14] On the other hand, post-operative type Ia endoleaks are quite rare with the Aorfix. The PYTHAGORAS study reported three cases of Type Ia endoleak detected on computed tomography (CT) scans. The first two occurred in the first year; one was treated by EndoAnchor and the second was left untreated. The third was diagnosed on postoperative follow-up between the third and fourth postoperative years and was treated with a fenestrated cuff.

Type II Endoleak

In Hinchliffe's study, of 24 patients receiving the Aorfix Stent-Graft, there were only two non-graft related (Type II) endoleaks. The first was detected at completion angiography in a patient with four paired lumbar arteries and the second was detected at discharge.[11] The endoleaks spontaneously sealed by 30 days. In the PYTHAGORAS trial, the incidence of Type II endoleaks was similar between standard-angle (<60 degrees) and highly angulated neck group at all time points (13%, 8%, and 9% at 1, 3, and 5 years respectively) (Table 9.1).

Type III and Type IV Endoleaks

There are no reported cases of Type IV endoleak or endotension with this device. On the other hand, one case of Type IIIa endoleak occurred at 12 months in the PYTHAGORAS trial. The investigator initially believed the leak to be a Type Ib and treated it with a distal extension endograft, which was unsuccessful. Lumbar arteries were then coiled and the endoleak was successfully treated. There are no known or reported Type IIIb endoleaks caused by device fabric defect (Box 9.3).

TABLE 9.1 Aneurysm size changes, endoleaks, graft migration, fractures and reintervention rates at 1, 3, and 5 years in the PYTHAGORAS Trial (Lombard Medical Inc., Irvine, California).

Variable	Aorfix (*N* = 218)	Aorfix, <60 degrees (*N* = 67)	Aorfix, ≥60 degrees (*N* = 151)	*P* value
Sac shrinkage (>5 mm)				
1 year	42 (69/165)	39 (20/51)	43 (49/114)	0.73
3 years	57 (74/129)	7 (26/43)	56 (48/86)	0.71
5 years	61 (52/85)	64 (16/25)	60 (36/60)	0.81
Sac expansion (>5 mm)				
1 year	1 (2/165)	0 (0/51)	2 (2/114)	1
3 years	7 (9/129)	7 (3/43)	7 (6/86)	1
5 years	12 (10/85)	4 (1/25)	15 (9/60)	0.27
Type I or III endoleak				
1 year	1 (2/149)	0 (0/46)	2 (2/103)	1
3 years	0 (0/114)	0 (0/38)	0 (0/76)	1
5 years	0 (0/72)	0 (0/25)	0 (0/47)	1
Type II endoleak				
1 year	13 (20/149)	15 (7/46)	13 (13/103)	0.67
3 years	8 (9/114)	5 (2/38)	9 (7/76)	0.47
5 years	9 (7/75)	11 (3/27)	8 (4/48)	0.69
Migration				
1 year	1 (2/165)	0 (0/51)	2 (2/114)	1
3 years	5 (6/128)	2 (1/42)	6 (5/86)	0.66
5 years	4 (3/85)	4 (1/25)	3 (2/60)	1
Fixation zone fracture				
1 year	6 (9/159)	5 (2/43)	6 (7/116)	1
3 years	19 (23/123)	13 (5/39)	21 (18/84)	0.32
5 years	23 (17/75)	21 (5/24)	24 (12/51)	1
Main body fracture				
1 year	2 (3/159)	0 (0/43)	3 (3/116)	0.56
3 years	1 (1/123)	0 (0/39)	1 (1/84)	1
5 years	1 (1/75)	0 (0/24)	2 (1/51)	1
Reintervention				
1 year	10 (22/218)	8 (5/67)	11 (17/151)	0.47
3 years	14 (31/218)	9 (6/67)	17 (25/151)	0.21
5 years	17 (38/218)	12 (8/67)	20 (30/151)	0.18

BOX 9.3 Tips to minimize the risk of endoleaks

- Preoperative imaging and proper patient selection with adequate proximal and distal seal zone length are crucial especially in cases with severe angulation.
- The importance of proper stent oversizing in reducing the incidence of Type I endoleak is clearly demonstrated.
- Proper deployment at the lowest renal or transrenal deployment in cases of short neck will provide adequate proximal seal and reduce the risk of Type I endoleaks.
- Proper limb overlap is crucial to avoid Type IIIa endoleaks.

In case of intraoperative and/or delayed proximal or distal Type I endoleaks, additional treatment options for Types Ia and Ib can be followed similar to any other endograft:

1. Compliant balloon dilation
2. Non-compliant balloon dilation
3. Extending the repair proximally or distally with aortic cuff or iliac limb, respectively, in cases where additional room is available
4. Placement of balloon-expandable stents
5. Use of Aptus Heli-Fx Endograft with EndoAnchors (Aptus Endosystems, Sunnyvale, California)
6. Use of the snorkel technique with proximal extension
7. Use of fenestrated cuff
8. Use of branched endograft for renal, SMA, or internal iliac arteries

BOX 9.4 Tips to avoid graft migration

- Based on the experience gained in the PYTHAGORAS trial, the instructions for use for Aorfix now warns against landing the device >8 mm below the distal renal artery and against implantation in necks that increase in diameter by 5 mm or more over a 15-mm length (reverse taper neck). Early outcomes of the PYTHAGORAS trial showed that grafts were landed at least 8 mm below the distal renal arteries in four subjects suffering migration. In two of these four cases, the diameters of the necks also increased by more than 5 mm over their 15 mm length.[13]
- If the sheath is accidentally withdrawn, the implant will prematurely deploy and may be incorrectly positioned.
- Use magnification when visualizing the renal landing zone to improve accuracy of placement.
- Inaccurate placement or an inadequate seal zone may result in an increased risk of leakage into the aneurysm or migration of the Stent-Graft.

BOX 9.5 Tips to avoid IIA occlusion

- Careful measurements and appreciation of the preoperative CTA images, especially centerline length measurements in tortuous iliac arteries and angulated necks, can help avoid IIA occlusion.
- Intraoperative measurement from the contralateral gate to the origin of the IIA with pigtail catheter placed in the iliac vessels over a moderate stiffness wire (for example, Ampalz Super Stiff Guidewire—Boston Scientific, Marlborough, Massachusetts) can confirm preoperative planning. The same steps should be repeated on the ipsilateral side if iliac limb extension is needed. Having a stiff wire will straighten the anatomy and could change the graft position after removal of the wire.
- Careful and slow deployment of iliac limb extensions with proper adjustment (accordion the limb if too long) will avoid inadvertent coverage of the IIA.

Stent-Graft Migration

No evidence of Stent-Graft migration was noted in many single institutional studies suggesting that the Aorfix stays in place and continues to function well despite increased forces caused by angulation. In the PYTHAGORAS trial, the high rates of device fracture reported in the trial (23% at 5 years) were initially a cause for concern. However, these reported fractures were entirely limited to the barbs, and did not involve the stent graft itself. There was no association between barb fracture and increased rates of stent migration. There was also no association between migration and neck angulation. However, proximal neck dilation greater than 10% at 5 mm above the proximal renal and 1 mm below the distal renal, increased the risk of graft migration fourfold (relative risk, 4.38, $P = 0.01$ and 4.33, $P = 0.002$, respectively)[7] (Box 9.4).

Despite the graft having no suprarenal component, the association between suprarenal dilatation and a higher relative risk of migration suggests that non-iatrogenic aortic dilatation (i.e., that arising from aging or disease progression) is a factor in increasing the risk of migration.[7] Moreover, since perirenal dilation is unusual, the increased risk of migration likely indicates loss of integrity of the proximal fixation site because of the poor quality of the aorta.[6] On the other hand, Aorfix showed increased relative risk of migration with dilation of the lower aortic neck, which highlights the robustness and compliance of the independent stent ring design.

Unplanned Internal Iliac Artery (IIA) Occlusion

Over-lengthy occlusion of the ipsilateral vessels particularly with light systemic anticoagulation can lead to vessel occlusion.[13] Single institutional studies have reported unplanned internal iliac artery occlusion in 5% to 25%, which was most likely accounted for by the learning curve of the various centers (Box 9.5).

There has been no major clinical sequela or major complications to date in the case of unplanned or intentional occlusion of an internal iliac artery (Grade 1 complication according to reporting standards for EVAR).[1] Postoperative transient buttock claudication in a patient with bilateral IIA occlusion has been reported but subsequently resolved without any further sequelae.

Iliac Limb Occlusion

Several factors can result in iliac limb occlusion such as placement of the implant in an aorta with a diameter of 18 mm or less in the region of the gate, use of a distal extender in a leg that has a smaller diameter than the distal extender, and failure to dilate fully the proximal end of a distal extender. In addition, insertion of a distal extender with more than 20 mm overlap into a leg graft risks compressing the proximal part of the extender with the tapered part of the leg graft can lead to stenosis or occlusion[13] (Box 9.6).

BOX 9.6 Tips to avoid iliac limb occlusion

- Proper ballooning of all overlap limbs is required for placement of all endografts.
- In the case of a narrow distal aortic neck, placement of self-expanding kissing stents with proper post-stent kissing ballooning should help minimizing the risk of limb occlusion.
- If the distal neck is less than 10 mm in diameter, conversion to aorto-uni-iliac endograft with femoral–femoral bypass is a safer approach.
- Avoidance of excessive iliac limb oversizing (suggested 1-mm oversizing by instructions for use) can minimize the risk of graft buckling and occlusion.

In the PYTHAGORAS trial, two stents were placed to treat compression of the ipsilateral limb at the level of the cannulation gate during the first postoperative months and no graft occlusions were reported after the first postoperative year.[12] The former patients had long and narrow terminal aortas. Poor dilation of the overlap region of three distal extenders caused limb occlusion and a grossly oversized limb caused a fourth occlusion.

Sac Expansion/Rupture

Sac expansion (>5 mm, per Society of Vascular Surgery guidelines) is device-dependent and is associated with endoleaks and the need for remedial endovascular or open procedures. In the PYTHAGORAS trial, overall sac expansion rate was 12% at 5 years, which is lower than that reported in prior studies. There was a trend toward a higher incidence of sac expansion in the highly angulated neck group but this was not statistically significant[5,12] (Box 9.7).

Five-year freedom from sac rupture was 99% in both groups. Five cases of sac rupture have been reported overall. The first case occurred intraoperatively after maneuvers, including lateral abdominal pressure, to negotiate a sharp neck angle (126 degrees). The second was a limited rupture of the proximal neck at 7 days postoperatively and was caused by ballooning to treat a Type Ia endoleak. This was managed with a surgically applied patch (open surgery without graft resection). In one patient, there was a contained rupture at the proximal neck at the sixth

BOX 9.7 Tips to avoid post-EVAR rupture

- Identify patients at high risk of sac rupture and follow them diligently with consideration given to more frequent follow-up.
- The main risk factors for sac rupture are challenging anatomy, particularly short aortic necks, in addition to high levels of calcified plaque at the transition of the aortic neck to the aneurysm sac.
- Other factors include aortic neck sizes that lie outside the indications of the Aorfix instructions for use, trapezoidal necks with a diameter change of 5 mm or more over 15 mm, patients in whom the proximal landing zone could not be juxtarenal (particularly if the lowest part of the fish-mouth is 8 mm or more distal to the distal renal artery) and over-ballooning.

postoperative week with no associated endoleak or excessive oversizing. Review of device sizing indicated that the proximal diameter of the graft was undersized and that the aortic neck had high levels of thrombus preoperatively. The patient was treated with proximal aortic cuff extension at 13 months postoperatively and continued to be well 6 years post-rupture. The other two cases occurred between the second and third postoperative years. In one, a 7-mm neck dilation resulted in migration and endoleak. All fixation hooks were intact. The patient was treated with open conversion. Finally, in the last case, the highly calcified inner curve of a 103-degree neck angle caused fretting damage to the graft giving rise to a Type III endoleak and sac rupture. The patient had an open conversion and subsequently died. On explant, a hole was found on the posterior wall of the Stent-Graft. CT analysis showed a large calcified deposit in the aorta, which corresponded in position with the hole. It was concluded that the hole was worn in the graft fabric secondary to rubbing against the calcified plaque.

Device Fracture

In the PYTHAGORAS trial, 24% of patients had fractures at 5 years, including 23% at the fixation zone (i.e., barb fractures) and 1% of the main body stents (Table 9.1). Both fixation zone and main body fractures occurred with similar frequency between the highly angulated and standard-angle neck groups.[12] Analysis of 10 subjects with hook fractures at 12 months showed that fractures were associated with subjects where the proximal sealing zone had dilated rapidly (mean 4.85 mm). In many cases, this dilation was associated with the device having been landed more than 1 cm below the distal renal artery, usually in an attempt to use an adequate infrarenal proximal landing zone for the device. Initial analyses of neck diameters indicated that dilation was not a consequence of radial force, however with long term results, the degree of oversize does appear to correlate with rate of neck dilation.[7]

The most likely consequences of hook fractures are migration and Type Ia endoleaks. A revised wire specification was introduced during 2010. The method of finishing the nitinol on the stent and barbs was modified and since then many fewer fractures have occurred in hooks manufactured with the revised wire specification.[12,13] Patients in whom barb fractures are detected should be followed up more frequently.

Visceral Vessels Complications

A number of implant complications have been reported with the Aorfix Stent-Graft. In the PYTHAGORAS 5-year outcomes study, nine implant complications involved the renal arteries, six of which were consequent to placing an additional aortic cuff, which was particularly common in aneurysms with neck angulation >90 degrees. Seven renal stents were used, of which three were placed during the index procedure; one of these was placed for concomitant treatment of a diseased renal artery.[12] In addition, one superior mesenteric artery (SMA) was impinged and stented during the index procedure. Many of the renal vessel-related complications were associated with improper low initial endograft deployment requiring additional proximal aortic cuff and accidental coverage of one of the renal artery. Proper initial deployment at the renal or transrenal can avoid this complication (Box 9.8).

BOX 9.8 Tips to avoid visceral vessel complications

1. Proper preoperative imaging with CTA 3D reconstruction is crucial to confirm adequate 20 mm distance from the lower end of the superior mesenteric artery (SMA) to the beginning of the aneurysm. If there is less than 10 mm separation between the distal margin of the SMA and the distal renal artery, care must be taken in placing the proximal end of the Stent-Graft. This can avoid accidental coverage of the SMA with the peak of the endograft in cases where transrenal fixation was used. Lateral views may be helpful in positioning the graft precisely below the SMA.
2. Operators should familiarize themselves with the deployment mechanism and the fish-mouth shape of the endograft. Initial experience with straight proximal anatomy may be helpful before embarking on treating patients with severely angulated necks.
3. When deploying the proximal cuff, ensure that its orientation and axial position are carefully controlled.
4. Ensure that the fish-mouth will not occlude any part of the renal arteries when fully deployed. Check that the SMA has not been covered by the anterior peak. If necessary, use a lateral view to confirm patency.
5. As a result of the fish-mouth shape at the proximal end of the stent graft, it is necessary to balloon parts of the aorta that are not completely covered with the Stent-Graft. When a balloon catheter is used, do not inflate to greater than the diameter of the aorta and do not balloon completely outside the Stent-Graft.[13]
6. Place the balloon so that the fish-mouth lies symmetrically along the length of the balloon, in other words so that the balloon lies half in and half out of the Stent-Graft. If the balloon is inflated from full within the Stent-Graft, the expanding proximal end of the balloon may have a tendency to push the Stent-Graft proximally.
7. When deploying the aorto-uni-iliac (AUI) converter, avoid accidental occlusion of branch vessels by ensuring that it lies completely below the top of the primary graft and that the fish-mouth of the AUI converter has the same orientation as the primary graft.
8. Leave the pigtail catheter in place suprarenally throughout deployment in order to check renal patency before final release of the implant from the delivery system. The pigtail can be safely recovered after straightening with a guide wire without risk of being impaled by a barb.
9. In cases of short angulated neck, having brachial access and selection of the lowest renal with Amplatz wire (Boston Scientific, Marlborough, Massachusetts) and 6 French Shuttle Select sheath (Cook Medical, Bloomington, Indiana) can allow for snorkelling technique in case of renal artery impingement.

GENERAL COMMENTS

- The success of EVAR using the Aorfix is based on appropriate patient selection, careful planning using multi-planar CT imaging, accurate selection of appropriate graft dimensions, and the high degree of flexibility and conformability of the graft.[10]

- **Oversizing:** High levels of oversizing are most commonly used in steeply conical or irregular necks. Therefore, it is important to be cautious with treatment of necks that change in diameter by ≥5 mm over their 15-mm length and to select oversizing from within the recommended range of 10% to 30%.
- **Neck diameter and seal zone virtual graft modelling:** The best predictors of complications related to Aorfix in patients with highly angulated neck anatomy have been shown to be proximal aortic neck diameter (hazard ratio, 1.14; 95% confidence interval, 1.03–1.27; $P < 0.05$) and the seal zone inner curve length (hazard ratio, 1.03; 95% confidence interval, 1.01–1.06; $P < 0.05$).[15] For every 1-mm increase in neck diameter, there is a 22% increase in the risk of endoleak, migration, or sac expansion, regardless of neck angle or endograft oversizing. Other measures of aortic aneurysm anatomy including distal neck diameter, seal zone centerline length, seal zone, and stent diameter were also significantly associated with complications after EVAR but to a lesser extent.
  - The success of EVAR is contingent upon a clear mental model of affected anatomy and thorough pre-operative planning; this is especially true with challenging anatomy. The commonly used proximal neck length measurements taken along the centerline may not capture the true length of vessel available for sealing in patients with highly angulated aortic necks. Highly angulated necks tend to have a sufficient centerline length but a very short seal zone based on the curvature (Fig. 9.3). Preoperative 3D virtual graft modeled seal zones can better capture the limitations of a short, angled neck and assess a patient's risk for endograft-related complications.[15] Therefore, in highly angulated necks, surgeons may consider 3D modeling the seal zone during preoperative planning to predict the expected seal zone, paying close attention to the inner curve length, as this is a predictor of complications independent of anle or oversizing.[15] However, this might not be applicable before every EVAR procedure.
- **Neck length and neck angle:** Neither neck angle nor neck length was found to be significant predictors of device-related complications.[5,15] The Aorfix endograft is able to handle severely angulated and short necks without kinking, which most likely reduces the influence of angle and length on post-EVAR outcomes.[12] Moreover, Aorfix's fish-mouth design may also reduce the radial force exerted at the proximal end of the aortic neck, thereby making neck diameter a more important factor with other endografts. This reduced radial force might also minimize post-EVAR neck dilation.
- In the case of marked angulation of the proximal neck, the key is to get the C-arm properly oriented, so that the entire length of the neck appears on the screen and therefore parallax phenomenon avoided.
- The appearance of a new endoleak, device migration, reduced blood flow through the graft, and/or decrease in renal function due to renal artery occlusion should prompt further investigation into the need for further patient treatment, including additional intervention or surgical conversion.[13]

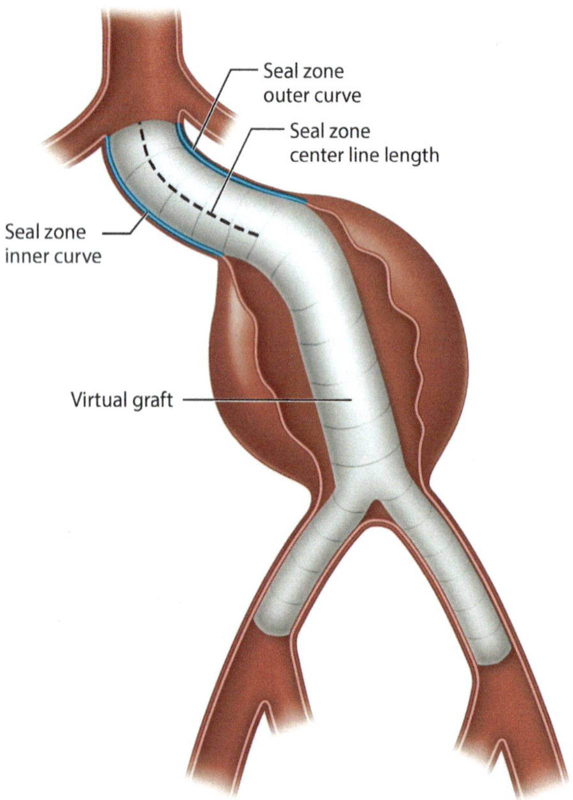

Fig. 9.3 Diagram of a virtual Aorfix graft and the seal zone parameters. (Wang S, Hicks CW, Malas MB. Neck diameter and inner curve seal zone predict endograft-related complications in highly angulated necks after endovascular aneurysm repair using the Aorfix endograft. *J Vasc Surg.* 2018;67(3):760–769. Permission obtained from publisher and authors.)

REFERENCES

1. Perdikides T, Georgiadis GS, Avgerinos ED, et al. The Aorfix Stent-Graft to treat infrarenal abdominal aortic aneurysms with angulated necks and/or tortuous iliac arteries: midterm results. *J Endovasc Ther.* 2009;16:567–576.
2. Malas MB, Ohki T, Veith FJ, et al. Absence of proximal neck dilatation and graft migration following endovascular aneurysm repair with Balloon expandable stent-based endograft. *J Vasc Surg.* 2005;42:639–644.
3. Aburahma AF, Campbell JE, Mousa AY, et al. Clinical outcomes for hostile versus favorable aortic neck anatomy in endovascular aortic aneurysm repair using modular devices. *J Vasc Surg.* 2011;54:13–21.
4. Candell L, Tucker LY, Goodney P, et al. Early and delayed rupture after endovascular abdominal aortic aneurysm repair in a 10-year multicenter registry. *J Vasc Surg.* 2014;60:1146–1152.
5. McGillicuddy EA, Fillinger M, Robinson WP, 3rd, et al. Lombard Aorfix high angulation device, sac behavior following implantation. *J Vasc Surg.* 2017;66:71–78.
6. Ouriel K, Tanquilut E, Greenberg RK, et al. Aortoiliac morphologic correlations in aneurysms undergoing endovascular repair. *J Vasc Surg.* 2003;38:323–328.
7. Malas MB, Jordan WD, Cooper MA, et al. Performance of the Aorfix endograft in severely angulated proximal necks in the PYTHAGORAS United States clinical trial. *J Vasc Surg.* 2015;62:1108–1117.
8. Hobo R, Kievit J, Leurs LJ, et al. Influence of severe infrarenal aortic neck angulation on complications at the proximal neck following endovascular AAA repair: a EUROSTAR study. *J Endovasc Ther.* 2007;14:1–11.
9. US Food and Drug Administration. Recently approved devices: Aorfix flexible Stent-Graft system - P110032. Updated 2013. Available at: https://www.accessdata.fda.gov/scripts/cdrh/cfdocs/cfpma/pma.cfm?id=P110032. Accessed June 25, 2020.
10. Balasubramaniam K, Hardman J, Horrocks M, et al. The advantages of Aorfix for endovascular repair of abdominal aortic aneurysm. *J Cardiovasc Surg (Torino).* 2009;50:139–143.
11. Hinchliffe RJ, Macierewicz JA, Hopkinson BR. Early results of a flexible bifurcated endovascular Stent-Graft (Aorfix). *J Cardiovasc Surg.* 2004;45:285–291.

12. Malas MB, Hicks CW, Jordan Jr WD, et al. Five-year outcomes of the PYTHAGORAS U.S. clinical trial ofthe Aorfix endograft for endovascular aneurysm repair in patients with highly angulated aortic necks. *J Vasc Surg.* 2017;65:1598–1607.
13. US Food and Drug Administration. Instructions for Use of the Aorfix™ AAA Flexible Stent-Graft System and Aorfix™ Plus AAA Flexible Stent-Graft System. Available at: https://www.accessdata.fda.gov/cdrh_docs/pdf11/P110032C.pdf. Accessed June 25, 2020.
14. Albertini JN, Perdikides T, Soong CV, et al. Endovascular repair of abdominal aortic aneurysms in patients with severe angulation of the proximal neck using a flexible Stent-Graft European multicenter experience. *J Cardiovasc Surg (Torino).* 2006;47:245–250.
15. Wang S, Hicks CW, Malas MB. Neck diameter and inner curve seal zone predict endograft-related complications in highly angulated necks after endovascular aneurysm repair using the Aorfix endograft. *J Vasc Surg.* 2018;67(3):760–769.

10

Nellix

Katherine K. McMackin, MD and Jeffrey P. Carpenter, MD

The Nellix device (Endologix, Irvine, CA) is a novel endovascular aneurysm sealing system (EVAS) designed to address some of the issues with current infrarenal endovascular aneurysm devices. Persistent flow in the aneurysm sac after deployment of a stent graft can lead to aneurysm sac expansion and ultimately rupture. The Nellix device utilizes polymer-filled EndoBags to seal the aneurysm sac space. This is designed to decrease persistent sac flow and potential for endoleaks. First introduced in 2008, it has since been approved for commercial use in Europe and New Zealand. In the United States, it remains an investigational device, with refinement of the indications for use in 2016 based on complications observed in the first two years of data collection.

As this new device continues to be used and the EVAS procedure evolves, subsequent complications have become better understood. The unique design of the Nellix device means complications seen with both EVAS and EVAR, such as device migration and endoleak, cannot be addressed with the same conventional techniques that are used in EVAR. This chapter will address the structure of the Nellix device and how that structure, in addition to patient-specific factors, can lead to device migration, endoleaks, and aneurysm expansion. Prevention of these complications and available treatment modalities will be addressed.[1]

ISOLATED MIGRATION

Migration of the Nellix device (>10 mm) has been found to be caused by bending of the central stents. The Nellix device's design means it is subject to downward flow forces not seen in traditional EVAR, ultimately leading to the foreshortening of the central stents. The polymer surrounding the stents creates a shelf against which blood flowing through the aorta impacts. This force of the blood contacting the polymer has been dubbed the "shelf force." With each impact the shelf force must be resisted by a combination of the strength of the stents, the surrounding polymer, and that which surrounds the polymer, thrombus, and aortic wall. A second drag force is present in any stent not perfectly straight, caused by lateral force, which further bends the stent (Fig. 10.1).

The strength with which the central stents resist the shelf and drag forces is not primarily caused by the rigidity of the stent itself, but from the surrounding polymer in the EndoBags. Understanding the aforementioned forces is paramount to prevention of device migration. Minimizing the distorting forces and maximizing the supporting forces can prevent this complication.

PREVENTION

Minimizing Distortion Forces

The shelf force is directly proportional to the area of the polymer shelf. As the diameter of neck in which the Nellix is deployed increases, so does the area of the polymer shelf. Therefore, limiting the aneurysm neck diameter decreases the area of the polymer shelf and thus the shelf force. Discovery of the shelf force as a primary cause of caudal migration led to refinement of the instructions for use (IFU) of the device, limiting neck diameter to 18–28 mm. Prior to the 2016 refinement of the IFU, aneurysms with neck diameters up to 32 mm had been included.

Maximizing Supporting Forces

The lateral force caused by drag slowly bends the stent into the surrounding thrombus, arresting only when coming in contact with the aortic wall. The stents themselves do not have the strength to resist this force and rely on the surrounding polymer for support. The amount of polymer able to be deployed in the EndoBags is limited by the amount of thrombus between the bag and the aortic wall. The refinement of IFU in 2016 created the "thrombus index," a new method for evaluating this relationship. The thrombus index is defined as the ratio of the maximal aneurysm diameter to maximal flow lumen diameter. A thrombus index <1.40 has been seen to allow for sufficient polymer in the EndoBag to prevent device migration.[1]

TREATMENT

Stent Relining

Those Nellix devices that have isolated migration, without endoleak or sac expansion, can undergo stent relining. This technique increases the

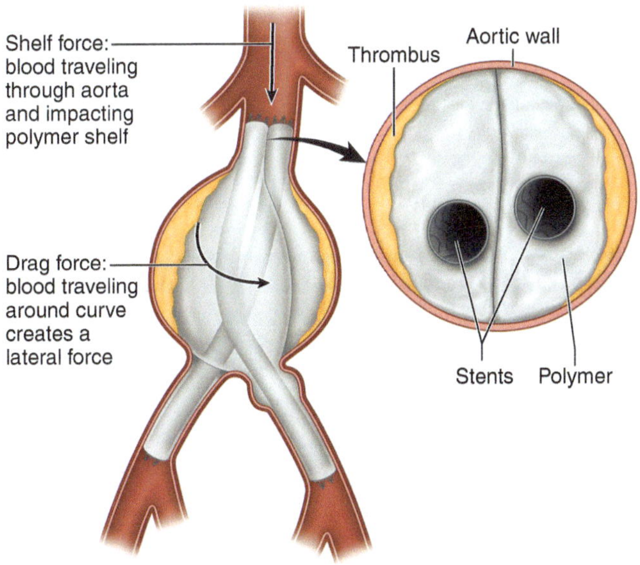

Fig. 10.1 Forces leading to migration and cross-sectional image of proximal aspect of Nellix device illustrating polymer shelf, stents, thrombus, and aortic wall.

overall stiffness of the system, thereby increasing the forces opposing the distortion forces. The stent-in-stent fix has the benefit of being a minimally invasive intervention, which does not preclude future interventions. Some technical considerations must be taken into account prior to relining the stent. It is the recommended technique in the absence of an endoleak and with at least 10 mm of remaining seal zone. The goal of treatment is to arrest migration and prevent the development of a Type 1A endoleak.

Relining can be achieved either with Nellix stents or an alternative balloon expandable covered stent. Balloon expandable stents are preferred because of the higher radial force during deployment. Using a Nellix to reline the Nellix has the benefit of requiring only a single stent, because of its long length. This avoids overlap required with multiple shorter stent deployment and prevents triple overlap, which optimizes lumen diameter.

Steps for Relining

1. Obtain retrograde access via bilateral common femoral arteries.
2. Use a standard technique to access the lumen of the Nellix stents.
3. Pre-dilate the Nellix stents with noncompliant PTA balloons 12 × 40 mm throughout the entire length of the stents.
4. Select a balloon expandable covered stent or Nellix stent.
5. Deploy the new stents.

> **TIP BOX 10.1**
>
> When selecting the Nellix stents, ensure an overlapping length of at least 35 mm between the original implanted Nellix stent and the new Nellix stents.

(Note: If using Nellix stents to reline, inject about 10 mL of saline through the EndoBag port of the console. Saline is used to reduce friction within the EndoBag, which will reduce the force required to detach the implant from the catheter.)

6. Perform a post-dilation of the stents after deployment with noncompliant PTA balloons 12 × 40 mm.
7. Perform a completion angiogram.

> **TIP BOX 10.2**
>
> The new stents should reline the entire length of the previously implanted Nellix device.

TYPE 1A ENDOLEAK

The overall incidence and persistence of a Type 1A endoleak with the Nellix device is extremely low. Published single-center studies as well as the Global Post Market Registry mark the incidence of Type 1A endoleak at 0%–4.3%, with early follow-up persistence of endoleak at 0%–0.4%. However, because of the unique design of the Nellix device, Type 1A endoleaks cannot be addressed as they are with traditional EVAR. The Nellix device is not compatible with proximal aortic cuffs or large balloon expandable stents, and therefore new technologies and adaptations of procedures currently in use can be used when this complication arises.

Understanding the anatomic and procedural risk factors that lead to Type 1A endoleaks can help the surgeon in the preoperative planning and during initial deployment of the Nellix device to prevent Type 1A endoleaks. Anatomic risk factors include: aneurysms with hostile infrarenal neck anatomy, including wide necks, severe calcification, significant thrombus, and neck angulation >60 degrees. "Stomach" shaped aneurysms, those with both angulation and large lateral diameters, can lead to stent bowing, loss of proximal stent alignment, and ultimately a Type 1A endoleak. Procedural factors can also contribute to the endoleak rate. During the initial deployment, low stent placement and stent misalignment forfeit available neck utilization and, therefore, increase the risk for this type of endoleak. These endoleaks may resolve spontaneously but should be closely surveilled every 3 to 6 months until sac stabilization or regression occurs, followed by annual check-ups. Those endoleaks associated with an increase in sac size may require intervention. Early diagnosis, continued monitoring, and, if necessary, endovascular treatment are key to prevent endoleak progression to aneurysm sac expansion and ultimately rupture (Table 10.1).[2]

Prevention

During initial deployment of the Nellix device, performing a contrast-enhanced, saline prefill of the EndoBag and keeping the Nellix balloons inflated during prefill and polymer injection can mitigate stent bowing and proximal stent misalignment, which are risk factors for Type 1A endoleak.

Performing a prefill of the EndoBag allows for an accurate estimate of both the definitive polymer volume required to achieve a seal as well as the fill pressure. The surgeon must examine both apposition of the EndoBag to achieve a seal as well as stent location, which can move slightly during polymer filling. Performing a prefill allows the surgeon to make corrections to positioning prior to polymer injection.

TABLE 10.1 Treatment options for Type 1A endoleak.

Intervention	Device migration?	Stent misalignment or low stent?	Distance between lowest renal artery and Nellix	Minimal proximal seal zone required
Coil and liquid embolics	No	No	n/a	10 mm infrarenal seal zone
Proximal extension with covered stents plus coil and liquid embolization	No	Yes	n/a	10 mm infrarenal seal zone
Proximal extension with Nellix system	Yes	Yes	≥30 mm	15 mm infrarenal seal zone
Nellix revisional ChEVAS: Proximal extension with Nellix system and parallel grafts	Yes	Yes	<30 mm Note: 30 mm extension is required for EndoBag unfurling and wall apposition	15 mm seal zone at variable locations dependent on parallel grafts

After prefill, but prior to polymer fill, it is essential to ensure the Nellix stents have not moved. If the stent does move during prefill, once the saline has been aspirated from the EndoBag, the stents may be repositioned. After this, the Nellix balloons can remain inflated within the stent during polymer fill. This stabilizes the stents and allows the EndoBag to fill while maintaining stent position.

Perform prefill.

1. Inject non-heparinized saline to the target pressure of 180 mmHg ± 10 mmHg.
2. Contrast in the prefill can be of a maximum concentration of 15% of the non-heparinized saline volume.
3. Perform an angiography in multiple views to assess aneurysm seal.
4. Completely aspirate the saline once complete aneurysm sealing has been achieved.

Treatment

Unlike with EVAR, Type 1A endoleaks in Nellix devices are not treated with a proximal extension via either large balloon expandable stents or aortic cuffs. Four main minimally invasive options for intervention are available. Those not amenable to endovascular intervention can undergo conversion to open repair.[3] The choice of treatment is dependent upon the anatomic characteristics of the leak and the aneurysm's anatomic relationship to the Nellix graft. When deciding which intervention is appropriate, the surgeon must evaluate for the presence of device migration, the position of the Nellix stents, and the distance between the lowest renal artery and the Nellix device.

COIL AND LIQUID EMBOLICS

For small to moderate Type 1A endoleaks without device migration and with correctly aligned stents, the surgeon can perform a minimally invasive deployment of a coil matrix with liquid embolics. To perform this, retrograde access via the bilateral femoral arteries and access from the brachial artery are obtained. Standard techniques are used to access each stent. Balloons are placed at each of the Nellix stents to allow partial or complete aortic occlusion proximal to the site of the endoleak and to avoid distal embolization of embolic material. A catheter is placed into the endoleak via brachial access. Angiography is performed to ensure placement. Coils are deployed taking care not to propagate the coils proximally. A scaffold is built in the endoleak with the coils. Liquid embolic agent is then deployed under continuous imaging into this scaffold, with Onyx being the most commonly reported embolic agent in the literature. A completion angiogram should be performed.

Reports of secondary intervention for proximal endoleak with Nellix are limited to case series. Harvey et al. and Ameli et al. described their institutions' experience with coils and liquid embolics for Type 1A endoleak following placement of the Nellix graft with three and nine patients respectively. In both series, no residual endoleak or sac enlargement was seen on follow-up.[4] In their series of 105 patients, Brownrigg et al. identified four patients with Type 1A endoleaks all treated with liquid and coil embolization. Following treatment there was complete endoleak resolution confirmed with postprocedure duplex.[5]

A potential pitfall of this technique, as with all coil or liquid embolization, is the migration of the coil or reflux of liquid out of the endoleak site. Ameli-Renani et al. described two such cases in their series where Onyx refluxed from the endoleak during deployment into the limb of the Nellix graft causing stenosis. In both instances the stenosis was successfully treated with placement of a stent.[6] To mitigate this risk, use of partial or complete aortic occlusion via balloon inflation within and/or proximal to the Nellix stents facilitate effective liquid embolic agent delivery with less risk of systemic embolization.

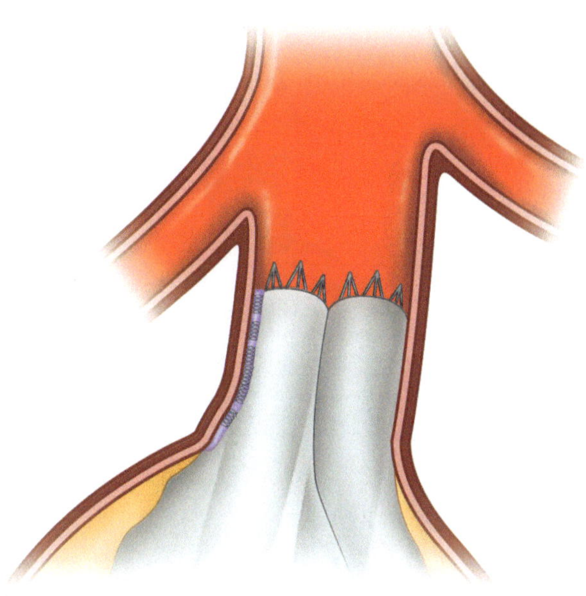

Fig. 10.2 Illustration of Nellix device after deployment of embolic coil matrix with liquid embolics to seal a Type 1A endoleak.

WARNING BOX 10.1

The catheter should be rapidly withdrawn to avoid adhesion to the aneurysm sac or coaxial catheter.

PROXIMAL EXTENSION WITH COVERED STENTS PLUS COIL AND LIQUID EMBOLIZATION

A Type 1A endoleak in the setting of stent misalignment or a low stent placement may require more than coil and liquid embolization. In this instance, proximal extension with covered stents is recommended for small to moderate proximal endoleak when the seal zone can be reconstituted.

Steps for Insertion of Proximal Extenders with Coil and Liquid Embolics

1. Obtain bilateral common femoral and brachial artery access.
2. Use standard techniques to gain access to each stent.
3. Perform angiogram.
4. Advance coaxially a micro catheter into the endoleak cavity from either an antigrade or retrograde approach.
5. Predilate the Nellix stents with noncompliant PTA balloons 12 × 40 mm prior to stenting or deploying embolics.
6. Deploy a 10 mm balloon or self-expanding covered stent below the ostium of the most caudal renal artery (Fig. 10.3).
7. Postdilate overlapping zones with a noncompliant PTA balloon 12 × 40 mm.
8. Perform coil and liquid embolization between newly placed stent and aortic wall. Balloon occlusion of the limbs during embolization may help prevent distal embolization of glue or coil material (Figs. 10.4 and 10.5).

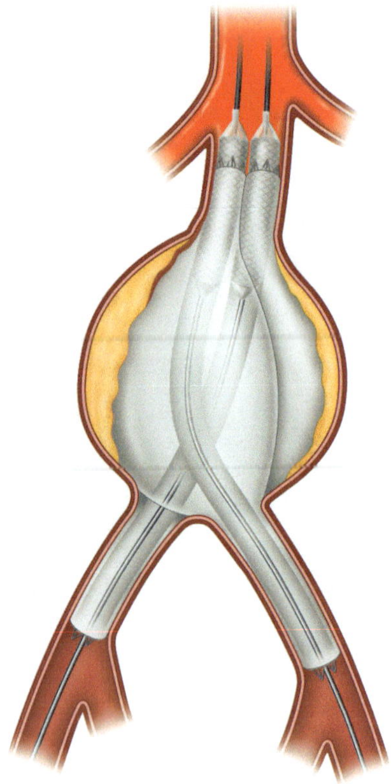

Fig. 10.3 Illustration of Nellix graft with bilateral covered stents deployed with PTA balloons in place (Step 6).

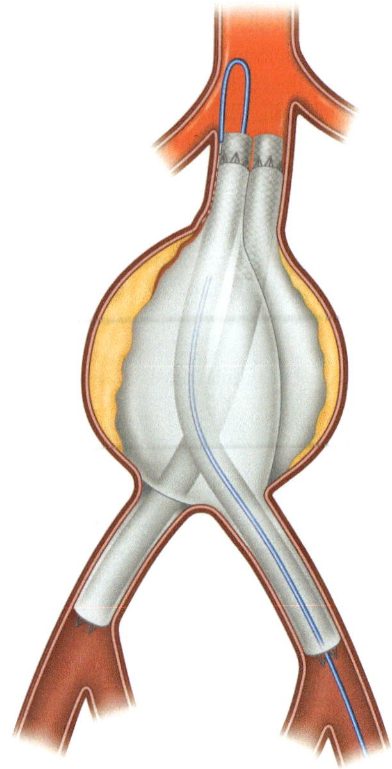

Fig. 10.4 Illustration of Nellix graft with micro catheter placement into endoleak cavity and adjacent to deployed covered stents to deploy coils and liquid embolic agent (Step 8).

> **TIP BOX 10.3**
>
> Ensure at least 30 mm of overlapping between the covered stent and the Nellix stent.

PROXIMAL EXTENSION WITH NELLIX SYSTEM

When the Type 1A endoleak is associated with migration of the Nellix device, the distance between the renal arteries and the Nellix device should be examined. If the distance is ≥30 mm (inclusive of a 15 mm proximal seal zone), proximal extension of the Nellix system with adjunctive Nellix devices is recommended. This "Nellix-in-Nellix" technique will treat both the endoleak and the migration by reestablishing the seal zone. This technique has so far only been described in small case series. A "too long distance" has not yet been defined (Fig. 10.6).

Steps for Proximal Extension with Nellix System

1. Obtain retrograde access of bilateral common femoral arteries.
2. Use standard technique to access the lumen of the Nellix stents.
3. Predilate the Nellix stents with noncompliant PTA balloons 12 × 40 mm throughout the length of the device.
4. Select adjunctive Nellix stent length to ensure maximum relining of index Nellix stent and positioning of first stent element at the most caudal renal artery ostium.

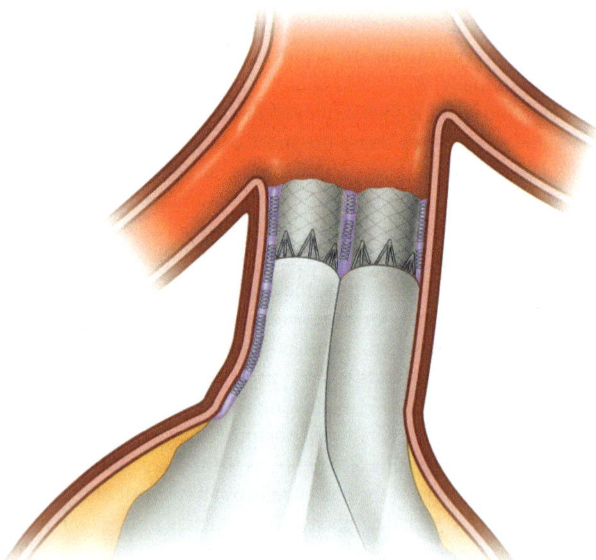

Fig. 10.5 Illustration of the Nellix device after deployment of proximal extenders with coils and liquid embolics to seal a Type 1A endoleak.

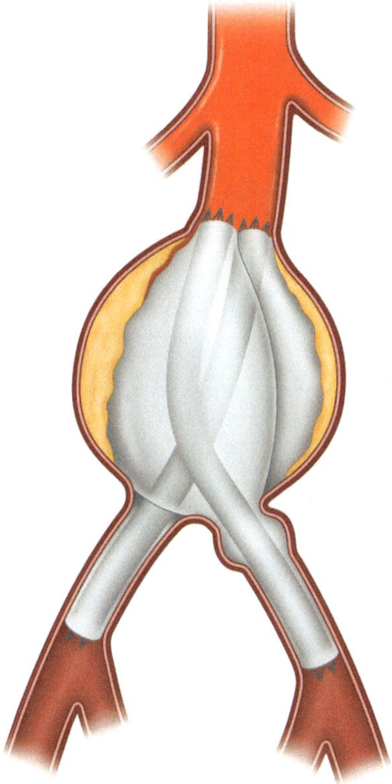

Fig. 10.6 Illustration of a Type 1A endoleak with a Nellix device amenable to proximal extension with an adjunctive Nellix system.

5. Introduce the adjunctive Nellix catheters, connect the console and unsheathe.
6. Unfurl the new EndoBags using saline through the EndoBag port prior to stent inflation, then remove unfurling prefill solution.
7. Inflate Nellix balloons up to 7 atm until both adjunctive Nellix stents are completely expanded, then deflate balloons.
8. Perform saline prefill, then aspirate.
9. Fill the EndoBags with polymer to a target pressure of 180 mmHg ± 10 mmHg (Fig. 10.7).
10. Once polymer fill has been completed, postdilate the Nellix balloons up to 7 atm until the polymer is cured.
11. Once the polymer is cured, deflate the Nellix balloons.
12. Perform a completion angiogram in multiple views to confirm complete seal.
13. If required, perform a secondary polymer fill.

WARNING BOX 10.2

Perform prefill and polymer fill slowly and carefully to avoid excessive pressure spikes and EndoBag rupture or prolapse.

NELLIX REVISIONAL CHIMNEY EVAS (ChEVAS): PROXIMAL EXTENSION WITH NELLIX SYSTEM AND PARALLEL GRAFTS

In patients with a Type 1A endoleak and significant device migration, adequate seal zone (minimum 15 mm) and extension length

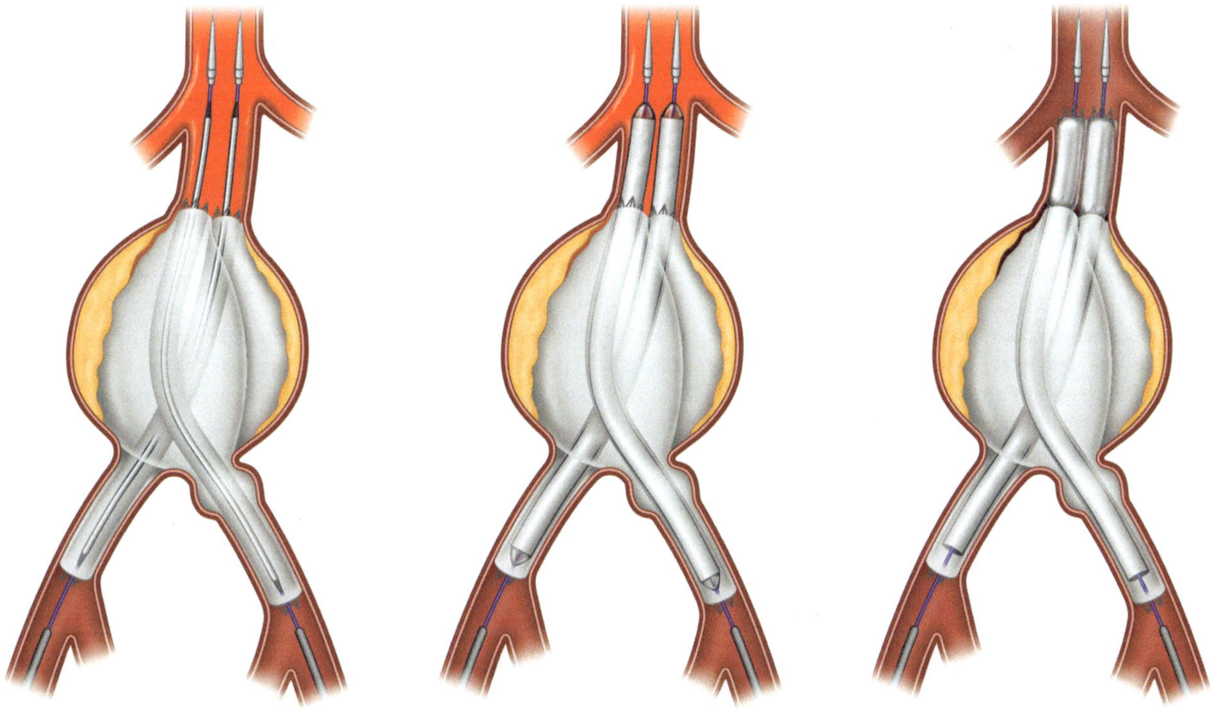

Fig. 10.7 Introduce the Nellix catheters (Step 5), inflate the Nellix balloons (Step 7), fill the EndoBags, (Step 9), effectively seal the Type 1A endoleak.

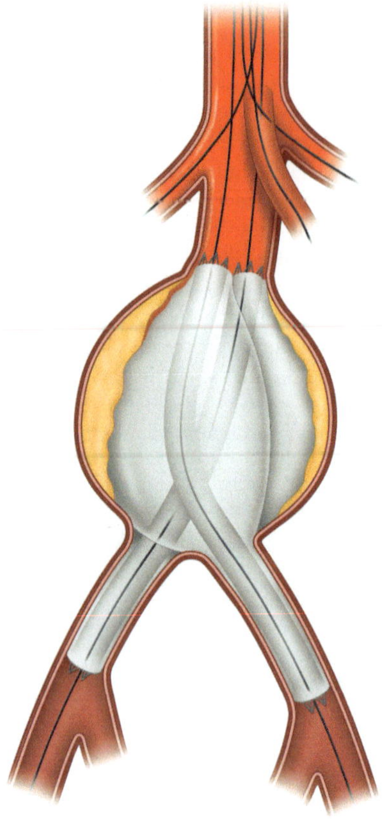

Fig. 10.8 Obtain wire access to visceral arteries (Steps 2a and 2b).

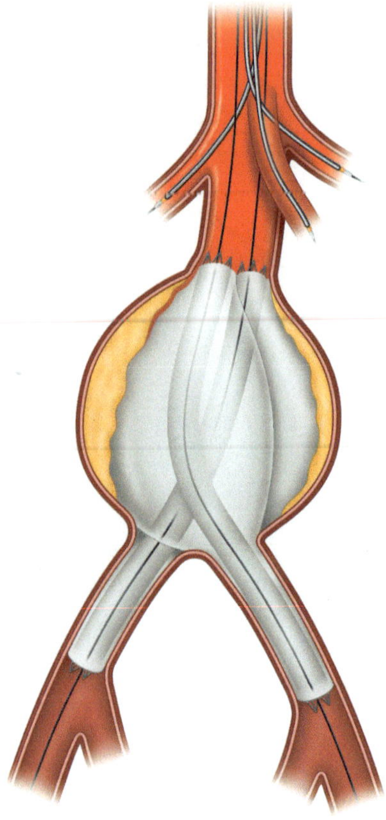

Fig. 10.9 Track covered stents through sheath and position within visceral arteries (Step 2g).

(minimum 30 mm of the proximal Nellix extenders needs to be exposed outside the primary Nellix implant) may not be available to allow for proximal extension with a second Nellix system alone. In such cases, a Nellix revisional ChEVAS can be performed by extending the Nellix system proximally and placing parallel grafts into the visceral and renal segments.

Steps for Nellix Revisional ChEVAS

1. Obtain bilateral femoral artery access and arm access (brachial or axillary).
2. Establish guide wire access to visceral arteries.
    a. Advance one upper extremity access sheath to a position proximal to the target artery.
    b. Use a pre-curved 5-French angiographic catheter and a soft guide wire to cannulate the target artery (Fig. 10.8).
    c. Exchange the soft guide wire for a support wire (e.g., Rosen).
    d. Perform diagnostic angiography to confirm placement.
    e. Advance the upper extremity access sheath into the target renal artery and then remove the dilator.
    f. Predilate the vessel using standard balloon angioplasty techniques, if required.
    g. Track the selected covered stent grafts through the sheath. Both balloon and self-expanding stents have been described (Fig. 10.9).
    h. Repeat steps b–g if other vessels have to be treated.
3. Position the Nellix stents (Fig. 10.10).
4. Predilate implanted Nellix stents with noncompliant PTA balloons 12 × 40 mm.
5. Deploy the Nellix stents, inflating the Nellix balloons to 7 atm.
6. Deploy the visceral stents (Fig. 10.11).
7. If using self-expanding visceral stents, introduce PTA balloons to maintain lumen patency during polymer filling.
8. Perform prefill as described while keeping the visceral balloons open to maintain luminal patency.
9. After polymer fill, reinflate the Nellix balloons up to 7 atm until polymer is completely cured (Fig. 10.12).
10. Postdilate the Nellix stents to ensure stent lumens are optimized.
11. Perform a completion angiogram to confirm successful treatment of the endoleak.

Donselaar et al. presented their case series of five patients with Type 1A endoleaks that were all secondary to caudal stent-graft migration. Four of the five index procedures were performed outside of the IFU. All patients required parallel grafts to the visceral segments to reestablish a proximal seal zone. This included 3-vessel ChEVAS to the superior mesenteric artery and bilateral renal arteries in two patients, bilateral renal chimneys were used in two patients, and a single renal artery in one patient. On follow-up examination, four of the five patients had no further caudal migration of the Nellix endograft.[7]

TYPE 1B ENDOLEAK

When a Type 1B endoleak is identified, the recommended treatment is distal extension with a covered stent. This technique has the benefit of being minimally invasive and does not preclude future interventions. This technique is limited in patients with insufficient distal seal zone,

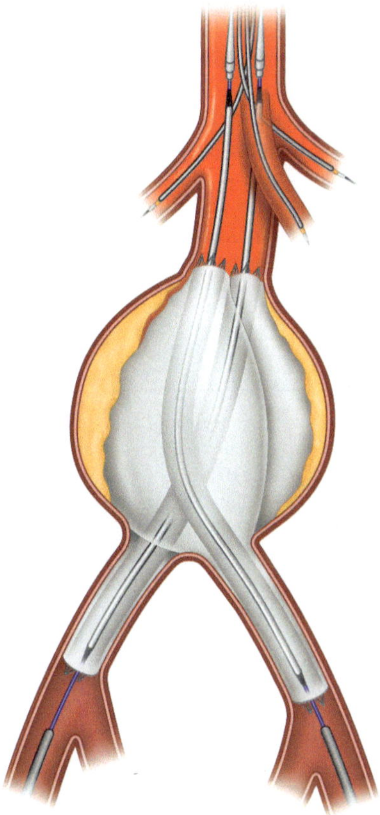

Fig. 10.10 Position the Nellix stents (Step 3).

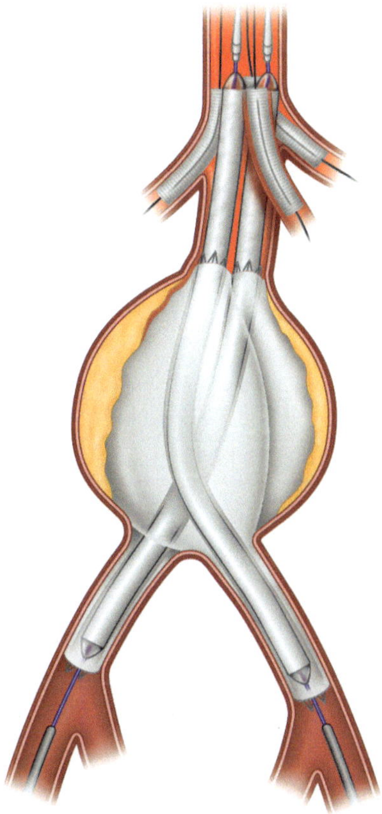

Fig. 10.11 Deploy the visceral stents (Step 6).

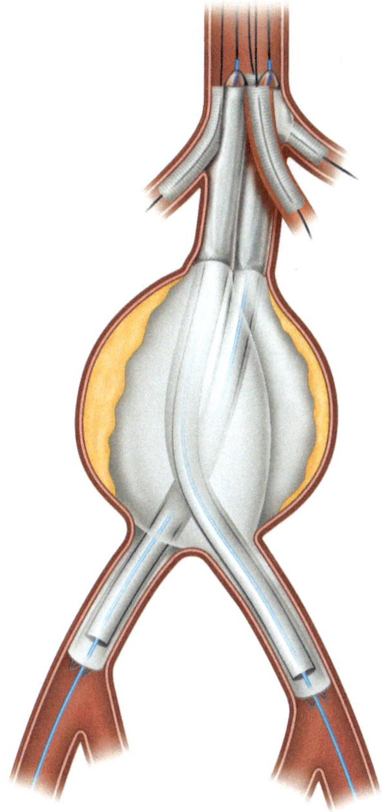

Fig. 10.12 Fill Nellix EndoBags with polymer while keeping a balloon inflated in visceral stents (Steps 7–9).

whereby hypogastric artery preservation is indicated. The occurrence of 1B endoleak is extremely low; 0.8% at one year has been reported.[1]

Steps for Treatment of Type 1B Endoleaks

1. Obtain retrograde access of the common femoral artery.
2. Use standard endovascular technique to gain access to the Nellix stent.
3. Perform retrograde angiography to mark the internal iliac artery.
4. Predilate the Nellix stent with a noncompliant PTA balloon, 12 × 40 mm.
5. Select and deploy the distal covered stent extension (Fig. 10.13).
6. Postdilate the overlapping zone with noncompliant PTA balloons, 12 × 40 mm and not exceeding iliac artery diameter.
7. Perform a completion angiogram to verify aneurysm exclusion.

TIP BOX 10.4

Ensure ≥30 mm of covered stent overlap with the Nellix stent.

ANEURYSM EXPANSION

During a root cause analysis looking at the EVAS FORWARD IDE Trial, absence of healthy distal seal zone was associated with aneurysm sac expansion. The proposed mechanism is transmission of pressure through thrombus around the EndoBag retrograde into the aneurysm

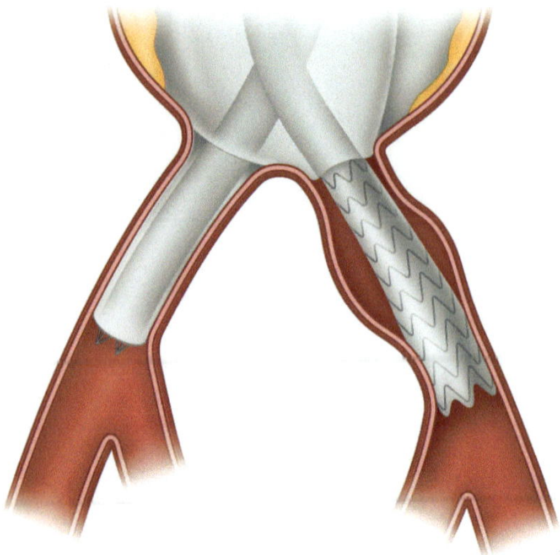

Fig. 10.13 Distal extension of the Nellix device.

sac. This discovery led to the addition of IFU criteria designed to address this issue. A distal seal zone of >10 mm in the iliac artery (9–20 mm diameter) is required. This IFU refinement reinforces exclusion of the distal thrombus, which eliminates the mode of pressure transmission and thus aneurysm expansion.

LIMB OCCLUSION

The complication of limb occlusion can be treated similarly to limb occlusion after traditional EVAR. Thrombolysis, thrombectomy, PTA ballooning, and either balloon or self-expanding covered stenting can be used. Few case series with limb occlusions have been published. The largest was by Böckler et al. in a multicenter analysis reporting 8 limb occlusions (5%) across 171 patients treated in a real-world, all-comer series. Writing early in the evolution of the EVAS procedure, the authors attributed limb occlusion to a combination of early learning curve and under-deployment of the Nellix stents. To decrease the rate of this complication, the authors recommend a retrograde "blow-back" completion angiogram to detect any incomplete seal.[8]

The Nellix device has brought new possibilities for the treatment of abdominal aortic aneurysms. With this novel system also comes a unique set of complications and innovative techniques by which to solve them. As further complications are identified, so too will the steps that can be taken to prevent them.

REFERENCES

1. Carpenter J, Lane J, et al. Refinement of anatomic indications for the Nellix System for endovascular aneurysm sealing based on 2-year outcomes from the EVAS FORWARD IDE trial. *J Vasc Surg.* 2018;68(3):720–730.
2. Antoniou G, Bashaeb K. Nellix stent graft migration after endovascular aneurysm sealing. *Vasa.* 2016;45(6):505–507.
3. Tolenaar J, van dem Ham L, et al. Late conversion after sac anchoring endoprothesis for secondary aortic aneurysm infection. *J Endovasc Therapy.* 2015;22(5):813–818.
4. Harvey J, Stefan B. Transcatheter embolization of Type IA endoleak after Nellix endovascular aortic aneurysm sealing with n-butyl cyanoacrylate: technique in three patients. *J Vasc Interv Radiol.* 2016;27(2):194–199.
5. Ameli-Renani S, Morgan R. Transcatheter embolisation of proximal Type 1 endoleaks following endovascular aneurysm sealing (EVAS) using the Nellix device: technique and outcomes. *Cardiovasc Intervent Radiol.* 2015;38(5):1137–1142.
6. Brownrigg J, de Bruin J, et al. Endovascular aneurysm sealing for infrarenal abdominal aortic aneurysms: 30-day outcomes of 105 patients in a single center. *Eur J Vasc Endovasc Surg.* 2015;50(2):157–164.
7. Donselaar E, Holden A. Feasibility and technical aspects of proximal Nellix-in-Nellix extension for late caudal endograft migration. *J Endovasc Therapy.* 2017;24(2):210–217.
8. Böckler D, Holden A, et al. Multicenter Nellix EndoVascular Aneurysm Sealing system experience in aneurysm sac sealing. *J Vasc Surg.* 2015; 62(2):290–298.

11

Vascutek (Bolton) TREO Endograft

Michael C. Stoner, MD, FACS, DFSVS and Matthew J. TerBush, MD

INTRODUCTION

Bolton Medical was founded in 1998 and is based in Sunrise, Florida, and Barcelona, Spain. The company was acquired in 2017 by Terumo (Tokyo, Japan), with Bolton Medical's products merged into Terumo's Vascutek line of vascular grafts. Bolton Medical manufactures Treovance and TREO, its EVAR endografts, with TREO being its newest. The company also manufactures an aorto-uni-iliac endograft and a customized endograft.

These endografts have been used for some time around the world, including Europe, China, South America, and Japan. In May 2020, the TREO endograft was approved by the FDA for use in the United States. This chapter will focus only on the TREO endograft.

DEVICE INFORMATION

TREO is currently indicated for treatment of infrarenal abdominal aortic aneurysms (AAAs). It is a three-piece modular device comprising nitinol stents sutured to a woven polyester fabric. The endograft should not be implanted in those with a nickel or polyester allergy. Permeability is low at 120 mL/min/cm^2, theoretically mitigating plasma diffusion and development of Type V endoleak (aneurysm endotension). Sizes available are shown in Table 11.1. The diameter of each leg of the main bifurcated stent-graft is always the same size (14 mm), regardless of proximal diameter or length. Leg extensions are always 15 mm in diameter proximally. Aortic cuffs can also be used to treat focal lesions in the aorta. If doing so, there must be proximal and distal aorta that fits the instructions for use (IFU) criteria for the proximal main body. Straight extension legs are also available, although sizes are more limited. Table 11.2 shows the IFU.

TREO has several unique features. There is dual proximal fixation with an open suprarenal fixation stent that extends 17 mm above the main body and infrarenal fixation barbs where the fabric begins proximally. This offers the theoretical advantage of mitigating Type I endoleaks and distal migration. Also unique to TREO are five rounded barbs within the main body legs to lock leg extensions in place (referred to as lock stent), theoretically mitigating the risk of Type III endoleaks and leg migration. Preliminary bench testing has demonstrated that it requires potentially 5 × the force to dislodge legs with lock stent versus a comparable system with no system to lock the legs in place. Testing with physiologic fatigue stresses remains unavailable. Longer term testing that examines impact of renal function with suprarenal fixation is also unavailable. The endograft is also unique in that it allows for variability in leg extension placement. Variability of 1 cm on the contralateral side and 3 cm on the ipsilateral side is possible.

The deployment mechanism is of the "pin and pull" variety, allowing the operator to unsheathe the endograft via a turn knob mechanism. The suprarenal fixation stent is constrained in a clasping mechanism, which simultaneously folds the polyester fabric to constrain the infrarenal barbs. The main body is unsheathed before this clasp is disengaged, allowing the operator to make cranial and caudal adjustments before final deployment, allowing for a more controlled deployment.

TREO is "MRI conditional", allowing patients to undergo MRI if the MRI is in normal or first level controlled operating modes with a 1.5 or 3 T magnetic field, a 720 G/cm or less magnetic field spatial gradient, and a maximum whole-body averaged specific absorption rate of 4 W/kg for 15 minutes of scanning. These recommendations are based on non-clinical trials.

Outcome data remain limited to short-term results. Most studies available are out of Europe and investigate the Treovance endograft. Few published studies are available for TREO. The ADVANCE trial was the first major study, which prospectively recruited 30 patients across five European centers. All deployments were successful, although one required an aortic cuff. No intraoperative Type I and Type III endoleaks were reported. There were no access site and endograft complications. No severe device complications occurred within 30 days.[1]

The ADVANCE trial was designed more to validate 30-day safety. Other investigators evaluated 1-year outcomes in smaller series. In a single center study of eight patients, one patient required an aortic cuff for Type Ia endoleak, which did not recur at 1 month. One patient required bilateral common femoral reconstructions after the device was removed because of access complications. Five patients had 6-month follow-up and two had 1-year follow-up, with no device or aneurysmal sac complications.[2] In another cohort of eight patients, all had technical successes with no 30-day device-related complications. At 3 months, one required surgical intervention for leg extension occlusion. At 1 year, six followed up and none had other device-related complications or Type I or III endoleaks.[3]

One of the larger studies recruited 46 poor open surgical candidates in two European centers. Intraoperatively, eight adjunctive procedures were performed in seven patients (four for Type 1a endoleaks, two for Type 1b endoleak, and two for leg-extension kinking). At 30 days, one required a leg extension for a Type Ib endoleak. Seven Type II endoleaks and an asymptomatic common iliac artery stenosis were found, which did not require intervention. At 1 year, no deaths or aneurysmal sac ruptures occurred. Eight were defined to have "hostile" necks, defined to be either a <15 mm neck, (n = 2) or >60 degrees angulation (n = 5). One patient had both. The number of adjunctive procedures, Type I and II endoleaks, graft stenoses, organ injuries, and reinterventions were not significantly different.[4]

Another five patient cohort was evaluated with implantation off of proximal neck IFU (which is not recommended by the authors and Bolton Medical). All five procedures were technical successes without need for adjuncts. At 12 and 18 months, no Type I or III endoleak, stent graft complication, or aneurysmal sac complication was noted.[5]

TABLE 11.1 Sizes available for TREO endograft.

Proximal main body diameter	20, 22, 24, 26, 28, 30, 33, and 36 mm
Lengths of main body (proximal end; ipsilateral end)	100, 120, and 140 mm
Leg extension diameter	All are 15 mm proximally Distally: 9, 11, 13, 15, 17, 20, and 24 mm
Leg extension lengths	80, 100, 120, 140, and 160 mm
Aortic cuff diameters	Same as main body
Aortic cuff lengths	40, 55, and 70 mm
Straight leg extension diameters	9, 11, and 13 mm
Straight leg extension lengths	80 mm only

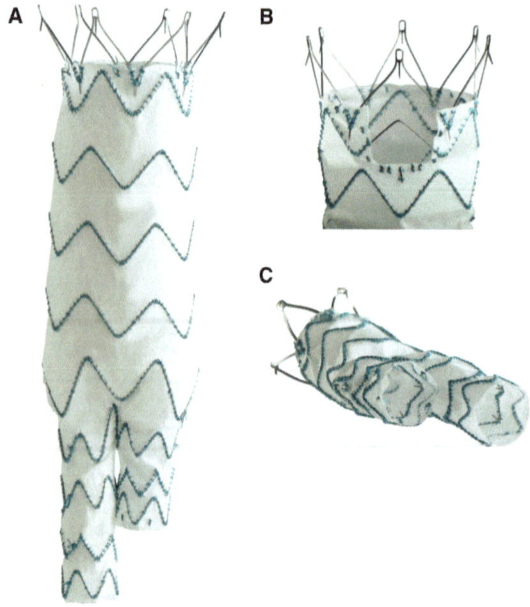

Fig. 11.1 (A) TREO endograft. (B) Dual proximal fixation of the TREO endograft. (C) Internal fixation barbs featured inside limbs of the main body. Courtesy Terumo Aortic, Sunrise, FL, USA.

TABLE 11.2 TREO Instructions for Use.

Pathology	Infrarenal abdominal aortic aneurysms
Aortic neck diameters	Infrarenal neck angle 0–60 degrees: 17–32 mm Infrarenal neck angle 61–75 degrees: 17–30 mm
Suprarenal neck factors	Suprarenal neck angulation less than 45 degrees
Proximal landing zone	Infrarenal neck angle 0–60 degrees: 10 mm Infrarenal neck angle 61–75 degrees: 15 mm
Distal landing zone	Iliac vessel diameter less than 13 mm: 10 mm Iliac vessel diameter greater than 13 mm: 15 mm
Other	Ability for iliofemoral system to accept 18–19 French sheaths

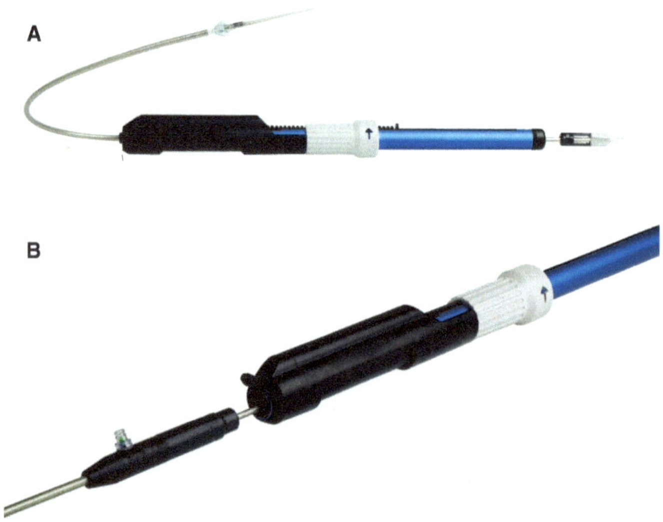

Fig. 11.2 (A) TREO endograft deployment mechanism for main body. (B) Deployment mechanism for limb extension. Courtesy Terumo Aortic, Sunrise, FL, USA.

PREOPERATIVE CONSIDERATIONS

All patients who are candidates for TREO implantation should have an arterial phase computer tomographic angiogram of the abdomen and pelvis, recommended to be done with at most 2 mm slices for more accurate measurements. When sizing for TREO, vessel diameter is measured from outer wall to outer wall. Whether this is done from manual measurements from axial images or through centerline 3D reconstructions is up to the discretion of the operator. Iliac and femoral arteries must be of an appropriate size to accept an 18 or 19 French main body system and a 13 or 14 French leg extension system. The main body side may be predicated on iliofemoral vessel size, tortuosity, and calcification. Leg extension length is an additional consideration. If leg extension length determination is more difficult on one side, consider placing the main body on that side; greater length variability will be available. Calcification of the intended proximal and distal landing zones will also be a consideration.

Be cognizant if internal iliac artery coverage is anticipated. Consider embolization to prevent Type II endoleaks if needed. Iliac branch devices are not available yet. Accessory renal arteries can usually be covered without complication. Consider an alternative procedure if proximal fixation will not be adequate or the renal arteries will need to be covered. If preoperative imaging shows a prominent meandering mesenteric artery, consider an alternate surgical strategy to avoid intestinal ischemia.

Special attention should be given to the IFU, as they do notably differ with angulation of the aortic neck and iliac artery diameter (Table 11.2).

INTRAOPERATIVE CONSIDERATIONS

The deployment steps for the TREO endograft are demonstrated in Fig. 11.3. In order to ensure adequate and safe deployment, all steps

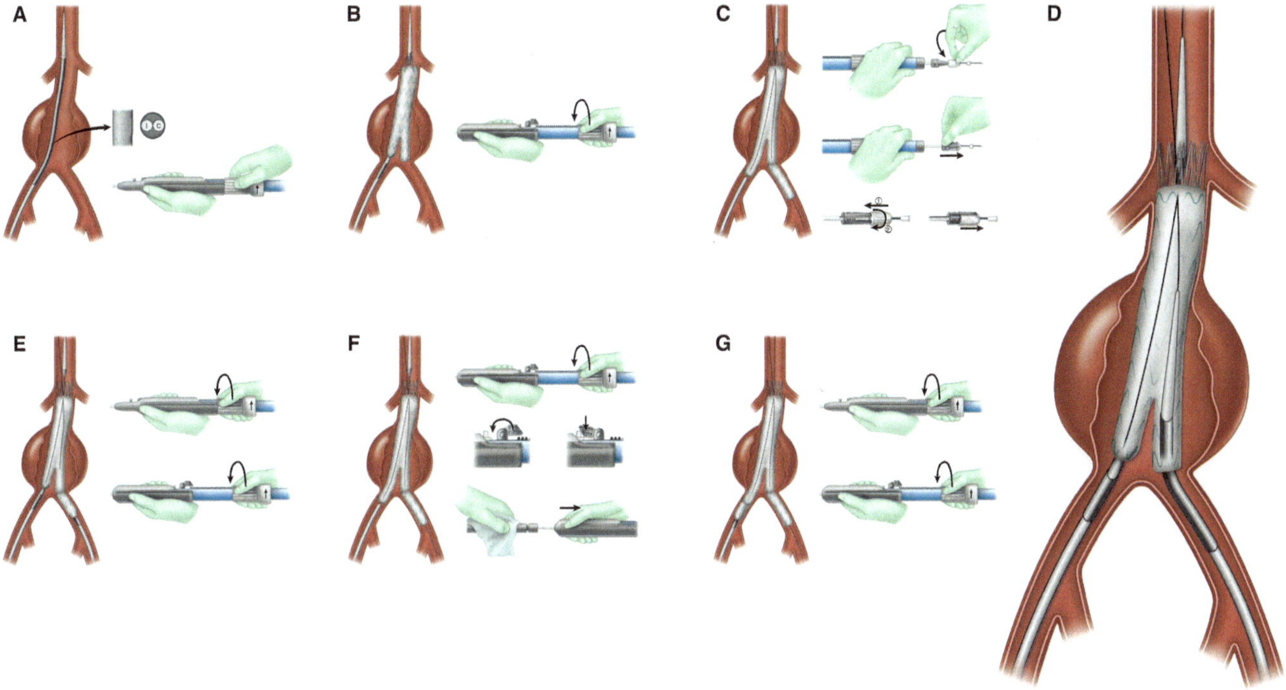

Fig. 11.3 (A–G) Steps demonstrating deployment of TREO endograft. See text for details.

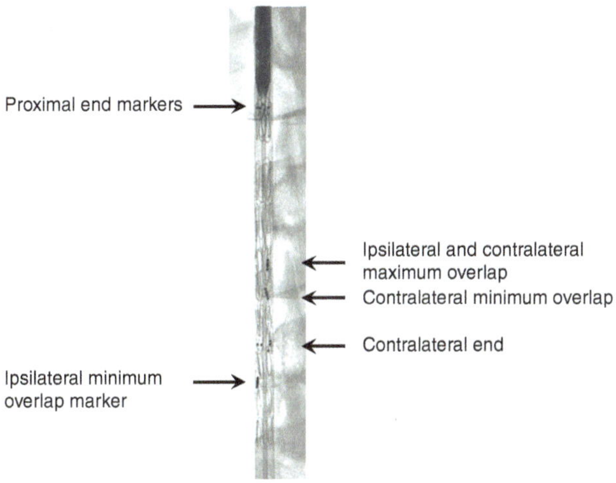

Fig. 11.4 Positional markers present under fluoroscopy. Courtesy Terumo Aortic, Sunrise, FL, USA.

should be followed closely and measures should be taken not to deviate from protocol. Potential complications during the procedure are best overcome by prevention and careful preoperative planning. Steps will be predicated on deploying the main body first, the contralateral leg second, and the ipsilateral leg last.

Bilateral common femoral vascular access can be obtained percutaneously with ultrasound or with direct surgical femoral exposure. A 0.035″, 260–300 cm long stiff wire (for example, Lunderquist (Cook Medical, Bloomington, Indiana), Amplatz Super Stiff (Boston Scientific, Boston, Massachusetts), or Glidewire Advantage (Terumo, Tokyo, Japan), is advanced into the descending thoracic aorta. After performing an initial aortogram, the main body 18 or 19 French deployment sheath should be advanced over wire so the proximal radiopaque markers are just below the renal arteries after wetting the hydrophilic surface (Fig. 11.3A). The sheath flush port should face medially to approximate the endograft's correct orientation. Under fluoroscopy, orientation can be confirmed by locating the contralateral minimal and maximal overlap markers, which are in line 1 cm apart, and the ipsilateral minimum overlap marker further distally. If these markers are in line, rotate the endograft until the markers are in the correct position, which can be done by rotating the black stationary grip. If this is difficult, move the sheath to a straighter portion of the aorta, rotate the sheath, and then place it back to the intended location. After initiating main body deployment, it can no longer be rotated safely without potentially damaging the graft and the aorta, so make any rotational adjustments now.

TIP BOX 11.1

When advancing the main body sheath, keep the flush port medial to approximate the correct orientation of the endograft.

TIP BOX 11.2

The ipsilateral side offers more length variability. Place the main body up the side where limb length is more uncertain, if able.

The main body is deployed by holding the black stationary grip firmly and turning the gray turn knob clockwise (in the direction of the arrow) (Fig. 11.3B). Continue until the first covered stent is exposed. Because the suprarenal and infrarenal barbs are still constrained by the clasping system, the device can be adjusted cranially and caudally. Once satisfied with proximal positioning, continue deployment until the contralateral leg is uncovered. The proximal fixation barbs are still constrained. This is the final opportunity to adjust the graft cranially or caudally.

Once longitudinal position is ensured, push the gray component that resides toward the distal end of the device forward, then turn it 90 degrees. The proximal endograft is still constrained. To release the clasp, retract the black piece until it attaches to the gray component with two clicks (Fig. 11.3C). At this point, never advance this clasp mechanism forward. It could reopen and when the system is withdrawn at the end of the case, it could catch on a bare stent barb, causing unintentional graft movement or damage to the aorta.

TIP BOX 11.3

Cranial and caudal position of the main body can be changed up until the proximal fixation barbs are no longer constrained.

Despite the more controlled deployment offered by this clasping system, improper placement can still occur. If the endograft is too distal, complete full deployment and consider placing an aortic cuff. If deployed too proximally with renal artery coverage, adjunctive procedures must be done expeditiously to minimize warm ischemia time to the kidneys. Access could be obtained up and over the main body bifurcation with a 6 French or 7 French sheath. With a wire snared contralaterally, the system can be pulled downward. With the endograft's dual fixation, this can injure the aorta and have an unpredictable outcome. Mechanical pullout force testing in bovine aorta has previously been performed using the Treovance endograft. The failure mode tends to be at the infrarenal barbs and is associated with intimal injury.[6] While at these tensile stresses the nitinol graft struts will most likely elastically deform, it is unclear whether plastic deformation could occur and hamper the effectiveness of the endograft's fixation. Use this adjunct with caution. Brachial access can be obtained (preferably left), using it to place a guide wire around the endograft to engage the renal arteries to attempt a balloon expandable renal stent placement (more details about snorkel EVARs can be found in Chapter 16). If these are unsuccessful, an open surgical repair may be required, exposing the patient to a significantly increased risk of morbidity and mortality. The best method to avoid this complication is prevention. It further emphasizes careful endograft deployment, patient selection per IFU, and preoperative planning.

CAUTION BOX 11.1

Do not rotate the endograft once the main body has begun to deploy!

CAUTION BOX 11.2

After the clasp mechanism is released, the endograft can no longer be adjusted cranially or caudally. Make final adjustments before releasing the clasp!

CAUTION BOX 11.3

Do not move the clasping mechanism and its associated metal rod forward after it is released!

Once the proximal fixation is deployed, obtain wire access into the contralateral leg via the contralateral groin. Utilization of an MP1 or vertebral catheter can be helpful. If this is difficult, adjusting the angle of the C-arm for a better view may be needed. From the ipsilateral groin, up-and-over access on the main body bifurcation can be obtained to snare the contralateral wire into the contralateral leg. Snaring can also be achieved via left brachial artery access. If the contralateral gate still cannot be cannulated, consider conversion to an aorto-uni-iliac configuration (a contralateral plug is manufactured) with a concomitant femoral–femoral bypass as a last resort.

Exchange the contralateral wire for a stiff wire, ensuring the wire does not get caught on the bare struts on advancement. If this does happen, back the wire out carefully and advance again, spinning the wire or using a torque device to prevent it from happening again. Before placing the contralateral leg extension on the wire, ensure the system is flushed and the delivery system is properly seated in the outer sheath. If it is not, use another leg.

Advance the contralateral leg extension under fluoroscopy and align the proximal leg extension markers between the contralateral minimum and maximum overlap markers. Ensure the distal marker is also in the proper location on the iliac artery (Fig. 11.3D). Be aware that the leg extension can drift distally up to 5 mm and therefore plan on deploying the limb slightly above the target. After confirming proper placement, turn the gray knob clockwise (in the direction of the arrow). Do not advance the leg cranially after the first covered stent is deployed; the leg can still be manipulated caudally during deployment. Once fully deployed, if the leg is below the minimum overlap marker proximally, consider placing another leg extension. If it is accidently deployed above the maximal overlap marker, take note of this and attempt to deploy the ipsilateral leg extension at the same level proximally. Once fully deployed, ensure that the sheath tip is distal to the distal leg extension before system removal (Fig. 11.3E).

The entirety of the contralateral leg delivery system can now be removed or the sheath can remain in place to serve as a catheter, depending on operator preference. To remove the system entirely, rotate the gray turn knob counterclockwise (in the opposite direction to the arrow) until it makes contact with the lead screw. Holding the black stationary grip firmly, bring the gray turn knob to the black stationary grip. The entire system can now be removed over the wire. To keep the sheath, start by holding the black stationary grip firmly and pull the gray turn knob toward the back end of the system as far as the lead screw can travel. Proximally next to a white check valve, a sheath release lever is exposed. Hold the blue portion of the system firmly instead; the black stationary grip will now serve a different function. Flip the sheath release lever over until a clicking sound is made (Fig. 11.3F). Remove the deployment device over the wire by pulling back on the black stationary handle. If separation is difficult, first check whether the proximal clasping mechanism is completely retracted. If it is, try pulling with more force. If unsuccessful, the whole system should be removed and an alternate catheter should be used instead.

TIP BOX 11.4

Deploy the extension limbs slightly more proximal than intended, as they can drift distally up to 5 mm.

TIP BOX 11.5

If the extension limbs are deployed too proximally, place kissing stents to prevent the extension limbs from being compressed.

To deploy the rest of the ipsilateral main body leg, hold the black stationary grip firmly and pull the gray turn knob towards the back end of the system as far as the lead screw can travel. Detachment is identical to what was done contralaterally (Fig. 11.3F). If the delivery system will not separate easily, remove the entire system and replace it with a 16 French introducer or the ipsilateral leg extension deployment system. Once separated, a sheath hub assembly is left behind. Once the tip of the delivery system passes the hemostasis valve, the valve can be closed by rotating the distal end of this assembly clockwise, if needed.

Prepare the ipsilateral leg extension and advance the delivery system into the sheath, ensuring that the hemostasis valve is open on the sheath (if closed, open it by rotating it counterclockwise). Position the proximal leg markers between the minimum ipsilateral overlap marker and the minimum contralateral overlap marker and ensure the distal leg extension markers are appropriately placed at the distal target. Deployment of the ipsilateral leg extension is identical to that of the contralateral leg (Fig. 11.3G). If the ipsilateral leg extension is deployed too low proximally, deploy another leg extension. If deployed too high, consider placing "kissing" stents to prevent radial force from affecting contralateral flow.

After the endograft is fully deployed, use a balloon to mold the seal zones. IFUs recommend going no higher than 1 atm in pressure. Be sure not to balloon the native vessel to avoid vessel perforation. The proximal leg extension seal zones are safe to balloon mold even with the rounded barbs. However, if the balloon does rupture, this usually has no ill effects. Carefully remove the balloon and replace with another. Perform an angiogram to rule out damage to the endograft and address as needed. If the balloon becomes ensnared on the barbs, a support sheath can be used to retrieve the balloon. Perform a completion angiogram. Balloon mold any locations where there may be a Type Ia, Ib, or III endoleak first. If ineffective, consider placing a proximal cuff (if Type Ia) or a new leg extension (if Type 1b or Type III). Type II endoleaks can be tolerated. If an aortic cuff is needed, the mechanism of deployment is the same as the main body, described previously. If the result is deemed satisfactory, remove all sheaths and close all arteriotomy sites as appropriate.

CONCLUSIONS

Bolton Medical's TREO EVAR endograft is another alternative for the repair of infrarenal abdominal aortic aneurysms. The device includes dual proximal fixation and internal extension leg barbs that can theoretically mitigate endoleaks and migration. The clasp deployment mechanism allows for more controlled deployment. Based on preliminary data, TREO can successfully treat a variety of aortic anatomies, potentially including more "hostile" anatomies. Short-term data are promising, but longer-term outcomes have yet to be studied. It is important to note that the device has yet to be approved for use in the United States and remains an investigational device. It is available in the United States since April 2020.

REFERENCES

1. Chiesa R, Riambau V, Coppi G, et al. The Bolton Treovance abdominal stent-graft: European clinical trial design. *J Cardiovasc Surg (Torino).* 2012; 53(5):595–604.
2. Georgakarakos E, Georgiadis GS, Argyriou C, Schoretsanitis N, Antoniou GA, Lazarides MK. Preliminary Single-Center Experience with the Bolton Treovance Endograft in the Treatment of Abdominal Aortic Aneurysms. *Ann Vasc Surg.* 2016;34(Supplement C):68–74.
3. Kahlberg A, Mascia D, Marone EM, Logaldo D, Tshomba Y, Chiesa R. The Bolton Treovance endograft: single center experience. *J Cardiovasc Surg (Torino).* 2014;55(1):77–84.
4. Thind A, Sarma D, Allouni AK, Abdallah F, et al. Preliminary Dual-Center Experience with the Bolton Treovance Endograft. *Vasc Endovascular Surg.* 2017;51(8):533–537.
5. Rossi U, Settembrini A, Dallatana R, et al. IP039. Abdominal Aorta Aneurysm With Hostile Neck: Early Outcomes in Outside Instructions for Use in Patients Using the Treovance Stent Graft. *J Vasc Surg.* 2016; 63(6, Supplement):68S–69S.
6. Rahmani S, Grewal IS, Nabovati A, Doyle MG, Roche-Nagle G, Tse LW. Increasing angulation decreases measured aortic stent graft pullout forces. *J Vasc Surg.* 2016;63(2):493–499.

12

Grafts Outside the United States

Giuseppe Asciutto, MD, PhD and Timothy Resch, MD, PhD

INTRODUCTION

The market of aortic endografts is in continuous development. Several endografts that have gained the CE mark are under investigation by the FDA before launching in the U.S. market. This chapter describes their peculiarities and the evidence acquired with the use of these endografts. Since the majority of the devices described in this chapter have been recently introduced, the evidence on the feasibility of their use in the treatment of aortic aneurysm is limited. The available data report of short-term results in terms of patency, freedom from Types I and III endoleak (EL), and freedom from aneurysm sac enlargement is comparable to those of devices that have been longer in use (Table 12.1).

DESCRIPTIONS OF THE DEVICES

Altura

Lombard Medical (Irvine, California) launched the Altura endograft system in 2016. The Altura endograft is designed to treat infrarenal abdominal aortic aneurysms (AAAs) with an aortic neck of 18–28 mm and distal iliac of 8–18 mm (only straight iliac legs available). The endograft consists of two parallel aortic grafts that can be placed at different heights. The ability to position and offset the aortic endografts independently with their bilateral D-stent design is thought to maximize sealing in infrarenal neck. The two aortic grafts are then extended into the iliac vessels.

Because of its 14-French low-profile design, the Altura endograft has the advantage of a minimally invasive approach. The use of two parallel aortic endografts eliminates contralateral limb cannulation, theoretically shortening procedures. The removal of the delivery system does not require any redocking. Furthermore, a built-in injection port simplifies the procedure, allowing precise endograft placement.

The presence of six different sealing zones (aortic neck, between the aortic endografts, two overlap zones between the aortic and the iliac endografts, and the two distal iliac landing zones) theoretically increases the risk of the occurrence of Type III EL.

There is in 2018, a published report on the efficacy of the system in treatment of AAA at 10 clinical sites in two prospective, controlled clinical studies.[1] Krievins et al. report 90 patients treated with a technical success rate of 99%. The procedure-related mortality and reintervention rates were 1% and 4%.

During a median follow-up of 12.5 months (range 11.5–50.9), there were no aneurysm ruptures, surgical conversions, or AAA-related deaths. Clinical success was 94% (84/89) at 30 days, 98% (85/87) at 6 months, and 99% (82/83) at 1 year.

BOX 12.1 Altura

- Treatment range: 18–28 mm aortic neck; 8–18 mm distal iliac landing zone
- Neck length: ≥15 mm
- Neck angulation: ≤60 degrees
- Iliac arteries length: ≥15 mm
- 14-French low-profile design

Anaconda

The Anaconda AAA Stent Graft System (Vascutek, Terumo, Inchinnan, Scotland) gained the CE mark in 2014. It is indicated for angulated infrarenal necks up to 90 degrees. A peculiarity of this three-piece system is the fully repositionable deployment, enabling relocation of the proximal ring stents for optimal positioning at the aortic neck. The bifurcated component and the aortic cuffs have a treatment range of 17.5–31 mm (20–23 French). Iliac legs sizes range from 8.5 to 21 mm (all 18 French) for straight, tapered, and flared configurations. The multiple independent leg ring stent design is intended to minimize potential for kinking and allowing treatment of isolated iliac artery aneurysms. Cannulation of the contralateral limb is accelerated by using magnetic forces.

The Anaconda endograft is also available as a fenestrated custom-made device. In comparison with other fenestrated endografts, the presence of two sealing rings and of the unsupported body at the proximal sealing zone allows a more flexible positioning of fenestrations. Furthermore, the Fenestrated Anaconda Custom AAA Stent Graft System is the only fully repositionable fenestrated endograft available on the market. The absence of a top cap allows access to fenestrations proximally and distally.

The widest single-center experience published[2] to date reports 177 patients who underwent implantation of an Anaconda endograft to treat unruptured AAA. Technical success was achieved in 98.9% of the cases. After a mean follow-up time of 33 ± 23.3 months, the late assisted clinical success was 97.7%. The overall survival at 12, 24, and 36 months was 96.4%, 89%, and 86.2%, respectively. Freedom from reintervention was 94%, 92%, and 85% at 12, 24, and 36 months, respectively. Three (1.7%) conversions to open surgery occurred during follow-up. There were 14.1% ELs at the completion angiography (EL Ia, 1.1%; EL II, 13%). Late ELs were 20.2% (EL Ia, 1.1%; EL Ib, 2.2%; EL II, 16.9%). Iliac leg complications occurred in 5.6% of the cases. An AAA shrinkage >5 mm was observed in 130 (73.4%) patients. In 7 (4%) cases there was an AAA enlargement >5 mm.

The widest experience[3] with the fenestrated Anaconda endograft is the result of a prospective study in eight Dutch institutions, where 25 patients were treated for juxtarenal (n = 23) and short-neck infrarenal AAA (n = 2). A total of 56 fenestrations were incorporated, and 53 (94.6%) were successfully cannulated and stented. On completion of

TABLE 12.1 Complication rates in comparison with devices already present on the United States market. Follow-up duration in brackets.

	Freedom from endoleak Type I/III	Endograft patency	Freedom from sac enlargement
Infrarenal devices			
Anaconda (33 ± 23 months)[2]	96.7%	94.4%	96%
Incraft (48 months)[6]	97.4%	97.6%	89.7%
E-vita/E-tegra (10 months)[8]	100%	94.7%	100%
Zenith Flex (60 months)[9] (COOK)	98.9%	99%	91%
Excluder AAA (60 months)[10] (Gore)	95.2%	99.6%	87.9%
Endurant (60 months)[11] (Medtronic)	100%	98.8%	94%
Fenestrated devices			
Anaconda fenestrated (11 months)[3]	100%	Not reported	100%[a]
Zenith fenestrated (60 months)[12] (COOK)	100%	100%	95.5%

[a]At 1 month.

angiography, three Type I ELs and seven Type II ELs were observed. One patient died of bowel ischemia caused by occlusion of the superior mesenteric artery in the immediate postoperative period. At 1 month of follow-up, all ELs had spontaneously resolved, while the primary patency of cannulated and stented target vessels was 96%. After a median follow-up time of 11 months (range 1–29 months) no aneurysm ruptures or aneurysm-related deaths and no reinterventions had occurred.

One of the claimed advantages of the Anaconda graft is the ability to treat AAA with severe angulated necks. The same Dutch research group previously cited conducted a prospective study on 36 patients treated because of infrarenal AAA with an aortic neck of >60 degrees (mean angulation: 82 degrees). In this study cohort, the primary technical success was achieved in 30 of 36 patients (83%).[4] There was no aneurysm-related death. Four-year primary clinical success was 69%. In the first year, eight clinical failures were reported including four leg occlusions that could be solved using standard procedures. After the first year, three patients with additional failures occurred; two of them were leg occlusions. Four patients needed conversion to open AAA exclusion. In six of 36 patients, one or more reinterventions were necessary. Three of them were performed for occlusion of one Anaconda leg and two were for occlusion of the body. The authors concluded that the use of the Anaconda endovascular graft in AAA with a severe angulated infrarenal neck can lead to clinical failures, mostly in the first year post-implantation, but midterm results have been considered acceptable.

BOX 12.2 Anaconda

- Treatment range: 17.5–31 mm aortic neck; 8.5–21 mm distal iliac landing zone
- Neck length: ≥15 mm
- Neck angulation: ≤90 degrees
- Iliac arteries length: ≥20 mm
- Profile: aortic component 20–23 French; iliac legs 18 French
- Available as full repositionable fenestrated custom-made device

INCRAFT

The INCRAFT AAA Stent-Graft System (Cordis Corp., Milpitas, California) is a low-profile endograft that was reengineered from a conventional bifurcated stent graft system. The device received FDA approval in December 2018.

The INCRAFT endograft is a three-component system that became available in Europe in September 2014. It was designed to address EVAR in patients with smaller, more diseased iliac vessels. The bifurcated component and the aortic extensions have a treatment range of 17–31 mm (14–16 French). Iliac legs in straight, tapered, and flared configuration with a treatment range of 7–22 mm (12–13 French) are also available.

The introduction of cap-free and partial proximal repositioning enhances the ability of the device to better match individual aortoiliac anatomy. Moreover, it allows customizing the implant during the procedure with bilateral in situ length adjustment features. In particular, the legs of the trunk are designed to allow intraprocedural length adjustment of up to 28 mm on ipsilateral leg and 19 mm on contralateral leg between the modular components. This helps the distal placement precision and potentially reduces the need for extensions. However, an issue in the use of this endograft is the cannulation of the contralateral gate. When the main body is deployed, there is not much space between the opening of the contralateral gate and the release of the ipsilateral leg. This means that in case of accidental opening of the ipsilateral leg, cannulation of the contralateral gate may be harder and even challenging, especially when iliac–femoral vessels are small and tortuous.

The INCRAFT endograft is under investigation in the joint United States–Japan multicenter, open-label, nonrandomized INSPIRATION trial, which began in July 2012 and completed the enrollment in 2013.

To date, the largest publication on the INCRAFT endograft is the INNOVATION study, a multicenter, open-label, prospective, nonrandomized study of the first in-human use of the INCRAFT system.[5] A total of 60 patients were enrolled and successfully treated. All-cause mortality at 4 years was 17.6% with no AAA-, device-, or procedure-related deaths. The 1-year secondary reintervention rate was 4.6%, primarily from stent thrombosis. In total, 10 patients required 13 post-procedure interventions within 4 years (2 Type I EL, 4 Type II EL, 1 for stent thrombosis, 1 renal stenosis, 1 aneurysm enlargement, 2 limb migration, and 2 prosthesis stenosis or occlusion). There were four cases (10%) of aneurysm enlargement reported at the 4-year follow-up. At 4 years, 38 of 39 patients were free from Types I and III EL.

Early results of a series of consecutive patients treated with the INCRAFT have been reported.[6] Prospectively collected data of 17 patients enrolled in the INNOVATION trial (group IT) and 24 consecutive patients from CE Mark (group CM) approval to April 2015 were retrospectively evaluated and compared. Patients included in group IT had a median follow-up time of 60.4 months (95% CI, 55–63), and patients in group CM had a median follow-up time of 12.5 months (6.6–13.5). Comorbidities were comparable between the groups. Adjunctive interventions for iliac artery disease were performed in eight patients (33%) in group CM, whereas no adjunctive was required in group IT. Major adverse events within 30 days were not significantly different. Survival and reintervention rates were also equivalent after a median follow-up of 13 months. The authors concluded that compared with the patients of the IT group, those treated after CE Mark approval had significantly more challenging access routes reflecting the difficulties of "real-world" conditions.

BOX 12.3 Incraft

- Treatment range: 17–31 mm aortic neck; 7–22 mm distal iliac landing zone
- Neck length: ≥15 mm
- Neck angulation: ≤60 degrees
- Iliac arteries length: ≥10 mm
- Profile: aortic component 14–16 French; iliac legs 12–13 French

E-vita and E-tegra

The E-vita ABDOMINAL XT (JOTEC GmbH, Hechingen, Germany) is an evolution of the original E-vita ABDOMINAL endograft. It consists of polyester with a nitinol skeleton. It has a modular design, consisting of the main body and contralateral leg. Iliac and aortic extensions are available. The delivery systems for main bodies and aortic extensions are 20–22 French, while for contralateral legs and iliac extensions, 16–18 French. The bifurcated components are available at a diameter of 24–34 mm and aortic extensions 26–36 mm. Contralateral leg are available in tapered, straight, and reversed tapered configurations (distal diameter 12–24 mm). Iliac extensions are available only in straight configurations, diameters of 14–26 mm.

The bimodular E-tegra is an evolution of the E-vita system. Its low-profile delivery systems start at 18 French for the main bodies, aortic extensions, and aorto-uni-iliac components and at 16 French for contralateral legs and iliac extensions.

Previous reports have shown encouraging results in patients treated with the initial E-vita abdominal endograft. In a case series of 19 patients treated with the initial E-vita, the technical success rate was 100% and the 30-day mortality was 0%.[7] No conversion to open surgery and no Type I EL were noted. Furthermore, the aneurysm diameter was reduced in 42% of cases and remained unchanged in 58%, while one patient required open surgery at 1 year for thrombotic occlusion of the stent-graft after a mean 10-month follow-up. No stent fractures, migrations, or secondary ELs were noted.

BOX 12.4 E-vita and E-tegra

- Treatment range: 21–33 mm aortic neck; 11–24 mm distal iliac landing zone
- Neck length: ≥15 mm
- Neck angulation: ≤60 degrees
- Iliac arteries length: ≥10 mm
- Profile: aortic component 20–22 French; iliac legs 16–18 French
- Available as iliac branched device and fenestrated custom-made device

E-liac

The E-liac endograft system is indicated in the treatment of both aortoiliac and isolated iliac aneurysms. Its low-profile configuration (18 French) allows the treatment of small iliac vessels. For isolated iliac aneurysms, the range of endograft available is 14–18 mm for the proximal landing zone and 10–14 mm for the distal landing zone. The total length covered varies between 109 and 121 mm. For aortoiliac aneurysms, the endograft is available with a proximal diameter of 14 mm and a distal diameter of 10–14 mm.

The efficacy of the E-liac has been tested in a prospective study which included 82 implants as a stand-alone procedure or in combination with AAA exclusion.[8] Technical success was achieved in 100% of the revascularized internal iliac arteries. Within 30 days, one symptomatic occlusion of a treated common iliac artery was observed. In two other cases, an asymptomatic kinking of the common iliac artery segment of the E-liac was revealed in the predischarge follow-up duplex ultrasound examination and corrected with relining. After a median follow-up time of 12 months (range 6–16 months), survival was 98.5% with all internal iliac arteries remaining patent, whereas two common iliac artery and two external iliac artery limb occlusions occurred. The freedom from occlusion was 92% at 1 year and freedom from Type I EL was 87% at 1 year.

REFERENCES

1. Krievins D, Krämer A, Savlovskis J, et al. Initial clinical experience using the low profile Altura endograft system with double D-shaped proximal stents for endovascular aneurysm repair. *J Endovasc Ther.* 2018;25(3):379–386.
2. Freyrie A, Gallitto E, Gargiulo M, et al. Results of the endovascular abdominal aortic aneurysm repair using the Anaconda aortic endograft. *J Vasc Surg.* 2014;60:1132–1139.
3. Dijkstra ML, Tielliu IF, Meerwaldt R, et al. Dutch experience with the fenestrated Anaconda endograft for short-neck infrarenal and juxtarenal abdominal aortic aneurysm repair. *J Vasc Surg.* 2014;60:301–307.
4. Rodel SG, Zeebregts CJ, Huisman AB, et al. Results of the Anaconda endovascular graft in abdominal aortic aneurysm with a severe angulated infrarenal neck. *J Vasc Surg.* 2014;59:1495–1501. e1491.
5. Pratesi G, Pratesi C, Chiesa R, et al. The INNOVATION Trial: four-year safety and effectiveness of the INCRAFT(R) AAA Stent-Graft System for endovascular repair. *J Cardiovasc Surg (Torino).* 2017;58:650–657.
6. Sugimoto M, Torsello GF, Torsello GB, et al. Postmarket clinical experience with the INCRAFT AAA Stent Graft System for challenging access routes. *Ann Vasc Surg.* 2017;40:120–127.
7. Zipfel B, Buz S, Dusterhoft V, et al. Initial experience with abdominal aneurysm repair using the E-vita abdominal stent-graft: a single-center study. *J Endovasc Ther.* 2009;16:577–589.
8. Mylonas SN, Rumenapf G, Schelzig H, et al. A multicenter 12-month experience with a new iliac side-branched device for revascularization of hypogastric arteries. *J Vasc Surg.* 2016;64:1652–1659. e1651.
9. https://www.cookmedical.com/data/resources/AI-D27262-EN_1467130791235.pdf.
10. Poublon CG, Holewijn S, van Sterkenburg SMM, et al. Long-Term Outcome of the GORE EXCLUDER AAA Endoprosthesis for Treatment of Infrarenal Aortic Aneurysms. *J Vasc Interv Radiol.* 2017;28:637–644. e631.
11. http://www.medtronic.com/content/dam/medtronic-com-m/mdt/endov/images/endurant_clinical_update_dec.pdf.
12. https://www.cookmedical.com/aortic-intervention/2016-zenith-fenestrated-clinical-update/.

13

Ruptured EVAR Complications

Jeffrey C. Hnath, MD, Andre R. Ramdon, MBBS and R. Clement Darling, III, MD

Endovascular repair of ruptured aneurysm continues to evolve since the advent of endovascular repair of abdominal aortic aneurysm (EVAR) in the 1990s. Prior to 1994 ruptured aneurysm mortality was 45%–60%.[1–5] There has been an increasing trend to treat ruptures endovascularly with evidence of improved outcomes[1,2,6,7] and reduced length of hospital stays.

In our experience time is of the essence and time to seal is imperative for best possible outcomes. Randomized trials have suggested no difference in long-term mortality.[6,7] Additionally, more than half of patients presenting with ruptures may not be anatomically amenable to EVAR.[6,7]

The first step is to develop established protocols and pathways to manage acute aortic emergencies. It is important to have a multidisciplinary center equipped with the necessary skills and armamentarium to be able to handle difficult situations and complex care in the preoperative to postoperative periods in order to minimize morbidity and mortality. Hospitals that do not have the device inventory or staffing required for the urgency of a ruptured aneurysm may consider transferring the patient to a specialty center equipped to deal with magnitude using a multidisciplinary and standardized approach.[1]

Time is of the essence. This presents a major obstacle that is sometimes out of the control of the surgeons. Hinchliffe et al. showed that computer tomography does not delay the time to the operating room (OR) compared with open to endovascular repair.[1] On the contrary, the earlier French randomized trial suggested the delayed time to surgery averaged 1.3 hours for open versus 2.9 hours for EVAR.[2] Our own institution has an average time to OR of 10–35 minutes with an average time of 20 minutes.[5] Lloyd et al. showed that more than 88% of patients died 2 hours after diagnosing a ruptured aneurysm.[8] An ideal management protocol for rupture fast tracks the patient to the CT scanner. Arguably, unstable patients can be taken directly to the OR and a treatment decision made after the initial aortogram; however, alternative and less deadly diagnosis should always be entertained. Additionally, an endovascular first approach allows for endovascular aortic control with an occlusion balloon. If the anatomy is not amenable to endovascular repair, the endovascular aortic control proves to be invaluable during the time required for aortic dissection and clamping.

Permissive hypotension or hypotensive hemostasis is important until aortic control is achieved and should be emphasized to limit rerupture and ongoing hemorrhage.

Arrival in the operating room is usually met with much disarray, and it is important to be prepared with a variety of endografts to allow for rapid deployment. Adjuncts, such as sheaths, wires, and catheters, should already be open on the field as well as the concomitant equipment for possible open repair. We advocate using an endograft with which the operator is familiar and comfortable, to decrease the chance of maldeployment and to decrease operative time. The IMPROVE trial showed that local anesthesia for the procedure may offer mortality benefit.[3] Our practice is to prepare and to drape the patient, and even to establish aortic balloon for control, prior to induction of anesthesia.

Rapid percutaneous femoral access is followed by the placement of a stiff wire into the descending thoracic aorta followed by a 12 French introducer sheath, and an occlusion balloon as described by Li et al. is appropriate for unstable ruptures.[6] In unstable patients, there may not be time for placement of closure devices prior to sheath placement, and the femoral arteries can be exposed and primarily repaired at the end of the case. It is not uncommon for iliac access vessel anatomy to be challenging. A stiff wire can be used to straighten tortuous iliac arteries, and there are a few techniques to cross small or heavily diseased iliac access arteries. Balloon angioplasty to create a passage for the device is usually the first option. Unusually small and calcified iliac vessels are the most problematic. The so-called "pave and crack" technique may allow the easier passage of stent graft after the initial lining of the iliac with balloon expandable covered stent. This will allow the endograft to seal within the covered stent. Access vessel injury is usually identified after the endograft is in place and the sheaths are being removed. Injury to the iliac bifurcation usually occurs as the large sheath is retracted through the external and the common iliac. Classically, resistance and then complete lack of resistance is felt as the sheath tears the external iliac off the common iliac artery at the origin of the hypogastric. Concurrently, a drop in blood pressure will be seen when the retroperitoneal hemorrhage occurs. Most importantly, wire access must be maintained at all times so that an occlusion balloon can be placed. A covered stent graft is used to bridge the gap and seal the hemorrhage. Again, the key is to maintain wire access so that an occlusion balloon can be placed and a stent graft can be used to bridge the gap. If there is the possibility of an iliac injury, placement of an occlusion balloon into the aorta from the contralateral side and imaging of the iliac as the sheath is removed may prevent significant blood loss. Fortunately, endovascular device technology has created lower profile devices and more flexible sheaths, making access vessel rupture a rarity (Fig. 13.1).

Once access is obtained and a stiff wire platform is established, a key maneuver is to place the sheath as far as possible into the aorta to support an occlusion balloon for unstable patients. This prevents downward displacement from improved blood pressure from the resuscitative efforts. The sheath needs to be left in place during the stent graft deployment so that the occlusion balloon can be safely withdrawn. The use of an exchange length wire for occlusion balloon support cannot be overemphasized as much as the fact that access can never be lost. The exchange length Lunderquist wire (Cook Medical, Bloomington, Indiana) will support the balloon in the descending aorta and limit the need for wire exchanges. Another option is to place the occlusion balloon from an upper extremity access to avoid downward displacement; however, the required sheath size increases the risk of upper extremity arterial injury. Disadvantages of a large brachial sheath are (1) the cut-down can deny a potential access point for anesthesia, (2) stiff wire around unknown arch anatomy may cause unnecessary trauma, and (3) the extended arm can impede imaging.

Great care should be taken to avoid the over-inflation of the compliant occlusion balloon, which may cause secondary rupture. Continued

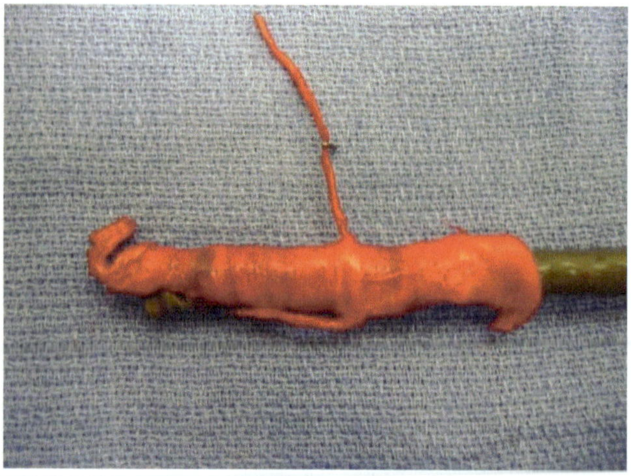

Fig. 13.1 Iliac on a Stick. Be careful when removing tight sheath.

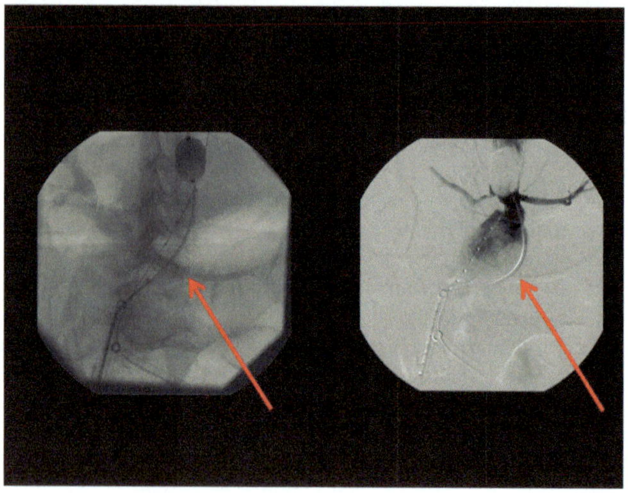

Fig. 13.2 Aortic Occlusion During EVAR. Requires forward tension and advancement of the sheath to prevent balloon migration *(arrows)*.

unstable hemodynamics after inflation of the occlusion balloon should trigger troubleshooting the occlusion balloon and may provide insight to either under-inflation or over-inflation with secondary rupture. The under-inflated balloon is recognized by mobility with each cardiac cycle. Additionally, confirming balloon apposition to the aortic sidewalls can confirm adequate inflation. When the balloon ruptures, it will obviously not be possible to instill any more half-and-half saline and dye solution, and blood may be retrieved from the port. The balloon should be inflated to the point that the balloon does not extend past the markers on its catheter. If rupture of the segment with the occlusion balloon occurs, additional coverage is necessary with a thoracic stent graft and reinflation of the balloon within the stent graft. Most balloons come with a stopcock in the package to maintain the desired pressure and to free the operator's hands. The balloon shaft is then securely clamped to the drapes and inspected at intervals to prevent migration. Once the occlusion balloon is appropriately placed, anesthesia may start aggressive resuscitation with blood and blood products to limit coagulopathy postoperatively (Fig. 13.2).

A useful tip and time-saving step is to use the sheath as an injection port with hand injections of contrast. The quality of the images can be adequate to allow the decision for EVAR versus open and angiographic locating of the lowest renal without needing to take the time for setting up power injection equipment. If flow is inadequate, the occlusion balloon can be gently deflated before repeat injection. Multiple earlier studies suggest 20%–47% of cases of ruptured abdominal aorta are amenable to off-the-shelf EVAR within the manufacturer's indications for use.[1,4,9] With the advancing stent graft technology and increasing outcome data for outside indications for use, it is estimated that EVAR can be used to treat up to 80% of ruptures with the application of adjunctive techniques.

Contralateral groin access is achieved and percutaneous methods can be used for larger sheath insertion. A second stiff wire is advanced into the aorta followed by a larger sheath and the endograft main body. If an occlusion balloon is used, it may be necessary to deflate it partially in order to pass the wire to the thoracic aorta. The graft is usually oriented so that the iliac limbs are crossed. Attention must be paid to the contralateral sheath as it is inserted and its relation to the ipsilateral sheath in order to identify where the contralateral limb should open so that cannulation of the contralateral limb is improved. Cannulation can be time-consuming if not performed correctly. Once the device is in the appropriate position, the occlusion balloon must be retracted into the sac to prevent impinging and entrapment, which can be deleterious. Some degree of hypotension is likely with deflation. Making your staff aware and prepared is a key step in allowing the rapid conduct of the case. One approach is to deploy the main body fully and to insert the occlusion balloon into the aortic neck from the main body side. A second option is to continue cannulating the gate and to proceed in the traditional fashion. A useful tip in large aneurysms is to leave the wire in the suprarenal aorta, because it allows for maintained conformation of the aortoiliac anatomy, and then double access the introducer sheath with a glide wire for cannulation of the gate. Another useful tip is to have a second aortic occlusion balloon primed and ready for use. Reintroduction of a previously inflated balloon into the smaller sheaths can be difficult. During the gate cannulation process, the occlusion balloon needs to be monitored to prevent distal migration from improving blood pressure. If the balloon is pushed down, this may cause endograft main body migration and loss of the seal zone. If this occurs, a cuff can be placed to improve the seal.

Gate cannulation is the most feared cause for interruption of the case progress; however, the increased number of elective endograft placements has made most operators more capable than in the past. It is important to have a variety of catheter shapes and tip conformation to assist with cannulation. The contralateral limb can often be cannulated without problem. However, if there is difficulty, a snare can be used to cannulate the gate. This can be done using the up-and-over technique with the wire, placing the snare at the base of the contralateral limb, and using multiple angles to place the wire in the body of the snare. If a snare is needed, it is preferable to finish the ipsilateral iliac stent graft deployment so that at least one aspect of the repair is completed. Alternatively, the gate can be crossed from a brachial puncture and then snared in the iliac. If unable to proceed with gate cannulation despite adjuncts, the bifurcated device can be converted to aorto-uni-iliac configuration by either deploying an aortic cuff over the gate orifice or simply deploying a second main body inside the first main body. The contralateral common iliac artery is then embolized and a cross-over bypass is performed. Most gates are usually cannulating in 5 minutes. For unstable ruptures, time of cannulation remains of the essence, and if not feasible with the options described, consideration for conversion to aorto-uni-iliac should be rapid. Reichart[9] suggested that 16% of gate cannulations will take longer than 20 minutes. Early in our experience, 15% of our patients required an aorto-uni endograft, but currently the vast majority can be treated with standard bifurcated devices.

Another important clinical issue is whether bifurcated or aorto-uni endografts are better. AJAX[4] randomized trial used only aorta-uni endografts with the advantage of an easy learning curve and rapid control of abdominal hemorrhage; however, this adds time for the femoral–femoral crossover and increases risk of infection. Additionally, general anesthesia is required to perform a bilateral groin cut-down in an emergency setting. It has also been found that bilateral groin incision may increase pain, therefore increasing pain requirements and contributing to postoperative respiratory issues. Fewer stent-graft resources are needed to support a rupture for aorto-uni devices. The most common device needed is usually the largest. In 2002, Verhoeven et al.[10] showed that bifurcated devices could be deployed under local anesthesia. Post hoc analysis of the IMPROVE trial suggested that bifurcated devices offer a survival advantage.[3]

Once the graft of choice is deployed and the proximal, distal, and connecting segments are ballooned, an aortogram is performed with specific emphasis on endoleak, kinking, or clot formation. For aortic necks outside of those indicated for use or persistent type Ia endoleak, special adjuncts may be useful to create a seal. Aptus endoanchor (Aptus Endosystem, Sunnyvale, California) has been found useful by delivering a stapling device to the site of leak, and it also only requires a 16-French sheath from the main body access site. Additionally, a Palmaz stent (Cordis Endovascular, Miami, Florida) may be used as a last-ditch effort to create a seal. Imaging is of key importance in decision making for open versus endovascular repair, but conversion rates are still 1%–2%. In a last-ditch effort for unstable patients with Type Ia endoleak, the risk and benefit of coverage of a low renal orifice with or without an attempt to snorkel and stent the renal will need to be assessed. For patients with end-stage renal failure, the renal artery orifices can be covered with impunity. Type Ib endoleaks are usually managed with extension to the external iliac with concomitant coiling or plugging the ipsilateral hypogastric artery. Care is taken to prevent coverage of both the hypogastric arteries with the concomitant coverage of patent inferior mesenteric artery. If this occurs, the importance of ensuring the patency of the superior mesenteric artery and celiac artery cannot be overemphasized in order to prevent bowel ischemia. A large persistent endoleak may require a conversion to open repair. Conversion to open is not without consequences, because conversion has higher mortality in an already morbid situation.

Thrombosis of the access vessels secondary to the presence of large-bore sheaths is a concern, especially because use of heparin is variable among surgeons. With ruptures, it is generally our practice not to anticoagulate. Unstable patients with massive transfusion and supraceliac occlusion are usually in a coagulopathic state, and anticoagulation contributes to the ongoing bleeding and worsening abdominal compartment pressures. It is not unreasonable to administer heparin and it is a common practice among many groups, especially after aortic control. There is the opposing school of thought that an occluded femoral can be thrombectomized at the end of the case, rather than to contribute to the continued massive exsanguination from the lumbar vessels and raw surfaces of the autodissected retroperitoneum with heparinization.

Access-site complications are relatively simple to control and to treat. For patients in whom closure devices were not placed prior to sheath insertion, cut-down and repair is safest. Heavily diseased or stenotic femoral arteries occasionally require some type of revascularization after sheath removal. In these situations, simplicity and expediency are best in order to get the patient out of the operating room. Most repairs usually involve only a patch angioplasty or a local endarterectomy.

Significant clinical challenge can occur in the postoperative period. Bowel ischemia after elective EVAR is less than 1%, compared with 6.4% after ruptures. The risk factors for this, apart from age and coverage of the hypogastric artery, are not controllable. The combination of inferior mesenteric artery coverage and systemic hypotension is enough to cause colonic ischemia. If undetected, this has been shown to increase mortality significantly. Bowel movements intraoperatively, or even in the immediate perioperative time, should raise suspicions of colonic ischemia. It is our practice that all ruptured aneurysms undergo sigmoidoscopy at the bedside postoperatively on day 1, or sooner, based on clinical suspicion. Treatment for colonic ischemia is based on the degree of ischemia. Mild ischemia is treated with IV antibiotics and bowel rest, and more severe forms with bowel resection. Bowel ischemia involving the small intestine can prove to be more difficult to diagnose. The combination of preexisting atherosclerosis and hypotension can lead to infarction of bowel in the celiac and superior mesenteric distributions. Use of occlusion balloons can also predispose to embolization or ischemia to the mesenteric vessels. Exploratory laparotomy is often the only way to diagnose the problem, and treatment usually involves bowel resection and, occasionally, arterial reconstruction.

Compared with open repair, EVAR has a higher abdominal compartment syndrome rate, affecting up to 20% of the ruptured abdominal aneurysms.[11] Large retroperitoneal hematoma with accompanying space-occupying effect, large volume fluid resuscitation, and the associated soft tissue edema result in high abdominal compartment pressures. These high pressures can result in reduced cardiac venous return, respiratory, renal, and cardiac dysfunction. Acute abdominal compartment syndrome is not only associated with increased mortality, but delayed diagnosis results in 100% mortality.[11] Coagulopathy, use of occlusion balloon, conversion to aorta-uni device, and massive transfusion are all associated with increased risk of abdominal compartment syndrome. Diagnosis is usually made by a combination of physical and physiological findings. The abdomen becomes distended and tense on examination. Pressures required for adequate tidal volumes on the ventilator increase and urine output decreases. Measuring bladder pressures may give some insight into the abdominal compartment pressure situation, but the diagnosis is usually based on clinical suspicion and a variety of subtle signs. Treatment involves laparotomy and open abdominal dressing without disruption of the retroperitoneum. This will require multiple OR trips for closure. Entry into the retroperitoneal hematoma is to be avoided.

Irrespective of the modality used for ruptured aneurysm, acute renal failure is more pronounced, accounting for up to 40% postoperatively. Use of larger doses of contrast coupled with hemodynamic instability contributes to acute renal impairments. The United States national inpatient sample database review of the years 2005–2012 suggests doubled mortality and incidence of acute renal failure with EVARs compared with open repair.[14] Additionally, ruptured EVAR is estimated to require 2 to 3 times the amount of contrast compared with routine EVAR. Aggressive and timely resuscitation is the only tool we have against contrast-induced nephropathy, because appropriate imaging is critical to appropriate sealing of the rupture. Use of intravascular ultrasound and carbon dioxide angiography in ruptured aneurysms has not been explored in the literature. The issue with using alternative imaging is that it may slow down the procedure in a patient with ongoing bleeding. The authors believe that contrast use should be judicious, but as much contrast as is necessary should be used to allow for necessary fluoroscopic images.

The IMPROVE trial reintervention after ruptured aneurysm showed the midterm interventions to be as much as twice as high for rupture. The majority of these were for endoleaks.[12] Our personal experience was different and suggested that Type II endoleaks were less common and Type 1 endoleaks were similar to elective EVAR.[13] In any event, these are mostly treated with translumbar or transfemoral routes in elective fashion.[13] The bigger picture is that even with the late finding of an endoleak, patients survive the acute event and can now be treated in a more elective and controlled setting.

Unpublished data from our institution have demonstrated that endografts placed for abdominal aortic aneurysm rupture are at a higher risk of infection. In this series, the microbiology was skin flora compared with the endografts placed for nonruptured aneurysms, which grew a wide variety of organisms. This may be the result of preoperative antibiotics not being given during less than ideal skin preparation or device handling.

EVAR for ruptured aneurysms offers a less invasive option, which if performed in the appropriate setting, may offer a mortality and morbidity advantage.

TIP BOX

- Always have a noncompliant aortic occlusion balloon readily available in ruptured abdominal aortic aneurysms with difficult access.
- In ruptured abdominal aortic aneurysms, maintain stiff wire access at all times.
- Maintain pressure on 12-French or bigger sheath under occlusion balloon at all times (to prevent migration).
- Always know where your occlusion balloon is.
- Beware of iliac rupture if sheath resistance gives; it could be the external iliac separating from the bifurcation.
- Never lose wire access.
- Remember that the position of the sheaths can direct how best to place contra limb for cannulation.
- Limit your time for contra access; remember snare, arm access, or aorto-uni if it is not working.

REFERENCES

1. Hinchliffe RJ, Bruijstens L, MacSweeney ST, Braithwaite BD. A randomised trial of endovascular and open surgery for ruptured abdominal aortic aneurysm – results of a pilot study and lessons learned for future studies. *Eur J Vasc Endovasc Surg*. 2006;32(5):506–515.
2. van Beek SC, Conijn AP, Koelemay MJ, Balm R. Editor's Choice - Endovascular aneurysm repair versus open repair for patients with a ruptured abdominal aortic aneurysm: a systematic review and meta-analysis of short-term survival. *Eur J Vasc Endovasc Surg*. 2014;47(6):593–602.
3. Powell JT, Hinchliffe RJ, Thompson MM, et al. Observations from the IMPROVE trial concerning the clinical care of patients with ruptured abdominal aortic aneurysm. *Br J Surg*. 2014;101(3):216–224. Discussion 224.
4. Hoornweg LL, Wisselink W, Vahl A, Balm R. The Amsterdam Acute Aneurysm Trial: suitability and application rate for endovascular repair of ruptured abdominal aortic aneurysms. *Eur J Vasc Endovasc Surg*. 2007; 33(6):679–683.
5. Mehta M, Taggert J, Darling RC, 3rd, et al. Establishing a protocol for endovascular treatment of ruptured abdominal aortic aneurysms: outcomes of a prospective analysis. *J Vasc Surg*. 2006;44(1):1–8. Discussion 8.
6. Li Y, Li Z, Wang S, et al. Endovascular versus open surgery repair of ruptured abdominal aortic aneurysms in hemodynamically unstable patients: literature review and meta-analysis. *Ann Vasc Surg*. 2016;32:135–144.
7. Ten Bosch JA, Teijink JA, Willigendael EM, Prins MH. Endovascular aneurysm repair is superior to open surgery for ruptured abdominal aortic aneurysms in EVAR-suitable patients. *J Vasc Surg*. 2010;52(1):13–18.
8. Lloyd GM, Bown MJ, Norwood MG, et al. Feasibility of preoperative computer tomography in patients with ruptured abdominal aortic aneurysm: a time-to-death study in patients without operation. *J Vasc Surg*. 2004;39(4):788–791.
9. Reichart M, Geelkerken RH, Huisman AB, et al. Ruptured abdominal aortic aneurysm: endovascular repair is feasible in 40% of patients. *Eur J Vasc Endovasc Surg*. 2003;26(5):479–486.
10. Verhoeven EL, Prins TR, van den Dungen JJ, et al. Endovascular repair of acute AAAs under local anesthesia with bifurcated endografts: a feasibility study. *J Endovasc Ther*. 2002;9(6):729–735.
11. Mehta M, Darling RC, 3rd, Roddy SP, et al. Factors associated with abdominal compartment syndrome complicating endovascular repair of ruptured abdominal aortic aneurysms. *J Vasc Surg*. 2005;42(6): 1047–1051.
12. Powell JT. Re-interventions after repair of ruptured abdominal aortic aneurysm: a report from the IMPROVE Randomised Trial. *Eur J Vasc Endovasc Surg*. 2018.
13. Quinn AA, Mehta M, Teymouri MJ, et al. The incidence and fate of endoleaks vary between ruptured and elective endovascular abdominal aortic aneurysm repair. *J Vasc Surg*. 2017;65(6):1617–1624.
14. Aziz F, Azab A, Schaefer E, Reed AB. Endovascular repair of ruptured abdominal aortic aneurysm is associated with lower incidence of postoperative acute renal failure. *Ann Vasc Surg*. 2016;35:147–155.

14

Complications of Fenestrated Endovascular Aneurysm Repair

Timothy A. M. Chuter, MD

STENT GRAFT DESIGN

Many of the complications of endovascular aneurysm repair result from a mismatch between the demands of the pathology and the capabilities of the device, and many can be avoided by proper patient selection and device selection, based on a thorough understanding of the differences between various alternatives.

The first branched stent grafts were of *unibody* design: inserted whole with the branches already attached. The implantation of an entire unibody multibranched stent graft was achieved using a complex system of catheters, all of which had to work in perfect synchrony. The resulting degree of irreducible complexity made the unibody approach unforgiving and complication prone.

These days, most multibranched stent grafts are of *modular* design: inserted in pieces and assembled in situ. Modular stent grafts fall into two main groups, fenestration-based and cuff-based, depending on the type of branch attachment site.

A fenestration-based branch exits the trunk of the stent graft through a small wire-reinforced hole (Fig. 14.1A). The entire ring of contact between the two is barely longer than the thickness of the graft wall. Secure hemostatic attachment depends on the transaxial orientation of the branch and the presence of a slightly overdilated flange at the proximal end of a balloon-expanded covered stent.

A cuff-based branch exits the trunk of the stent graft through a short axially oriented branch (Fig. 14.1B) and runs between the wall of the stent graft and the wall of the aorta before turning into the lumen of the corresponding target artery. A 14–18 mm long zone of contact between the inner aspect of the cuff and the outer aspect covered stent helps stabilize the inter-component connection. The curved path of the branch calls for some flexibility in the covered stent, which is usually of the self-expanding variety.

The first step in branch deployment is the same regardless of whether the branch attachment site is a fenestration or a cuff: a catheter is directed from the lumen of the stent graft, through the perigraft space, and into the lumen of the target artery.[1] This bridging catheter is then exchanged, over a stiff guidewire, for the delivery system of a covered stent (the branch). However, there the similarities end. Fenestration-based and cuff-based multibranched stent grafts are selected differently, planned differently, and implanted differently. They fail in different ways, and their failure modes require different remedies. Although most users have a distinct preference for one or the other, the choice often depends on arterial anatomy. As a rule, nondilated, or mildly dilated, segments of the aorta call for fenestration-based branches, whereas truly aneurysmal segments of the aorta call for cuff-based branches. Most experienced centers plan complex endovascular repairs accordingly.

FAILURE TO INSERT THE TRUNK OF A MODULAR STENT GRAFT

The original multibranched stent grafts were bulky devices, especially those that had long helical cuffs.[2] It used to be relatively common for the delivery sheath to be too wide, or too inflexible, to traverse the external iliac arteries, especially in women.[3,4] This has become less of a problem since thin-walled fabrics, nitinol stents, and low-profile cuffs have reduced the caliber of the delivery system (Fig. 14.2A,B). The low-profile version of the most widely used multibranched stent graft (t-branch, Cook Medical Inc., Bloomington, Indiana) now has an 18-French sheath.[5]

Nevertheless, very small, calcified, stenotic external iliac arteries sometimes impede or prevent transfemoral insertion of even a low-profile delivery system. Under these circumstances, a surgically created route of access is sometimes needed in the form of iliofemoral bypass. We prefer to do this at a separate operation prior to definitive aneurysm repair, thereby minimizing the blood loss that would otherwise be associated with prolonged heparin anticoagulation (during the remainder of a long complicated multibranched stent graft insertion) and allowing the patient to recover in the interval between the two operations. Before embarking on surgical bypass, a close look should be taken at the state of the common iliac arteries, which may be too narrow to admit the delivery system or too calcified to clamp. When the obstructing lesion is confined to the external iliac artery, it may be possible to perform an endovascular bypass of the external iliac artery by aggressive balloon dilatation of the offending artery with a covered stent already in place in case of iliac artery rupture.[6] This is fairly straightforward if the internal iliac artery is already occluded. Otherwise, the proximal end of the covered stent has to be positioned very carefully to preserve flow through internal iliac collaterals to the spine.[7,8]

FAILURE TO POSITION THE TRUNK OF THE STENT GRAFT AT THE CORRECT LEVEL

Even when the iliac artery disease is not severe enough to prevent insertion, it can still complicate deployment by generating friction between the iliac arteries and the delivery system. Applying caudally direct traction to the entire aortoiliac segment results in high deployment of the stent graft.

Cuff-based stent grafts are quite forgiving of small errors in stent graft position because they run down the outside of the aorta for a variable distance. High deployment of the stent graft just lengthens the

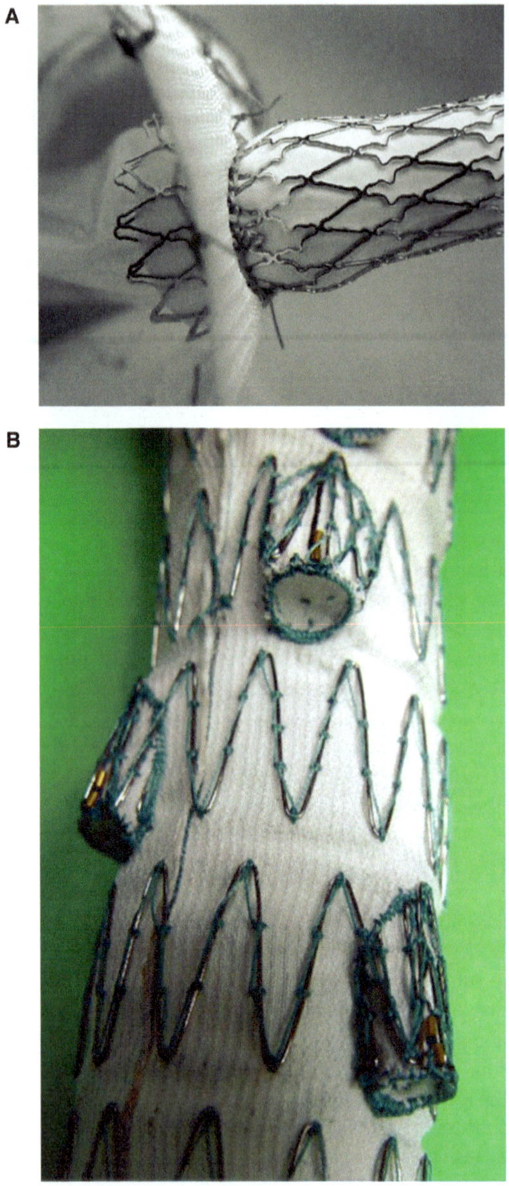

Fig. 14.1 (A) A balloon-expanded covered stent traversing a fenestration in the wall of a stent graft. Note the flaring of the covered stent on either side of the stent graft, which helps to create secure hemostatic attachment of one component to the other. (B) Multiple caudally oriented cuffs in the wall of a stent graft.

necessary stent graft. Low deployment is a different matter. If the outer orifice of a caudally oriented cuff comes to lie *below* the orifice of the corresponding artery, it can be difficult, if not impossible, to turn the tip of the catheter upward.

Fenestration-based stent grafts are less forgiving of stent graft malposition because the branches run a short distance straight across the perigraft space in a transaxial plane, leaving little room for corrective rerouting.

Failure to Position the Trunk

Continuous corrective torque is applied to the outer part of the delivery system as it is withdrawn and re-advanced as many times as necessary, taking care to keep the guidewire in place. Unfortunately, the correct degree of rotation of one end is not necessarily matched by the same degree of rotation at the other. If this happens, focus should be on the proximal markers while applying slow sheath withdrawal. If the proximal stents open in the correct orientation, they will tend to impose their orientation on the distal stents through the fabric of the open stent. The correct orientation can be determined *before* device insertion by rotating the delivery system clockwise. The maintenance of a partially expanded state by the constraining ties allows some fine-tuning of stent graft orientation and position, which may be helpful in the deployment of a fenestration-based stent graft, but less so when implanting (a more forgiving) cuff-based stent graft.

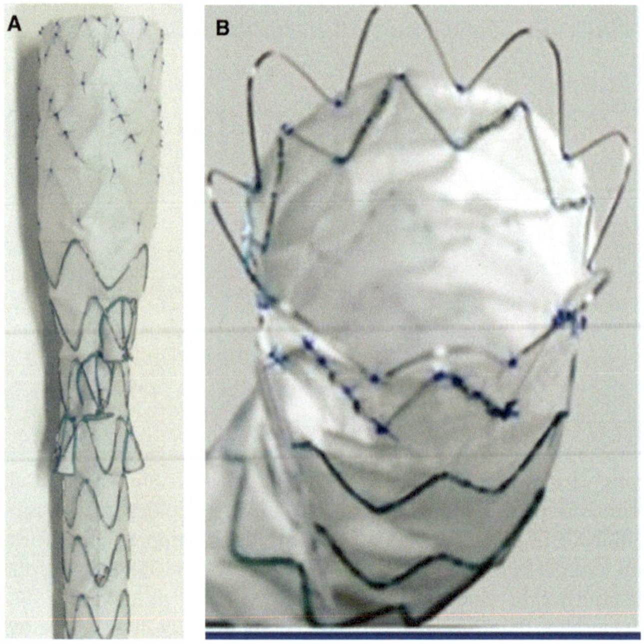

Fig. 14.2 (A) The cuff-bearing portion of a low-profile 4-branch stent graft. Note the distribution of the cuffs, which approximates the distribution of branches radiating from the typical thoracoabdominal aorta. (B) The Zenith Alpha low-profile stent graft, which serves as a proximal extension to the cuff-bearing portion in cases of Crawford Types II and III thoracoabdominal aortic aneurysms.

FAILURE TO CATHETERIZE THE TARGET ARTERY

In an ideal world, all stent grafts would be customized to achieve a perfect match between the distribution of branch attachment sites on the stent graft and the distribution of branches on the aorta. In reality, this is often difficult to achieve. Branch attachment sites are confined to the spaces between the struts of the stent graft. They cannot always go exactly where wanted. Moreover, it is not always possible to predict the exact orientation of the stent graft, especially in cases of aortic tortuosity. Sometimes the stent graft deploys in alignment with the aorta, sometimes in alignment with the delivery system.

In fenestration-based repairs, the catheter is usually introduced into the stent graft through an access site in the femoral artery and directed out of the stent graft through each fenestration, and constraining ties prevent full stent graft expansion. The resulting preservation of a limited perigraft space allows the catheter enough freedom of movement to accommodate moderate degree of misalignment (see earlier description of failure to orient the stent graft). In addition, the partially deployed stent graft is free to move a little in response to externally

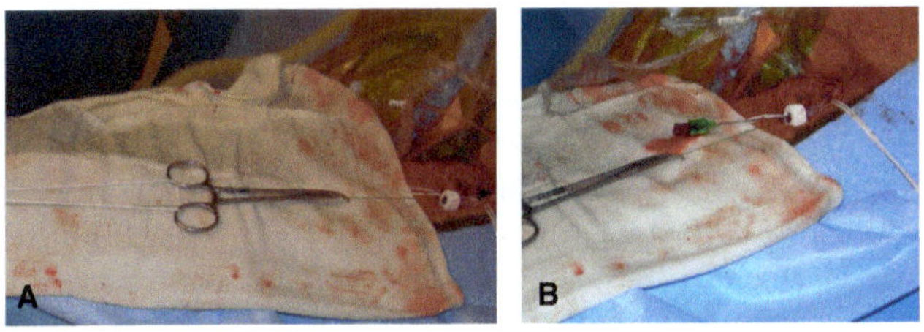

Fig. 14.3 (A) A small (0.014″) brachiofemoral buddy wire is placed under tension by rubber loops to help stabilize a 12-French brachial sheath. (B) Puncture of the sheath valve establishes a second line of access to be used for branch insertion in cases of cuff-based multibranched thoracoabdominal aortic aneurysm repair.

applied torque and traction. Most experienced users have learned how to tweak stent graft position during deployment and how to use a range of catheters, in conjunction with a repertoire of catheter manipulations, to bridge the gap in case of less than perfect alignment. The VanSchie range of catheters (numbers 1–5, Cook Medical Inc., Bloomington, Indiana), with its range of acutely angled radiopaque tips, was developed specifically for this purpose. When a particularly wide degree of misalignment cannot be corrected by reorienting the stent graft, it may be necessary to reform a recurved (visceral selective or Sos) catheter in the perigraft space. The preoperative CT will show the proper viewing angle. In most cases, the best angle is at right angles to the arterial ostium, but intermittent views down the long axis of the branch artery help to show the relative positions of the catheter tip, the fenestration, and the arterial ostium.

In cases where some (usually the renal) branches arise from a nonaneurysmal segment of the aorta, the perigraft space can be so compressed as to limit the free movement of a catheter. Under these circumstances the catheter, guidewire, and sheath need to be stiff enough to push the offending stent graft aside. Any tendency for the sheath to form redundant loops at bends in often tortuous pathways from the brachial artery to the cuff can generally be overcome by the tension in a small (0.014) brachiofemoral buddy wire (Fig. 14.3A).

In patients who have undergone renal stenting with a portion of the uncovered stent sticking out into the lumen, the catheter tip sometimes finds its way between the fabric and a stent attached to its outer surface; although the guidewire slips through this gap into the target artery, the catheter will not follow. The only remedy is to withdraw both the catheter and guidewire to the outer orifice of the cuff and start again. Under these circumstances, the wire passes easily into the artery through the wall, not the end, of the stent. Catheterization is even more difficult if the end of the stent protrudes from the target artery orifice and impinges on the wall of the stent graft. Under these circumstances, it is sometimes possible to deflect the tip of the wire through the short acutely angled catheter off the wall of the stent graft into the lumen of the stent.

Most experienced users have learned a range of more radical maneuvers for use when all else fails. The piggy-back technique of Ferreira, is an example in which,[9] in which a transbrachial guidewire is carried by a snare over a previously placed transfemoral wire into the target artery. Alternatively, a wire can be introduced into the surgically exposed distal renal artery, retrieved by a snare, and brought out through the usual transfemoral or transbrachial access site.

FAILURE TO DEPLOY THE BRANCH

The covered stent and its delivery system face two main impediments to smooth trauma-free insertion: the angle between the long-axis of the stent graft (or cuff) and the long-axis of the target artery; and areas of compression, kinking, or stenosis that obstruct the path from the lumen of the stent graft to the lumen of the target artery.

In fenestration-based repairs, the line of insertion has to make a turn of at least 90 degrees to achieve the proper alignment for secure hemostatic attachment between the balloon-expanded covered stent and the margin of the fenestration, unless the vessel is cranially oriented, in which case it will be less than 90 degrees. Assuming the typical transfemoral line of insertion, caudally oriented branches and large aneurysms require the support of stiff guidewires and/or sheaths. Unfortunately, the stiffer the wires and sheaths, the more likely they are to bow and fall out. It may be difficult to insert a stiff wire without the support of a stiff catheter and difficult to insert a stiff catheter (or sheath) in the absence of a stiff wire. There is no universal solution to this particular catch 22. An incremental approach often has to be adopted, using a succession of wires and sheaths of gradually increasing stiffness. Directional sheaths provide robust support and controllable angulation. They are available in an ever-increasing range of lengths and tip curvatures for the insertion of Endoanchors and in the electrophysiology lab for cardiac ablation.

Sometimes, in cases of 3- and 4-branch fenestration-based repair, a large occlusion balloon above the branches will serve to buttress the transfemoral line of insertion. When the renal arteries are very caudally oriented, it may be preferable to use a transbrachial approach (rather than the usual transfemoral approach). A scallop in the proximal margin of the stent graft provides access to the stent graft catheter with the assistance of an indwelling catheter.

BRANCH ARTERY INJURY

The wires that guide branch insertion often have to be very stiff, because the line of insertion is tortuous, and the arteries, especially the renal arteries, are short. Any uncontrolled movement of such a wire has the potential to perforate distal renal branches or dissect proximal renal branches, with dire consequences. Distal arterial perforation, in a heavily anticoagulated patient, may cause sufficient bleeding to require coil embolization, reversal of heparin, and cessation of the procedure. Although extravasation is usually confined by the perinephric capsule, the resulting capsular pressurization can cause a complete, if temporary, loss of renal function. Arterial dissection occurs when the tip of the guidewire moves back and forth through the primary branch point. Left untreated, the resulting dissection can cause total permanent loss of renal function. The best remedy involves the placement of a short self-expanding stent over a guidewire in the true lumen, which is one reason to perform completion angiograms through a 5-French sheath with a guidewire in place.

As always, an ounce of prevention is worth a pound of cure. If the renal artery is long enough and wide enough, a Rosen guidewire (Cook Medical Inc., Bloomington, Indiana), with its atraumatic tip, can be substituted for some of the more dangerous straight-tip alternatives. Regardless of guidewire choice, the real culprit is uncontrolled wire tip movement, resulting from poor fluoroscopic guidance, an unstable sheath, or a highly curved (or otherwise obstructed) path of branch insertion.

For proper fluoroscopic control of guidewire position, the tip of the wire has to be in the field of view and the X-ray beam directed at right angles to the trunk of the renal artery. This is not necessarily the same beam angle used for catheterization of the cuff and renal orifice. The right renal artery, for example, often originates from the anterolateral aorta (requiring a left anterior oblique [LAO] view), before turning posteriorly and laterally (requiring a right anterior oblique [RAO] view).

KINKING OR COMPRESSION OF THE BRANCH

Kinking or compression of the branch is easy to correct at the time of implantation, less easy to correct once the guidewire has been removed from the branch, and difficult, or impossible, to correct months later when the branch occludes. Kinking occurs more often in cuff-based repairs, in which the proximal end of a self-expanding branch must share the same axial orientation as the cuff and the distal end must share the same axial orientation as the target artery, resulting in an unavoidable bend. The branches of a fenestration-based branch are less susceptible to kinking because they are straight at the time of balloon-driven deployment and robust enough to stay that way, at least in the short to medium term.

VISCERAL ISCHEMIA

The modular approach to multibranched aneurysm repair is designed to avoid interruption of flow to the visceral arteries within the field of repair. Both fenestrations and cuffs provide a path for blood flow through the wall of the stent graft into the perigraft space, and through the perigraft space into any as-yet-vacant target arteries. Under normal circumstances, this pathway maintains visceral perfusion right up to the point at which branch deployment bridges the gap, excludes the perigraft space, and provides a more direct source of perfusion through the lumen of the branch itself. Furthermore, in fenestration-based repair, the stent graft is maintained in a state of partial compression by a series of constraining ties until all the target arteries have been catheterized and prompt branch deployment assured.

The proximal superior mesenteric often gives rise to a couple of indispensable arteries: the middle colic and right hepatic. Careful preoperative computerized tomography angiography (CTA), intraoperative angiography, and precise deployment are mandatory to avoid inadvertent coverage.

Early fenestrated stent grafts usually had one stented fenestration for each renal artery and one unstented scallop for the superior mesenteric artery.[2,3] The renal fenestrations were positioned over the corresponding renal orifices using balloon-expanded stents, first covered then uncovered. This pattern remains the norm in the United States, mainly because of the glacial pace of regulatory approval. Elsewhere, there has been a shift toward the use of stent grafts with fenestrations and covered stents for the superior mesenteric and celiac arteries.[3,4,10] One factor driving this shift is the potential for the margins of the unstented scallop to cover part, if not all, of the superior mesenteric artery, a cause of late-occurring superior mesenteric occlusion.[11]

EMBOLISM

Postoperative CTA reveals splenic and renal infarcts, presumably the result of intraoperative embolism, in many cases of multibranched endovascular aneurysm repair. This is hardly surprising, given the complexity of aortic instrumentation and the prevalence of extensive mural thrombus in many of these patients. What is surprising is the low overall rate of serious embolic complications such as stroke, paraplegia, renal failure, and intestinal perforation. Some of this disparity may be attributed to aspects of standard implantation technique that isolate much of the aortic wall from the disruptive effects of endovascular instrumentation. Nearly all the aorta within the field of the repair is covered early in the operation by the deployment of a stent graft, and any uncovered aorta between the left subclavian artery and the top of the stent graft is protected by a sheath. Once the sheath is in place and its position stabilized by a brachiofemoral wire, no guidewire, catheter, or branch delivery sheath touches the thoracic aorta.

The disparity between the rate of embolism seen on postoperative CT versus the rate of clinical complications is partly attributable to organ tolerance for small isolated emboli. CT proven embolism to the small intestine rarely causes ischemic necrosis and perforation. Often the only manifestation of localized embolism to the small intestine is a self-limiting ileus. Although the central nervous system is generally considered to be intolerant of ischemia, embolism-related stroke and paraplegia are rare, even when postoperative CTA shows localized areas of hypoperfusion. Lower body embolism, as evidenced by the typical cutaneous mottling, rarely causes serious morbidity unless associated with embolism to upstream intraabdominal organs. The typical course is relatively benign with spontaneous resolution within days. Even in the presence of digital gangrene, a policy of benign neglect results in the least amount of tissue loss.

PARAPLEGIA

To understand the treatment of paraplegia, an understanding is required of the role played by a network of spinal and paraspinal arteries that receive and distribute blood from multiple feeding arteries, including the vertebral, internal mammary, costocervical, internal iliac arteries, segmental (lumbar and intercostal) branches of the aorta (Fig. 14.4), and the anterior spinal artery.[7] Spinal ischemia occurs when this network is unable to provide a sufficient net (minus CSF pressure) perfusion pressure to the spine. Assuming the arterial pressure is high enough and the CSF pressure low enough, the loss of one feeding artery, even the great radicular artery (artery of Adamkiewicz), is generally well tolerated. The impact is much greater in the absence of normal flow through feeding arteries such as the left subclavian artery and internal iliac arteries.[8,12]

There is an important difference between fenestration-based versus cuff-based repairs in the risk of lower extremity weakness following multibranched endovascular repair of pararenal aortic aneurysm (PAA) and Type IV thoracoabdominal aortic aneurysm (TAAA). The presence of a cuff prevents apposition between the wall of the stent graft and the wall of the aorta. Since the uppermost cuff (to the celiac artery) sits 1–3 cm above the celiac artery and the seal zone sits 2–4 cm above the celiac cuff, the proximal margin of the stent graft is often 7 cm, or more, above the celiac artery (Fig. 14.3A). A fenestration-based stent graft occupies far less proximal aortic territory. Assuming the uppermost fenestration occupies nondilated aorta (PAA and TAAA), the sealing zone seldom needs to extend more than 15 mm proximal to the upper fenestration. In theory, this should result in a higher rate of paraplegia for cuff-based repair. In practice, the difference may not be enough to matter because adjunctive measures such

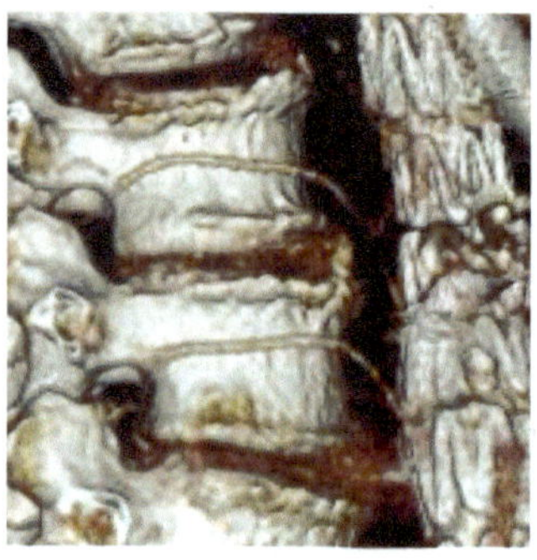

Fig. 14.4 Postoperative computerized tomography angiography, showing collateral-fed intercostal arteries adjacent to an excluded segment of the aorta.

as collateral preservation, spinal drainage, euglycemia, various types of staging, and blood pressure support (see later) have reduced the rate of permanent lower extremity weakness to a very low level in cases of pararenal and Type IV TAAA.

Very few patients wake from anesthesia with signs of spinal ischemia. The development of lower extremity weakness usually occurs hours later, presumably as anticoagulation is reversed and endoleaks resolve, closing collateral paths of spinal perfusion. Treatment, in the form of CSF drainage and measures to support blood pressure, can be titrated to symptoms. Aggressive management is reserved for those who need it, thereby minimizing the rate of drain-related complications such as intracranial hemorrhage. However, there is still a role for routine preoperative spinal catheterization because the spine can go rapidly from normal to irreversible ischemic injury. There is no time to call in a suitably trained anesthesiologist to insert a spinal drain. Besides, most patients are mildly coagulopathic and thrombocytopenic in the early postoperative period when lower extremity weakness typically develops.[13]

Our routine practice is to drain 10 mL/h for at least a day to make sure we have a patent catheter when we need it. After that, the drain is capped for a day and removed only when the patient leaves the ICU. If symptoms develop, the first thing to do is to drain 20 mL of CSF and an additional 20 mL every 10 minutes until the weakness resolves or the patient develops a headache. Most patients exhibit some response to these measures. Moreover, even a partial response, is predictive of a complete response. The goal is to help the at-risk spine through the first few days, by which time a reorientation of paraspinous arterioles provides sufficient collateral flow to make spinal drainage redundant. Having observed that high glucose levels within blood and CSF were associated with high rates of lower extremity weakness, we adopted routine insulin infusion titrated to maintain euglycemia. So far, the results have been very promising.

Since most patients wake with normal spinal function, it is difficult to see much of a role for intraoperative monitoring. Intraoperative changes in evoked potentials are most often caused by interruption of flow to the internal iliac arteries. Sheath withdrawal generally restores internal iliac flow and returns monitoring to normal.

Although paraplegia occasionally occurs weeks or months after repair, such cases are rare. The at-risk period seems to be self-limited, presumably because of the rapid reorientation of arterioles within the paraspinous muscles and the rather less rapid development of collateral arteries. With this in mind, several groups have adopted a strategy of staged repair, intended to isolate some of the aorta at one operation, leaving the rest to be treated when the repair is completed later.[13,14]

EARLY ENDOLEAK

The typical modular branched stent graft is assembled in situ from many components, and each individual component adds at least two potential sites for leakage: the intercomponent junction where the branch joins the stent graft; and the distal implantation site where the branch enters the corresponding arterial lumen. Of the two, the intercomponent junction is more of a concern, especially in fenestration-based branches, which lack a zone of overlap. Secure hemostatic implantation at the ring of apposition depends on exactly the right orientation and exactly the right amount of flaring. Balloon-expanded stents (the kind used to form fenestration-based branches) are somewhat fragile. If the branch is somehow distorted during removal of the delivery system or balloon dilatation of the aorta, it will stay that way and so will the resulting endoleak.

Angiography and CTA have different roles in the detection of endoleak. Angiography is more specific in locating the route of leakage, whereas CTA is more sensitive in detecting the presence of leakage.

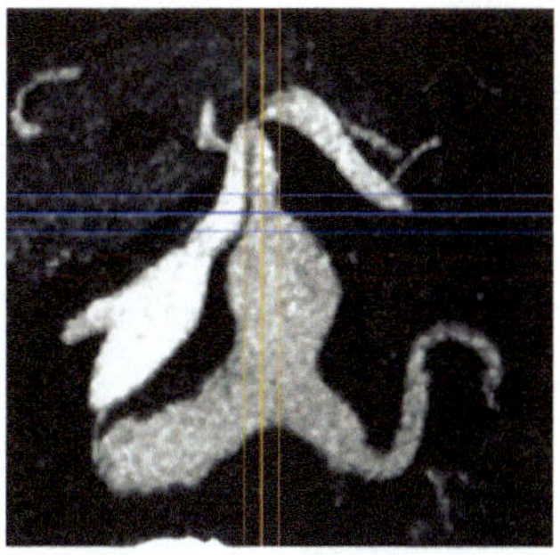

Fig. 14.5 Postoperative computerized tomography angiography, showing flow through the superior mesenteric branch of a multibranched stent graft into the distal portion of a dissected superior mesenteric artery, across the distal fenestration, and back into the aneurysm. The net result, despite attempted catheter based treatment, was persistent perfusion, aneurysm dilatation, and eventual rupture.

Postoperative CT scans often identify endoleaks of indeterminate type (or site), many of which resolve. Those that are clearly direct (Type I or III), persistent, or associated with aneurysm dilatation require angiographic study and transcatheter treatment. That said, it is always easier to treat an endoleak at the time of stent graft insertion than later, when the catheters and wires have been removed and arterial access sites have been closed. Flush aortograms have a low yield and a high contrast load. Selective angiography is more revealing, especially in patients with dissection of the target arteries themselves (including the common iliac arteries) beyond the implantation site, because the false lumen may undermine the repair by allowing retrograde flow (Type Ib endoleak) to the aneurysm (Fig. 14.5).

LATE-OCCURRING TYPE I ENDOLEAK

A late-occurring Type I endoleak is caused by stent graft migration, or by dilatation of the aorta at the implantation site, or by some combination of the two. Long-term follow-up shows that a fenestrated repair in healthy pararenal aorta is more stable than a standard repair in a short, conical, or thrombus-lined neck. Similarly, a 4-branch (cuff-based or fenestration-based) repair is more stable that a 2-fenestration repair.[2–4,10,11] Moreover, the surgically repaired arch may be the only stable proximal implantation site in a patient with connective tissue disease. Endovascular rescue of late-occurring endoleak can be difficult or impossible when remnants of the failed repair litter the field.

Long-term data show cuff-based repairs to be very stable in this regard. Cuff-based stent grafts migrate less often than fenestration-based stent grafts.[2,15] The difference is attributable in part to the more extensive nature of the cuff-based repair, and in part to the effect of branch type. The self-expanding branches of a cuff-based repair are more resilient, more securely connected to the trunk of the stent graft, and better oriented to provide support to the trunk of the stent graft. Migration of a fenestration-based stent graft is often accompanied by branch fracture, distortion, and dislocation.[16]

LATE-OCCURRING TYPE III ENDOLEAK

As a relatively recent addition to the endovascular toolbox, multibranched stent grafts have benefited from the lessons of early experience with infrarenal stent grafts, many of which were structurally unstable. Modern devices of all types are more robust. The same tightly woven fabrics, properly polished Nitinol stents, and long intercomponent overlaps have largely eliminated structural failure of the multibranched stent graft.

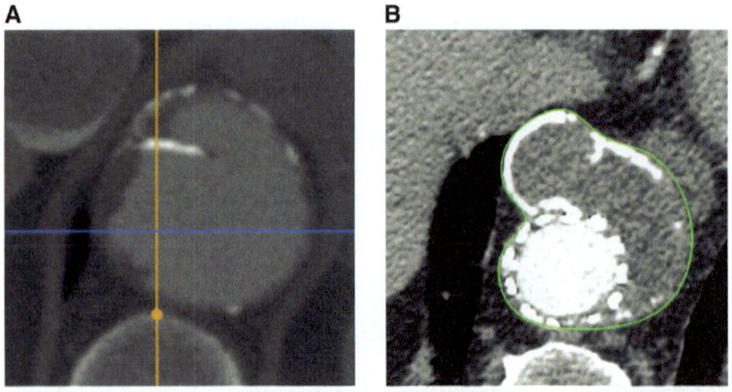

Fig. 14.6 (A) Preoperative computerized tomography angiography (CTA), showing a spicule of calcium, poking into the aneurysm. (B) CTA of the same patient a little over a year later after implantation of a second stent graft to close a hole in the first stent graft.

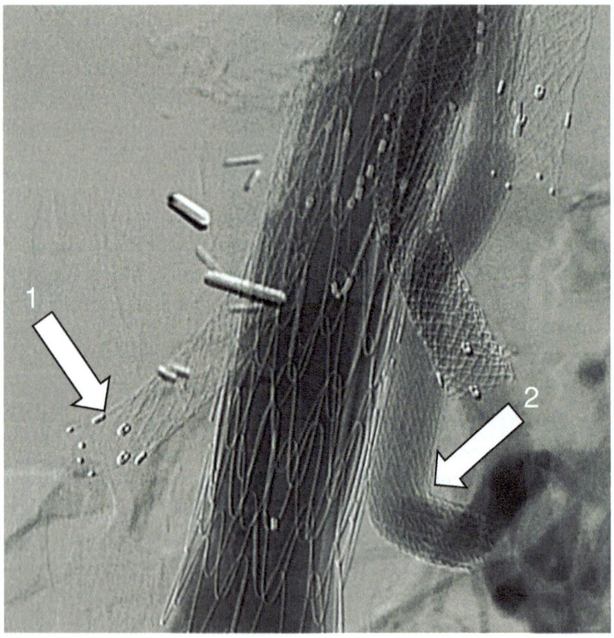

Fig. 14.7 Angiography showing occlusion of a stiff straight Fluency-based branch *(arrow 1)* and patency of a flexible bent Viabahn-based branch *(arrow 2)*.

The typical pulsatile forces of the endovascular environment are not sufficient to degrade stent graft structure unless coupled with some other source of injury, such as a spicule of calcium (Fig. 14.6A,B). In addition, the self-expanding branches of cuff-based stent grafts are also relatively robust. They rarely fracture, separate, or leak.

LATE-OCCURRING BRANCH OCCLUSION

Late-occurring renal branch occlusion is by far the most common late failure mode of cuff-based stent grafts. The probable cause is microtrauma to the soft, flexible, mobile renal artery where it meets a hard unyielding inflexible Fluency-covered stent. Indeed, the rate has fallen significantly since the substitution of a flexible Viabahn-covered stent (Fig. 14.7).

The branches of a fenestration-based stent graft are much less prone to occlusion, perhaps because they do not extend as far into the renal artery. They fail in other ways, including fracture and dislocation.

BOX 14.1 Traumatic stent graft insertion.

Note

- The combination of iliac tortuosity, calcification, and stenosis is far more dangerous than each in isolation.
- Iliac artery injury usually becomes apparent on delivery system removal, not insertion. If in doubt, leave the wire in place for a minute or two following sheath removal, and be ready with a balloon and a covered stent to make repairs.

Prevention

- Substitute a low-profile alternative (e.g., Cook Alpha)
- Test iliac straightening during a first-stage operation

Treatment

- Create a surgical bypass/conduit to provide a low resistance alternative to the diseased iliac artery, bearing in mind it may be impossible to bypass proximal common iliac disease in the presence of an aortic aneurysm.
- Endovascular bypass (crack and pave) taking care to preserve the internal iliac artery.
- Consider separating the access and implantation parts of the procedure, especially if access preparation involves an limited abdominal operation.

BOX 14.2 Failure to align branch attachment sites (cuffs or fenestrations) with target arterial orifices.

Note

- This is more of a problem for fenestration-based branches, which are less forgiving than cuff-based branches, because they take a less direct route to the target artery.
- Beware of tortuosity of the pararenal aorta, which makes it difficult to predict the lie of the stent graft.
- Once bent (by a tortuous heavily calcified iliac artery), the delivery system will rotate, rather than bend again, when it encounters differently oriented bends in the aorta.
- Beware the symmetrical stent graft, which looks just fine even though it may be back-to-front.
- The distal check mark is not an entirely reliable indicator of stent graft orientation.

Prevention

- Study CT-based 3-D imaging
- Before stent graft insertion, rotate the delivery system under fluoroscopy to determine orientation and front/back position

Correction

- Focus on the orientation of the top end. Once that is secured in the proper position, you can adjust the distal half as it leaves the delivery system one stent at a time.
- Small disparities can be corrected by dynamic rotation (twisting the delivery system while moving the delivery system back and forth), but take care not to lose guidewire position.
- If orientation changes markedly during insertion, withdraw the stent graft back into the iliac, rotate it, and reinsert.

BOX 14.3 Failure to insert cuff-based branches.

Note

- A narrow (<25 mm) pararenal aorta is a relative contraindication to the use of cuff-based renal branches: fenestration-based branches are preferred.
- Target artery stenosis is the most common indication for staged repair with an interval of weeks between the first procedure (angioplasty) and the second (stent graft implantation).
- Upward cuffs may look fine, but, for some unknown reason, they often cause the kidneys to shrink.
- The catheter and wire occasionally get caught between the outer surface of the graft and the stent. If in doubt, inflate a balloon within any site that seems to impede sheath or catheter passage.

Prevention

- Tension on the ends of a 0.014″ brachiofemoral buddy wire stops the brachial sheath coiling into the ascending TA, helps stabilize the transbrachial route of branch insertion, and prevents paradoxical movement of catheters and wires.
- Preoperatively placed stents should not protrude from the target artery into the aorta.

Treatment

- Use a stiff short-lead guidewire to direct branch insertion.
- Bend the wire to match the curved line of insertion.
- Bend the wire into a Z to carry the tip away from a lop-sided lesion.
- Slowly deflate and apply traction to a small balloon in the target artery while simultaneously advancing a narrow sheath.
- Use a Wallstent to smooth and widen the path to the target artery.
- Use a tip-deflecting sheath to support passage of the branch into a caudally oriented target artery.
- Use a snare to carry the wire, catheter, and sheath over a separately inserted wire into the target artery.

BOX 14.4 Failure to insert fenestration-based branches.

Note

- A narrow pararenal artery rarely impedes the insertion of a fenestration-based branch.
- The fenestrated stent graft delivery system available in the United States lacks several of the aids (in-dwelling catheter and wire, for example) that feature in the version available outside the United States.
- The constraining ties allow small positional adjustments of the stent graft.

Prevention

- Tortuosity of the pararenal aorta can interfere with stent graft orientation and fenestration/branch alignment.
- Beware severe caudal orientation (down-going) of the renal arteries.

Treatment

- Before poking away with the catheter tip in the region of the markers, make sure the fenestration and target artery are properly aligned, using oblique views both parallel and perpendicular to the target artery.
- The following may help sheath insertion in difficult (caudally oriented) anatomy: use a stiff guidewire; reorient the stent graft; bounce the catheter off the top cap; bounce the catheter off a large balloon; pass the branch through a tip-deflecting sheath; bend the distal segment of a stiff guidewire.

BOX 14.5 Paraplegia.

Note

- Very few patients wake with lower extremity weakness or numbness. The usual cause is embolism.
- Most symptoms of spinal ischemia develop later (hours to days) as coagulation normalizes and endoleaks resolve.
- Untreated weakness soon becomes permanent.
- CSF drainage can cause serious complications such as intracranial bleeding.
- Partial recovery of lower extremity movement predicts full recovery.
- Intraoperative changes in evoked potentials are usually caused by big sheaths in the iliac arteries, obstructing flow into the internal iliac arteries.
- Hypotension is the most common cause of late onset (>24 h) weakness.

Prevention

- Preserve flow into the left subclavian artery
- Preserve flow into both internal iliac arteries
- Correct hypotension, and hyperglycemia (under 120 mg/dL), even in the absence of weakness

Treatment

- Drain CSF until symptoms start to resolve, or the patient develops a headache.
- Routine preoperative drainage, although this remains controversial and some advocate a wait-and-see policy, especially in lower risk cases
- Pressors provide an immediate rise in BP, but, given time, IV fluid and blood are more effective.

CONCLUSION

As a rule, the more complicated the stent graft, the more opportunities there are for failure, and, if one part of the stent graft fails to function as intended, the whole repair fails. Given that the typical multibranched stent graft is constructed from over 20 parts, all introduced through long catheters and implanted under two-dimensional fluoroscopic guidance, it is remarkable that the results are as good as they are. A big part of that success derives from an operator's ability to get out of trouble. Stent grafts rarely behave quite as intended and preoperative imaging rarely depicts all the potential anatomic obstacles. Consequently, the learning curve is long and unforgiving. The best results are obtained by a dedicated team of experts. This is not something that needs to be part of every vascular surgery practice.

REFERENCES

1. Browne TF, Hartley D, Purchas S, Rsenberg M, Van Schie G, Lawrence-Brown M. A fenestrated covered suprarenal aortic stent. *Eur J Vasc Endovasc Surg*. 1999;18:445–449.

2. Mastracci TM, Eagleton MG, Kuramochi Y, Bathurst S, Wolski K. Twelve-year results of fenestrated endografts for juxtrarenal and group IV thoracoabdominal aneurysms. *J Vasc Surg*. 2015;61:355–364.
3. Sveinsson M, Sobocinski J, Resch T, et al. Early versus late experience in fenestrated endovascular repair for abdominal aortic aneurysm. *J Vasc Surg*. 2015;61:895–901.
4. Austermann M, Donas KP, Panuccio G, Troisi N, Torsello G. Pararenal and thoracoabdominal aortic aneurysm repair with fenestrated and branched endografts: lessons learned and future directions. *J Endovasc Ther*. 2011;18:157–160.
5. Ramanan B, Fernandez C, Sobel JD, et al. Midterm results of the use of low profile multibranched thoracoabdominal aortic stent grafts. *Vasc Surg*. 2015;62:527–528.
6. Asciutto G, Aronici M, Resh T, Sonesson B, Kristmundsson T, Dias NV. Endoconduits with "pave and crack" technique avoid open ilio-femoral conduits with sustainable mid-term results. *Eur J Vasc Endovasc Surg*. 2017;54:472–479.
7. Etz CD, Kari FA, Mueller CS, et al. The collateral network concept: a reassessment of the anatomy of spinal cord perfusion. *J Thorac Cardiovasc Surg*. 2011;141:1020–1028.
8. Eagleton MJ, Shah S, Petkosevek D, Mastracci TM, Greenberg RK. Hypogastric and subclavian artery patency affects onset and recovery of spinal cord ischemia associated with aortic endografting. *J Vasc Surg*. 2014;59:89–94.
9. Ferreira M, Katsargyrus A, Rodrigues E, et al. "Snare-Ride": A bailout technique to catheterize target vessels with unfriendly anatomy in branched endovascular aortic repair. *J Endovasc Ther*. 2017;24:556–558.
10. Katsagyris A, Oikonomou K, Kouvelos G, Mufty H, Ritter W, Verhoeven ELG. Comparison of outcomes for double fenestrated endovascular aneurysm repair versus triple or quadruple fenestrated endovascular aneurysm repair in the treatment of complex abdominal aortic aneurysms. *J Vasc Surg*. 2017;66:29–36.
11. Ullery BW, Lee GK, Lee JT. Shuttering of the superior mesenteric artery during fenestrated endovascular aneurysm repair. *J Vasc Surg*. 2014;60:900–907.
12. Sobel JD, Vartanian SM, Gasper WJ, Hiramoto JS, Chuter TA, Reilly LM. Lower extremity weakness after endovascular aneurysm repair with multi-branched thoracoabdominal stent grafts. *J Vasc Surg*. 2015;61:623–628.
13. Liouspis C, Corriveau MM, Mackenzie KS, et al. Paraplegia prevention branches: a new adjunct for preventing or treating spinal cord injury after endovascular repair of thoracoabdominal aneurysms. *Vasc Surg*. 2011;54:252–257.
14. O'Callaghan A, Mastracci TM, Eagleton MJ. Staged endovascular repair of thoracoabdominal aortic aneurysms limits incidence and severity of spinal cord ischemia. *J Vasc Surg*. 2015;61:347–354.
15. England A, Garcia-Finana M, Fisher RK, et al. Migration of fenestrated aortic stent grafts. *J Vasc Surg*. 2013;57:1543–1552.
16. Mastracci TM, Greenberg RK, Eagleton MJ, Hernandez AV. Durability of branches in branched and fenestrated endografts. *J Vasc Surg*. 2013;57:926–933.
17. Hongku K, Resch T, Sonesson B, Kristmundsson T, Dias N. Applicability and midterm results of branch cuff closure with vascular plug in branched endovascular repair for thoracoabdominal aortic aneurysms. *J Vasc Surg*. 2017;66:367–374.
18. Chuter TA, Hiramoto JS, Park KH, Reilly LM. The transition from custom-made to standardized multi-branched thoracoabdominal aortic stent grafts. *J Vasc Surg*. 2011;58:660–667.
19. Chang C, Chuter TA, Nieman CU, et al. Systemic inflammation, coagulopathy and acute renal insufficiency following endovascular thoracoabdominal aortic aneurysm repair. *J Vasc Surg*. 2009;49:1140–1146.

15

Complications With Branched Endovascular Devices

Piotr M. Kasprzak, MD, Kyriakos Oikonomou, MD and Karin Pfister, MD

POINTS OF ATTENTION IN BRANCHED EVAR

Branched endovascular aortic aneurysm repair (B-EVAR) was developed for the treatment of thoracoabdominal aortic aneurysms (TAAA). With increasing physician experience and device evolution we can at the moment treat almost all types of aneurysms extending from the aortic arch to the iliac bifurcation. In connective tissue disease, open reconstruction remains the first choice of treatment. There is a multitude of different configurations for branched devices, including downward- or upward-oriented branches, internal or external configurations, and a combination of branches and fenestrations. A typical branched-only device has four downward-facing branches intended for the celiac artery (CA), the superior mesenteric artery (SMA), and two renal arteries (RA). This common design has led to the development of the single currently available off-the-shelf branched device (T-branch, Cook Medical, Bloomington, IN, USA). Other companies (WL Gore & Associates, Newark, DE, USA; Jotec GmbH, Hechingen, Germany) are developing comparable systems that will enable physicians to treat patients even in an acute setting. Despite increasing standardization, applicability of off-the-shelf endografts is not universal, and a significant proportion of patients with TAAA will still require treatment with custom-made devices (CMD) to address specific anatomical characteristics. This underlines the need for meticulous planning of this complex endovascular procedure, which is the first step to avoid intraoperative complications. Nevertheless, a number of technical challenges can arise during B-EVAR, requiring experience with specific endovascular techniques and bail-out measures to achieve technical success.

DEVICE PLANNING

Preoperative planning of B-EVAR requires good-quality imaging with thin cut (≤1 mm) spiral computerized tomography angiography (CTA) from the chest to the groin with the option of axial, coronal, and three-dimensional reconstructions. To this purpose, physicians have an increasing software arsenal for multiplanar reconstructions and center-line measurements enabling precise placement and orientation of side branches as well as selection of proximal and distal components in composite systems. If a tube graft is required proximally in the descending thoracic aorta, it should be designed to land 3 cm above the orifice of the CA. This facilitates catheterization of the target arteries, while ensuring sufficient overlap between components. In compromised proximal neck, additional fixation with endoanchors can be considered.[1] Typical branch orientation includes clock positions of 01:00 for the CA, 12:00 for SMA, 09:00–11:00 for the right RA and 01:00–03:00 for the left RA. Usually, the endograft main body consists of 10–12 bare metal stents covered with graft material. Branches originate at the midportion of the endograft, and each single stent can accommodate up to two branches; this means that in cases of three or more vessels originating at the same level, one branch has to be positioned higher and the target vessel secured with a longer bridging stent. In situations when the aorta has an hourglass shape, with narrowing of the renomesenteric segment or narrow true lumen in postdissection TAAA, fenestrations or branches can be an option. Specific points of attention are supraaortic artery anatomy in association with proximal landing and intraoperative stroke risk, shaggy aorta, which is the main contraindication for B-EVAR, and access vessels that may restrict endovascular solutions or mandate use of low-profile devices.

- Landing zone: Maximal diameter is 40 mm. In hostile anatomy, adequate sealing length is mandatory with possible additional fixation with endoanchors.
- Access-vessels tortuosity, calcification, or stenosis: surgical exposure for conduit.
- Kinked anatomy (aorta, target vessels): Plan longer overlap and consider ways for accurate device deployment.
- Focally narrow aortic segment: Consider a combination of branches and fenestrations to accommodate individual anatomy.
- Shaggy aorta: Main contraindication for B-EVAR.

In order to exclude the aneurysm completely with endovascular methods, physicians need to extend the level of repair well above and below the aneurysm to a parallel segment of the aorta to achieve a safe and durable seal. A problem arising particularly in the case of B-EVAR is the risk of spinal cord ischemia (SCI) with increasing length of covered aorta.[2] Preservation of the left subclavian artery and pelvic circulation should always be targeted. Proximally, this can be achieved with the use of carotid–subclavian or carotid–carotid–subclavian bypass and debranching or arch stent grafts with branch fenestrations and, in some cases, chimneys for supraaortic vessels. In cases of common iliac artery involvement, the distal sealing zone can be extended below the iliac bifurcation with iliac branched devices that preserve flow to the external and internal iliac arteries. Despite these measures, published studies have demonstrated that extensive TAAA repair is associated with considerable SCI rates.[3–6] It is therefore advisable to try to reduce the length of covered descending aorta to the minimum required for an adequate seal. In the case of descending aortic diameters of 32–38 mm, where the branched component usually has to be extended proximally with deployment of a tapered tube-graft and additional aortic coverage of approximately 10 cm, we now have the option to use a double-barrel "2-in-1" CMD device (Cook Inc.). This consists of two coaxial stent grafts with a maximal outer diameter of 44 mm, allowing for adequate seal at the level of the branched component, without extension of the proximal landing zone. Aside from stent graft planning, prevention of SCI requires care with operative timing, pre-, intra-, and postoperative management.

An additional consideration during TAAA repair is the risk of bowel and liver ischemia, caused by embolic complications or malperfusion of main tributaries and important collaterals. Studies have reported an estimated risk of 2%–3% for bowel ischemia in aortic endovascular repair, with a respective mortality of 50%.[7] Specific planning to avoid this in extensive TAAA repair can include additional branches or fenestrations in case of separate orifices of intestinal vessels, an additional branch to prominent (≥4 mm) inferior mesenteric arteries (IMA) when mesenteric circulation is compromised, and branches for the preservation of the internal iliac arteries.[8]

- SCI Prevention: Preserve flow to LSA and IIA, do not unnecessarily extend aortic coverage.
- Bowel ischemia: Preserve all important tributaries.

PROCEDURAL PLANNING

Although B-EVAR is considered a less invasive procedure than open TAAA surgery, it still constitutes a major and extensive procedure and therefore requires thorough preoperative medical assessment and evaluation of overall patient status and life expectancy, e.g., in our experience, significantly comorbid patients (ASA IV) have a higher rate of midterm all-cause mortality.[9]

Preoperative patient management should maintain preexisting medication with the exception of aggressive antihypertensive treatment to avoid perioperative hypotension that could increase the risk of SCI. Preoperative antiplatelet therapy with aspirin is standard.

Recent studies have demonstrated that patients with extensive thoracoabdominal disease benefit from staged exclusion of the TAAA.[7,10] There are several staging strategies that can be applied in atherosclerotic and postdissection TAAA. One consists of primary TEVAR and deployment of the branched device at a second stage. The advantage of this method in patients treated with CMD is that a standard off-the-shelf thoracic device can be implanted immediately while the branched component is in production. An additional benefit in postdissection TAAA with narrow true lumen is to expand the thoracic aorta and create more space prior to implantation of the branched device. A possible disadvantage of this method in atherosclerotic aneurysms is the free-floating distal end of the stent graft, which may interfere with the aortic thrombus and cause embolization. Alternatively, staging can be carried out by means of temporary aneurysm sac perfusion (TASP) either through an open branch for the celiac artery or by iliac extension, which is secured in a second stage following the initial procedure. The PAPA-ARTIS study which is currently being carried out, with preemptive coiling of spinal arteries prior to TAAA repair, might provide further insights to possible SCI prevention protocols. Despite the obvious advantage of staging strategies in relation to SCI, it has to be noted that any continuing perfusion of the aneurysm sac may be associated with an unclear rupture risk in the time interval to completion.

In order to reduce time to complete aneurysm exclusion, intraoperative monitoring of motor evoked potentials (MEPs) may play an important role.[11] Our strategy is to monitor MEPs intraoperatively during the initial procedure, after deployment of the stent grafts. Following removal of sheaths and restoration of flow to the limbs, the remaining open branch and the respective target vessel are selectively occluded with a balloon from 30–40 min, while sack pressure is monitored. Uneventful MEPs in normotension and induced hypotension indicate that completion of the procedure in a single stage is feasible. If MEPs decline during induced hypotension and recover in normotension, the procedure is staged, 7–10 days after initial procedure, during the same hospital stay. On the contrary, a significant decrease in MEPs with recovery only after balloon deflation indicates that the completion interval should be extended. We have observed reduction of perfused aneurysm sac volume and visible intercostal arteries during the TASP interval, but the exact delay to maximize TASP protection while minimizing the risk of rupture is still not precisely defined.[12]

- Preoperative evaluation: General status and comorbidities should play an important role in patient selection.
- Staging: Lowers paraplegia risk in extensive TAAA repair. MEPs monitoring may determine time of completion.

OPERATIVE BASICS, TIPS, AND TRICKS

As a result of the long procedural duration, B-EVAR is usually carried out under general anesthesia. Regional or local anesthesia can be an option in staged procedures, especially during the TEVAR stage or during TASP completion. If local anesthesia is applied for the branch/iliac completion step, monitoring of MEPs is not necessary. Cerebrospinal fluid (CSF) drainage is generally indicated for patients with extensive TAAA. Monitoring of spinal fluid pressure and drainage should be carried out with an automated system (e.g., LiquoGuard, Möller Medical GmbH, Fulda, Germany) and is usually continued for 72 hours postoperatively. Monitoring of intraoperative lower limb perfusion is advisable because of the use of occluding sheaths in the femoral arteries and can be carried out with somatic oximetry sensors (INVOS).

ISCHEMIA MONITORING: APPLY INVOS AND MEPS

Standard access for B-EVAR includes one or both common femoral arteries and, in our center, the left axillary artery in order to avoid crossing of the aortic arch and apply shorter sheaths for branches and target vessels. In some centers the subclavian/brachial artery is used instead, alternatively left- or right-sided. Percutaneous access can be applied in patients without atherosclerotic lesions; alternatively, cutdown access is used.

If repair extends to the level of the left subclavian artery or further proximally, the first thoracic component is introduced over a superstiff wire (e.g., Lunderquist, Cook Medical, Bloomington, IN, USA), placed in the ascending aorta. In all other cases, a through-and-through wire from the common femoral to the axillary artery is used. The patient is heparinized aiming for an activated clotting time equal to or in excess of 300 seconds. During introduction via the through-and-through wire, tension has to be applied and a sheath or catheter advanced through the axillary artery to prevent damage of the left subclavian artery and the proximal descending aorta from the wire.

In cases of angulation or kinking of the aorta or iliac vessels, with difficulty advancing, the wire can be fixated at the distal end of the deployment system and the device pulled via the transaxillary end of the wire. In case stent graft advancement through heavily calcified or stenosed iliac arteries is not possible, different methods to facilitate passage have been described.[13] These include balloon dilatation of the iliac stenosis, the "paving and cracking" technique, or our method of preference, which consists of gradual dilatation of the access vessel using dilators of increasing sizes. Regardless of the method used, the risk of iliac artery rupture should not be ignored and appropriate covered stents should therefore be readily available. To minimize blood loss, these maneuvers should be carried out under temporary proximal balloon occlusion. In some patients a proximal surgical conduit may be necessary.

- Access problems: Specific endovascular techniques (i.e., gradual sheath dilatation, PTA, "paving and cracking") may be required to avoid open surgical exposure/conversion.

Correct alignment of the branches needs to be controlled under X-ray prior to introduction, and the stent graft needs to be advanced correspondingly. Further corrective maneuvers might need to be undertaken to achieve the same orientation during advancement, especially in kinked anatomies. Rotation of the delivery system over 90 degrees should be avoided, otherwise there is a risk of "candy-wrap" torsion of the endograft between two stents (Fig. 15.1). In cases where

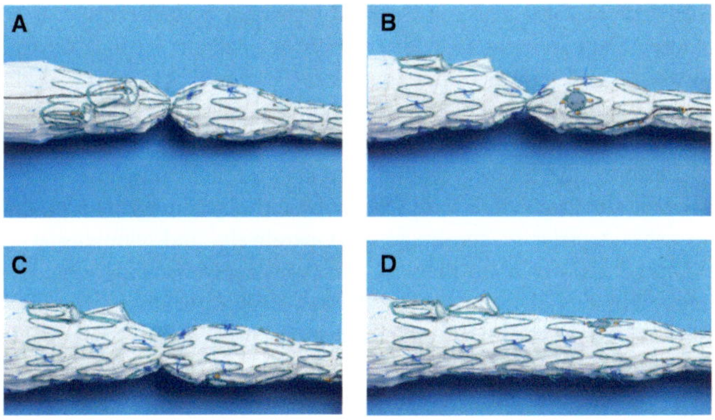

Fig. 15.1 Excessive rotation of the deployment system during corrective maneuvers can lead to "candy-wrap" torsion of the branched graft (A, B) and should be corrected prior to release (C, D) (Cook Medical, Bloomington, IN, USA).

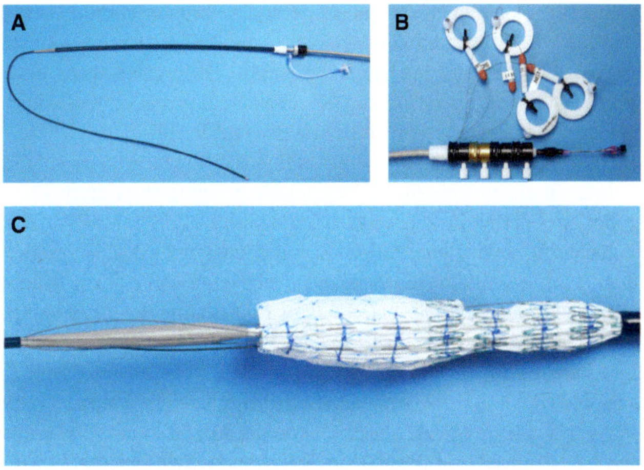

Fig. 15.2 Preloaded CMD device (Cook Medical, Bloomington, IN, USA) (A) with through-and-through wires (B) in two branches and two fenestrations (C).

extensive rotation of the device is required, the system should be retracted and reintroduced in adjusted orientation.

Stent graft deployment is always performed either following digital subtraction angiography (DSA) or using fusion imaging. It is important to adjust position of the C-arm to the length axis of the aorta. The branched component usually features different intended distances between the end of each branch and the upper edge of the respective target vessel. Prior to deployment, stent graft position has to be adjusted according to the branch with the shortest intended distance to its target vessel. In this way, all branches are securely deployed above their target vessels. During gradual deployment, orientation of the stent graft and height of the branches have to be maintained with slight immediate corrections if necessary. If "candy-wrap" distortion of the device occurs, deployment should be stopped immediately and the wrap resolved by counter-rotating the whole system with the distal part of the device inside the sheath. An overlap of three stents between components is typically planned. This overlap should not be reduced below two stents. In cases of severe aortic kinking, accurate positioning of the thoracic tube graft and the branched graft might be difficult, because the distal edge of the component might shift upward after release, adjusting to the aortic anatomy, possibly compromising overlap or/and increasing distance to target vessels. The distal component is deployed according to the standard for infrarenal aortic aneurysm repair.

Following deployment of all aortic components, immediate removal of occluding sheaths should be carried out, to restore flow to the internal iliac arteries and the lower limbs, maintaining the through-and-through wire. Prompt sheath removal facilitates collateral flow to the spinal cord and plays a preventive role for SCI and lower limb ischemia.[5]

- Positioning and orientation: Meticulous gradual stent graft deployment and immediate corrections are imperative to achieve accurate placement. Femoral sheaths should be removed and blood flow restored prior to target vessel catheterization.

Target vessels in B-EVAR are typically secured with bridging stents via the axillary access. To this purpose, a 12-French sheath is advanced to the supraceliac segment over the through-and-through wire. Access to each branch is achieved with the help of an angiography catheter. It is advisable to begin with the most challenging target vessel. Branch catheterization can be facilitated with the use of preloaded systems featuring through-and-through wires in branches/fenestrations (Fig. 15.2). Following branch catheterization, the respective target vessel is visualized with angiography, selectively catheterized, and a stiff wire for bridging stent placement (e.g., Rosen) is advanced. A coaxial 8-French sheath can be helpful in cases of narrow anatomy or branch apposition to the aortic wall or for protection during advancement of a balloon-expandable stent graft. Target vessel catheterization can be one of the most challenging aspects of B-EVAR. Particularly in postdissection TAAA with target vessels originating from different lumina, crossing the dissection membrane may be necessary. To this purpose different methods can be used to switch to the appropriate lumen. In our experience, a steerable transfemoral sheath can be placed against the dissection flap under fusion control or fluoroscopy in multiple projections. Perforation of the dissection membrane can subsequently be carried out with the use of a stiff wire followed by balloon dilatation. In atherosclerotic and in postdissection TAAA, a wide range of different wires and catheter configurations may be required, especially in kinked anatomy, stenotic target vessels, or misalignment of the branch and the respective vessel. In some cases, direct antegrade catheterization through the branch may nevertheless not be feasible. Several techniques to achieve target vessel access in such cases have been described.

For renal arteries, especially when upward oriented, the "snare-ride" technique can be applied.[14] The branch of the graft is catheterized from an axillary access. The respective target vessel is then catheterized via a femoral access. An Indy snare (Cook Inc.) is advanced over the transfemoral wire and positioned near the entrance of the target vessel. The transaxillary wire inside the branch of the graft is then advanced, snared, and pushed inside the target vessel with the snare. The procedure is thereafter continued with antegrade bridging of the target vessel in routine fashion. Another bail-out measure is retrograde access to the branch through the distal segment of the target vessel, which can be carried out via open surgical exposition or in cases of renal arteries via CT-guided puncture.[15,16] After gaining access to the vessel, a soft wire is retrogradely advanced into the aneurysm sac and snared through the branch. This wire is retrieved over the branch using a snaring device to obtain a through-and-through wire. Subsequently the corresponding target vessel is stented with a balloon-expandable or self-expanding covered bridging stent. Particularly for the SMA and the CA, the loop technique can be applied.[17] This consists of catheterization of one of two vessels, advancement of the soft wire over the gastroduodenal artery in retrograde fashion into the second vessel (i.e., CA or SMA), and then snared back to the left brachial artery forming a loop. Finally, in cases where target vessel stenting through the branch cannot be achieved, the respective vessel can be perfused by other endovascular techniques (i.e., chimney, periscope in standard or "sandwich" technique), or by open bypass surgery. The branch should then be occluded with plugs and coils after placement of a covered stent into the branch, to extend the occlusion length. Performing these procedures at a second operation can be considered, provided perfusion of the target vessel through the open branch is sufficient.

Following successful stiff-wire placement in the target vessel, different balloon-expandable or self-expandable bridging stent grafts can be applied. Currently, no dedicated bridging stent grafts for B-EVAR are available. A recent publication has demonstrated similar midterm patency for self- and balloon-expandable covered stents.[18] For balloon-expandable covered stents, placement of a sheath into the target vessel is required. Sheath advancement can sometimes be tedious, especially in kinked anatomies and wire instability. In these cases, advancement can be facilitated with the use of a balloon that is inflated in the target vessel, acting as a dilator for the sheath. Upon gradual balloon deflation, the sheath is advanced over the balloon. Following bridging stent graft placement, endolining might be necessary in the event of kinking or compression of the stent graft. This can be carried out by deployment of a self-expanding stent. If kinking occurs at the distal end of the bridging stent graft, endolining should extend further distally into the target vessel.

Target vessel catheterization and stent grafting can result in severe complications such as dissection, perforation, or vessel thrombosis. Such issues should be immediately identified and treated accordingly. In the case of vessel dissection, the bridging stent graft should be extended with a self-expandable stent to ensure adequate flow. Distal vessel perforation should be treated with coil embolization, proximal covered with a bridging stent graft. In cases of thrombosis or embolization, aspiration thrombectomy or local thrombolysis can be applied. The cause of thrombosis should be identified and treated.

- Target vessel catheterization and sheath advancement may require use of multiple catheters, wires, and sheaths as well as additional techniques such as the "snare ride," retrograde access via puncture/surgical exposure, the "loop technique," or use of a balloon as dilator.
- Endolining of bridging stent grafts may be necessary in narrow or kinked target vessel anatomy.
- Complications such as vessel dissection, perforation, and thrombosis should be immediately identified and treated.

POSTOPERATIVE MANAGEMENT

Postoperatively, patients are monitored in the intensive care unit for 48–72 hours. Arterial blood pressure is continuously measured invasively. Intravascular volume and hemoglobin levels are aggressively corrected with a targeted hemoglobin level of $\geq$9 g/dL. Vasoactive medications are used if needed to maintain a mean arterial blood pressure $\geq$90 mmHg until neurologic status is evaluated. For this purpose, every effort is made for prompt postoperative extubation of the patients. The CSF drainage is removed after 48–72 h in patients who are hemodynamically stable and do not present neurologic symptoms after a 6-h clamping period. In cases where placement of CSF drainage is not possible, spinal cord pressure can be controlled indirectly with the use of orbital duplex sonography, as an indicator of intracranial pressure changes.[19] In cases of SCI symptoms, aggressive blood pressure regulation and spinal fluid drainage are carried out with a mean arterial blood pressure goal of $\geq$90 mmHg and spinal pressure of $\leq$10 cm H_2O. Therapeutic heparinization is applied to prevent thrombosis of additional intercostal and lumbar arteries. In our institution, administration of high-dose corticosteroids is used as a pharmacological adjunct in selected cases to improve neurological recovery: there is, however, no published evidence supporting its use as standard. Finally, a possible direct approach to reverse spinal cord ischemia, in cases where the aneurysm sack has not completely thrombosed postoperatively, is to induce a Type Ib endoleak by deployment of a balloon-expandable stent between the distal end of the aortic stent graft and the aortic wall. In this way, flow into the aneurysm is partially reestablished, which can increase spinal cord perfusion and possibly reverse paraplegia.[20]

Postoperative antiaggregation consists of double antiplatelet therapy and anticoagulation with low molecular heparin agents subcutaneously. Aspirin is continued perioperatively and clopidogrel is stopped 7 days prior to the procedure and readministered after safe removal of the CSF drainage. Despite lack of high-quality evidence specifically for branched stent grafts, our group proposes life-long double antiplatelet therapy if tolerated.

- Blood pressure and hemoglobin level regulation and CSF drainage play an important role in paraplegia prevention.
- In cases of SCI symptoms, blood pressure, hemoglobin management, and CSF drainage are more crucial. Additional measures include heparinization, possibly corticosteroid application, and consideration of sac reperfusion.
- Life-long double antiplatelet therapy after B-EVAR can be considered.
- Postoperative imaging and follow-up.

Postoperative evaluation includes B-mode, continuous wave duplex and contrast-enhanced sonography, abdominal radiography in four planes, and CTA. Intraoperative cone beam CT can replace the initial postoperative CTA. One or more modalities are usually performed within 3 to 5 days of the endovascular procedure, before and after secondary side-branch completion, after 6 months, and yearly thereafter, or in any case of suspected organ malperfusion or dysfunction. Duplex and contrast-enhanced ultrasonography are used postoperatively to differentiate between intended TASP side branch perfusion and non-intended Type I or III endoleaks, especially in patients with acute or chronic renal failure. If CTA at 1 year demonstrates no endoleak and no aneurysm progression, the time interval between CTAs can be increased to 2 years, with annual contrast-enhanced ultrasonography and abdominal radiography in four planes.

CONCLUSION

Thoracoabdominal aneurysms represent one of the most challenging vascular pathologies. Open surgery is associated with high perioperative mortality and morbidity, prohibitive for high-risk patients. The use of endovascular TAAA repair, planned and performed in high-volume centers, is feasible and provides high technical success rates and low perioperative mortality rates.[21,22] It has to be stressed, however, that this type of endovascular procedure represents the pinnacle of minimal invasive aortic repair and is associated with multiple challenges in planning, execution, and perioperative management. High-quality imaging and hybrid operating rooms are prerequisites. Extensive experience with standard aortic endovascular procedures and renovisceral vessel interventions is required prior to extending operator spectrum to branched thoracoabdominal stent grafting, and a learning curve has to be accepted. A multitude of catheters, wires, and endovascular devices should be readily available to address intraoperative technical issues and to carry out bail-out maneuvers when necessary. The role of perioperative management by a dedicated surgical and anesthesiologic team should be underlined.

The risk of spinal cord ischemia, with increasing aortic coverage, is a valid concern. With increasing experience, better management of hypovolemia and hypotension, as well as use of adjunct measures, clinical outcome has improved; however, the risk of SCI is still considerable. TAAA repair is usually an elective/preventive procedure, and SCI is a grievous complication, severely limiting quality of life and life expectancy.

Regarding follow-up, overall, midterm safety and durability as reflected by the absence of late aneurysm rupture and target vessel stent patency are excellent. The need for reintervention currently seems to represent the main deficit of the technique over open repair.[9,21,22] Branched devices consist of multiple components featuring many connections and zones of overlapping. Endoleaks may be the result of device fatigue, disconnections, and device migration or a result of postoperative aortic remodeling, with changes in vessel diameter and angulation. In the vast majority, endoleaks can be successfully addressed by minimal invasive means. They do not necessarily constitute a "failure to treat"; they do, however, underline the need for rigorous follow-up. To this purpose, use of different modalities, including CTA, contrast-enhanced ultrasound sonography, and plain radiography, is imperative to differentiate accurately between endoleak types and to plan reintervention. The role and fate of Type II endoleaks in extensive TAAA repair, as well as the role of preventive lumbar artery and IMA coiling, remain unclear.

Despite its shortcomings and technical challenges, this technology offers a less invasive treatment option to patients with extensive aortic aneurysm disease, with outcomes that challenge those of open repair. It allows treatment of patients who would otherwise be considered unfit for open repair. Because of the rarity and complexity of this type of pathology, centralization of treatment is important. Long-term results are still sparse and will ultimately be the defining factor for a possible paradigm shift in treatment of TAAA. To this end, pooling of results from high-volume centers would be advisable.

REFERENCES

1. Ongstad SB1, Miller DF, Panneton JM. The use of EndoAnchors to rescue complicated TEVAR procedures. *J Cardiovasc Surg*. 2016; 57:716–729.
2. Dias NV, Sonesson B, Kristmundsson T, Holm H, Resch T. Short-term outcome of spinal cord ischemia after endovascular repair of thoracoabdominal aortic aneurysms. *Eur J Vasc Endovasc Surg*. 2015;49:403–409.
3. Katsargyris A, Oikonomou K, Kouvelos G, et al. Spinal cord ischemia after endovascular repair of thoracoabdominal aortic aneurysms with fenestrated and branched stent grafts. *J Vasc Surg*. 2015;62:1450–1456.
4. Bisdas T, Panuccio G, Sugimoto M, et al. Risk factors for spinal cord ischemia after endovascular repair of thoracoabdominal aortic aneurysms. *J Vasc Surg*. 2015;61:1408–1416.
5. Maurel B, Delclaux N, Sobocinski J, et al. The impact of early pelvic and lower limb reperfusion and attentive peri-operative management on the incidence of spinal cord ischemia during thoracoabdominal aortic aneurysm endovascular repair. *Eur J Vasc Endovasc Surg*. 2015;49:248–254.
6. Kasprzak PM, Gallis K, Cucuruz B, et al. Editor's choice—Temporary aneurysm sac perfusion as an adjunct for prevention of spinal cord ischemia after branched endovascular repair of thoracoabdominal aneurysms. *Eur J Vasc Endovasc Surg*. 2014;48:258–265.
7. Becquemin JP, Majewski M, Fermani N. Colon ischemia following abdominal aortic aneurysm repair in the era of endovascular abdominal aortic repair. *J Vasc Surg*. 2008;47:258–263.
8. Pfister K, Kasprzak PM, Apfelbeck H, et al. Inferior mesenteric artery side branch for selected patients with endovascular aortic aneurysm repair. *EJVES Short Rep*. 2016;31:1–5.
9. Oikonomou K, Kopp R, Katsargyris A, et al. Outcomes of fenestrated/ branched endografting in post-dissection thoracoabdominal aortic aneurysms. *Eur J Vasc Endovasc Surg*. 2014;48:641–648.
10. Amr G, Sobocinski J, Koussa M, et al. Staged procedure to prevent major adverse events in extensive aortic aneurysm repair. *J Vasc Surg*. 2013;57:1671–1673.
11. Banga PV, Oderich GS, Reis de Souza L, et al. Neuromonitoring, cerebrospinal fluid drainage, and selective use of iliofemoral conduits to minimize risk of spinal cord injury during complex endovascular aortic repair. *J Endovasc Ther*. 2016;23:139–149.
12. Gallis K, Kasprzak PM, Cucuruz B, Kopp R. Evaluation of visible spinal arteries on computed tomography angiography before and after branched stent graft repair for thoracoabdominal aortic aneurysm. *J Vasc Surg*. 2017;65:1577–1583.
13. Hinchliffe RJ, Ivancev K, Sonesson B, Malina M. "Paving and cracking": an endovascular technique to facilitate the introduction of aortic stent-grafts through stenosed iliac arteries. *J Endovasc Ther*. 2007;14:630–633.
14. Ferreira M, Katsargyris A, Rodrigues E, et al. "Snare-Ride": A bailout technique to catheterize target vessels with unfriendly anatomy in branched endovascular aortic repair. *J Endovasc Ther*. 2017;24:556–558.
15. Oikonomou K, Katsargyris A, Brinster CJ, et al. Retrograde target vessel catheterization as a salvage procedure in fenestrated/branched endografting. *J Endovasc Ther*. 2015;22:603–609.
16. Hertault A, Clough RE, Martin-Gonzalez T, et al. Translumbar puncture for retrograde catheterization of a kinked left renal stent after fenestrated endograft repair. *J Endovasc Ther*. 2016;23:976–981.
17. Erben Y, Oderich GS, Gloviczki P. The loop technique: addressing celiac artery dissection in a branched and fenestrated endograft for the treatment of a type III thoracoabdominal aneurysm. *J Endovasc Ther*. 2016;23:614–617.
18. Mastracci TM, Carrell T, Constantinou J, et al. Editor's choice - effect of branch stent choice on branch-related outcomes in complex aortic repair. *Eur J Vasc Endovasc Surg*. 2016;51:536–542.
19. Ertl M, Barinka F, Torka E, et al. Ocular color-coded sonography—a promising tool for neurologists and intensive care physicians. *Ultraschall Med*. 2014;35:422–431.
20. Reilly LM, Chuter TA. Reversal of fortune: induced endoleak to resolve neurological deficit after endovascular repair of thoracoabdominal aortic aneurysm. *J Endovasc Ther*. 2010;17:21–29.
21. Eagleton MJ, Follansbee M, Wolski K, et al. Fenestrated and branched endovascular aneurysm repair outcomes for type II and III thoracoabdominal aortic aneurysms. *J Vasc Surg*. 2016;63:930–942.
22. Verhoeven EL, Katsargyris A, Bekkema F, et al. Editor's Choice - Ten-year experience with endovascular repair of thoracoabdominal aortic aneurysms: results from 166 consecutive patients. *Eur J Vasc Endovasc Surg*. 2015;49:524–531.

16

Complications of EVAR With Snorkels, Chimneys, and Sandwich Techniques

Gianluca Faggioli, MD, PhD, Enrico Gallitto, MD, PhD and Mauro Gargiulo, MD, PhD

BACKGROUND

The chimney technique (Ch-EVAR) allows off-the-shelf endovascular repair of complex aortic pathologies involving the visceral arteries, such as aneurysms involving the juxtarenal (Fig. 16.1), pararenal, and thoracoabdominal aorta and the aortic arch (Fig. 16.2). First described by Greenberg et al.[1], Ch-EVAR was reported as a bailout procedure to maintain renal artery patency in case of unintended coverage during standard endovascular aneurysm repair. Bare or covered stents are deployed into visceral branches parallel to the main aortic endograft in order to achieve a cranial extension of the proximal sealing zone with preservation of renal or splanchnic arteries.[1,2] A periscope graft is a distally oriented Ch-EVAR that allows retrograde flow into an aortic side branch.[3] The sandwich technique first deploys a tubular endograft to create an artificial proximal neck, which is intended to accommodate the proximal end of the Ch-EVAR in its lumen.[3] A second aortic endograft is then overlapped to the first in order to repair the underlying diseased aorta.[3] With this technique, Ch-EVAR remains eventually sandwiched between the two aortic endografts.[3] It was initially described to preserve the hypogastric artery and later for visceral arteries in thoracoabdominal aortic aneurysm.[3,4]

Urgent aortic cases unfit for open repair and fenestrated-branched endografting because of manufacturing delays[5,6] can be managed by these techniques, if an adequate sealing zone is absent. In some centers, Ch-EVAR is considered a possible first-line treatment, even in elective cases.[3] The available literature on chimney/periscope/sandwich techniques is mainly about case reports and single-center series with a limited number of patients and little follow-up data. Furthermore, patients have been treated with a variety of off-the-shelf devices and different follow-up protocols, leading to a difficult overall analysis of the procedure.[7] The largest worldwide Ch-EVAR experience was published in 2015 by Donas et al. with data on 898 snorkel stents placed in 517 patients, resulting in a technical success rate of 97.1%, elective 30-day mortality of 3.6%, and primary branch vessel patency of 94% at a mean follow-up of 17.1 months.[7]

PREOPERATIVE ISSUES

Choice of Device

A variety of combinations of different materials have been used to achieve satisfactory results with this technique. Mestres et al. have shown that results in terms of apposition, stent compression, and in-folding may vary between different combinations. Endografts with a low radial force behave better in terms of apposition and stent compression but are at higher risk of in-folding. As a matter of fact, the risk of endograft in-folding is maximum if a 40% oversize is applied to a low-radial force endograft, such as the Excluder (Gore, W. L. Gore, Flagstaff, Arizona) endograft. On the other hand, this kind of endograft allows lower stent compression, and this is particularly evident when parallel stent grafts with low radial force (Viabahn, W. L. Gore, Flagstaff, Arizona) are used. By using a greater radial force main endograft, such as the Endurant (Medtronic, Santa Rosa, California) together with the Viabhan device, a significant stent compression is more likely to occur. The best combination in terms of endograft and stent apposition is achieved with an oversize of 30% of the Excluder endograft, with the Advanta V12 (Atrium/Maquet, Hudson, New Hampshire) parallel stent graft, which are characterized by a greater radial force.[8]

Recently, the CE mark for Ch-EVAR procedures has been assigned to the Endurant device, following publication of the PROTAGORAS study.[9] In that study, 128 patients were treated with a combination of Endurant device and Advanta or Viabahn parallel stent grafts, with a technical success of 100% and only 1.6% Type I endoleak needing a second procedure. At a mean follow-up time of 24.6 ± 17.4 months, a 93.1% freedom from chimney graft-related reinterventions was achieved[9], indicating that this technique may be effective in the mid-term, even if the long-term outcome is yet to be assessed.

INTRAOPERATIVE/EARLY COMPLICATIONS

Technical Failure: Target Visceral Vessels Loss/Lesions/Early Occlusions

Inability to cannulate and stenting target visceral vessels (TVVs) cause an intraoperative TVV loss. As a result of manipulations with guidewires, catheters, balloons, and stent/stent graft, TVVs lesions such as dissection, rupture, or thrombosis are possible.[3] The use of stiff guidewires with a short soft tip (i.e., Rosen or Amplatz guidewire: Cook, Bloomington, Indiana) is advantageous once access has been obtained in order to gain sufficient stability for insertion of the stent graft in the visceral arteries, without causing excessive endothelial trauma to their distal segment.[3] Ruptures or dissections of distal renal artery branches with subsequent hemorrhage or parenchymal infarct may occur, as well as intestinal bleeding or ischemia.[3] The consequences of these complications are variable but clearly can be fatal. Undesired coverage of aortic side branches can also occur in case of imprecise planning or intraoperative technical problems. Accidental coverage of target visceral vessels by stent graft can occur as a result of planning or intraoperative errors (Fig. 16.3).

A recent literature[3] review reports a risk of 1% TVV-loss in Ch-EVAR for abdominal/thoracoabdominal aneurysms and arch pathologies, leading to an overall early TVV-patency of Ch-EVAR of 97%–99%. Acute TVV occlusion can be either symptomatic or asymptomatic; however, when occurring in the superior mesenteric artery, it can easily cause fatal massive bowel ischemia. Alternatively, renal

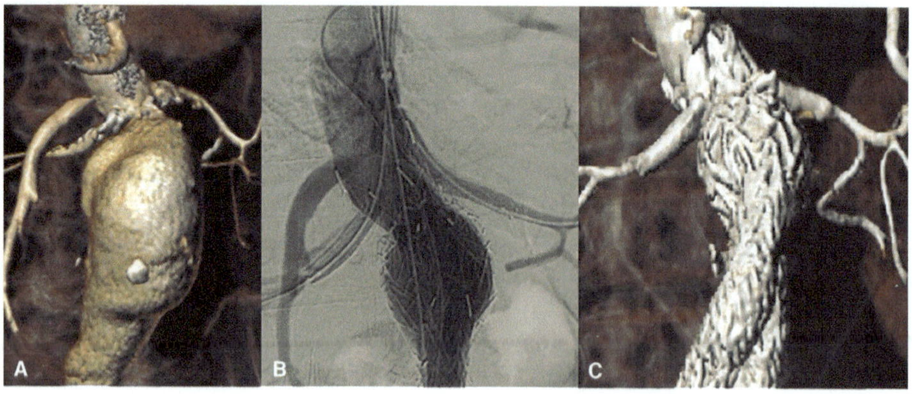

Fig. 16.1 Example of double chimney technique for endovascular treatment of a juxtarenal aneurysm. (A) Preoperative computed tomography angiography with volume rendering reconstruction of the juxtarenal aneurysm. (B, C) Completion angiography and of volume rendering reconstruction of the double chimney technique for renal arteries perfusion and complete aneurysm coverage.

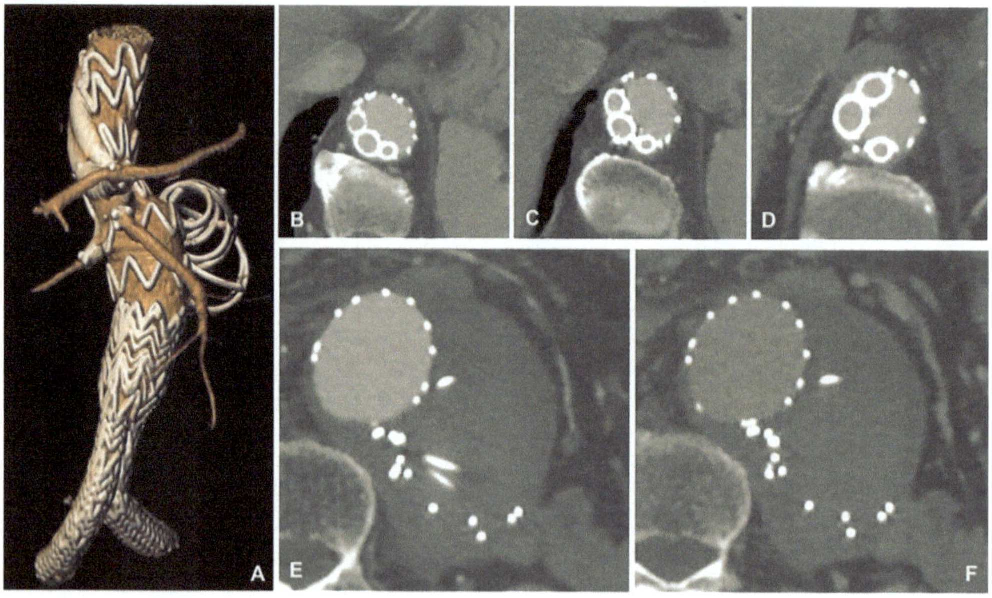

Fig. 16.2 Postoperative computed tomography angiography of a pararenal aneurysm repair with triple chimney for the celiac trunk, the superior mesenteric the artery, and right renal artery. (A) Volume rendering reconstruction. (B, C, D) Axial cuts show patency of the chimney stent grafts and the absence of gutters. (E, F) Axial cuts show the aneurysm exclusion in both arterial and venous acquisition.

artery occlusion may cause worsening of the renal function and necessitate permanent dialysis when occurring bilaterally or in patients with single kidneys, or it may remain completely asymptomatic.[3] Extraanatomic bypass has been extensively reported in the treatment of target visceral failures.[3,14]

GUTTERS/PROXIMAL TYPE I ENDOLEAK

A critical issue for Ch-EVAR is the presence of gutters, defined as channels between the visceral and the main aortic endografts, causing Type I–III endoleak and failure of excluding the aneurysm sac.[10] Gutters are described as a lack of apposition between the main body of the endograft, the chimney stent graft, and the aortic wall, and can be classified according to their location.[11] Type A gutters originate at the proximal fabric of the endograft, Type B are determined by apposition failure between the chimney stent graft and the branch vessel and Type C are those starting below the fabric of the endograft.[9]

Independently of their origin, postprocedural Type I–III endoleaks are frequently reported and can be considered the Achilles' heel of all parallel graft strategies. Proximal Type I endoleaks occur in approximately 13% of cases (range 0%–33%) of juxtarenal or pararenal and TAAA and 11% (range 0%–44%) of thoracic arch treated with Ch-EVAR.[3] They can be stratified into high-flow endoleaks, which appear immediately after contrast injection, and low-flow endoleaks, which appear after some delay[10] (Fig. 16.4). The latter may be compatible with hemorrhage control even in patients with ruptured aneurysms and usually disappear during early follow-up when normal coagulative parameters are restored. Visceral Type I endoleaks have been observed in as many as 70% of cases, with subsequent spontaneous sealing.[3,12] High flow Type I–III endoleaks are potentially fatal in cases of aortic

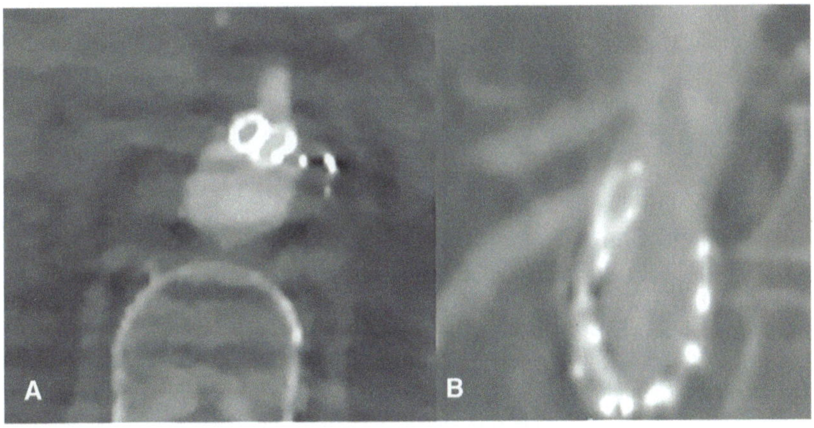

Fig. 16.3 Postoperative computed tomography angiography of a double chimney for the renal arteries. In axial (A) and sagittal (B) views, one of the main possible drawbacks of this technique is shown: the stent grafts for renal arteries lie directly in front of the origin of the superior mesenteric artery, with possible lumen obstruction.

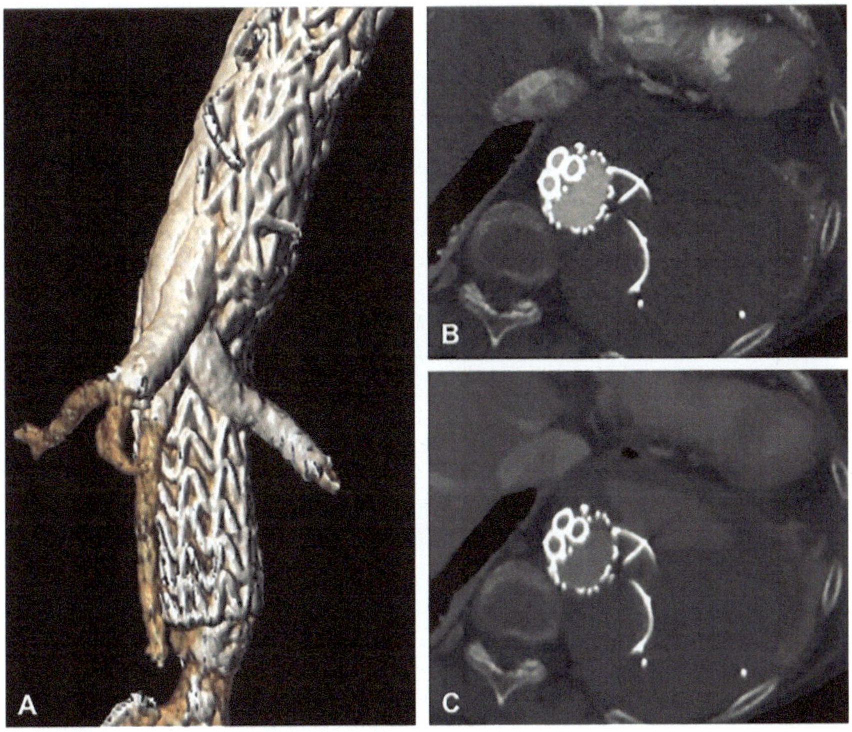

Fig. 16.4 Postoperative computed tomography angiography of a triple chimney for celiac trunk, superior mesenteric artery, and left renal artery. The volume rendering reconstruction (A) and the axial cut in arterial acquisition (B) do not show any endoleak; however, an axial cut in venous acquisition shows a low-flow endoleak originating from the chimney's gutters (C).

rupture, as demonstrated by cases of AAA-related mortality after Ch-EVAR repair. Up to 30% of early postoperative imaging studies show the presence of gutter-related Type Ia endoleaks[12], with spontaneous resolution in 44.3%, 65.2%, and 88.4% of patients after 6, 12, and 18 months respectively, with secondary intervention required in only 3% of cases.[12] At a mean radiologic follow-up of 20.9 months, there were no differences in mean aneurysm sac size change between cases, with or without early Type Ia gutter endoleak.[12] The low number of gutter-related reinterventions required and the low rate of endoleaks associated with aneurysm sac growth lead to speculation that the natural history of Type I endoleak in Ch-EVAR may be more benign than initially expected.[3,12]

ACCESS-RELATED COMPLICATIONS/STROKE

Of patients submitted to Ch-EVAR, 6% to 8% have access related complications.[3] Complications include intraoperative stroke, iliac artery problems, bleeding, or pseudoaneurysm at the puncture site.[3] For a Ch-EVAR implant, an aortic arch navigation through an axillary/subclavian/brachial access is necessary. The presence of floating plaques or arch disease near the origin of supraaortic trunks enhance the perioperative risks of stroke and should be considered a contraindication to this technique. A postoperative stroke rate of 10% after Ch-EVAR was reported by Katsargyris et al.[13] in a literature review on juxtarenal aneurysm repair, significantly higher than that of fenestrated endograft (4%) or open surgery (0%).

Stenosis or Kinking of Visceral Stent Graft

Any visible stenosis or kinking of the visceral stent graft should be addressed aggressively at the time of implant, since it may lead to early or late acute thrombosis, with subsequent visceral ischemia. Ideally, wire access should be maintained in all visceral vessels treated until completion imaging confirms adequacy of seal and lack of kinking of stent grafts. If kinking or stenosis is seen, the parallel graft and the main aortic endograft should be treated with adjunctive dilatation performed with a kissing technique. If there is difficulty advancing the sheath with the dilator, a small balloon (i.e., 4 × 2) may be inflated and used as a dilator for the sheath by slowly deflating as the sheath is advanced. The main body is best addressed by compliant balloons such as Coda (Cook, Bloomington, Indiana) or Reliant (Medtronic, Santa Rosa, California), and the visceral chimney grafts are dilated simultaneously with semicompliant balloons, such as (Armada, Abbott, Illinois, or Evercross, ev3 Inc., Irvine, California).[14]

By this maneuver, both the main endograft and the chimneys can adapt to the aortic and visceral vessel anatomy and any possible extrinsic compressions eliminated or greatly reduced. Additionally, the risk of Type I endoleak is greatly reduced. A liberal use of adjunctive self-expandable bare metal stents (i.e., Protegé, ev3 Inc., Irvine, California, or Luminex, Murray Hill, New Jersey) should be considered in cases of residual stenosis or kinking of TVV after dilatation. Again, wire access should be maintained in all vessels until satisfactory imaging is achieved.

Stenosis of Native Visceral Vessels

Any stenosis of the native visceral vessel distal to the visceral stent graft should also be addressed aggressively with balloon angioplasty, either with or without drug eluting devices, and stent-graft relining, in order to maintain the patency of the chimney stent graft.

EARLY MORTALITY

According to a recent literature review[3], the 30-day mortality was 4% for juxta/pararenal/thoracoabdominal aneurysm (range 0%–10%) and 4% for thoracic arch (range 0%–17%).

FOLLOW-UP/LATE COMPLICATIONS

Large studies with long-term follow-up after Ch-EVAR are lacking. In a recent literature review, the mean follow-up ranged from 1 to 27 months, with a median of 17 months.[3] The reported overall mortality during follow-up differs among the studies, with a mean of 14% for visceral and 11% for thoracic arch Ch-EVAR.[3] Late proximal Type I endoleak was detected in 2% and 4% for visceral and aortic arch Ch-EVAR, respectively.[3]

Aneurysm shrinkage or stable aneurysm size was seen in 90% (range 71%–100%) and sac increase was reported in 11% (range 0%–29%).[3] Aneurysm rupture and TVV-occlusions are possible late complication of Ch-EVAR, but long-term data are presently not available.[12] The PERICLES registry reported a mean follow-up of 17 months, with an estimated patient survival and target visceral patency of 74.9% and 87.0%, respectively.[5]

Endoleak from Gutters

If a gutter connected with the aneurysm sack is detected, a guide and a 4- or 5-French catheter can be advanced from above in the space between the main aortic endograft and the visceral stent grafts. Through this route, micro-coils (Concerto, ev3 Inc., Irvine, California) and/or glue (Onyx, ev3 Inc., Irvine, California) can be released directly in the aneurysm sac. Additionally, this maneuver can be performed not only in the nidus, but along the gutter while retrieving the catheter, filling the space among the endografts, thus reducing the gutter space and the relative risk of low flow endoleaks.

ACUTE OCCLUSION OF VISCERAL STENT GRAFT

The critical issue in addressing this complication is to advance a guidewire in the target visceral vessel beyond the occlusion. Several options are possible dependent on the anatomy, timing of thrombosis onset, and the available materials. A 0.035, 0.018, or 0.014 guidewire can be used, according to the extension and firmness of the thrombus. A 4- or 5-French angiographic catheter can then be advanced into the occluded stent graft in order to infuse fibrinolytic drugs, such as urokinase or rtPA. The injection should be performed with an initial bolus of 100,000 IU, followed by continuous infusion for up 72 hours, with different infusion protocols according to the patient clinical characteristics. After lysis of the thrombus, it becomes quite easy to advance the guide in the native vessel and to reline all the stent graft with a new device. It is always preferable to use a new stent graft rather than a bare metal stent in order to trap all the residual thrombus. A critical issue is to detect the cause of the occlusion (stenosis of the TVV below the stent graft, acute angle between stent graft and native TVV) and to correct it.

Another available option, if the thrombosis is limited to a short segment and the guide can be advanced directly in the TVV, is to reline the whole previous stent graft directly with a self-expandable new stent graft, without the need for thrombolysis. With this approach, predilatation with a 3–4 mm balloon is usually necessary, but this should be done with extreme caution to minimize the risk of distal embolization.

Nowadays, different systems of thrombus-aspiration are also available, which are intended for the treatment of acute and subacute occlusions of arterial and venous vessels. The Angio-jet (Boston Scientific, Boston Scientific, Marlborough, Massachusetts) and Indigo (Penumbra, Alameda, California), although developed over different working principles, are both very effective in addressing this type of complication. The devices can be carefully advanced inside the occluded graft to remove the thrombus partially or totally inside the stent graft. After that, a complete relining is always recommended, because hidden clot material may lead to an acute early restenosis.

DISCONNECTION OF THE VISCERAL STENT GRAFT

This type of complication may occur when the origin of the visceral target vessel is at an excessive distance from the endograft and long or multiple stent grafts are necessary to achieve the revascularization. In these cases, if the aneurysm sac does not allow sufficient external support, the stent grafts can disconnect either distally or in their overlap zone, if multiple segments were used. The most difficult task in the relining procedure is to gain new access to the visceral vessel or to the disconnected stent grafts, because the misalignment may be very severe and stability of the guidewire and catheter may be a major issue. A high level of expertise with the use of coaxial sheaths or steerable guiding sheaths (Oscor, Destino 7 or 9 French, Palm Harbor, Florida) may be necessary in these cases because they overcome the instability of guide and simple catheters engaged in tortuous vessels.

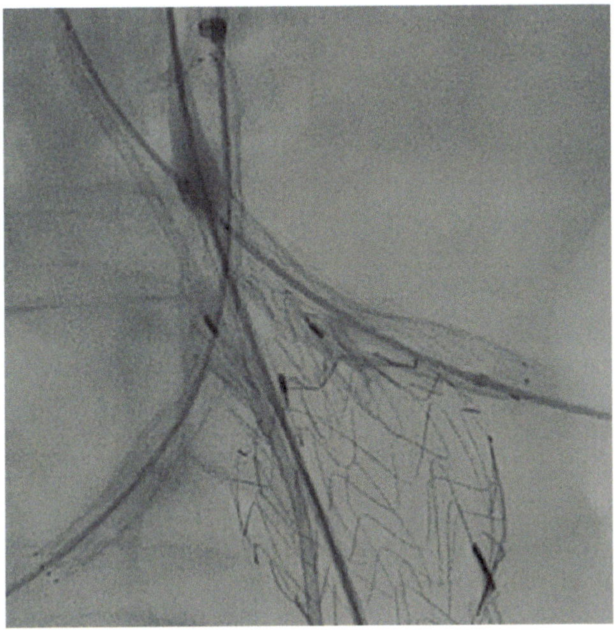

Fig. 16.5 Intraoperative image of a double chimney for the renal arteries. After deploying balloon-expandable stent graft as chimney for the renal artery, a bilateral relining was performed with self-expandable bare metal stents in order to avoid stenosis or kinking and ensure long-term patency.

PREVENTION AND TREATMENT

The most important recommendation is to prevent complications. In this sense, accurate and meticulous planning is crucial. While a certain degree of arterial branch disease can be accepted when planning this technique, a target artery should be free from major disease and have a minimal diameter of 4 mm and a safe landing zone of at least 1 cm. The choice of adequate materials, with different combinations depending on the surgeon's preferences, and appropriate sizing are also of paramount importance. Conformable endografts such as ePTFE covered nitinol stents (i.e., Gore C3 Excluder or Tag +Viabahn, Gore, W. L. Gore, Flagstaff, Arizona) are usually preferred in our experience because, despite their lesser radial force, they are more adaptable in difficult anatomies. Measurement and planning of a chimney graft can be performed with a variety of methods, considering elliptic models, vessel areas (especially for a barrel/sandwich technique) or simply calculating an oversize of about 30%.[15–18] The overlap length between the CPGs and the main aortic graft is another important issue.[15–18]

To achieve adequate sealing between the CPGs, the main aortic graft, and the aortic wall, an overlap of ~4 cm is required in order to minimize Type I endoleaks and gutters, although this may not always be anatomically feasible.[15–18] The number of chimney grafts should be kept to a minimum because the risk of gutters and ELI is directly correlated with it. Procedures with four chimney grafts are associated with a risk of ELI significantly greater compared with 3, 2 or 1 chimney grafts.[15–18] Relining of visceral stent grafts by self-expandable bare metal stents is required in cases of stenosis or kinking in order to maintain the patency (Fig. 16.5). Again, conformable nitinol stents are preferred in order to achieve a good adaptability, although extrinsic compression by calcified plaques may require the use of higher radial force stents.

TIP BOX 16.1

- Accurate planning with adequate oversizing
- Appropriate material choice
- Possible interaction with the origin of other visceral vessels should be considered

WARNING BOX 16.1

- Consider access-related risks particularly when approaching from the aortic arch
- Be prepared to extend both the visceral stent and the aortic endograft
- A greater number of visceral artery stent grafts increases the risk of gutters and endoleaks

REFERENCES

1. Greenberg RK, Clair D, Srivastava S, et al. Should patients with challenging anatomy be offered endovascular aneurysm repair? *J Vasc Surg.* 2003;38:990–996.
2. Criado FJ. Chimney grafts and bare stents: aortic branch preservation revisited. *J Endovasc Ther.* 2007;14:823–824.
3. Lindblad B, Bin Jabr A, Holst J, Malina M. Chimney grafts in aortic stent grafting: hazardous or useful technique? Systematic review of current data. *Eur J Vasc Endovasc Surg.* 2015;50. 722e731.
4. Lobato AC, Camacho-Lobato L. A new technique to enhance endovascular thoracoabdominal aortic aneurysm therapy—the sandwich procedure. *Semin Vasc Surg.* 2012;25(3):153–160.
5. Gallitto E, Gargiulo M, Freyrie A, et al. The endovascular treatment of juxta-renal abdominal aortic aneurysm using fenestrated endograft: early and mid-term results. *J Cardiovasc Surg (Torino).* 2015.
6. Gallitto E, Gargiulo M, Freyrie A, et al. Endovascular repair of thoracoabdominal aortic aneurysm in high-surgical risk patients: fenestrated and branched endografts. *Ann Vasc Surg.* 2017;40:170–177.
7. Donas KP, Lee JT, Lachat M, Torsello G, Veith FJ. PERICLES investigators. Collected world experience about the performance of the snorkel/chimney endovascular technique in the treatment of complex aortic pathologies: the PERICLES registry. *Ann Surg.* 2015;262(3): 546–553.
8. Mestres G, Uribe JP, Garcia-Madrid C, et al. The best conditions for parallel stenting during EVAR: an in vitro study. *Eur J Vasc Endovasc Surg.* 2012;44:468–473.
9. Donas KP, Torsello GB, Piccoli G, et al. The PROTAGORAS study to evaluate the performance of the Endurant stent graft for patients with pararenal pathologic processes treated by the chimney/snorkel endovascular technique. *J Vasc Surg.* 2016;63:1–7.
10. Donas KP, Criado FJ, Torsello G, Veith FJ, Minion DJ. PERICLES Registry Collaborators. classification of chimney evar-related endoleaks: insights from the PERICLES registry. *J Endovasc Ther.* 2017;24(1): 72–74.
11. Overeem SP, Boersen JT, Schuurmann RCL, et al. Classification of gutter type in parallel stenting during endovascular aortic aneurysm repair. *J Vasc Surg.* 2017;66(2):594–599.
12. Ullery BW, Tran K, Itoga NK, Dalman RL, Lee JT. Natural history of gutter-related type Ia endoleaks after snorkel/chimney endovascular aneurysm repair. *J Vasc Surg.* 2017;65:981–990.
13. Katsargyris A, Oikonomou K, Klonaris C, Töpel I, Verhoeven EL. Comparison of outcomes with open, fenestrated, and chimney graft repair of juxtarenal aneurysms: are we ready for a paradigm shift? *J Endovasc Ther.* 2013;20(2):159–169.
14. Usai MV, Torsello G, Donas KP. Current evidence regarding chimney graft occlusions in the endovascular treatment of pararenal aortic

pathologies: a systematic review with pooled data analysis. *J Endovasc Ther.* 2015;22(3):396–400. Epub April 15, 2015. Review.
15. Lachat M, Veith FJ, Pfammatter T, et al. Chimney and periscope grafts observed over 2 years after their use to revascularize 169 renovisceral branches in 77 patients with complex aortic aneurysms. *J Endovasc Ther.* 2013;20(5):597–605.
16. Schiro A, Antoniou GA, Ormesher D, Pichel AC, Farquharson F, Serracino-Inglott F. The chimney technique in endovascular aortic aneurysm repair: late ruptures after successful single renal chimney stent grafts. *Ann Vasc Surg.* 2013;27(7):835–843.
17. Tolenaar JL, Zandvoort HJ, Moll FL, van Herwaarden JA. Technical considerations and results of chimney grafts for the treatment of juxtarenal aneursyms. *J Vasc Surg.* 2013;58(3):607–615.
18. Moulakakis KG, Mylonas SN, Avgerinos E, et al. The chimney graft technique for preserving visceral vessels during endovascular treatment of aortic pathologies. *J Vasc Surg.* 2012;55(5):1497–1503.

17

Endoleaks

Marc L. Schermerhorn, MD, FACS and Thomas F.X. O'Donnell, MD

OVERVIEW

Endoleaks, or persistent flow into the aneurysm sac, are the most common complication of EVAR, occurring in up to a third of cases.[1] They occur at the time of graft implantation, or arise during followup, with varying implications. The Society for Vascular Surgery classifies endoleaks into five categories (Fig. 17.1)[2]:

Type I. Attachment site endoleak
- IA. Proximal attachment site endoleak
- IB. Distal attachment site endoleak

Type II (the most common). Back-filling of the aneurysm sac through branch vessels of the aorta
- IIA. Single causative vessel (often referred to as a "to-and-fro" endoleak)
- IIB. Multiple involved vessels

Type III. Graft defect or component misalignment
- IIIA. Leaks from junctions of the endograft components
- IIIB. Leak from fabric tear/disruption

Type IV. Leakage through the graft itself caused by the porosity of some endografts

Type V. Also called endotension, Type V endoleaks are poorly understood, but thought to result from aortic pressure transmitted through the graft or thrombus to the aneurysm sac.

Most endoleaks seen on completion angiogram mandate attempts at correction prior to leaving the operating room. Notable exceptions are most Type II endoleaks, which often resolve as the vessels thrombose over time, and Type IV endoleaks, which resolve with cessation of heparinization. However, surgeons must pay particular attention to completion angiograms, as Type IV endoleaks appear very similar to Type I. Type II endoleaks discovered at follow-up can often be observed as long as they are not associated with significant sac expansion (defined as ≥5 mm).[3] Late Type I or Type III endoleaks, however, almost universally require intervention. While the aneurysm sac remains excluded from aortic pressure, it weakens and atrophies. This atrophic sac is at increased risk of rupture from a high-pressure leak such as a Type I or Type III.

TYPE IA ENDOLEAKS

Intraoperative

Type Ia endoleaks result from inadequate seal at the proximal attachment site (the neck). Type Ia endoleaks that occur at the time of the operation usually result from unsuitable anatomy. Consequently, careful preoperative planning may help avoid many of these complications (Box 17.1). Surgeons should ensure an adequate neck length of at least 15 mm, preferably without significant calcification (>50% of the diameter of the vessel), neck angulation (>60 degrees), or conical shape (increase in size from proximal to distal). Short or angulated necks, or segments of aorta without parallel walls, benefit from fenestrated, custom-made, surgeon-modified endografts, or open repair. Although the instructions for use (IFU) of many devices include neck lengths as short as 10 mm, the advent of fenestrated devices obviated the need to push the tolerances of prior devices. As such, we rarely deploy standard endografts in these marginal cases, even within the IFU. In addition, although the IFU for many devices include neck diameters of up to 32 mm, such wide necks represent early aneurysmal degeneration (Box 17.2). Even if no Type Ia occurs at the time of implant, one often develops over time as the neck continues to expand, creating a potentially life-threatening leak. Fortunately, surgeons can rely on a range of alternative strategies to deal with unsuitable necks, from fenestrated, snorkel, custom-made, or surgeon-modified devices to traditional open repair. Short or wide necks are situations in which other options such as open surgery or fenestrated, scalloped or snorkel devices should be considered. In our practice, we rarely place grafts wider than 32 mm below the renal arteries.

If a Type Ia endoleak does occur at the time of the initial procedure, many will resolve with ballooning of the seal zone using a compliant, molding balloon such as a Coda (Cook Medical, Bloomington, Indiana) or Reliant (Medtronic, Santa Rosa, California). If ballooning is unsuccessful, the next step is to place an aortic cuff if there is an adequate landing zone (>5 mm). Some advocate placing a giant Palmaz stent (Cordis Corp., Bridgewater, New Jersey) if a cuff fails to resolve the leak, but many centers (including ours) now avoid placing Palmaz stents except in special circumstances such as an incompletely deployed stent. A Palmaz rarely succeeds long-term. In addition, should the Palmaz fail to resolve the leak, its tight mesh complicates further endovascular maneuvers such as deploying a fenestrated cuff. Placement of an aortic cuff or a giant Palmaz stent should be followed by additional ballooning of the landing zone. In our practice, if ballooning and/or an aortic cuff are unsuccessful, we reinforce the landing zone using the Heli-FX EndoAnchor (Aptus Endosystems, Sunnyvale, California). EndoAnchors (also known as screws) should be avoided in heavily calcified necks, because the screws will not penetrate the calcium and will actually push the graft away from the aortic wall.

At this point, should a leak persist, the surgeon must assess the quality of the leak and consider whether the leak requires immediate action. After the above maneuvers, the only option available during the index procedure (although almost never used) is open conversion, as any further endovascular therapies require planning time. Fortunately, most leaks can be observed for a limited time while further action is planned and we avoid open conversion during the index case except for the rarest of circumstances. One particularly challenging scenario is an undersized graft. If the initial graft is undersized, then unfortunately screws (and likely most endovascular maneuvers) rarely succeed. To deal with a proximal endoleak with an undersized graft, some surgeons place a new cuff and parallel grafts in chimney fashion, although we prefer custom-made or surgeon-modified fenestration. Some may require conversion to open. Large or even moderate leaks need further intervention, but

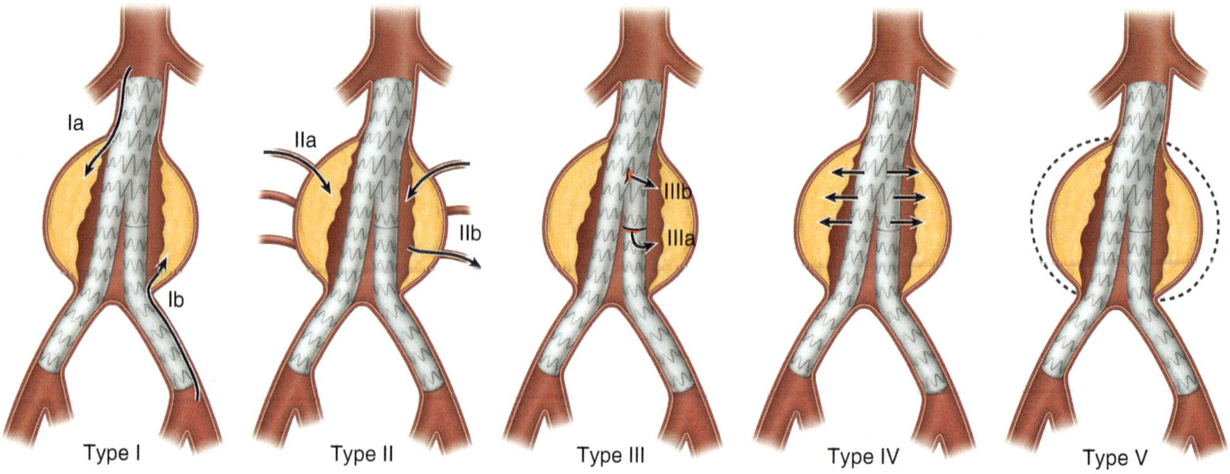

Fig. 17.1 Endoleak types. Type Ia (proximal attachment site); Type Ib (distal attachment site); Type IIa (single back-bleeding vessel); Type IIb (multiple back-bleeding vessels); Type IIIa (graft junctions); Type IIIb (fabric tear); Type IV (graft porosity); Type V (endotension).

TIP BOX 17.1

The most important factor in the prevention of endoleaks is careful preoperative planning.

WARNING BOX 17.1

Although the instructions for use for many devices allow up to a 32 mm neck, we do not advise sealing into a neck this size because it probably represents early aneurysmal degeneration and carries significant risk of late Type IA endoleak.

many small gutter leaks will resolve after reversal of heparinization.[4] Some surgeons will follow these smaller leaks with serial computed tomography (CT) scans at frequent intervals (1 month, 6 months, and 1 year if the endoleak persists). Moderate to large leaks, or those that fail to resolve in serial followup, require further intervention.

In recent years, the armamentarium of the modern vascular surgeon increased dramatically. Subsequent efforts to correct a proximal endoleak should take into account the surgeon's familiarity with these novel techniques, as well as the anatomy of the surgical neck. If there is an adequate seal zone above the newly-placed endograft or cuff, the surgeon can place another cuff or place a second EVAR device. If there is no seal zone below the renal arteries, the Cook Z-Fen (Cook Medical, Bloomington, Indiana) can extend the seal zone above the renal arteries. However, commercially available Z-Fen devices taper to 24 mm and extend at least 5 cm distally toward the bifurcation (and longer lengths for grafts greater than 24 mm to allow for a flaring cuff), which limit its ability to deploy within most pre-existing EVAR. An alternative strategy is placement of a Z-Fen cuff and then an aorto-uni-iliac (AUI) device. This avoids the space issue, but requires a subsequent femorofemoral bypass. Consequently, the most commonly applied therapy in our hands is the physician-modified endograft (PMEG). A custom-modified body of a Cook Alpha device (Cook Medical, Bloomington, Indiana) avoids the aforementioned problems with the Z-Fen, because it is shorter and does not taper down. However, these devices are still experimental and should be only be used by surgeons experienced in their use and with approval from their institution's Institutional Review Board. Currently, PMEGs are performed under an Investigational Device Exemption and/or after a thorough discussion with the patient concerning the off-label modification of an endograft. In limited series and anecdotal reports, perioperative mortality following PMEG is lower than open conversion, but long-term durability remains unknown.

If these rescue maneuvers fail to resolve the leak, the surgeon can convert to open repair (Fig. 17.2). Open conversion should not be undertaken lightly, as it carries substantial morbidity and mortality (10% rate of death within 30 days).[5] The two primary approaches are to explant the device and perform a traditional open repair or to band the proximal neck with felt pledgets. Often the iliac limbs are left in place at the time of open conversion.

Late

Late Type Ia endoleaks result from graft slippage or aneurysmal degeneration at the seal zone. Consequently, the surgeon should approach such a late endoleak as if it were a second aneurysm. These endoleaks are high risk for rupture. While the EVAR successfully excluded the aneurysm sac from aortic pressure, the sac atrophies. If this weakened sac is exposed to the high pressure of a proximal leak, aortic rupture may result. Most of these late Type Ia endoleaks require the placement of an aortic cuff; conversion to fenestrated, snorkeled, or branched device; or conversion to open repair.

TYPE Ib ENDOLEAKS

Type Ib endoleaks result from an inadequate seal at the distal landing zone (the common iliac artery in the case of a nonaneurysmal common iliac artery or the external iliac artery in the case of a common iliac artery aneurysm). Most Type Ib endoleaks occur in common iliac aneurysms. As with proximal endoleaks, preoperative planning is crucial. Surgeons must familiarize themselves with the anatomy of the patient's pelvic circulation including the patency of their hypogastric arteries in case one or more need to be occluded during the case.

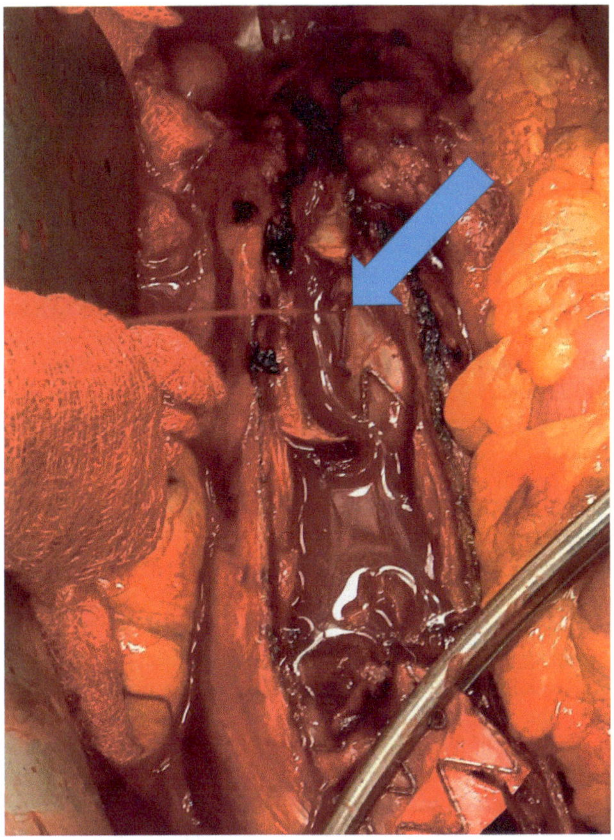

Fig. 17.2 Open conversion with graft explantation for Type III endoleak *(blue arrow)*.

In patients with common iliac aneurysms, we advocate placing an iliac branch device or endoprosthesis (IBD/IBE) whenever possible. The decision to place these devices needs to occur preoperatively. The IFU limits their applicability to a small proportion of patients and once another iliac limb is placed, conversion to an IBE is quite difficult. If a patient's anatomy is unsuitable for a branched device, surgeons should coil/plug the ipsilateral hypogastric artery and extend down into the external iliac artery. As with large (32 mm) proximal necks, iliac arteries over 2 cm should be considered aneurysmal and surgeons should avoid sealing into them if possible (despite the availability of iliac limbs up to 27 mm). Bilateral common iliac artery aneurysms present a challenge if neither side meets the IFU for an IBE, as bilateral hypogastric artery coiling should be avoided if at all possible. In patients who may rely on their pelvic circulation, such as patients undergoing coverage of a substantial portion of aorta, or those who previously underwent TEVAR, sealing into the iliac aneurysm with a larger iliac limb (such as a 27 mm) preserves flow into the hypogastric artery. Although this strategy risks a late Type Ib endoleak and is not a long-term solution, it remains preferable to inciting pelvic or spinal cord ischemia. These patients warrant close monitoring and may eventually need reintervention.

If a Type Ib endoleak occurs at the time of initial implantation, the first adjunctive maneuver should be ballooning with a compliant balloon. Surgeons should take care to balloon gently if the graft limb is placed into aneurysmal iliac artery. If more than 5 mm of distal landing zone remains, an extension should be placed. Without an adequate landing zone, the surgeon must consider the patency and adequacy of the contralateral hypogastric artery. If the cross-pelvic circulation is sufficient, the ipsilateral hypogastric artery can be sacrificed and the landing zone extended into the external iliac artery. Most surgeons prefer to place an Amplatzer II plug (St. Jude Medical, St. Paul, Minnesota) and/or a series of coils.

For patients reliant on their ipsilateral hypogastric artery and not eligible for IBE, we prefer to seal into the aneurysmal common iliac artery and follow the patients closely. They may eventually require reintervention, but Type Ib endoleaks and eventual reintervention are easier to manage than pelvic insufficiency or spinal cord ischemia. For particularly challenging anatomy, the next step is to deploy an AUI device with femorofemoral bypass and contralateral common iliac occlusion. Contralateral common iliac occlusion can be achieved through use of an Amplatzer II plug (St. Jude Medical, St. Paul, Minnesota) and/or coils. For larger iliac arteries (the largest Amplatzer available is 22 mm), you can make your own by tying off the end of a stent graft or making a "candy plug." A candy plug is a stent graft in which the middle portion of the graft is sutured in purse-string fashion using a permanent suture to narrow the lumen, leaving adequate room to remove the delivery system. This modified stent graft is then deployed into the iliac artery and an Amplatzer deployed into the narrowed region. Usually this can be avoided by extending into the external iliac artery. Alternatively, if the contralateral hypogastric artery is important for pelvic blood flow, a flexible stent graft (e.g. Viabahn, W.L. Gore, Flagstaff, Arizona) may be placed retrograde from the external iliac artery into the hypogastric artery, excluding the common iliac artery while maintaining hypogastric patency. Although historically considered benign, buttock claudication and pelvic insufficiency, even unilaterally, are often disabling and associated with poor patient-reported outcomes. For patients who develop disabling pelvic insufficiency, surgeons can consider an external iliac artery to hypogastric artery bypass.

TYPE III ENDOLEAK

Type III endoleaks should be considered a technical failure and require immediate intervention. The most important factor in avoiding Type III endoleaks is careful preoperative planning ensuring adequate component overlap. Junctional Type III endoleaks usually result from inadequate overlap. If a Type IIIa endoleak occurs despite adequate component overlap, we balloon the junction with a compliant balloon and then a noncompliant balloon. If this fails to resolve the leak, we typically adopt a watchful waiting approach and follow this at the 1-month scan as long as we are confident there is enough overlap. In the case of marginal overlap, the treatment consists of placing an additional component to bridge and to reinforce the junction. Rarely, we would consider placing a balloon-expandable stent at the junction if the flow is such that we are confident it will not thrombose. Alternatively, this could be done as a secondary intervention at a later time if the leak persists. Similarly, fabric defects (Type IIIb endoleaks) require deployment of additional components inside the endograft in the defective region. Sometimes, Type IIIb endoleaks occur at areas that preclude relining, such as the bifurcation. In these situations, surgeons can convert to an AUI bypass. If a Type IIIb occurs but the origin cannot be easily localized, we place a new cuff and then advance the bifurcation with two new iliac limbs essentially to reline the endograft. Advancing the bifurcation allows improved coverage and additional overlap. Before relining a graft, surgeons must ensure that doing so would still allow adequate room to convert to an AUI if the relining process fails to address the endoleak adequately. If this occurs, an AUI is the next bailout maneuver and surgeons must therefore ensure they keep their options open.

TYPE IV ENDOLEAK

Many modern endografts, such as the Medtronic Excluder II (Medtronic Vascular Inc, Santa Rosa, California), are slightly porous and commonly demonstrate Type IV endoleaks on completion angiogram. These endoleaks resolve with cessation of heparinization, but must be distinguished from Type I or Type III endoleaks before concluding they are benign. By definition, Type IV endoleaks do not persist and a leak seen at one month should be considered a Type I or Type III.

TYPE V ENDOLEAK (ENDOTENSION)

Type V endoleaks are sac enlargement without evidence of an endoleak. This poorly understood phenomenon is thought to be caused by aortic pressure transmitted through either the graft or thrombus to the sac. At our institution, we treat these leaks as if they were Type Ia endoleaks if the seal zone appears marginal, using aortic cuffs, PMEG, or open conversion if necessary. Often, these endoleaks are Type I or II, but poorly visualized.

TYPE II ENDOLEAK

Type II endoleaks are the most common endoleak seen on either completion angiogram or at followup, complicating up to 20% of cases. These endoleaks almost never require intervention at the time of initial implant, but require intervention at follow-up if associated with aneurysm sac growth of at least 5 mm. The most common vessels involved are the inferior mesenteric artery (IMA), lumbar arteries, and accessory renal arteries. Occasionally, in the setting of a large, patent vessel, surgeons may elect to embolize prophylactically one or more of these vessels prior to deploying their graft. In our practice, we embolize accessory renal arteries if they come off the sac itself or close to the seal zone. Accessory renal arteries coming off the neck rarely require embolization because they will likely thrombose once excluded by the proximal seal zone. Occasionally, we elect to embolize a large IMA or particularly large lumbar, but more often these can be monitored because many will thrombose on their own. Alternatively, some surgeons opt to embolize the sac pre-emptively in patients with multiple large branches (>4 lumbar, patent IMA >3 mm, large patent aortic lumen), deemed high risk for developing Type II endoleak. This is accomplished by leaving a wire/catheter in the sac at the time of graft deployment and then deploying coils through the catheter once the endograft has been fully deployed, but not yet ballooned.

Ongoing research examines the potential benefit of eliminating the aneurysm sac with endovascular aneurysm sealing (EVAS) using devices such as the Nellix (Endologix, Irvine, California). The Nellix obliterates the aneurysm sac by deploying hydrogel-filled (*see* Chapter 10: Nellix) EndoBags, which may reduce the rate of Type II endoleaks, as well as blunt the postimplantation inflammatory response associated with sac thrombosis.[6]

If a Type II endoleak associated with an expanding aneurysm sac is present, the modern vascular surgeon has a dizzying array of potential solutions. Importantly, however, one must diligently rule out Type I or III endoleaks prior to intervening on what may appear to be a Type II. Even with patent lumbar arteries, accessory renal arteries, or IMA, if the nidus of the leak abuts the graft, it is crucial to rule out a Type I or III leak prior to assuming the leak is from the patent vessel. Indeed, intervening on a Type II leak in the setting of a Type I or III leak can precipitate rupture, because the patent feeder vessel may have been providing antegrade decompression of the sac. Typically, this is best done through catheter-based aortography. One helpful diagnostic maneuver is to balloon-occlude the iliac arteries to obstruct the outflow. This often helps identify leaks that are not readily identifiable on standard antegrade angiography.

Although novel therapeutic options increased the number of approaches to treat these endoleaks, the advent of fusion imaging represents the most important advance. CT road-mapping technology allows surgeons to identify the nidus of the endoleak, precisely plan their interventions and guide therapeutic maneuvers (Fig. 17.3).

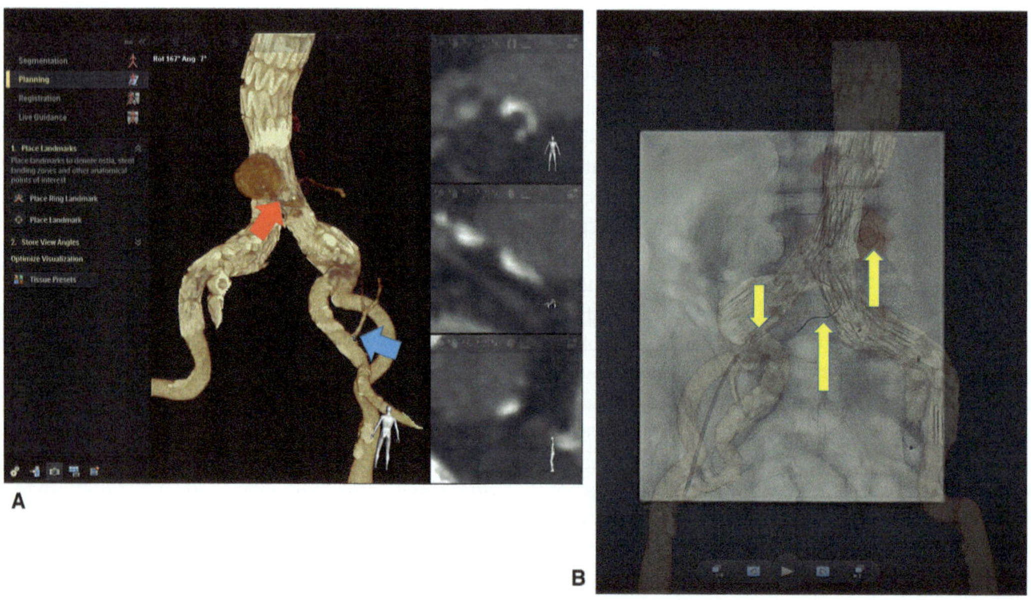

A

B

Fig. 17.3 Use of CT road mapping to embolize a Type II endoleak from a lumbar artery. (A) Fusion imaging demonstrates the endoleak *(red arrow)* and allows the surgeon to chart preoperatively an approach through the left hypogastric artery *(blue arrow)* and iliolumbar artery. (B) Intraoperative imaging using fusion technology. *Yellow arrows* show the culprit lesion accessed via the preplanned route, ready to deploy coils. We place a 5-French Ansel sheath into the hypogastric artery with a 4-French angled Glidecath aiming superiorly to enter the posterior branch of the hypogastric artery and use the iliolumbar, superior gluteal, or lateral sacral artery to follow up to the segmental lumbar artery. In a telescoping fashion, a microcatheter and a 0.014″ wire were advanced into the sac.

TIP BOX 17.2

Transcaval approach

For transcaval coiling of Type II endoleaks, use CT road mapping to select an area where the cava, but not the endograft, is well opposed to the aneurysm sac, and advance the needle SLOWLY. We use the Rosch-Uchida Transjugular Liver Access Set (Cook Medical, Bloomington, Indiana) and apply extra curvature near the tip using the metal stiffening cannula in place to facilitate orthogonal penetration of the cava and aorta. We first shape the stiffening cannula with the Check-Flo introducer and 10-French catheter mounted on it. After obtaining wire access, we place the stiffening cannula, introducer, and catheter and remove the wire. We direct the stiffening cannula toward the aorta, then insert the 5-French catheter and trocar stylet through the stiffening cannular to the end of the dilator and carefully advance the catheter and trocar stylet through the caval and aortic walls. Exquisite care must be taken to avoid puncturing the graft. We then remove the trocar stylet and blood return indicates successful engagement of the nidus, which can be confirmed with gentle hand contrast injection. 3D road mapping allows us to aim towards the nidus. At this point a microcatheter with 0.014″ wire can be advanced into the nidus and coils deployed. We do not recommend a coil exiting the aorta into the cava.

TIP BOX 17.3

Translumbar puncture

We use a long 19-gauge Yueh Centesis catheter needle (Cook Medical, Bloomington, Indiana) or a Chiba needle to access the sac with the patient in prone position and advance an 0.035″ wire. Again, CT road mapping provides the most efficient path to the nidus. Using CT image fusion, we identify both the point on the skin and the point on the aorta we want to enter. We line up those two points to determine the location on the skin to puncture and the aorta to enter. This is the pathway view. We then use a 90-degree view to check the depth intermittently. We place a 4-French sheath into the sac if we failed to access the nidus directly and use catheters and wires to enter the nidus and place coils. Alternatively, the patient can be placed on the side opposite to that being accessed, which decreases radiation exposure and is also more comfortable for obese patients.

Alternatively, CEUS has been shown to be very effective for identifying and categorizing the type of endoleak in centers in which it is available. For the purpose of embolization, we prefer to deploy a combination of coils and Onyx glue (Covidien, Mansfield, Massachusetts).

For large, lower lumbar arteries, we prefer to approach through the hypogastric artery (Fig. 17.3). The hypogastric artery allows for intervention on the lower lumbar arteries, but not usually the upper lumbar arteries. However, as lower lumbar arteries are more likely to be the causative vessel, this approach is often successful. As with most interventions for endoleak, CT road mapping and fusion technology are crucial. They allow surgeons to plan preoperatively a successful route from the hypogastric artery to the lumbar artery of interest and then implement that plan in the operating room.

For cases where we cannot approach through the hypogastric artery, a transcaval approach is often successful (Box 17.3). A large gap between the inferior vena cava and aorta or an endograft opposed to the aortic wall next to the cava preclude this approach, but it is feasible in many cases. Again, careful preoperative planning with CT road

TIP BOX 17.4

Before attempting graft-preserving open interventions for endoleaks, the crucial step is to secure the proximal seal zone (preferably with endoanchors prior to incision).

mapping is paramount to achieving success. The road map allows the surgeon to select the optimal location to cross over from the vena cava to the aorta and enter the causative vessel. The best location is an area where the aorta and inferior vena cava are well apposed but the endograft is separated from the wall of the aneurysm sac.

For endoleaks that persist despite the above maneuvers, or if these approaches are unavailable, other endovascular options include translumbar coiling (Box 17.2), or snaking a catheter retrograde around the outside of the iliac limb and into the sac. In some centers, experienced surgeons can laparoscopically clip or ligate the IMA or lumbar arteries, although it can often be difficult to find a willing surgeon.

For endoleaks that persist after exhausting the aforementioned options, we prefer to perform a sacotomy. We deploy endoanchors to reinforce the proximal neck and secure the graft in its position. We then expose the aneurysm sac through an open approach, open the sac, remove the debris from prior interventions, and oversew any bleeding vessels. This approach ensures direct visualization and intervention on bleeding vessels, while avoiding the added morbidity of an aortic crossclamp because the graft is left in situ. The key to this maneuver is ensuring the graft is secure and will not slip once the sac is opened (Box 17.4). We prefer to use endoanchors, but the other option is to reinforce the neck with a felt pledget after exposing the aneurysm but prior to opening the sac. We previously used this approach, but after the advent of endoanchors, we reserve this for calcified necks or suspected concomitant Type Ia endoleaks. The latter approach is especially useful if surgeons suspect a Type Ia endoleak as well as Type II. In rare cases, full open conversion with graft explantation represents the definitive solution.

REFERENCES

1. Lal BK, Zhou W, Li Z, et al. Predictors and outcomes of endoleaks in the Veterans Affairs Open Versus Endovascular Repair (OVER) trial of abdominal aortic aneurysms. *J Vasc Surg*. 2015;62(6):1394–1404.
2. Chaikof EL, Brewster DC, Dalman RL, et al. The care of patients with an abdominal aortic aneurysm: The Society for Vascular Surgery practice guidelines. *J Vasc Surg*. 2009;50(4):S2–S49.
3. Deery SE, Ergul EA, Schermerhorn ML, et al. Aneurysm sac expansion is independently associated with late mortality in patients treated with endovascular aneurysm repair. *J Vasc Surg*. 2017.
4. O'Donnell TF, Corey MR, Deery SE, et al. Select early Type 1A endoleaks after EVAR will resolve without secondary intention. *J Vasc Surg*. 2017.
5. Ultee KHJ, Soden PA, Zettervall SL, Darling J, Verhagen HJM, Schermerhorn ML. Conversion from endovascular to open abdominal aortic aneurysm repair. *J Vasc Surg*. 2016;64(1):76–82.
6. Berg P, Stroetges RA, Miller LE, Schoefferle J. A propensity score-matched analysis of inflammatory response with endovascular aneurysm sealing vs endovascular aneurysm repair. *J Endovasc Ther*. 2017; 152660281772201.

18

Complications in Endovascular Thoracoabdominal Aortic Aneurysm Repair

Brant W. Ullery, MD, FACS, FSVS and Kenneth Tran, MD

Endovascular repair of thoracoabdominal aortic aneurysms requires long segment stent graft coverage with concomitant revascularization of the renovisceral and potentially supraaortic arch segments. Such procedures represent the highest extent of complex endovascular therapy and are associated with increased technical demand, as well as the potential for iatrogenic injury to the target vessels and endoleak formation. Risk factors for intraprocedural loss of branch vessel patency include unstented vessels, high aortic angulation, dense intramural thrombus, multiple planned branch vessel involvement, and stenotic and/or small caliber (<4 mm) branch vessels. This chapter focuses on various intraprocedural complications associated with endovascular thoracoabdominal aortic aneurysm repair, including those related to target vessel events, retrograde type A aortic dissection, and bird-beak configuration.

TARGET VESSEL DISSECTION AND OCCLUSION

Lack of contrast opacification in renal or mesenteric branch vessels often indicates primary thrombotic occlusions or secondary occlusions caused by arterial dissection. Loss of branch vessel patency may be associated with sheath cannulation of a target vessel containing significant native ostial occlusive disease or prolonged sheath cannulation time.

Prevention

Frequent flushing of in-dwelling sheaths with heparinized saline will aid in minimizing thrombus formation around or within long sheaths. In cases of challenging target vessel catheterization owing to small vessel diameter, ostial occlusive disease, or target vessel angulation, careful attention is advised in order to engage the target vessel origin and safely cannulate the vessel. Predilation of the target vessel origin, utilization of the sheath dilator during advancement into the branch vessel, and working over an intermediate to heavy stiff wire platform (e.g., Rosen [Cook Medical Inc., Bloomington, Indiana] or Amplatz wire [Boston Scientific Corp, Maple Grove, Minnesota]) will facilitate a smooth and atraumatic branch vessel cannulation. Excess wire manipulation within target vessels or advancement of the sheath without aid of a dilator increases the risk of intimal disruption and may lead to associated thrombus formation and/or flow-limiting dissection within the target vessel.

Treatment

If target vessel occlusion or dissection is identified, the first step is to ensure maintenance of wire access to the distal target vessel. If wire access has been lost, it will be necessary to reestablish access using a combination of a soft hydrophilic wire and low-profile directional catheter. Once wire access into a distal branch is restored and exchanged for a stiffer wire platform, a flexible 6- or 7-French sheath can be advanced distal to the occlusion. Verification of patent outflow of the target vessel is performed using contrast angiography via the sheath side port. In cases of branch vessel thrombosis, balloon-expandable covered stent grafts may be used to exclude the thrombus and restore intraluminal patency of the vessel (Fig. 18.1). If arterial dissection is present, confirmation of true lumen wire access can be obtained with use of intravascular ultrasound and/or contrast angiography. Self-expanding bare-metal stents are the preferred treatment modality in cases of dissection to minimize the risk of distal progression of the intimal flap.

Occlusion of target vessels after they have already been stented can also occur. In these cases, it is important not only to restore vessel patency but also to determine the cause of the occlusion. Anatomic and mechanical variables to assess include presence of untreated or unrecognized arterial dissection, a kink at the transition of the distal branch vessel stent as it transitions to the native vessel, or improper sizing of the stent graft relative to the native branch vessel diameter. Placement of an additional self-expanding bare-metal stent, frequently overlapping with the initial branch vessel stent that was originally placed, may be required to treat any residual arterial dissection or to reduce significant branch vessel angulation at the distal end of the stent.

The above techniques generally lead to effective treatment in the renal arteries because occlusions and dissections tend to be limited to a short segment and occur proximal to renal artery branches. While uncommon, iatrogenic dissection or occlusion of the superior mesenteric artery (SMA) warrants immediate revascularization. In cases of dissection, entry into the true lumen can similarly be facilitated with intravascular ultrasound, contrast angiography, or advancement of the wire through the tip of a balloon angioplasty catheter with the balloon inflated at the orifice of the target artery. Dissection flaps within the SMA are treated with bare-metal stents that are sized 1:1 relative to the native vessel diameter (Fig. 18.2). In cases of thrombotic occlusion, it is important to assess the length and extent of occlusion relative to main branches of the SMA (e.g., middle colic, jejunal) prior to treatment. Extension of thrombus into the mid and distal SMA branches warrants consideration for adjunct procedures such as percutaneous pharmacomechanical thrombolysis or percutaneous mechanical thrombectomy. If there is difficulty obtaining antegrade access, some reports have described successful retrograde cannulation via celiac collaterals and using a snare to establish a through-and-through wire for sheath and stent advancement.[1] If percutaneous options fail to restore visceral patency adequately, other reports have described laparotomy and exposure of the SMA at the root of the mesentery with open thrombectomy and possible patch angioplasty repair as indicated.

Embolization

Distal embolization may occur in the setting of subtherapeutic intraprocedural systemic heparinization, aggressive wire or sheath

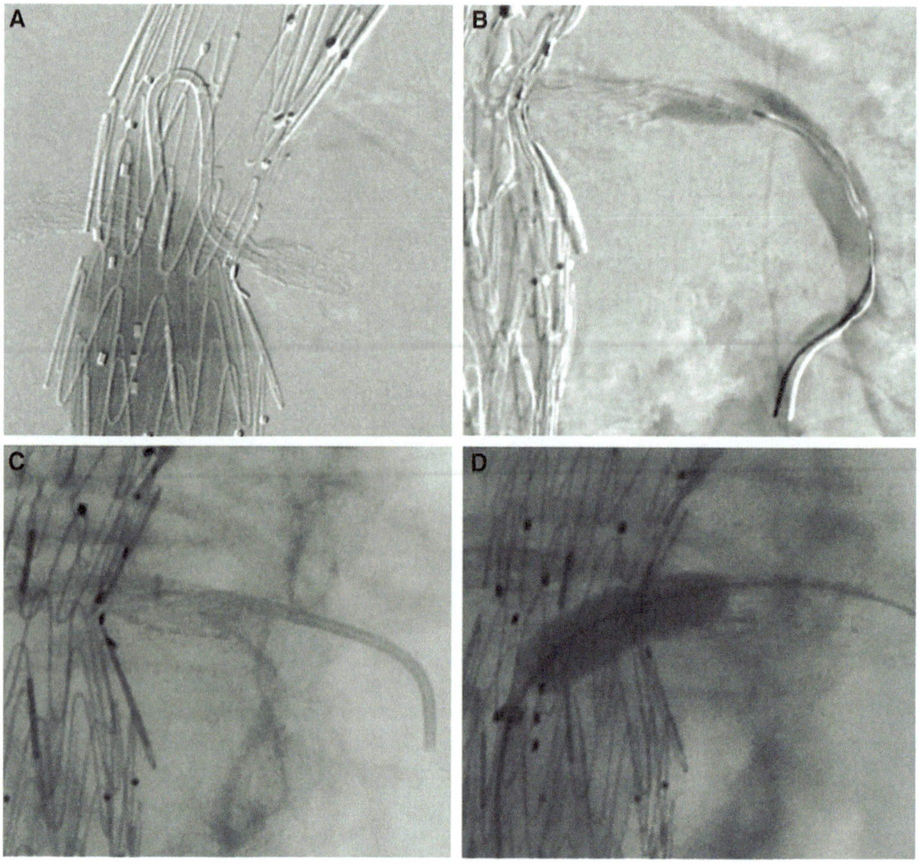

Fig. 18.1 Target Vessel Occlusion. (A) Angiographic evidence of complete in-stent occlusion of the left renal artery. (B) Successful subintimal cannulation past the occlusion. (C) Sheath and catheter placement between the native arterial wall and previously placed stent. (D) Balloon angioplasty of newly placed balloon-expandable covered stent with evidence of complete collapse of the prior renal stent.

manipulation, or as a result of dissection or occlusion in the more proximal target vessel. Less commonly, thrombus may form in distal side branches during stent deployment, particularly with balloon-expandable stents requiring prolonged inflation times.

In all cases of embolic events, the target vessel can often be salvaged with use of a variety of techniques. Catheter-directed thrombolysis can be successfully used for cases involving extensive thrombus burden or in those extending into smaller target vessel branches. Clot retrieval devices (e.g., Export Advance aspiration catheter [Medtronic AVE, Santa Rosa, California], Indigo [Penumbra, Inc, Alameda, California]) are used in cases involving thrombus in the larger caliber primary target vessel or in cases with residual thrombus following thrombolysis (Fig. 18.3). These devices typically use an 0.014- or 0.018″ system and can be easily advanced to distal branch vessels, if needed. Pharmacomechanical devices (e.g., AngioJet system [Boston Scientific Corp, Malborough, MA]) have also been described for salvage therapy of target vessels.

Perforation

Excessive wire manipulation, unnecessary wire advancement, and use of stiff wires within renovisceral vessels increase the risk of perforation. Initial management includes identifying the exact site of injury with contrast angiography and, if possible, attempting to achieve initial hemostasis via tamponade from prolonged gentle balloon inflation. Continued extravasation following attempts at balloon tamponade warrants definitive treatment and varies depending on the location of the perforation within the target vessel. Proximal perforation prior to the take-off of named branch vessels may be treated by placement of either a balloon-expandable or self-expandable covered stent graft with proximal extension of the stent into the main body of the device. Distal perforations can often be treated with coil embolization if it will not sacrifice significant end-organ perfusion (Fig. 18.4). A useful technique in such cases is to deliver coils through inflated balloon angioplasty catheters placed proximally to ensure hemostasis during coil delivery. Renal branch vessels may be sacrificed with the known consequence of ischemic injury to the supplied territory of renal parenchyma, whereas distal branches of the SMA may often be coil embolized without ischemic complications as a result of redundant collateral supply.

Stent Dislodgement/Migration

Although uncommon, distal migration may occur during deployment of stent grafts within target branch vessels. This often occurs in the setting of undersized stent grafts. For this reason, it is important to use balloon-expandable stents that are 15%–20% oversized relative to the native vessel diameter. This most commonly involves 6–7-mm stents in the renal arteries and 8–9-mm stents in the SMA. Distal migration may also occur during sheath manipulation, particularly if sheaths within target vessels are advanced without appropriate protection. If the surgeon discovers that this has occurred, recovery of migrated grafts can be achieved through a combination of a long flexible sheath placed immediately adjacent to the migrated stent graft. A 10-mm goose-neck snare (Medtronic AVE, Santa Rosa, CA) can then be advanced through the sheath and over the distal end of the stent graft (Fig. 18.5). An

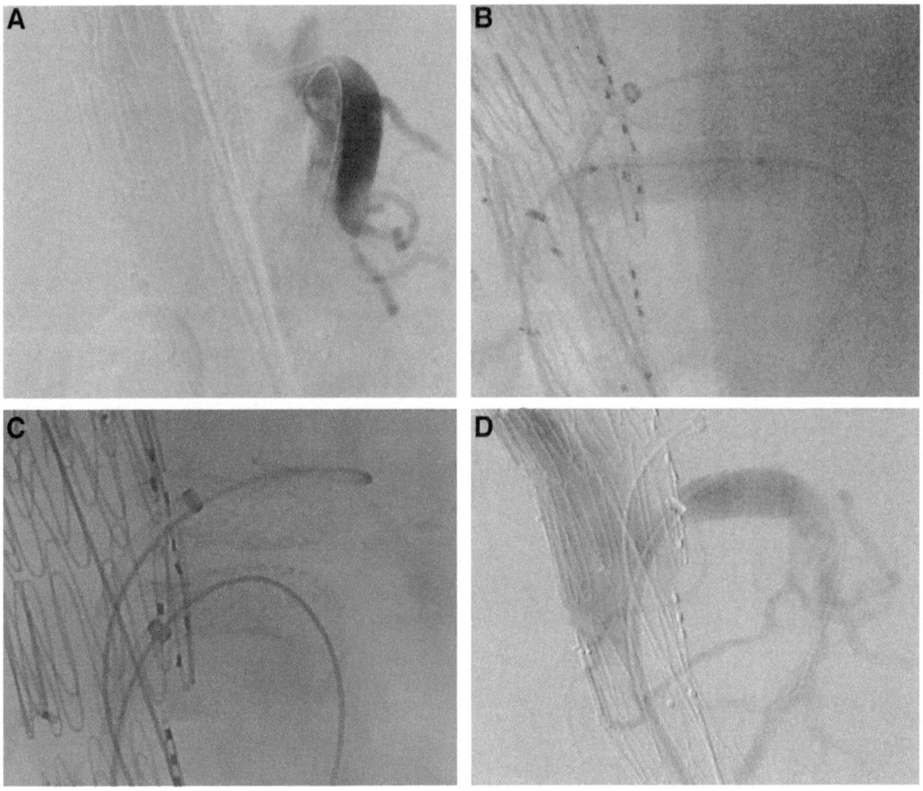

Fig. 18.2 Target Vessel Dissection. (A) Angiographic evidence of complete occlusion of the proximal superior mesenteric artery (SMA) because of iatrogenic dissection. (B) Successful wire canalization in the true lumen, facilitated by use of a 10-mm angioplasty balloon. (C) Deployment of a bare-metal stent into the proximal SMA. (D) Restored patency of the mid-distal SMA.

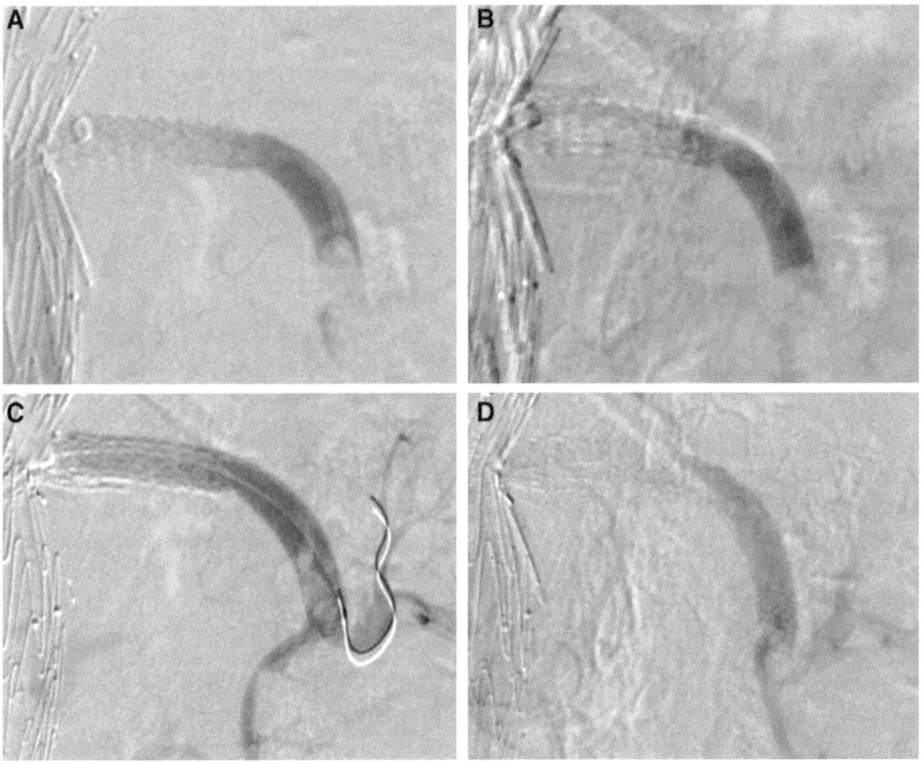

Fig. 18.3 Target Vessel Embolization. (A) Angiographic evidence of embolic debris in the distal left renal artery. (B) Partial resolution of thrombus after catheter-directed thrombolysis. (C) Successful wire cannulation and advancement of clot retrieval catheter. (D) Patent renal artery outflow after successful thrombolysis.

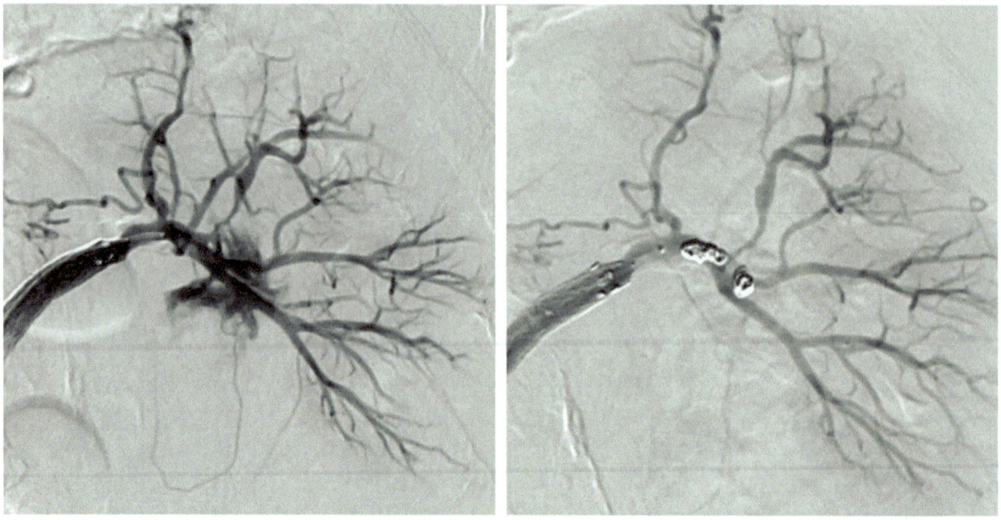

Fig. 18.4 Target Vessel Perforation. Wire perforation of an inferior segmental renal artery *(left)* and successful coil embolization with resolution of active extravasation *(right)*.

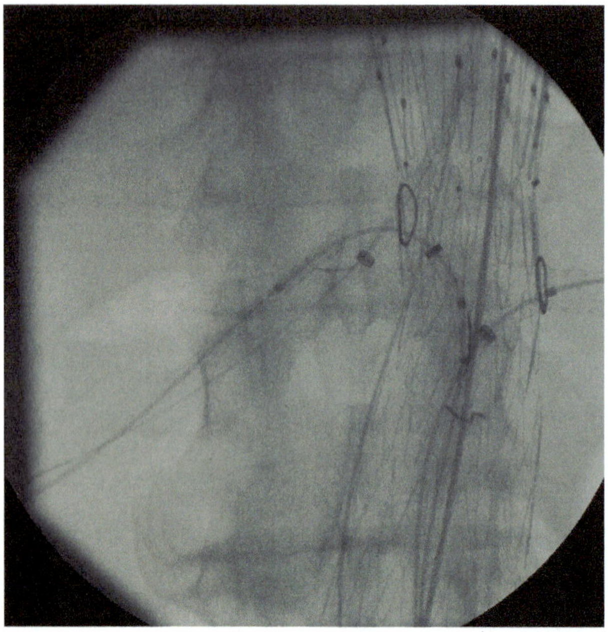

Fig. 18.5 Target Vessel Stent Dislodgement. Double cannulation of the target vessel with one wire within the dislodged stent graft, and a second system consisting of a guidewire, 7-French sheath, and 10-mm goose-neck snare encircling the target vessel. This system can be pulled back to reposition the dislodged stent graft into a more favorable location.

angioplasty balloon may then be advanced through the stent graft and partially inflated. The entire apparatus is then pulled back until the stent graft is at an appropriate position, the adjacent snare and sheath removed, and the stent graft balloon inflated to profile, with use of additional bridging stents as required.

In cases of proximal graft migration (i.e., "pull-out"), the dislodged stent may be reseated to a neutral, safe position (e.g., within a limb). This is achieved by recannulation of the dislodged stent, followed by advancement of an appropriately sized angioplasty balloon to encompass the entire length of the stent. The balloon is then inflated and steady retrograde pressure applied to the balloon/stent apparatus until released from the branch orifice. The inflated balloon and stent may then be advanced into a neutral arterial segment (e.g., external iliac or within a limb graft for larger stents) and deployed without major consequences.

Bird-Beak Configuration

Bird-beak configuration, or simply "bird-beaking", is defined as incomplete apposition of the proximal stent graft to the aortic wall, with a wedge-shaped gap between the undersurface of the proximal stent graft and the aortic wall along the lesser curvature of the aortic arch (Fig. 18.6). Previous studies using earlier generation thoracic aortic stent grafts noted that bird-beak configuration occurred in 44% of TEVAR cases performed for a heterogenous group of thoracic aortic pathologies.[2] Hsu et al.[3] hypothesized that when a stent graft lands in the distal aortic arch, especially in zones 2 and 3, the inner curve of the aortic arch acts as a fulcrum by which the proximal sealing segment hinges at the first or second interstent junction. The rigidity of the proximal stent graft combined with the "wind-sock" effect of blood flow in the aortic arch may predispose pulsatile blood flow to be directed between the proximal stent graft margin and the aortic wall, thereby lifting the leading edge of the stent graft off the inner curve and generating a bird-beak configuration. The clinical importance of the compromised proximal seal and turbulent flow dynamics in the bird-beak configuration is demonstrated by the significant increase in both Type Ia and Type II endoleak formation observed in these patients, as well as the potential increased risk for stent graft in-folding or collapse.

Both anatomic and device-specific variables are believed to predispose to bird-beaking. In their analysis of 80 patients undergoing TEVAR, Boufi and colleagues[4] detected bird-beak configuration in 57% of patients and their multivariate analysis identified the aortic angle of the deployment zone with a cut-off value of 51% to be the only independent risk factor for malposition leading to bird-beaking. Conventional aortic stent grafts are uniformly cylindrical in shape, which facilitates conforming to the traditionally straight thoracic and thoracoabdominal aorta. As such, these devices may not be ideally suited for the curvature and hemodynamic forces associated with the aortic arch. While bird-beak configuration appeared more common with earlier generation devices, the tendency for this suboptimal positioning of the thoracic aortic stent graft may be associated with differences in device design. Stent segment lengths, longitudinal support spines, fabric thickness, and proximal fixation mechanisms (e.g., covered flares, bare stents, barbs). Newer generation devices are being customized for the proximal thoracic aorta by incorporating enhanced flexibility and conformability, as well as preshaped curves to augment precision of deployment and prevent bird-beak configuration.

Prevention

Recommendations for reducing the risk of bird-beak configuration centers on proper selection of the proximal landing zone with specific consideration of the length, diameter, and aortic angulation. Proximal landing zones with aortic angulation of greater than 50 degrees should prompt deployment of the stent graft distal to the bend if there remains sufficient sealing length or, alternatively, more proximal deployment may be considered in such cases since mild (<2 cm in length) bird-beaking appears to be tolerated with low risk of associated complications. Regardless of the device used, stent graft deployment should follow the outer rather than inner curve to allow better accommodation to the aortic arch. Additional strategies to prevent bird-beak configuration center on moving the stent graft more proximally to overcome landing in a sharp curve. Devices with proximal bare springs facilitate a more proximal seal zone as they allow coverage of aortic branch vessels and provide better alignment of the proximal sealing stent. Although technically more demanding, a more proximal seal zone can also be achieved with arch debranching, use of branched devices, chimney techniques, and in situ fenestrations.

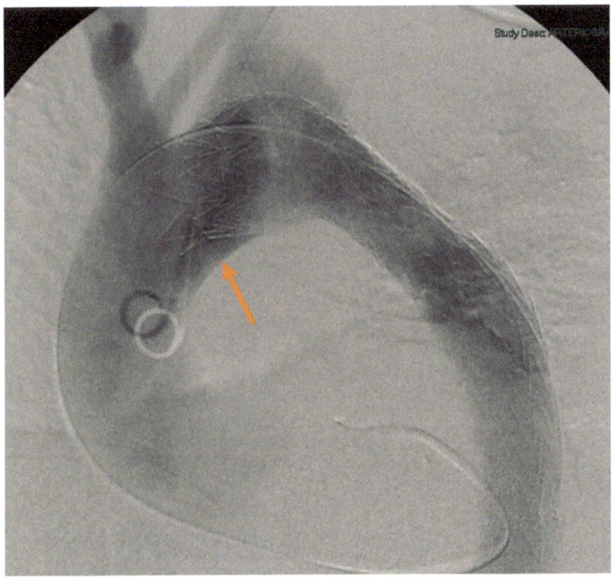

Fig. 18.6 Bird-Beak Configuration. Bird-beak configuration following thoracic aortic stent graft placement. *Arrow* indicates lack of apposition of the inferior aspect of the stent graft with the lesser curve of the aortic arch.

Treatment

Multiple options exist aimed at improving the apposition of the proximal edge of the aortic stent graft along the inner curve of the aortic arch. The first and simplest option is to augment expansion of the proximal thoracic aortic stent graft by use of simple balloon angioplasty of the proximal stent graft. Repeated and more aggressive balloon molding may be required in select cases. If a bird beak persists, the next step depends on whether there is residual uncovered thoracic aorta distal to the supraaortic arch vessel in the planned proximal seal zone. The presence of 3 mm or more of residual uncovered aorta in the proximal seal zone provides the opportunity for placement of a thoracic aortic proximal cuff extension to cover the bird-beak area and to achieve improved proximal fixation in a less angulated area of the aortic arch. If there is no residual uncovered aorta in the proximal seal zone or if placement of a cuff would fail to yield improved geometry in the proximal seal zone, deployment of a balloon-expandable bare metal Palmaz stent (Cordis Corporation, Bridgewater, New Jersey) overlapping the proximal seal zone may be used to increase the centrifugal force and to optimize molding of the stent graft to the intimal surface of the aorta. The bare-metal stent configuration reduces the risk of side-branch vessel compromise that is associated with the use of proximal aortic cuff extensions. An additional adjunctive maneuver in this situation includes utilization of Aptus Heli-Fx Endoanchors (Medtronic, Santa Rosa, California) to facilitate apposition of the inferior edge of the stent graft to the lesser curve.

Excessively hostile aortic arch anatomy may compromise the ability of balloon-expandable bare-metal stents or proximal cuff extensions to remedy bird-beak-associated Type Ia endoleaks adequately. In such cases, embolization of the aneurysm sac or the feeding endoleak tract along the bird-beak area may curtail sac pressurization. Endovascular access into the sac is commonly accomplished with a reverse-curve catheter such as a Cobra (Cordis Corporation, New Jersey) or SOS Omni (AngioDynamics Inc., Queensbury, New York) hooked over the proximal edge of the stent graft, with a microcatheter subsequently advanced through the tract and more distally into the aneurysm sac (Fig. 18.7). A variety of embolic agents, including coils, fibrin glue, and

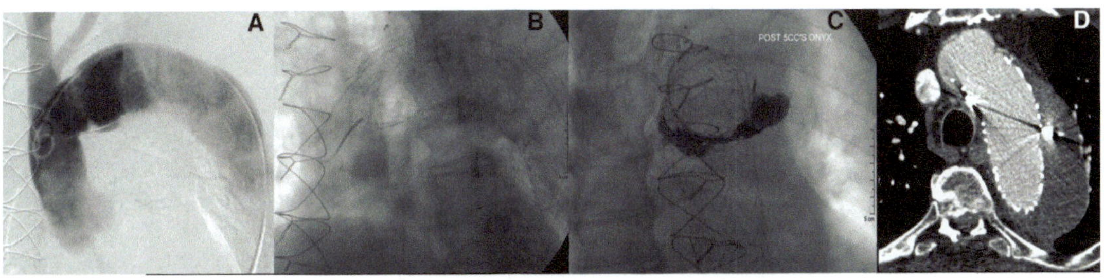

Fig. 18.7 Management of Bird-Beak Associated Type Ia Endoleak. Bird-beak morphology with associated Type Ia endoleak noted along lesser curve of aortic arch (A). Catheterization of inferior aspect of stent graft (B) with subsequent peri-graft glue embolization (C). Postembolization cross-sectional imaging noting resolution of proximal endoleak (D).

(Images courtesy Michael D. Dake, MD)

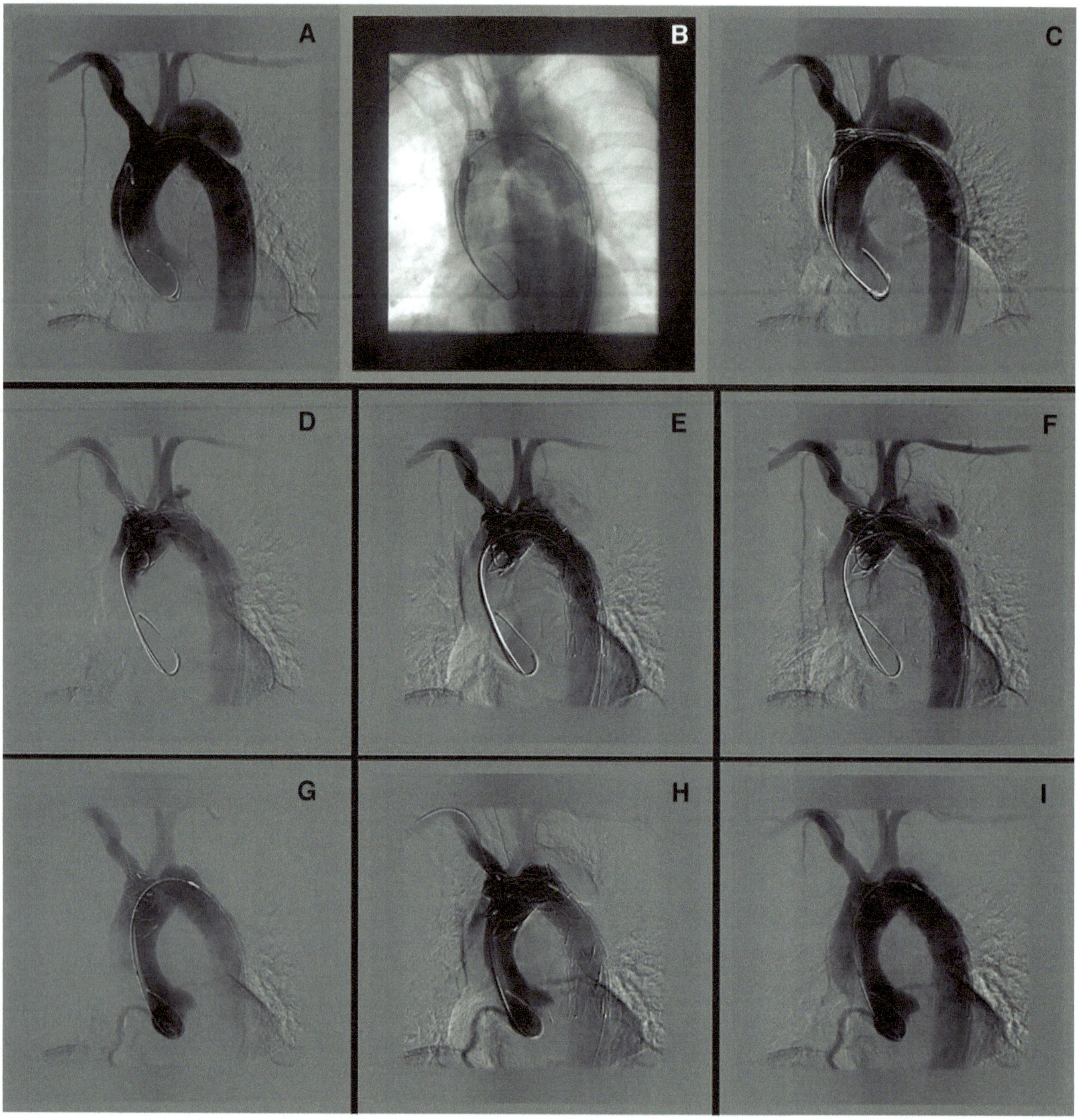

Fig. 18.8 Retrograde Type A Aortic Dissection. Predeployment angiography showing Type B aortic dissection with associated aneurysmal dilatation (A–C). Series of postdeployment angiograms demonstrating interval development of intraprocedural retrograde Type A aortic dissection (D–I).
(Images courtesy Michael D. Dake, MD)

n-butyl 2-cyanoacrylate, may be used to obliterate the tract and sac; however, liquid embolics such as Onyx (Covidien, Mansfield, Massachusetts) may facilitate more distal embolization than is possible with coils or adhesive agents.

If the aforementioned maneuvers fail to address the bird beak and/or associated Type Ia endoleak, the final consideration involves extraanatomic bypass in order to establish a proximal landing zone in a more favorable area of the aortic arch. This decision may be made intraoperatively but is more commonly deferred to a second staged procedure in elective cases.

Retrograde Type A Aortic Dissection

Along with stroke and spinal cord ischemia, retrograde Type A dissection (RTAD) represents one of the most feared complications of endovascular repair of pathologies involving the thoracic aortic segment (Fig. 18.8). A recent systematic review and meta-analysis surveyed 50 publications that included a total of 8969 patients undergoing TEVAR and reported a pooled incidence of RTAD of 2.5%, with a corresponding mortality of 37.1%.[5] Etiologic factors that have been proposed to be associated with RTAD generally include those that are device-related and procedure-related, patient specific, or natural progression of initial aortic dissection. The MOTHER registry, comprising the combined data from 5 prospective trials and institutional data from a single UK center, identified both aortic dissection indication and device oversizing as important contributors to the development of RTAD.[6] Multiple studies have similarly noted a significantly higher incidence of RTAD in those treated with TEVAR for aortic dissection, particularly among those treated in the acute phase, compared with those treated for degenerative aneurysmal disease.[5–7] In addition, the MOTHER registry determined that each percentage increase in endograft oversizing above 9% resulted in a relative increased risk of RTAD by 14%. Proximal landing zone in the ascending aorta or arch (zones 0–2) and proximal bare stent configuration are two additional variables that have been implicated by others as potential etiologic factors for RTAD[7]; however, the contribution of these factors has not been reliably demonstrated by others.[6,8]

In a review of 63 RTAD cases identified from the European Registry on Endovascular Aortic Repair Complications, 60% of these cases were classified by the investigators as being induced by the stent graft itself with direct evidence of stent graft-induced aortic injury observed during surgery or necropsy.[7] The remaining cases were related to guidewire or device manipulation during the procedure or progression of underlying aortic disease. From a procedural standpoint, RTAD may be associated with manipulation of the guide wire, catheter, or aortic stent graft delivery system in the aorta during TEVAR. The passage of these wires and devices, particularly across anatomically challenging areas of the aorta (e.g., excessive angulation, atheroma, calcification), generates friction along the inner aortic wall and may predispose to intimal injury and subsequent arterial dissection. Procedure-related small localized intimal tears may extend proximally into the ascending aorta acutely or even weeks or months after the procedure. The notably higher incidence of RTAD in those treated with acute and chronic type B aortic dissections compared with other aortic pathologies and in those with connective tissue diseases suggests an increased propensity for iatrogenic aortic injury in patients with baseline aortic fragility.

Prevention

Minimizing risk of RTAD is aimed at addressing the presumed etiologic factors and identified risk factors for this complication. Whereas the rigidity of earlier generation devices predisposed to aortic injury during deployment or as a result of subtle movement during the cardiac cycle, newer generation devices are increasingly conformable to navigate in the aortic arch with minimal manipulation of the adjacent aortic tissue. Careful wire catheterization, sheath advancement, and stent graft deployment are critical to the safety and efficacy of all endovascular aortic repairs and is particularly pronounced when treating pathologies involving the aortic arch and proximal descending thoracic aorta. All manipulations of the aorta with wires, catheters, or stent grafts must be performed under direct fluoroscopic guidance in order to minimize risk of inadvertent arterial injury. Moreover, intravascular ultrasound may serve as a useful adjunct to aid in correct device sizing, identifying origins of supraaortic arch vessels, confirming presence of true and false lumens, and locating entry site tears. Avoidance of routine balloon molding following stent graft deployment in the curved area of the aortic arch, unless there is presence of endoleak on angiography and especially in cases involving Type B aortic dissection, may also serve to decrease the potential for localized aortic injury in the highly dynamic aortic arch. Aggressive oversizing of stent grafts (>10% in dissections and >20% in aneurysms) should also be avoided to minimize excessive radial force on the aorta. Finally, recognizing the increased tendency for intimal injury in patients with aortic wall friability, all efforts should be made to avoid endovascular intervention in high-risk patients such as those with acute Type B dissection or connective tissue disease unless required based on inability to tolerate open procedure, presence of malperfusion, or aortic rupture.

Treatment

While RTAD serves as a relatively uncommon complication, it is life-threatening and generally requires emergency surgical repair. The reverse frozen elephant trunk procedure or total arch replacement are often performed in cases involving a dissection in the aortic arch, whereas ascending and hemiarch reconstruction is commonly sufficient in patients with dissection limited to the proximal aorta.[8] Interestingly, the presumed cause of RTAD in the European registry data reported by Eggebrecht et al.[7] significantly influenced their treatment approach. Dissections related to wire or device manipulation were limited to the distal ascending aorta or proximal aortic arch in one-half of patients and were generally treated conservatively (83%), whereas stent graft-induced dissections proved to be more extensive and prompted emergency open surgery (81%). Perioperative mortality remained universally high in their report but was no different between the stent graft induced and wire-related dissection groups (45% versus 43%). The majority (57%) of patients with progression of aortic disease underwent elective surgical repair and were noted to have improved perioperative mortality compared with the other groups (14%, $P = 0.22$).

Inadvertent branch vessel coverage

Inadvertent partial or complete branch vessel coverage may occur from malposition of the proximal or distal extent of the aortic endograft or may occur within the mid portion of the stent graft in cases involving branched or fenestrated technology. During fenestrated cases, "shuttering" occurs when a scallop or fenestration does not align perfectly with the target vessel ostium. Shuttering can theoretically range from 0% (perfect alignment) to 100% (complete coverage of the scallop/fenestration). The issue of branch-vessel malalignment in endovascular surgery has not been well described in the literature. We have previously explored this topic and, despite the custom design of currently available fenestrated technology, identified one-half of patients in our series to have shuttering of the SMA of any degree (range of shuttering, 12%–40%) on postoperative imaging.[9] Notably, no clinical events were noted during follow-up. Celiac artery shuttering/coverage has not been explored but, by extension, is also likely to be well tolerated given several recent reports demonstrating that planned celiac coverage during TEVAR is safe in select patients with SMA-celiac collaterals.[10,11]

Prevention

As with complex endovascular aortic repair, careful preoperative case planning is critical to technical success. Use of three-dimensional reconstructive imaging software facilitates accurate device selection and manufacturing, particularly in cases involving fenestrated technology. Increasing use of sophisticated fusion imaging technology may also aid in operative efficiency and reduction in associated vascular complications. Several strategies can be used to assist in minimizing the risk for inadvertent branch vessel coverage in select cases. First, prewiring of the branch vessels can be useful to confirm position of proximal and distal landing zones (e.g., marking the left subclavian or celiac artery). This technique adds an additional benefit as it may reduce fluoroscopy time because of the lack of additional angiograms to identify the proper proximal or distal landing zones. Prewiring of the renovisceral vessels may also be of great benefit to assist in optimal

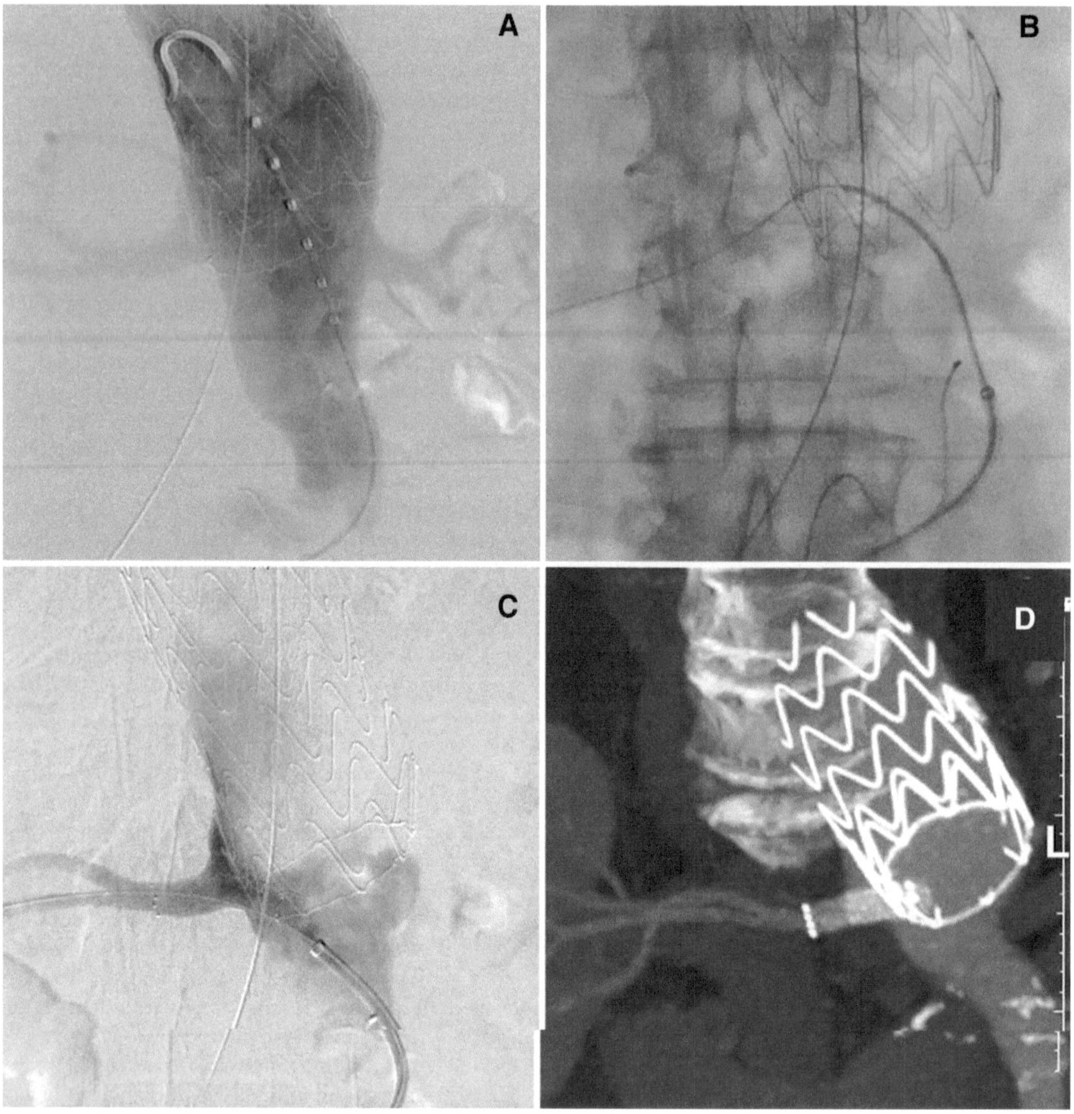

Fig. 18.9 **Management of Inadvertent Target Vessel Coverage Using Encroachment Technique.** Inadvertent right renal artery coverage after aortic stent graft placement (A). Transfemoral catheterization of right renal artery (B) followed by placement of a self-expanding stent to preserve flow into the right kidney (C–D).

alignment of scallops and fenestrations prior to stent graft deployment. Second, in cases with particularly challenging anatomy of the renovisceral segment, prewiring of the branch vessels can not only aid localization of the branch vessels but also allow the opportunity to perform balloon angioplasty to address any ostial stenosis that would otherwise hinder alignment of the stent graft or catheterization of the branch vessel through fenestrations. Third, in cases involving branched graft technology, it is important to ensure that the branch is positioned a minimum of 1–2 cm proximal to the target vessel origin to allow adequate room for catheterization. Branch grafts positioned too close to the target vessel may severely limit renovisceral catheterization efforts and result in unintended branch vessel coverage or endoleak as a result of retrograde filling of the sac from a noncatheterized target vessel.

Treatment

Multiple open and endovascular options exist to address inadvertent branch vessel coverage during endovascular thoracoabdominal aortic aneurysm repair. The initial approach in such cases involves attempted manual repositioning of the stent graft. If the graft is positioned too proximal such that it invades the supraaortic arch vessel origins, gentle caudal traction may be applied by either an intraaortic balloon placed at the aneurysm neck or transfemoral wire positioned across the graft bifurcation. Second, if inadvertent coverage of the branch vessels is detected at the proximal or distal extent of the stent graft, salvage of the branch vessel may be accomplished by stenting. If branch vessel coverage is minimal, stenting may proceed utilizing the encroachment technique whereby a stent is deployed above (e.g., left subclavian) or below (e.g., celiac) the main aortic stent graft in such a way as to facilitate improved perfusion of the branch vessel origin (Fig. 18.9). In cases involving more severe or complete inadvertent branch vessel coverage, a chimney stent is commonly required and is placed in a position parallel to the main aortic stent graft (Fig. 18.10). Technical success of chimney stents for branch vessel salvage is high and is improved in cases where prewire catheterization of the branch vessels is used

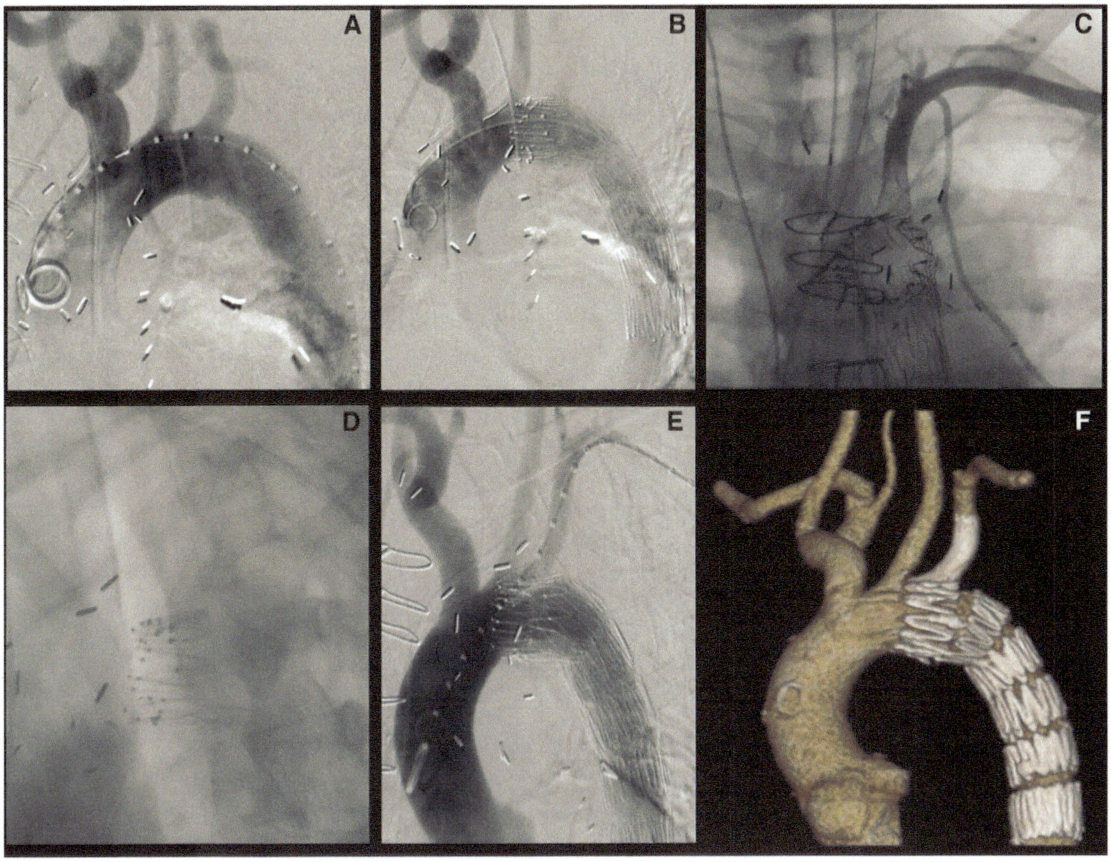

Fig. 18.10 Management of Inadvertent Left Subclavian Artery Coverage Using Chimney Technique. Initial angiography prior to thoracic aortic stent graft placement (A). Delayed contrast filling of left subclavian artery after inadvertent coverage by the stent graft (B). Transbrachial retrograde catheterization of the ascending aorta (C, D) followed by left subclavian chimney stent graft placement (E, F).
(Images courtesy of Michael D. Dake, MD)

because the feasibility of this technique depends on some space between the aorta and the main body of the stent graft in order to advance a wire and catheter into the target vessel. A third endovascular technique involves in situ fenestration of the aortic stent graft using a transseptal needle or assistance with radiofrequency or laser technology. Although such maneuvers are not performed commonly and are considered off-label use of technology, a recent systematic review highlighted these techniques to be safe, efficacious, and associated with minimal morbidity.[12] In fenestrated cases, "shuttering" of the branch vessels may occur and is best treated by early identification and stenting to facilitate realignment of the fenestration with the target vessel ostium.

While the aforementioned endovascular techniques provide an effective strategy and should be considered the initial therapy to restore branch-vessel patency in cases involving inadvertent coverage, conversion to open surgery remains a safe and reliable option in such cases where endovascular salvage attempts fail. Extraanatomic bypasses such as carotid–carotid and left carotid–subclavian bypasses are commonly used in elective cases prior to planned coverage of the supraaortic vessels but can also be pursued in cases of inadvertent aortic arch coverage. In the abdominal segment, both open and hybrid revascularization efforts can be pursued, including open exposure and retrograde catheterization of branch vessels (e.g., SMA and renal arteries) to facilitate parallel stent graft (chimney) placement. Additional open surgical options following inadvertent coverage of the renovisceral segment include hepatorenal, splenorenal, ileorenal, and iliomesenteric bypasses.

REFERENCES

1. Robken J, Shammas NW. Treatment of a totally occluded superior mesenteric artery facilitated by retrograde crossing via collaterals from the celiac artery. *J Endovasc Ther.* 2007;14:745–747.
2. Ueda T, Fleischmann D, Dake MD, et al. Incomplete endograft apposition to the aortic arch: bird-beak configuration increases risk of endoleak formation after thoracic endovascular aortic repair. *Radiology.* 2010;255:645–652.
3. Hsu H, Chen C, Chen P, et al. The impact of bird-beak configuration on aortic remodeling of distal arch pathology after thoracic endovascular aortic repair with the Zenith Pro-Form TX2 thoracic endograft. *J Vasc Surg.* 2014;59:80–88.
4. Boufi M, Guivier-Curien C, Deplano V, et al. Risk factor analysis of bird beak occurrence after thoracic endovascular aortic repair. *Eur J Vasc Endovasc Surg.* 2015;50:37–43.
5. Chen Y, Zhang S, Liu L, et al. Retrograde type A aortic dissection after thoracic aortic endovascular aortic repair: A systematic review and meta-analysis. *J Am Heart Assoc.* 2017;6(9). pii: e004649.
6. Canaud L, Ozdemir BA, Patterson BO, et al. Retrograde aortic dissection after thoracic endovascular aortic repair. *Ann Surg.* 2014;260:389–395.

7. Eggebrecht H, Thompson M, Rousseau H, et al. Retrograde ascending aortic dissection during or after thoracic aortic stent raft placement: insight from the European registry on endovascular aortic repair complications. *Circulation*. 2009;120:276–281.
8. Idrees J, Arafat A, Johnston DR, et al. Repair of retrograde ascending dissection after descending stent grafting. *J Thorac Cardiovasc Surg*. 2014;147:151–154.
9. Ullery BW, Lee GK, Lee JT. Shuttering of the superior mesenteric artery during fenestrated endovascular aneurysm repair. *J Vasc Surg*. 2014;60:900–907.
10. Rose MK, Pearce BJ, Matthews TC, et al. Outcomes after celiac artery coverage during thoracic endovascular aortic aneurysm repair. *J Vasc Surg*. 2015;62:36–42.
11. Mehta M, Darling III RC, Taggert JB, et al. Outcomes of planned celiac artery coverage during TEVAR. *J Vasc Surg*. 2010;52:1153–1158.
12. Glorion M, Coscas R, McWilliams RG, et al. A comprehensive review of in situ fenestration of aortic endografts. *Eur J Vasc Endovasc Surg*. 2016;52:787–800.

19

TAA Endoleaks

Maciej L. Dryjski, MD, PhD, FACS, DFSVS, Dimitrios Koudoumas, MD, PhD and Brendon Reilly, MD, RPVI

INTRODUCTION

Thoracic endovascular aortic repair (TEVAR), first performed in 1992, has become the treatment of choice for the majority of thoracic aortic pathologies, including thoracic aortic aneurysms (TAAs) and complicated Type B aortic dissections (TADs).[1]

Presence of an endoleak is one of the most common reasons for early or late reinterventions and/or treatment failure following TEVAR. Endoleaks can be classified into four categories. A fifth category, called endotension, refers to aneurysmal sac pressurization without documented evidence of endoleak (Fig. 19.1). Endoleaks after TEVAR have been reported in 15%–30% of cases.[2,3] TEVAR failure in TAAs is most often a result of endoleaks, and failures in TADs are mainly because of persistent false lumen perfusion. The key element in prevention of endoleak formation is careful preoperative planning. However, once endoleaks develop, it is important to understand the cause of the endoleak as well as the anatomy of the aorta.

This chapter focuses on different techniques for treating endoleaks following TEVAR.

TYPE I ENDOLEAKS

Type I endoleaks originate from the sealing zones of the endograft and are further subdivided into proximal (Type Ia) or distal (Type Ib). Early Type I endoleaks are most often a result of an inadequate sealing zone in severely angulated, highly calcified aortic arches with increased thrombotic burden and vessel wall irregularity.[4] Graft in-folding secondary to more than 30% oversizing and bird-beak configuration (Fig. 19.2) are two very common reasons for Type Ia endoleaks. Progression of aortic disease is the cause of late Type I endoleaks.[5,6]

If Type I endoleak is identified on completion angiogram, the first step is balloon angioplasty. This corrects potential in-folding of oversized grafts. Nonetheless, this is not a simple maneuver and requires caution, particularly in dissection cases, where there is a risk of retrograde dissection. In addition, during balloon inflation, graft migration can occur as a result of windsock effect. This can be prevented by lowering blood pressure and ensuring good support from an introducer sheath. Rapid ventricular pacing is occasionally necessary.

Bird-beak formation was more frequently seen in early generation devices. This can potentially lead to complete collapse of the stent graft, with the risk correlating to the length of the beak. The endoleak secondary to bird beak is approached with a combination of interventions. Proximal stent-graft placement in conjunction with coverage and coil embolization of the left subclavian artery is often sufficient to correct the condition. However, placement of a proximal extension can be hazardous, because it may interfere with the left carotid artery. To minimize the risk of carotid coverage and to optimize stent graft placement, a sheath or a guidewire is introduced from the left carotid into the ascending aorta. This can be very helpful for bail-out stenting if unintentional coverage of the carotid occurs or intentional coverage is necessary for snorkel placement.

If a Type Ia endoleak results from insufficient neck length and placement of an extension cuff is not possible without cervical debranching, the use of Heli-FX EndoAnchor has been occasionally successful.[7,8] Use of the active fixation prevents graft migration in cases of complex aortic anatomy. Placement of a Palmaz stent in a short neck to eliminate Type I endoleak is unlikely to be successful. The treatment of perioperative Type Ib endoleak is balloon angioplasty and, if not successful, placement of an extension cuff. If coverage of the celiac trunk is needed, we use the sandwich technique to maintain celiac patency. However, if the celiac orifice is stenotic, it can be covered. The chimney or sandwich techniques are becoming more common procedures, allowing creation of prolonged proximal and distal landing zones without compromising perfusion of the branches.[9,10]

Another option is transcatheter embolization of the Type I endoleak. Published experiences include endoleak embolization using coils, cyanoacrylate, and Onyx.[11,12]

Open conversion, with partial or full extraction of the stent graft, allows easy access to the site of the endoleak but carries a particular high risk in old, frail patients who represent the majority of the population with aortic disease. In addition, the presence of the stent graft can complicate the repair, and hypothermic circulatory arrest may be necessary with modification of standard exposure.[13]

TYPE II ENDOLEAKS

Type II is the most frequent form of endoleak following TEVAR. Common sources of Type II endoleaks include the intercostal and bronchial arteries. Intraoperative Type II endoleaks are not routinely treated, since most resolve spontaneously. Nonetheless, endoleak from the subclavian artery may require special attention because of the large diameter of the vessel and its relationship to the aortic arch. The vessel can be easily accessed via a retrograde approach from the left brachial artery, and embolization with an Amplatzer plug or coils can be performed. A transthoracic approach for embolization of the subclavian artery can be used if a transbrachial approach is not possible (inadvertent ligation of subclavian artery distal to vertebral artery orifice, Fig. 19.3). The subclavian artery can be covered with a low incidence of side effects. However, revascularization with carotid–subclavian bypass is mandatory in patients with prior CABG with LIMA bypass, dominant left vertebral artery, or pre-existing incomplete posterior circulation.[14]

Type II endoleaks originating from the bronchial arteries are much less common, and it is often significantly more difficult to determine the exact location of the endoleak.

Special consideration should be given when approaching a Type II endoleak after endovascular repair of a thoracoabdominal aneurysm, because collateral vessels may play an important role for spinal cord

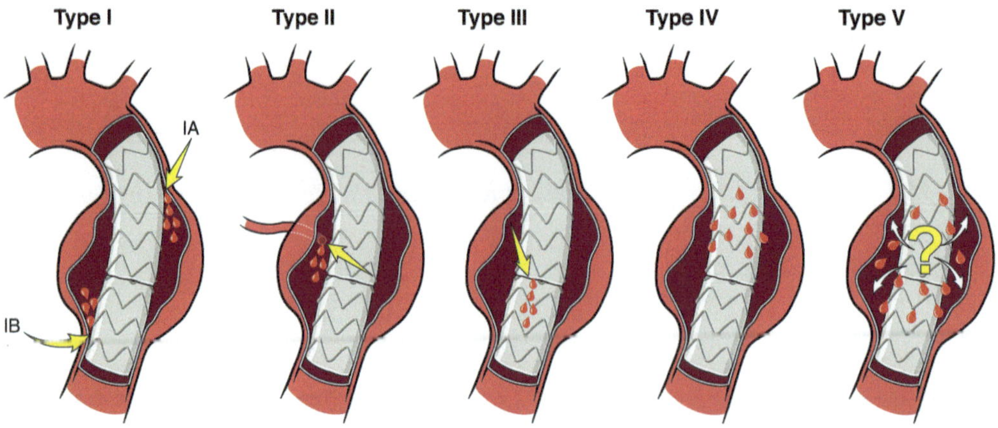

Fig. 19.1 **Types of Endoleaks.** Type I: inadequate fixation at the proximal (Ia) or distal (Ib) end of the graft to vessel wall, creating incomplete seal. Type II: retrograde filling of aneurysm sac from branch vessels. Type III: leak through a defect in graft fabric or inadequate opposition or separation of the modular components. Type IV: oozing through graft material. Type V: endotension. Aneurysm sac expands without any evidence of leak.

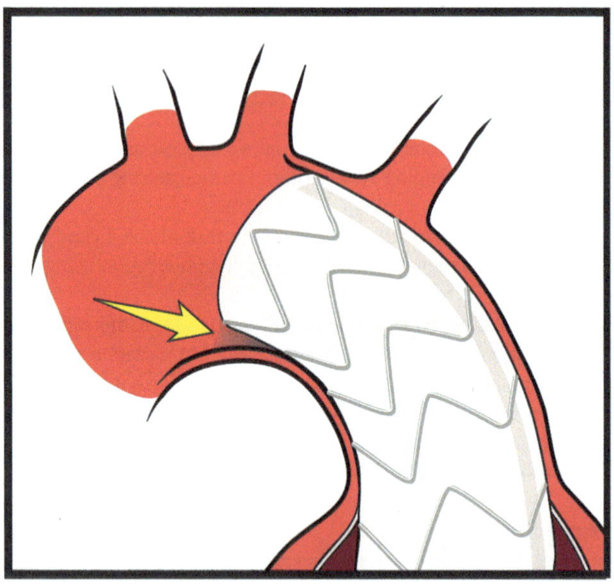

Fig. 19.2 Bird-beak configuration is created by an incomplete apposition of the proximal end of the graft with a wedge-shaped gap between the device and the aortic wall. Bird-beaking deformity has been associated with Type Ia endoleak and endograft compression and collapse.

circulation. Thus, embolization carries a risk of causing critical spinal cord ischemia. Spinal cord protective measures during and after embolization should be considered in patients with extensive stent graft of the aorta, or occlusion of the subclavian or hypogastric collaterals, such as cerebrospinal fluid drainage and strict blood pressure control management.

Even when treatment of a Type II endoleak is successful, close followup is warranted because patients are at risk of recurrence requiring reintervention.[15]

GUTTER ENDOLEAKS

Multiple parallel stent-graft combinations are being used nowadays for the management of complex TAAs and TADs. This may result in gutter endoleaks, the natural history of which still remains unknown. Literature data suggest that pressure transmission to the aneurysmal sac via nonthrombosed endoleak channels remains unchanged regardless of the length or diameter of the channel. On the other hand, in the presence of endoleak thrombosis the pressure reduction is directly proportional to the length and inversely proportional to the diameter of the channel. Catheter-based embolization techniques can be used to approach persistent gutter endoleaks.[16] To address the arch gutter endoleaks, the right brachial artery access is utilized. A long 6-French sheath (preferably Flexor Shuttle Guiding Sheath, Cook Bloomington, Indiana) is advanced to the arch and the gutter cavity is accessed using a 0.014″ wire and a microcatheter. The cavity is embolized with coils.

TYPE III ENDOLEAKS

A Type III endoleak occurs as a result of graft damage, tears, fatigue, or a disconnect between graft components. Type III endoleaks can be subdivided into Types IIIa and IIIb depending on whether the leak is related to a modular disconnect or to a fabric tear. They are at higher risk of sac enlargement and progression to rupture relative to other endoleaks, and early intervention is therefore advised.[17] The incidence of a Type III endoleak following endovascular thoracic aneurysm repair is variable. This is because of differences in graft selection and the reporting standards from the available literature. Regardless, the incidence of Type III endoleak is low, around 2%.[17] Early Type III endoleaks are identified on intraoperative completion angiography. These are usually related to misalignment of stent-graft components or inadequate postdeployment angioplasty. Late Type III endoleaks are, by definition, found on surveillance.

The best way to avoid a Type III endoleak is careful preoperative planning and adherence to instructions for use (IFU) with regard to minimum recommended overlap between components. Compromising overlap can predispose to disconnect between graft components. This is especially true in thoracic aortas with tortuous anatomy creating complex force vectors that are acting on the graft. Maximizing overlap is recommended to prevent the occurrence of a Type III endoleak.[4] Occasionally, oversizing of the distal component may result in in-folding of the graft and formation of a Type III endoleak.

If the endoleak is visualized on completion angiogram, angioplasty with compliant balloon is performed and, if unsuccessful, relining with an additional component will reinforce the junction. Management of a late Type III endoleak, regardless of etiology is accomplished with

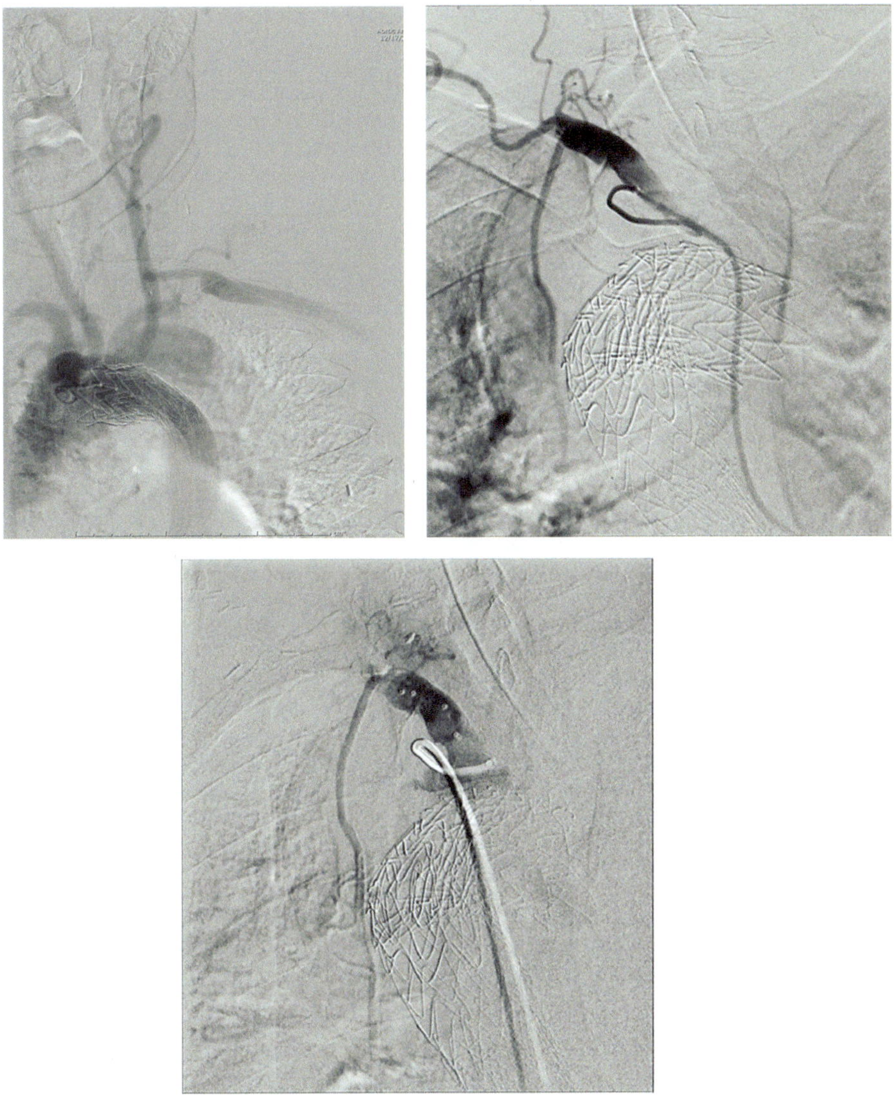

Fig. 19.3 Type II endoleak after TEVAR as a result of ligation of the subclavian artery distal to the internal thoracic artery (internal mammary artery), thyrocervical trunk, and costocervical trunk (A) at the time of carotid–subclavian bypass. The left vertebral artery had anomalous origin from the aortic arch; it was ligated and transposed to the left carotid artery. The endoleak was repaired by accessing the aneurysm transthoracically (B) and deploying an Amplatzer plug (C).

relining with a new device of the same size or 5%–10% larger. Heli-FX EndoAnchors (Medtronic, Minneapolis, Minnesota) can also be used to create graft-to-graft fixation. Finally, open repair is an option, but rarely necessary.

TYPES IV AND V ENDOLEAKS

Types IV and V endoleaks are rare. A Type IV is defined as flow through the graft material as a result of the native porosity of the graft. It is usually related to intraoperative anticoagulation with heparin and resolves without intervention. There are case reports of persistent type IV endoleaks that have gone on to rupture and to require emergency open intervention.[18–20]

Type V endoleaks are defined as an enlarging aneurysm sac with no visible endoleak, also referred to as endotension. There are no tips to prevent a Type V endoleak. However, some Type IV and V endoleaks are, in fact, Type I or III, but too small to be visualized using standard imaging techniques. Some go on to require repair because they lead to sac enlargement. A series of two cases from the University of Vienna, Austria, describe Type V endoleak following TEVAR. They were both treated with relining, which resulted in resolution of the endoleak and sac shrinkage in followup.[21] We had a similar experience with two cases, and both were successfully treated with relining.

PERSISTENT FALSE LUMEN PERFUSION FOLLOWING TEVAR FOR THORACIC AORTIC DISSECTION

Thoracic endograft placement in the case of complicated Type B dissection is performed to exclude the entry tear and thus eliminate perfusion of the false lumen. Perfusion may persist via distal re-entry tears. Reintervention may be required to avoid long-term disease progression and associated morbidity and mortality. It has been suggested that a partially thrombosed false lumen has an increased risk of aortic-related mortality in comparison with a fully thrombosed lumen. Thus, attempts should be made to achieve complete thrombosis of the false lumen whenever possible. The simplest way to address persistent false lumen perfusion is extension of coverage with additional stent-graft components. However, the benefits of doing so must be weighed against the increased risk of spinal cord ischemia and potential paralysis. Other ways to achieve false lumen thrombosis include sealing of re-entry tears with occlusive plugs or coil embolization of the false lumen.[16,22]

REFERENCES

1. Dake MD, Miller DC, Semba CP, Mitchell RS, Walker PJ, Liddell RP. Transluminal placement of endovascular stent-grafts for the treatment of descending thoracic aortic aneurysms. *The New England journal of medicine.* 1994;331(26):1729–1734. PubMed PMID: 7984192.
2. Parmer SS, Carpenter JP, Stavropoulos SW, et al. Endoleaks after endovascular repair of thoracic aortic aneurysms. *Journal of vascular surgery.* 2006;44(3):447–452. PubMed PMID: 16950414.
3. Preventza O, Wheatley GH 3rd, Ramaiah VG, et al. Management of endoleaks associated with endovascular treatment of descending thoracic aortic diseases. *Journal of vascular surgery.* 2008;48(1):69–73. PubMed PMID: 18486425.
4. Nakatamari H, Ueda T, Ishioka F, et al. Discriminant analysis of native thoracic aortic curvature: risk prediction for endoleak formation after thoracic endovascular aortic repair. *Journal of vascular and interventional radiology.* 2011;22(7):974–979 e2. PubMed PMID: 21570875.
5. Fairman RM, Tuchek JM, Lee WA, et al. Pivotal results for the Medtronic Valiant Thoracic Stent Graft System in the VALOR II trial. *Journal of vascular surgery.* 2012;56(5):1222–1231 e1. PubMed PMID: 22832267.
6. Kamman AV, Jonker FH, Nauta FJ, Trimarchi S, Moll FL, van Herwaarden JA. A review of follow-up outcomes after elective endovascular repair of degenerative thoracic aortic aneurysms. *Vascular.* 2016;24(2): 208–216. PubMed PMID: 26002781.
7. Garland BT, Singh N, Starnes BW. Endovascular repositioning of a migrated stent graft using "endoanchor capture". *Annals of vascular surgery.* 2015;29(1):123 e1–5. PubMed PMID: 24929051.
8. Ongstad SB, Miller DF, Panneton JM. The use of EndoAnchors to rescue complicated TEVAR procedures. *The Journal of cardiovascular surgery.* 2016;57(5):716–729. PubMed PMID: 27465392.
9. Cires G, Noll RE Jr., Albuquerque FC Jr., Tonnessen BH. Sternbergh WC, 3rd. Endovascular debranching of the aortic arch during thoracic endograft repair. *Journal of vascular surgery.* 2011;53(6):1485–1491. PubMed PMID: 21498028.
10. Kawatani Y, Hayashi Y, Ito Y, et al. A case of ruptured aortic arch aneurysm successfully treated by thoracic endovascular aneurysm repair with chimney graft. *Case reports in surgery.* 2015;2015:780147. PubMed PMID: 25815238; PubMed Central PMCID: PMC4359878.
11. Bangard C, Franke M, Pfister R, et al. Thoracic type Ia endoleak: direct percutaneous coil embolization of the aortic arch at the blood entry site after TEVAR and double-chimney stent-grafts. *European radiology.* 2014;24(6):1430–1434. PubMed PMID: 24643498.
12. Katada Y, Kondo S, Tsuboi E, Nakamura K, Rokkaku K, Irie Y. Type IA endoleak embolization after TEVAR via direct transthoracic puncture. *Japanese journal of radiology.* 2015;33(3):169–172. PubMed PMID: 25626572.
13. Coselli JS, Spiliotopoulos K, Preventza O, de la Cruz KI, Amarasekara H, Green SY. Open aortic surgery after thoracic endovascular aortic repair. *General thoracic and cardiovascular surgery.* 2016;64(8):441–449. PubMed PMID: 27314956.
14. Morales JP, Greenberg RK, Lu Q, et al. Endoleaks following endovascular repair of thoracic aortic aneurysm: etiology and outcomes. *J Endovasc Ther.* 2008;15(6):631–638. PubMed PMID: 19090634.
15. Sarac TP, Gibbons C, Vargas L, et al. Long term follow-up of type II endoleak embolization reveals the need for close surveillance. *Journal of vascular surgery.* 2012;55(1):33–40. PubMed PMID: 22056249.
16. Mehta M, Ohki T, Veith FJ, Lipsitz EC. All sealed endoleaks are not the same: a treatment strategy based on an ex-vivo analysis. *European journal of vascular and endovascular surgery: the official journal of the European Society for Vascular Surgery.* 2001;21(6):541–544. PubMed PMID: 11397029.
17. Leszczyński J, Macioch W, Chudziński W, Gaøåzka Z. Late type III endoleak after thoracic endovascular aneurysm repair and previous infrarenal stent graft implantation - a case report and review of the literature. *Wideochir Inne Tech Maloinwazyjne.* 2017;12(3):320–324. Epub July 31, 2017. PubMed PMID: 29062457; PubMed Central PMCID: PMC5649506.
18. Filis K, Zarmakoupis C, Karantzikos G, Sigala F, Bazigos G, Galyfos G. Late sac rupture due to a Type IV endoleak after previous endovascular aortic aneurysm repair: a case report. *Front Surg.* 2017;4:45. eCollection 2017. PubMed PMID: 28848736; PubMed Central PMCID: PMC5554120.
19. Wachal K, Szmyt K, Oszkinis G. Diagnosis and treatment of a patient with type IV endoleak as a late complication after endovascular aneurysm repair. *Wideochir Inne Tech Maloinwazyjne.* 2014;9(4):667–670. Epub 2014 Nov 28. PubMed PMID: 25562013; PubMed Central PMCID: PMC4280431.
20. Törnqvist P, Resch T. Endoleaks after EVAR and TEVAR: indications for treatment and techniques. *J Cardiovasc Surg (Torino).* 2014;55(2 Suppl 1): 105–114, Review. PubMed PMID. Available from: 24796903.
21. Zimpfer D, Schoder M, Gottardi R, et al. Treatment of type V endoleaks by endovascular redo stent-graft placement. *Ann Thorac Surg.* 2007; 83(2):664–666. PubMed PMID: 17258007.
22. Nienaber CA, Kische S, Rousseau H, et al. Endovascular repair of type B aortic dissection: long-term results of the randomized investigation of stent grafts in aortic dissection trial. *Circ Cardiovasc Interv.* 2013;6: 407–416.

20

Complications of TAG and Conformable TAG (CTAG) Thoracic Endoprosthesis

Tze-Woei Tan, MD, MPH, FACS and Wayne W. Zhang, MD, FACS

INTRODUCTION

The Conformable TAG (CTAG) endoprosthesis (WL Gore and Associates, Flagstaff, Arizona) is the third-generation thoracic endograft approved for treatment of aneurysm, traumatic transection, and Type B dissection in the descending thoracic aorta. The second-generation TAG endoprosthesis was the first stent graft approved for thoracic endovascular aortic repair (TEVAR) of descending aortic aneurysm by the US Food and Drug Administration (FDA) in 2005. More than 40,000 TAG devices were distributed worldwide prior to its discontinuation in 2013. These devices have been studied extensively in various clinical trials and real-world use clinical series and are associated with significantly lower short-term mortality and morbidity than open surgery for thoracic aortic aneurysm.[1,2] The efficacy of the newer CTAG device has been further studied for the treatment of Type B aortic dissection and traumatic aortic transection.[3,4]

The expansion of the use of the TAG and CTAG devices in treating thoracic pathologies have led to a unique set of device-related complications, which will be summarized in this chapter. The complications can be divided into intraoperative (maldeployment, retrograde dissection, branch occlusion), early events, and late events (stent graft collapse, stent fracture).

TAG ENDOPROSTHESIS

The TAG thoracic endoprosthesis is a self-expanding device comprising of an expanded polytetrafluoroethylene (ePTFE) and fluoroethylpropylene (FEP) tube graft, which is supported externally by a nitinol stent. There are flared covered scallops and a radiopaque gold marker at each end of the device (Fig. 20.1). An ePTFE sleeve is used to constrain the stent graft on the delivery catheter and remains in place between the external surface of the device and the aorta after deployment. The TAG endoprosthesis was available in sizes ranging from 26 to 45 mm for use in intended aortic inner diameters of 23–42 mm, with the recommended oversizing window of 8%–17%.

The phase II pivotal study was a prospective, nonrandomized, multicenter study, which enrolled 142 patients who underwent TEVAR of descending thoracic aortic aneurysms with the first generation TAG device.[5] The enrollment was between 1999 and 2001 and a total of 139 patients (98%) underwent successful implantation of the device. Three patients had procedural failure (2%) resulting from access issues secondary to iliac artery size and tortuosity. Two patients had misplacement of the device, resulting in unplanned coverage of subclavian and/or visceral arteries. The patient with coverage of visceral vessels underwent open removal of the displaced device. Major adverse events (MAE) within 30-days occurred in 32% of patients, including bleeding (9%), cardiac event (3%), pulmonary event (10%), and vascular complications (14%). The overall operative mortality was 2% and five patients (3.5%) suffered a perioperative stroke. Four patients developed spinal cord ischemia and the subsequent placement of spinal drain was beneficial in three out of those four patients. Five patients developed early endoleak, including one Type I and four Type II endoleaks. The patient who had early Type I endoleak was treated with placement of an additional proximal endograft.

The all-cause mortality and aneurysm-related mortality for the pivotal trial was 75% and 79% respectively at 2 years.[5] There were three proximal migrations and four component migrations during 2-year follow-up. Three patients underwent endovascular interventions and one had conversion to open surgery. No aneurysm rupture was reported during the follow-up. The cumulative rate of endoleak was 15% (21 patients) during the first 2 years after surgery. There were 20 stent fractures, which were identified in 19 patients. Up to 90% of the stent fractures occurred in the longitudinal spine and two in the apical nitinol support ring. The majority of patients with stent fracture in this cohort were asymptomatic (18 patients) and only one patient developed a Type III endoleak, which was treated successfully with extension of the pre-existing stent graft.

The complication of stent fractures in the initial pivotal trial led to voluntary withdrawal of the device in May 2001 and the development of the second generation TAG device.[6] The first generation TAG device was constructed with two ePTFE layers and was supported by two longitudinal columnar spines (Fig. 20.1A). The modified second generation TAG device was constructed with three ePTFE layers and the longitudinal wires, which were susceptible to fracture, were removed (Fig. 20.1B). The modified device was evaluated in the confirmatory trial, which enrolled 51 patients from 11 clinical sites. The MAE was 12% at 30-day follow-up and there was no device-related MAE reported.[6]

The intermediate and long-term results for the TAG pivotal trial were published in 2007 and 2008.[1,2] The rate of aneurysm-related mortality was significantly lower in the TAG group when compared with the open surgical group (2.8% versus 11.7%, $P = 0.008$). Endoleaks developed in 10.6% of TAG patients and the majority were Type Ia endoleak at the attachment site. Five TAG patients required aneurysm-related endovascular and open reinterventions (3.6%): one arch aneurysm repair for Type I endoleak and migration, five endovascular interventions in three patients for endoleaks, and one open conversion for aortoesophageal fistula. There were no additional spine fractures other than the previously reported 20 fractures (19 patients) after 24 months.

Structurally the TAG device was not as flexible as the newer generation CTAG device (described later). In patients with deep arch curves or so-called gothic arches, suboptimal placement resulted in a "bird-beak" appearance as a result of incomplete inner aortic curve apposition to the aortic arch (Fig. 20.2). This theoretically increased the risk of Type Ia endoleak and/or endograft collapse.[7,8] The less flexible TAG

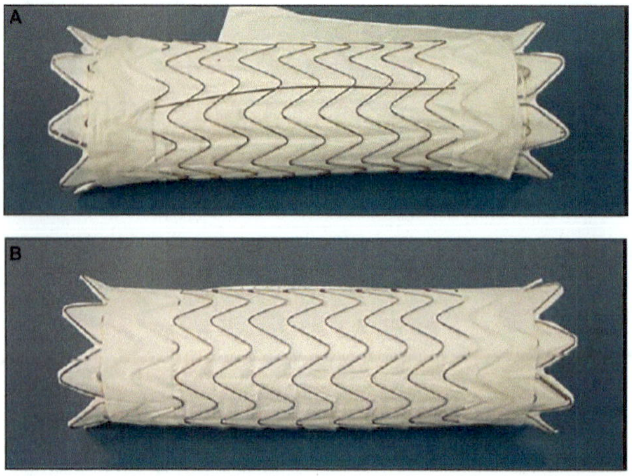

Fig. 20.1 The Gore TAG endoprosthesis. (A) The first-generation Gore TAG endoprosthesis with two longitudinal support wires. (B) The modified Gore TAG device without any longitudinal support wire. (Permission from Elsevier.)

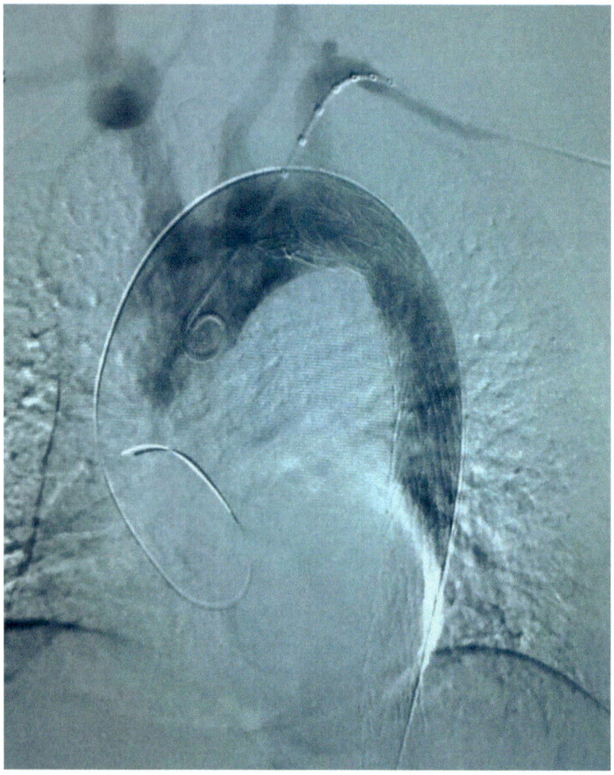

Fig. 20.2 "Bird-beak" appearance resulting from poor alignment of a TAG endoprosthesis in a patient with Type II aortic arch who underwent endovascular repair of descending thoracic aortic aneurysm.

endograft was also found in other off-label use to cause new antegrade intimal tears when it was used to treat aortic dissection (Fig. 20.3).[8,9] In our practice we recommend the placement of an extension endograft to correct the "bird beak" to eliminate the pressure onto the membrane of dissection. This type of graft-related complications have fortunately been minimized with the more flexible new generation CTAG endoprosthesis (Fig. 20.4).[10]

CTAG ENDOPROSTHESIS

Similar to the TAG endoprosthesis, the CTAG device is a self-expanding ePTFE/FEP graft which is supported by a nitinol stent and is constrained on the delivery catheter by a sewn ePTFE sleeve. In the CTAG the flared scallops on the proximal TAG device were eliminated and replaced by uncovered stent apices (Fig. 20.4A). The stent apices on the distal device are covered with graft material. The construction of the CTAG device has been optimized to allow for improved comfirmability to accommodate various aortic anatomies better. The structural changes from eight to nine stent apices and the increased wire diameter on the nitinol stent allow for improvement in compression resistance. The CTAG device is available in sizes between 21 and 45 mm and in 10, 15, and 20 cm length. The device is intended to be used in the inner aortic landing zone diameter between 16 and 42 mm, and the oversizing window for the CTAG has been expanded to 6%–33%. Two tapered devices are also available (26 × 21 and 31 × 26 mm).

The effectiveness of the CTAG device for the treatment of blunt thoracic aortic injury was evaluated in a company-sponsored trial published in 2013.[4] Fifty-one patients were enrolled between 2009 and 2011 at 21 sites. The majority were victims of motor vehicle collision (84.3%). The mean age for the cohort was 44.1 years, and the mean aortic diameter at the proximal implantation zone was 24.1 mm. Technical success for this cohort was 100%, and the mean time from injury to endovascular repair was 21 hours. Up to 88% of patients received one CTAG device. Six patients (12%) received two devices, including three patients with maldeployment distal to intended location and a patient who required a second implant because of a Type III endoleak. Mortality at 30-days was 7.8%, and the majority was caused by the injury and not procedure- or device-related. Although there was a 39% serious adverse event rate, there were no major device events reported in this trial. There was one reported stent migration of more than 10 mm on repeat imaging, but there were no cases of wire fracture or device collapse in this cohort. The data from this trial led to FDA approval for the use of the CTAG endoprosthesis for the treatment of traumatic aortic transection.

MALDEPLOYMENT

Endograft maldeployment is one of the operator's worst nightmares that fortunately happens infrequently. The TAG and CTAG devices have a single-step deployment mechanism that is appealing to operators because of its simplicity. The device is deployed by unlocking and pulling on the deployment knob at the distal end of the delivery catheter. The knob is connected to the deployment sleeve, which is used to constrain the stent graft on the delivery catheter. The pulling of the knob allows delivery of the device with expansion from the middle toward both ends of the stent graft simutaneously (Fig. 20.5A). The rapid expansion of the device during deployment minimizes the intraluminal movement related to arterial blow. There is, however, no backup deployment mechanism in the event the primary manoeuvre fails.

Lee et al. first described two cases of TAG thoracic endograft maldeployment (total of three devices) in 2007.[11] In both patients, the proximal end of the TAG endograft remained constricted after complete pulling of the deployment knob. The deployment strings in these cases were intact without any evidence of break or damage. The complication was addressed successfully using endovascular techniques. Through a contralateral femoral access, the authors used a smaller 0.014″ wire to pass through the constrained end of the stent graft from the open distal end. The wire was subsequently exchanged for a stiffer 0.035″ wire over a catheter. Various angioplasty balloons were used successfully to dilate and to expand the constrained portion. Two TAG devices failed to

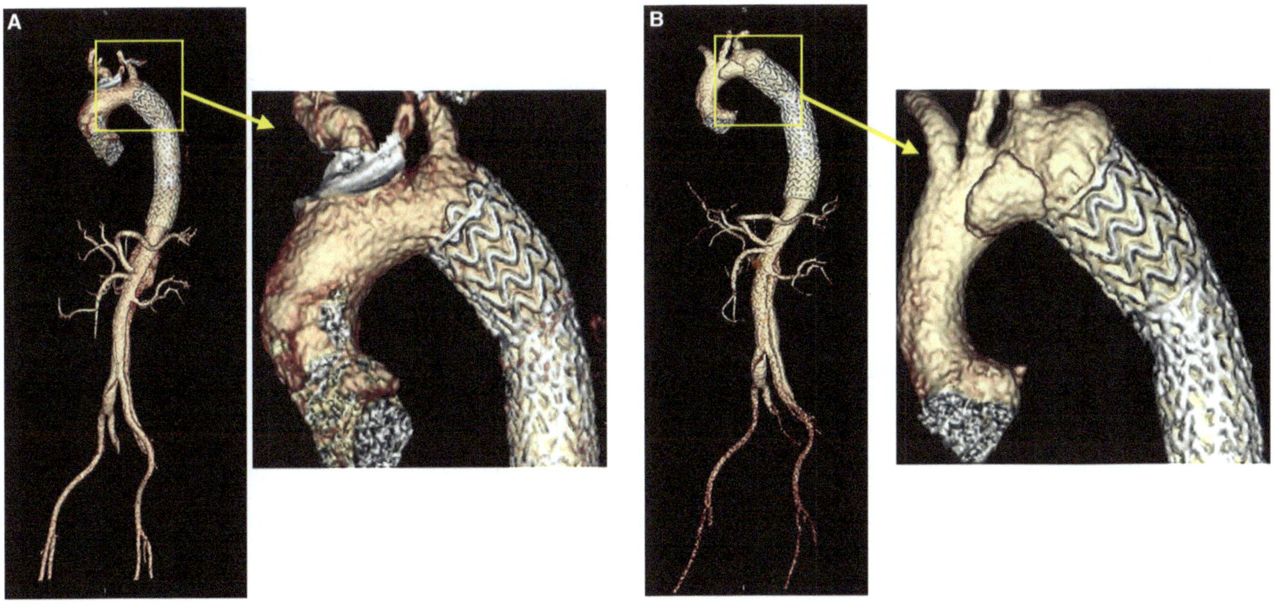

Fig. 20.3 Antegrade dissection in a patient who underwent endovascular repair of Type B aortic dissection because of poor angulation. CT angiogram of the chest (A) 1 month and (B) 8 months after surgery.
(Images provided by W-G Fu, Shanghai, China)

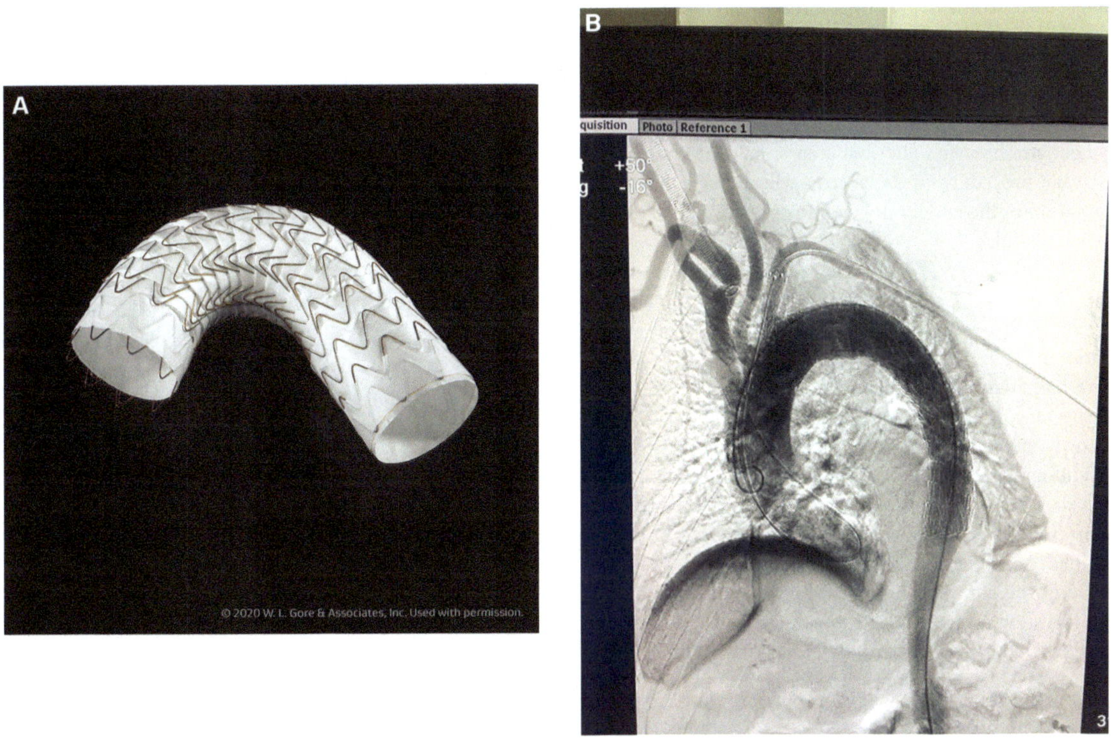

Fig. 20.4 (A) Gore Conformable TAG (CTAG) endoprosthesis; (B) Aortogram during placement of CTAG endograft and left subclavian stent graft for endovascular repair of acute Type B aortic dissection. Adequate alignment of the CTAG device in a patient with Type III aortic arch.

deploy at its proximal end in the same patient. The salvage procedure described earlier was used successfully. Unfortunately, one of the patients suffered a fatal intraoperative stroke.

In September 2017, the company issued a safety notification after four reported cases of incomplete or partial deployment among its newest generation CTAG endograft. In these events, half of the CTAG devices remained constrained to the delivery catheter after deployment. At least two of the deployment failures were secondary to issues with the deployment line stitch pattern or line damage. Almost all the reported cases required intraoperative open surgical conversion, which

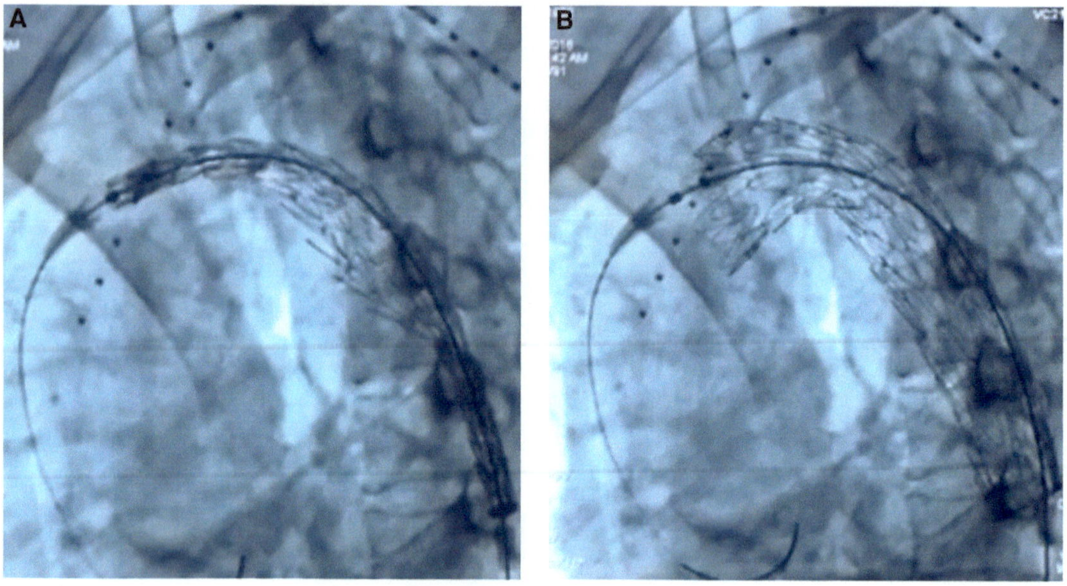

Fig. 20.5 (A) The TAG device expands from the middle toward both ends of the stent graft silmutaneously during deployment. (B) Approximately 5-mm distal migration occurred after deployment.

resulted in death or significant morbidities. The company estimated that the incidence of partial maldeployment in the CTAG device to be 0.03% (4 of 12,865 devices distributed) and has no current plans to remove this device from the market.

Although it is uncommon, the maldeployment of the TAG and CTAG devices can be a severe complication because of the lack of a backup deployment mechanism. The first step should be the use of endovascular salvage procedure as described earlier. Open thoracotomy with explantation of the endograft is required if the endovascular maneuver is not successful.

MIGRATION

Endograft migration may occur during and after deployment (Fig. 20.5B). The risk factors associated with migration may include high blood pressure during deployment, pulling the deployment knob too fast or too slowly, deploying over the floppy portion of the wire, or deploying with endograft protruding into a large aneurysmal sac, as well as anatomical risk factor such as aortic tortuosity.[12] Endograft migration can result in unplanned coverage of branch vessels or endoleaks because of inadequate sealing. To minimize this complication, we recommend pushing the stiff wire against the greater curvature and deploying the endograft while it is in contact with the outer aortic curve (Fig. 20.6). We typically use the extended double curve Lunderquist extra-stiff wire (Cook Medical, Bloomington, Indiana) and the wire is carefully pushed antegrade against the aortic valve for additional support. Temporary reduction of mean arterial pressure can be helpful to minimize "windsock" effect and migration. Others have also used rapid ventricular pacing and adenosine-induced asystole to achieve zero pressure deployment.[13,14]

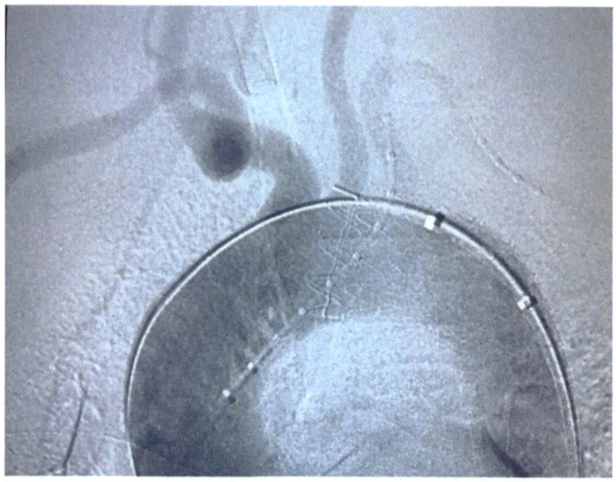

Fig. 20.6 The extra-stiff wire was pushed against the greater curvature to ensure direct contact between the device and the wall of the aorta during deployment.

COMPRESSION AND COLLAPSE

Thoracic stent graft compression and collapse are rare but potentially devastating complications.[15,16] Although it has been reported with all thoracic devices, it is most commonly described with the earlier generation TAG endoprosthesis (Fig. 20.7).[15,16] This could be partially related to the used of TAG endograft in young trauma patients with smaller inner aortic diameters. The smallest available TAG endograft was 26 mm and aggressive oversizing was inevitable because of the smaller aortic diameters in trauma patients when compared with the patients with thoracic aneurysms.[17] Thoracic endograft collapse can lead to acute aortic occlusion, which can result in malperfusion and multiorgan failure. The causes of endograft collapse are frequently multifactorial and might be related to excessive oversizing or native aortic anatomy and aortic arch curvature.[18,19]

In their meta-analysis, 60 cases of endograft collapse were identified and analyzed by Jonker et al.[19] Endograft collapse most frequently occurred when the initial TEVAR was performed for traumatic aortic injury (65%), followed by Type B aortic dissection (15%) and thoracic aortic aneurysm (12%). The TAG device was the most frequently used endograft (77%) in these patients. Patients with endograft collapse had

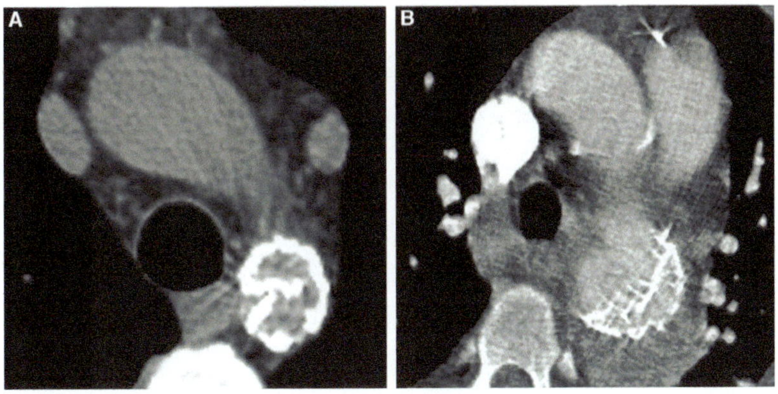

Fig. 20.7 Endoprosthesis collapse may cause mild to severe flow lumen occlusion.
(Cho JS, Haider SE, Makaroun MS. Endovascular therapy of thoracic aneurysms: Gore TAG trial results. Semin Vasc Surg 2006;19:18-24.).

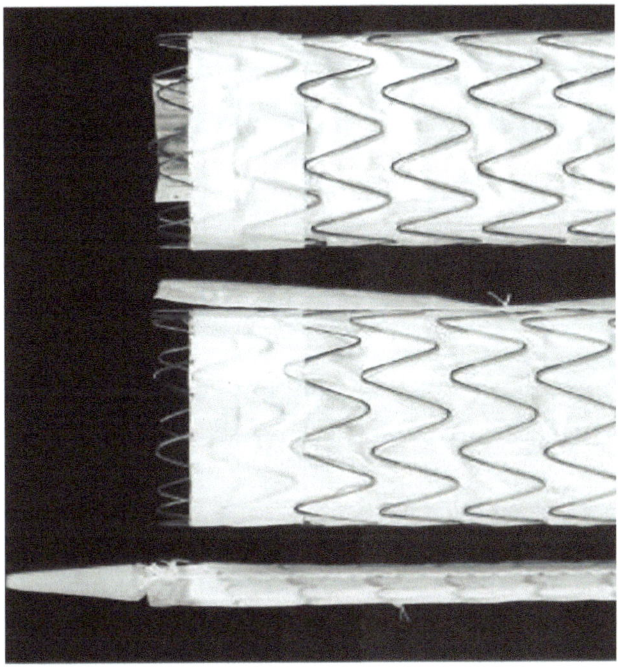

Fig. 20.8 The ePTFE wrapping sleeve of CTAG device is approximately 5 mm beyond the proximal end of the PTFE membrane.

significantly more oversizing than those without (26.7% versus 16.8%, $P < 0.001$). More than 20% oversizing was present in 67% of endograft collapse in this series, which was outside the recommended oversizing window for the TAG device. A large proportion of collapse was at proximal endograft (66%), followed by distal endograft (16%), and entire endograft (18%).

Endograft collapse was symptomatic in 41% of patients, while 59% was asymptomatic and discovered during follow-up imaging. The symptoms were absent or weak femoral pulses, chest pain, new onset or worsening hypertension, or acute renal failure. The median time for diagnosis of endograft collapse was 15 days after the initial procedure, and more than 65% were diagnosed within 30 days postoperatively. The majority of patients underwent additional interventions after the diagnosis. Endovascular intervention was used in 68% of patients and most commonly involved deployment of additional devices ($n = 36$; 60%). Balloon dilatation alone without additional device ($n = 3$) and coil embolization of the left subclavian artery ($n = 2$) for the thrombosis of the aneurysm sac or false lumen were also used. Around 18% of patients underwent open surgery including explantation and axillofemoral bypass. Eight of 60 patients however did not undergo any intervention.

Significant numbers of endograft collapse occur during the first month of deployment and most often after treatment for a blunt aortic injury. Excessive oversizing and small inner radius of curvature are the main reasons leading to endograft collapse. Oversizing, especially in young trauma patients, should be kept at less than 20% to minimize the risk of device collapse.

UNINTENDED BRANCH VESSEL OCCLUSION

Accidental branch vessel coverage can occur with inaccurate deployment or stent graft migration. Occlusion of a branch vessel by the proximal ePTFE wrapping sleeve is an infrequent event, and it is unique to the CTAG endoprosthesis design. As seen in Fig. 20.8, the wrapping sleeve is approximately 5 mm beyond the proximal end of the device. If this sleeve is positioned at the orifice of a branch vessel, it can obstruct the blood flow even if the endograft is placed and deployed accurately. Fig. 20.9 shows a TEVAR performed to treat thoracic aortic aneurysm with planned left subclavian artery coverage for adequate proximal sealing zone. The endograft was placed at the premarked position, which was immediately distal to the left common carotid artery, and was deployed accurately. Interestingly, a postdeployment angiogram demonstrated the occlusion of the left common carotid artery, although the covered portion of the endograft was distal to the branch artery. Immediate revascularization to restore blood flow with endovascular or open approach is mandatory for accidental coverage of the carotid artery. Selective revascularization of covered left subclavian artery might be required depending on the patient's clinical presentation and anatomy. Endovascular revascularization of carotid or subclavian artery can be performed with retrograde stent graft placement utilizing chimney/snorkel or in situ fenestration technique. Open surgical options include carotid–carotid artery bypass, carotid–subclavian artery bypass, or carotid–subclavian artery transposition.

SUMMARY

The CTAG endoprosthesis is the latest generation currently available of Gore thoracic endoprosthesis and has been shown to be effective for endovascular treatment of aneurysm, traumatic transection, and type B

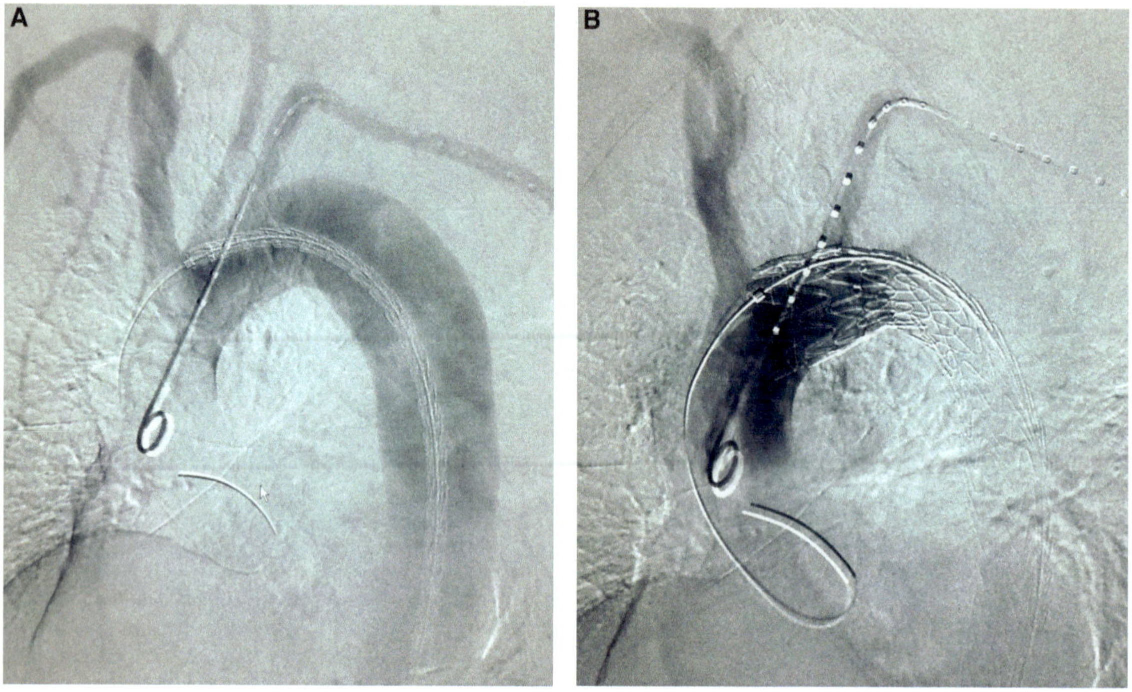

Fig. 20.9 A TEVAR with planned left subclavian artery coverage for proximal sealing zone extension was performed to treat thoracic aortic aneurysm. (A) The endograft was placed at the premarked position and deployed immediately distal to the left common carotid artery. (B) Post-deployment angiogram showed occlusion of left common carotid artery most likely by the wrapping ePTFE sleeve.

dissection in the descending thoracic aorta. The design modifications that led to improved comformability and the expansion of the oversizing window reduced complications such as graft collapse/compression and wire fracture seen in older-generation TAG endoprosthesis. Current modifications and next-generation devices are related to allowing the CTAG device to deploy in a more curved or angled landing zone.

REFERENCES

1. Makaroun MS, Dillavou ED, Wheatley GH, Cambria RP, Gore TAGI. Five-year results of endovascular treatment with the Gore TAG device compared with open repair of thoracic aortic aneurysms. *J Vasc Surg.* 2008;47:912–918.
2. Bavaria JE, Appoo JJ, Makaroun MS, et al. Endovascular stent grafting versus open surgical repair of descending thoracic aortic aneurysms in low-risk patients: a multicenter comparative trial. *J Thorac Cardiovasc Surg.* 2007;133:369–377.
3. Cambria RP, Conrad MF, Matsumoto AH, et al. Multicenter clinical trial of the conformable stent graft for the treatment of acute, complicated type B dissection. *J Vasc Surg.* 2015;62:271–278.
4. Farber MA, Giglia JS, Starnes BW, et al. Evaluation of the redesigned conformable GORE TAG thoracic endoprosthesis for traumatic aortic transection. *J Vasc Surg.* 2013;58:651–658.
5. Makaroun MS, Dillavou ED, Kee ST, et al. Endovascular treatment of thoracic aortic aneurysms: results of the phase II multicenter trial of the GORE TAG thoracic endoprosthesis. *J Vasc Surg.* 2005;41:1–9.
6. Cho JS, Haider SE, Makaroun MS. Endovascular therapy of thoracic aneurysms: Gore TAG trial results. *Semin Vasc Surg.* 2006;19:18–24.
7. Ueda T, Fleischmann D, Dake MD, Rubin GD, Sze DY. Incomplete endograft apposition to the aortic arch: bird-beak configuration increases risk of endoleak formation after thoracic endovascular aortic repair. *Radiology.* 2010;255:645–652.
8. Nienaber CA, Kische S, Ince H. Thoracic aortic stent-graft devices: problems, failure modes, and applicability. *Semin Vasc Surg.* 2007;20:81–89.
9. Williams JB, Andersen ND, Bhattacharya SD, et al. Retrograde ascending aortic dissection as an early complication of thoracic endovascular aortic repair. *J Vasc Surg.* 2012;55:1255–1262.
10. Kasirajan K. New C-TAG device and overcome of compression events. *J Cardiovasc Surg (Torino).* 2012;53:169–172.
11. Lee WA, Martin TD, Hess PJ, Beaver TM, Huber TS. Maldeployment of the TAG thoracic endograft. *J Vasc Surg.* 2007;46:1032–1035.
12. Boufi M, Guivier-Curien C, Dona B, et al. Risk Factor Analysis for the Mal-Positioning of Thoracic Aortic Stent Grafts. *Eur J Vasc Endovasc Surg.* 2016;52:56–63.
13. Nienaber CA, Kische S, Rehders TC, et al. Rapid pacing for better placing: comparison of techniques for precise deployment of endografts in the thoracic aorta. *J Endovasc Ther.* 2007;14:506–512.
14. Qu L, Raithel D. Techniques for precise thoracic endograft placement. *J Vasc Surg.* 2009;49:1069–1072; discussion 72.
15. Tadros RO, Lipsitz EC, Chaer RA, Faries PL, Marin ML, Cho JS. A multicenter experience of the management of collapsed thoracic endografts. *J Vasc Surg.* 2011;53:1217–1222.
16. Kasirajan K, Dake MD, Lumsden A, Bavaria J, Makaroun MS. Incidence and outcomes after infolding or collapse of thoracic stent grafts. *J Vasc Surg.* 2012;55:652–658; discussion 8.
17. Alberta HB, Secor JL, Smits TC, Farber MA, Jordan WD, Matsumura JS. Differences in aortic arch radius of curvature, neck size, and taper in patients with traumatic and aortic disease. *J Surg Res.* 2013;184:613–618.
18. Muhs BE, Balm R, White GH, Verhagen HJ. Anatomic factors associated with acute endograft collapse after Gore TAG treatment of thoracic aortic dissection or traumatic rupture. *J Vasc Surg.* 2007;45:655–661.
19. Jonker FH, Schlosser FJ, Geirsson A, Sumpio BE, Moll FL, Muhs BE. Endograft collapse after thoracic endovascular aortic repair. *J Endovasc Ther.* 2010;17:725–734.

21

Device-Specific Issues With EVAR: Cook

Michael R. Hall, MD and Mark A. Farber, MD, FACS

INTRODUCTION

Since the advent of endovascular abdominal aortic aneurysm repair (EVAR) for abdominal aortic aneurysms (AAA), the rate of technical proficiency has reached impressive levels, with modern reports reaching 99%–100% of endografts successfully placed during initial treatment.[1] However, despite technical success and exceedingly low perioperative mortality, the need for reintervention continues to be the crux of EVAR and is most often related to endograft-specific complications. Although complications may be universal to all devices, a significant proportion of devices are being used outside their instructions for use (IFU) guidelines, leading to concern for device-specific complications when used in this manner. Being aware of and knowing how to mitigate or to prevent these complications will help provide better outcomes for patients undergoing EVAR.

Although patient selection is often critical in achieving good outcomes, procedural/device-related issues can occur. Technical complications directly associated with endograft placement during EVAR include: device delivery and deployment issues; access-related complications; lack of fixation or poor sealing of the graft leading to endoleak or aneurysm expansion; stent fractures, graft material breakdown, or component separations. Despite these issues, EVAR has become the standard of care for the surgical treatment of AAA, and multiple devices share these common limitations.

Zenith endografts (Cook Medical Inc., Bloomington, Indiana), one of the most implanted endografts in the United States today, consist of a woven polyester and stainless steel main body. It is a modular, long-bodied, three-piece, self-expanding system with an active suprarenal fixation. It comes with an integrated sheath for delivery and its push-pull method of deployment allows accurate repositioning until the top cap is released. It is approved for 15-mm infrarenal necks and ≤60 degree angulation. Because it is one of the earliest and most used endografts, there is a relatively abundant amount of data on outcomes with use of this device. Here we review the complications that may arise with EVAR results associated with the use of Cook's Zenith endografts for the treatment of AAA.

ENDOLEAK

Early results using the Zenith AAA endovascular graft, reported in 2004 by Greenberg and colleagues[2], demonstrated a safe and effective treatment for AAA in both groups of patients, either deemed too high risk for open repair or those considered safe for open repair. Despite technical success being near 99% or higher for both groups, the rate of endoleak in the perioperative period was upward of 17%, the majority of perioperative endoleak being type II. On follow-up, the endoleak rate diminished to 7.4% and 5.4% at 12- and 24-months, respectively. No patient had persistent Type I or III endoleak by 24 months. This was counter-balanced by the standard risk group (for open repair) undergoing more secondary interventions, most of which were for endoleaks. Follow-up to this in 2008 for the same group concluded the long-term durability of the graft to be acceptable in both groups.[3] However, the rate of endoleak continued to be of concern. The rate of late endoleak development (first appearing 6 months after repair and surveillance) was reported between 12% and 14%, most of which were Type II. While generally considered benign, 80% of the endoleaks attributed to causing aneurysm sac enlargement were Type II. Moreover, the majority of secondary interventions were a result of these Type II endoleaks during the study period. Notably, in either group, no Type I or III endoleak was identified at the 5-year follow-up period.

Most recently, Verzini and colleagues have reported the 14-year outcomes of patients treated with Zenith endograft for AAA in Italy.[4] They treated 610 patients over a longer than 10-year period. Overall endoleak of any type at any time was 22.9%, 74% of which were Type II endoleaks. Endoleak of any type was attributed to 9 of the 11 conversions to open repair and 56 of the 80 patients requiring reintervention. While endoleak contributed to a large proportion of the reinterventions for these grafts, the results compare favorably in comparison with other reports, both remote and recent.[3,5]

Technical Considerations

The majority of endoleaks are Type II endoleaks; these are nonspecific to the device used for repair. However, to obviate the risk of Type Ia and Type Ib endoleaks with the Zenith endograft, close attention to preoperative device planning and sizing is paramount. The IFU, for the Zenith Flex for example, states the aneurysm neck to be no shorter than 15 mm and angled no more than 60 degrees relative to the long axis of the aneurysm. In addition, the device is approved for an aortic fixation site diameter of between 18 mm and 32 mm. It is important to note the measurement for the Cook device is outer wall to outer wall, regardless of the imaging software used to obtain this measurement. Finally, for proper deployment, familiarity with the proximal markers (gold radiopaque markers located 2 mm from the most proximal aspect of the graft material) is important in positioning and deploying the endograft for proximal seal.

ACCESS SITE COMPLICATIONS

Insertion of devices for deployment, most commonly the common femoral arteries as the access vessels for EVAR and TEVAR, but also brachial artery access for branched and fenestrated endograft placement, requires either direct vessel cut-down or percutaneous access. Complications during this portion of the procedure is one of the most common group of adverse events in most reports. As the case difficulty and anatomic complexity increases, so does the incidence of these complications.

Complications include acute bleeding during the procedure caused by sheath-size mismatch or vessel laceration, rupture or avulsion of the vessel, hematoma (developing during or after the procedure), thrombosis around the sheath, and dissection or embolization of the vessel distal to the access point. This may require open repair of the vessel in some cases.

Planning and evaluating access sites for device delivery is vital to minimizing these problems. Moreover, small common or external iliac arteries may be difficult to traverse with the large sheaths needed for device delivery. The caliber of the vessels, location and extent of calcification at any point in the vessel, and the tortuosity of the vessel are all characteristics of the access vessels that should be analyzed preoperatively.

Percutaneous Access

Percutaneous access for EVAR has been demonstrated to be safe and effective in multiple studies.[6,7] This technique contributes to decreased surgical pain experienced by patients and has been shown to decrease overall surgery time. The improvement of closure devices has facilitated this approach. Despite this, limitations remain because of sheath size for device delivery.

The introducer sheath diameters for the Zenith Flex device vary with the size of the endograft. The 22–26 mm proximal diameter devices are introduced on 18-French inner diameter systems (outer diameter 7.1 mm); 28–32 mm proximal diameter devices are introduced on 20-French inner diameter systems (outer diameter 7.7 mm); and the 36-mm proximal diameter device is introduced on 22-French inner diameter system (outer diameter 8.5 mm). Careful attention to femoral and iliac vessel diameters, calcifications or stenoses, and tortuosity of the vessel is important in determining whether the patient's anatomy is suitable for these devices, whether percutaneous or open femoral delivery.

A lower-profile thoracic device (Zenith Alpha), first used in Europe and Canada, is now available in the United States. This 18-French outer diameter delivery system can enable easier percutaneous delivery with more suitability in patients with challenging iliac anatomy, such as smaller diameters or more tortuous vessels. Results in Europe demonstrated success in smaller vessels, using the device in 22% of patients with external iliac arteries <7 mm, and with overall similar results with regard to limb occlusion, access complications, and reintervention and overall survival rates when compared with standard size Zenith systems.[8] Couchet and colleagues demonstrated similar efficacy with the Zenith Low Profile bifurcated body device in conjunction with the Zenith Spiral-Z limbs in treating 50 patients.[9] Endoleak rates were no higher than acceptable reported rates, with only proximal Type I endoleak and a 20% Type II endoleak rate. They reported one asymptomatic external iliac artery thrombosis distal to the iliac limb of the device requiring no intervention, in a small vessel (6 mm). Most importantly, there were no iliac limb occlusions and minimal access site complications. The study is limited by the fact that the patient population treated was 98% male but the surmised advantage would be the treatment of small iliac vessels that more commonly occur in female patients.

LIMB KINKING AND OCCLUSION

Limb kinking and occlusion are more commonly seen with endografts following EVAR (2.3% versus 0.2%) compared with open repair and have been associated with a significant increase in endoleak, graft thrombosis, and graft migration.[10] Moreover, graft kinking and occlusion can cause acute limb ischemia. When patients present with symptoms of occlusion, they are often subject to multiple interventions, including thrombolysis, angioplasty and stenting, or ultimately surgical bypass to restore limb perfusion. The rates of limb kinking and limb occlusion, however, are evolving with new devices and delivery systems.

Zenith Spiral-Z iliac limbs are composed of a continuous spiral nitinol stent, between two Z-stents at each end, which delivers kink resistance and flexibility. The rates of limb occlusion with Zenith devices ranges from 2.3% to 3.4%.[3–5] Concerns of significantly increased rates of limb occlusion with the Zenith LP device, report of upward of 35%[11], have been dulled by subsequent studies demonstrating minimal limb and access complications when used with Spiral-Z limbs, as mentioned earlier.[9]

DEVICE MIGRATION

Device migration is one of the major causes of secondary intervention after endovascular aneurysm repair. Migration is a time-dependent complication that requires close surveillance and consideration of serial assessments of the endograft. In general, migration of the endograft of 10 mm or more or any displacement requiring a secondary intervention should be considered a serious consequence. Most commonly, proximal aortic aneurysmal degeneration and dilatation or poor patient selection is attributed to device migration. Feared consequences of aneurysm expansion and ultimate rupture lead providers to aggressive intervention in most cases.

Early analysis of the Zenith endograft demonstrated promising results, with 98% freedom of migration (defined as >10 mm endograft movement or any migration related to a clinical event) at 4 years, compared with the AneuRx device, which was reported at 72%.[12] This durability has been further demonstrated by Greenberg, who reported no clinically relevant migrations of >10 mm at 5 years; of 19 patients who were found to have migration distance of 5 to 10 mm, none required secondary intervention or had associated adverse events.[3]

SEPARATION OF COMPONENTS

Endograft component separation is a consequence of modular endograft design or with more complex branched and fenestrated devices. In general, inadequate sizing or overlap may lead to separation or may be related to device-specific integrity. Most of these complications require intervention as a Type III endoleak and may require balloon angioplasty, additional stent placement for bridging the separation, or surgical revision. Component separation with the Zenith graft has been reported to be as low as <0.01% (3 of 736 endografts by Greenberg and colleagues).[3]

ADDITIONAL TECHNICAL CONSIDERATIONS

The top cap on the Zenith endograft device delivery system is a key component of deployment. The top stent is restrained by a trigger wire mechanism that is the limiting factor in deployment location and accuracy. Once the top cap is released, the barbed suprarenal fixation stent is released. The top cap must be advanced proximally into the aorta to deploy fully. If there is difficulty retrieving the top cap, the user should rotate the grey pusher to reorient the smooth edge to aid in advancement. In some cases, it may be difficult to release the trigger wire attached to the top cap. In those instances, inspection of the delivery system under fluoroscopy is mandated to ensure that the system has not been rotated excessively and needs to be untwisted. If difficulty still exists, then the top cap pin vise should be loosened and the top cap pulled down onto the grey pusher. Once the pin vise is retightened, attempts should be made to pull the trigger wire.

CONCLUSION

EVAR has revolutionized the treatment of AAA. Despite significant improvement in perioperative morbidity and mortality, EVAR is not flawless. Knowing the complications associated with vessel access, device delivery, short- and long-term endograft issues such as endoleak, migration, and component separation, or limb kinking and occlusion, will help providers to maintain the immediate and long-term success of EVAR for the treatment of AAA. The Cook Zenith endograft remains a safe and reliable option in the armamentarium of the vascular surgeon.

REFERENCES

1. Zarins CK, et al. Endovascular aneurysm repair at 5 years: does aneurysm diameter predict outcome? *J Vasc Surg.* 2006;44(5):920–929.
2. Greenberg RK, et al. Zenith AAA endovascular graft: intermediate-term results of the US multicenter trial. *J Vasc Surg.* 2004;39:1209–1218.
3. Greenberg RK, et al. Zenith abdominal aortic aneurysm endovascular graft. *J Vasc Surg.* 2008;48:1–9.
4. Verzini F, et al. Fourteen-year outcomes of abdominal aortic endovascular repair with the Zenith stent graft. *J Vasc Surg.* 2017;65(2):318–329.
5. Vaaramaki S, et al. Long-term experience of endovascular aneurysm repair with Zenith prosthesis: diminishing graft-related complications over time. *Ann Vasc Surg.* 2012;26(6):845–851.
6. Buck DB, et al. Percutaneous versus femoral cutdown access for endovascular aneurysm repair. *J Vasc Surg.* 2015;62(1):16–21.
7. Gimzewska M, et al. Totally percutaneous versus surgical cut-down femoral artery access for elective bifurcated abdominal endovascular aneurysm repair. *Cochrane Database Syst Rev.* 2017;2: CD010185.
8. Sobocinski J, et al. Evaluation of the Zenith low-profile abdominal aortic aneurysm stent graft. *J Vasc Surg.* 2015;62:841–847.
9. Couchet G, et al. An optimal combination for EVAR: low profile endograft body and continuous spiral stent limbs. *Eur J Vasc Endovasc Surg.* 2013;46:29–33.
10. EVAR trial participants. Endovascular aneurysm repair versus open repair in patients with abdominal aortic aneurysm (EVAR trial 1): randomised controlled trial. *Lancet.* 2005;365(9478):2179.
11. Urlings TA, et al. Thromboembolic complications after Zenith® Low Profile Endovascular Graft for infrarenal abdominal aneurysms. *Cardiovasc Intervent Radiol.* 2015;38:600–605.
12. Tonnessen BH, et al. Mid- and long-term device migration after endovascular abdominal aortic aneurysm repair: a comparison of AneuRx and Zenith endografts. *J Vasc Surg.* 2005;42(3):392.

22

Terumo Aortic Relay TEVAR

Michael C. Stoner, MD, FACS, DFSVS and Matthew J. TerBush, MD

INTRODUCTION

Bolton Medical (Sunrise, Florida), now owned by Terumo (Tokyo, Japan), introduced the Relay thoracic endovascular aortic repair (TEVAR) endograft in 2005, with Phase II trials for approval in the United States beginning in 2007. In 2009, RelayPlus was introduced, which is now one of Bolton Medical's main TEVAR endografts. While the endograft itself remained the same, the delivery system was updated. RelayPlus is the company's only endograft approved for use in the United States by the Food and Drug Administration (FDA), receiving this approval on September 21, 2012.

Bolton Medical also manufactures RelayNBSPlus, an alternative to RelayPlus. Although the delivery system is the same, the RelayNBSPlus does not feature an uncovered fixation portion proximally. The company also offers customizable options for unique anatomy. As these two endografts lack FDA approval, this chapter will only focus on RelayPlus.

DEVICE INFORMATION

RelayPlus (Fig. 22.1) is indicated for the treatment of thoracic aorta aneurysms (TAAs) and penetrating atherosclerotic ulcers (PAUs). Treatment of aortic dissections or traumatic aortic injuries is currently an off-label use. The endograft consists of nitinol stents sutured to a polyester fabric. More unique to RelayPlus is a curved bar of nitinol, called an "S-bar", which runs along the length of the graft. This provides longitudinal and torsional stability, theoretically allowing for better graft apposition along the aortic arch. In the literature, it remains unclear whether this S-bar translates to lower endoleak and migration rates. Proximally, the device has a bare stent that provides alignment to the graft and is 13–21 mm long, depending on endograft length. Radial force is primarily achieved through the first and last covered stents, with additional radial force achieved by the second covered stent. Sizes for the endografts are shown in Table 22.1.

Tapered endografts are also available, with the distal end 4 mm narrower than the proximal end. Sizes are more limited, however, and can accommodate proximal necks from 24 to 42 mm. Instructions for use (IFU) for the endograft are shown in Table 22.2. Be cognizant that proximal and distal sealing zone lengths differ depending on endograft size.

The delivery system (Fig. 22.2) is a hydrophilic coaxial construct with the endograft mounted inside a secondary sheath, which is mounted inside a primary sheath. The secondary sheath can be left behind if additional procedures (balloon angioplasty, angiography, etc.) are needed after deployment. The system is available from 22 to 26 French outer diameter, comparable to other TEVAR delivery systems. The endograft is deployed by retracting the secondary sheath over the endograft (a "pin-and-pull" deployment system). The proximal bare-stent portion is attached to a tip-capture mechanism, mitigating bare stent eversion on deployment.

RelayPlus is MRI conditional, allowing patients to undergo MRI if the MRI is in normal or first level controlled operating modes, with a 1.5 or 3 T magnetic field, a 720 G/cm or less magnetic field spatial gradient, and a maximum whole-body averaged specific absorption rate of 4 W/kg for 15 minutes of scanning. These recommendations are based on nonclinical trials.

The main study evaluating outcomes is the Bolton Relay Thoracic Aorta Endovascular Pivotal Trial, which evaluated 133 patients treated with the original Relay endograft (with the RelayTransport delivery system) for TAAs and later for PAUs. Between January 2007 and May 2010, 120 patients received surgery, with an additional 13 recruited between May 2010 and FDA approval. For the final 38 patients RelayPlus was used instead. Patients were also compared with 60 open surgical control patients. The two groups were statistically similar, although in the Relay group there were more patients with saccular aneurysms and PAUs.

Successful endograft deployment was achieved in 96.9% without damage to the endograft, intraoperative deaths, or the need for conversion to an open procedure. One patient had kinking and twisting of the endograft without compromised flow. Of the four patients who had an unsuccessful implantation, three were unsuccessful because of severe atherosclerotic disease, and one because of the inability to rotate endograft to correct alignment per IFU. After 30 days, there were 5.3% aneurysm related deaths in the Relay group, with 10% in the surgical group. A total of 20.3% of Relay patients and 48.3% of surgical patients suffered from a major adverse event (defined as stroke, paralysis, myocardial infarction, respiratory failure, renal failure, wound healing issues, and aneurysm related mortality). Over 1 year, 25.6% of Relay patients and 50% of surgical patients had at least one of these events. Over a 5-year postoperative period, freedom from major adverse events was higher in the Relay group (65.7% versus 44.7%). The surgical group also experienced higher rates of respiratory failure and procedural bleeding.

Outcomes for the endograft itself were also good. Among the RelayPlus subset, there was a 0% stroke rate at 30 days and a 2.6% overall stroke rate, no Type I or III endoleaks, no migrations, and no stent fractures. All endografts remained patent during the study period. Only 15% of patients had an increase of their aneurysm size of more than 5 mm. Of these patients, only one underwent another procedure 2 years later, with no further expansion. Overall, 7.5% of patients required a secondary intervention.[1]

PREOPERATIVE CONSIDERATIONS

Planning for placement of the RelayPlus endograft follows the same general principles for the placement of any thoracic endograft, described in Chapter 18. Specific to this device, aortic diameter should be measured from outer wall to outer wall.

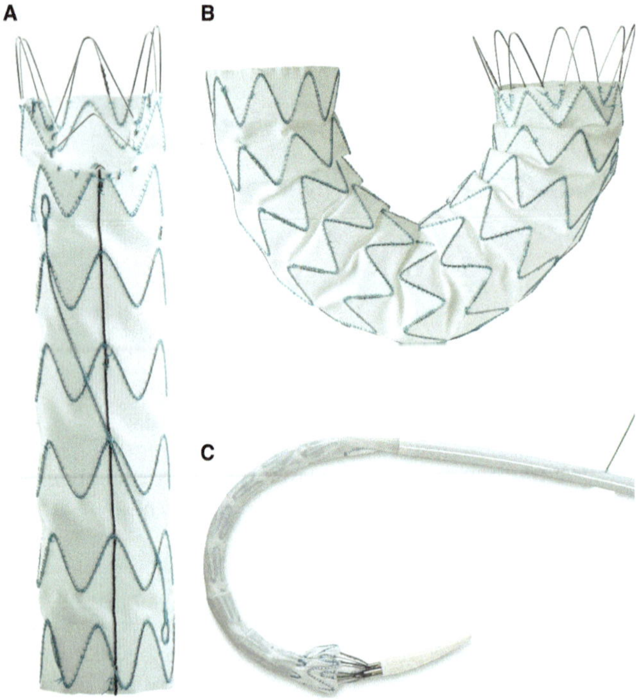

Fig. 22.1 (A, B) RelayPlus endograft. (C) Tip capture mechanism for endograft.

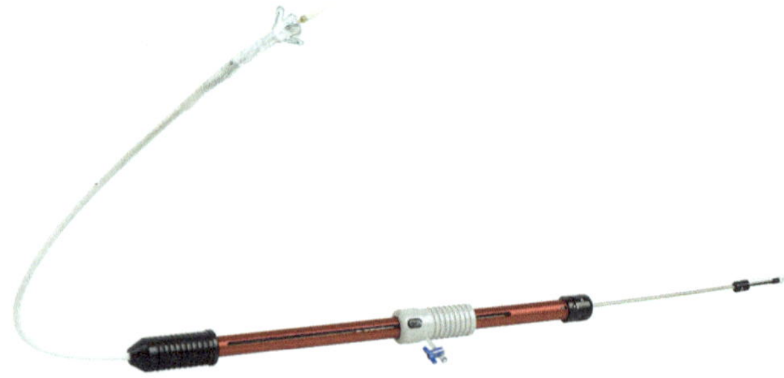

Fig. 22.2 RelayPlus deployment system.

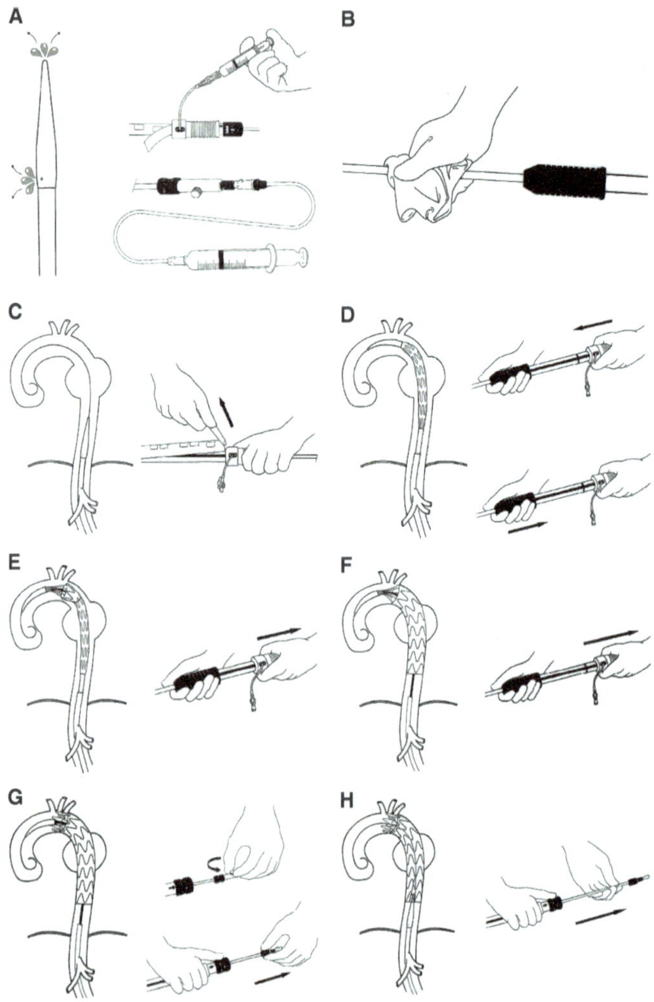

Fig. 22.3 (A–H) Steps demonstrating deployment of RelayPlus endograft.

TABLE 22.1 Sizes available for RelayPlus endografts.

Endograft lengths	100, 150, 200, 250 mm
Endograft diameters	22–46 mm with diameters available every 2 mm
Tapered endograft lengths	150, 200, 250 mm
Tapered endograft diameters	28–46 mm proximally, with proximal diameters available every 2 mm. Distally, diameter is 4 mm less than proximal end.

TABLE 22.2 US instructions for use for RelayPlus.

Pathology	Thoracic aorta aneurysms and penetrating atherosclerotic ulcers
Proximal aortic diameter	19–42 mm
Proximal landing zone	22–28 mm endografts: 15 mm 30–38 mm endografts: 20 mm 40–46 mm endografts: 25 mm
Distal landing zone	22–38 mm endografts: 25 mm 40–46 mm endografts: 30 mm
Other	Ability for iliofemoral system to accommodate 22–26 French sheaths

INTRAOPERATIVE CONSIDERATIONS

The deployment steps for the RelayPlus endograft are demonstrated in Fig. 22.3. To ensure adequate and safe deployment, all steps should be followed closely and measures should be taken not to deviate from protocol.

Obtaining common femoral access is similar to other endografts and can be done percutaneously using ultrasound or with surgical exposure. Obtain wire access with a stiff 0.035″ wire (for example, a double curved Lunderquist wire; Cook Medical, Bloomington, Indiana) into the ascending aorta. Inspect the deployment system and note any defects. Ensure the delivery system tip is seated properly in the outer sheath and the side hole is not covered by the outer sheath. Familiarize yourself with the device, noting the gray deployment grip distally, the black stationary grip proximally, and the black controller on the distal end of the device. Be aware of the position of the black controller on the distal end of the device at all steps of deployment and ensure that the controller is in position 1 before placing device into patient to avoid accidental deployment. If the position of the controller needs to be changed, push the controller toward the proximal end of the delivery device and rotate to the proper position while holding forward. Release the controller to set the position. Be aware of an orange shipping retainer placed between the black stationary and gray deployment grips. Do not remove this until ready to deploy the endograft because early removal risks accidental deployment.

CAUTION

Do not remove the orange shipping retainer until you are ready to begin deploying the endograft!

Before placing the device into the patient, be sure to flush the system with heparinized saline. Once complete, close the flush port under pressure to avoid air from entering the system. Be sure to remove the extension tubing once complete to begin accommodating wire access (Fig. 22.3A). Wet the introducer sheath before device introduction because it and the sheath tip are hydrophilic (Fig. 22.3B). Before introducing the sheath tip into the patient, rotate the device so that the tip faces upward, to optimize mechanical advantage.

The primary sheath is advanced over wire until the tip is at the anticipated distal landing zone. If the distal landing zone is at the level of the celiac origin, advance the primary sheath another 2 cm proximally to account for distal migration of the graft that could take place upon deployment. If proximally the aorta is seen to be tortuous, advance the primary sheath past this tortuosity instead, even if it needs to be in the aneurysm itself. If this cannot be done, the procedure should be aborted because from this point on it cannot be completed safely. Do not advance the primary sheath into the aortic arch to avoid aortic perforation.

In tortuous anatomy, increased force may be required to advance the primary sheath forward. Advance while holding the sheath close to the patient's body to avoid the system kinking. Use a piece of gauze if a better grip is needed. Manual pressure can be placed over the abdomen to straighten the iliac vessels. Serial dilations of the iliac arteries can be attempted. A "body floss" technique using transbrachiofemoral wire access can be used to stiffen the system, using a long brachial sheath to add trackability to the system. Overdilating a covered stent in the iliac vessels can also be done. Because the smallest outer diameter available for the system is 22 French, Terumo's Solopath balloon-expandable sheath is not compatible (this is because the largest inner diameter available is 21 French).

One of the most feared complications is a complete iliac vessel avulsion, known more informally as an "iliac on a stick". Should this happen, establish balloon occlusion of the iliac in-flow and perform an emergency retroperitoneal surgical exposure of the iliac vessels with the sheath remaining in place to mitigate bleeding. Remove the sheath in a controlled fashion once vessel control is achieved and reconstruct the iliac artery. Anticipate placing an iliofemoral bypass with a 10-mm Dacron graft to serve as a conduit in a future endograft implantation attempt. Focal rupture of the vessel can be fixed using a covered stent and can in itself serve as an adjunct as an endovascular endoconduit.

Once the primary sheath is in place, perform an angiogram to define the aortic anatomy while in a left anterior oblique position. Ensure the black controller is still set to position 1. Now is the proper time to remove the orange shipping retainer. Advance the secondary sheath to the intended proximal landing zone by holding the stationary grip firm and advancing the deployment grip to the stationary grip (Fig. 22.3C). Position the endograft's proximal markers to the intended proximal landing zone (Fig. 22.3D). Note that when exposed the secondary sheath expands slightly. Because of this, once the secondary sheath is advanced, the endograft is committed to be deployed. Be sure you are confident in deploying the graft before removing the orange shipping retainer. While advancing the secondary sheath, take note of the position of the more proximal D-shaped marker on the secondary sheath and two S-bar markers on the graft. These should face the outer curvature of the aortic arch. There are also two proximal markers, one facing the inner curve and the other facing the outer curve of the aortic arch. These markers ensure the S-bar is in the correct location to offer optimal mechanical advantage. Fig. 22.4 demonstrates the general placement of these markers under fluoroscopy.

CAUTION

Because the secondary sheath expands, once the secondary sheath is advanced, you are committed to deploying the graft! You cannot retract the secondary sheath.

Once the endograft is in the intended position, the gray deployment grip should be at or past the black line on the stationary sheath. This ensures the secondary sheath has been fully removed from the primary sheath. If this is not the case, hold the gray deployment grip firmly and pull back on the black stationary grip until the gray deployment grip meets the black line.

Once the device is in an adequate position, take an angiogram in the left anterior oblique position. The secondary sheath can then be adjusted cranially or caudally if needed. Ensure the S-bar markers face the greater curvature. If the endograft needs to be rotated, retract the

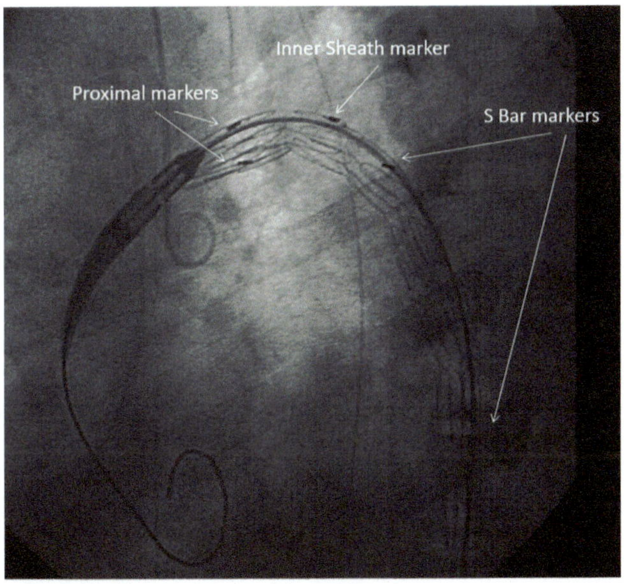

Fig. 22.4 Positional markers present under fluoroscopy.

entire deployment system into a straight portion of aorta by pulling the gray deployment grip back. Do not retract the distal end of the graft into the primary sheath; doing so can potentially damage the graft while rotating the graft. The whole system may need to be retracted distally in order to bring the entire endograft to a straight portion of aorta. Take note of the orientation of the "D" marker. If the round end of the marker faces the greater curvature, rotate clockwise. If facing the lesser curvature, rotate counterclockwise. To rotate the endograft, rotate the gray deployment grip while holding the black stationary grip firm. One to three full rotations may be needed before the graft is seen to rotate under fluoroscopy.

Ensure the controller is now set to position 2. Under fluoroscopy, pull back on the gray deployment grip while holding firm on the black stationary grip to uncover up to the first covered stent (Fig. 22.3E). This is the final opportunity to make any final cranial or caudal positioning changes. To do so, change the controller back to position 1 and use the gray deployment grip to make any changes. Turn back to position 2 when complete. If satisfied with positioning, pull back on the gray deployment grip in a continuous motion (to avoid distal migration of the graft) until the graft is fully deployed. Delay in final deployment may cause proximal blood pressure to rise rapidly, therefore some forward pressure may need to be applied to the black stationary grip to overcome this wind-socking effect. If this proves too difficult, adenosine can be given to momentarily pause the heart. Another adjunct is using transvenous pacing wires to pace the heart rapidly, momentarily lowering the blood pressure to keep the endograft stationary.

CAUTION

When uncovered stent and first covered stent are deployed, be sure to turn the controller to position 1 to readjust. Once entire graft is unsheathed, you can no longer readjust!

Unintended coverage of the aortic arch branch vessels can be a devastating complication. A particular advantage for the Relay endograft is that as the first covered stent is deployed, if an unintended vessel is covered, the operator can simply change the controller to position 1 and move the graft as appropriate. If, for any reason, the endograft unintentionally covers aortic arch vessels, other strategies can be used. However, as no accidental coverage of these vessels had occurred during clinical trials, there are currently no specific data that compare this graft with others in this aspect. A Coda balloon (Cook Medical, Bloomington, Indiana), can be inflated at the proximal or distal end and pulled back aggressively to move the graft distally. If the left subclavian artery needs to be revascularized, endovascular access to the left brachial artery can be obtained to facilitate access for a chimney graft or to perform an in situ fenestration. The patient can also receive a carotid–subclavian bypass or transposition. Coverage of the left carotid artery needs to be addressed in an expeditious fashion, as the patient is exposed to a high risk of stroke. The left common carotid can be surgically exposed and a sheath can be placed antegrade, which can accept arterial perfusion from the femoral artery sheath. From this access, a chimney graft or in situ fenestration can also be performed in a retrograde fashion. If all else fails, an emergent right to left carotid–carotid bypass may need to be performed. All of these adjuncts may need to be used, including doing so while obtaining right carotid surgical access, if all aortic arch vessels are covered.

To release the proximal bare stent, find the thumbscrew near the guidewire luer on the distal end of the delivery system. Rotate the thumbscrew counterclockwise two or three times and remove the cover plate attached to the thumbscrew. Locate the black release grip labeled 3 and pull it toward the luer (Fig. 22.3G). Turn the controller to position 4. Under fluoroscopy, pull back on the stainless steel rod to retract the delivery system tip to the outer sheath, making sure not to catch the endograft and alter its position. If the tip does not reseat easily, more force may need to be applied. Once done, remove the entire delivery system.

Consider balloon molding the proximal and distal covered stents if appropriate given the clinical situation (for example with a Coda balloon, Cook Medical, Bloomington, Indiana). Perform a completion angiogram, assessing for endoleaks. Type II endoleaks can be tolerated and do not require intervention. Address Type I endoleaks with balloon molding first. If unsuccessful, extension proximally or distally should be considered. However, as the company does not manufacture extension cuffs, placement of another endograft should be considered. As initial clinical trials did not experience Type I or III endoleaks, limited data exist for outcomes doing this. If the final result is satisfactory, remove all sheaths and close all arteriotomies.

CONCLUSIONS

Bolton Medical's RelayPlus endograft is another option in the American market for treatment of descending thoracic aorta aneurysms. It is unique to other endografts in that it features a support bar to provide greater stability and a deployment mechanism that offers more controlled deployment. Midterm results demonstrate that there is a greater freedom from adverse outcomes compared with open aortic surgery. With the endograft's ability to conform to more tortuous anatomy, RelayPlus is a viable option for the vascular surgeon's armamentarium for the endovascular repair of thoracic aortic aneurysms.

REFERENCE

1. Farber MA, Lee WA, Szeto WY, Panneton JM, Kwolek CJ. Initial and midterm results of the Bolton Relay Thoracic Aortic Endovascular Pivotal Trial. *J Vasc Surg.* 2017;65(6):1556–1566.e1.

23

Complication With Medtronic Thoracic Stent Endograft

Michael Sywak, MD, DABS and Paul Anain, MD

INTRODUCTION AND BACKGROUND

The introduction of thoracic stent grafts into clinical practice over the past two decades and the ability to image the thoracic aorta in high definition have offered a paradigm shift in the way we have been able to diagnose and to treat thoracic aortic pathologies. Looking at national registry data from 2002–2012, Wang et al. described a majority shift toward endovascular treatment of thoracic aortic aneurysms and dissections.[1] Given the number of products available to date to treat thoracic pathology, it is increasingly important that the vascular surgeon understands the capabilities and limitations for each device used. In 2009, Medtronic introduced the Valiant thoracic stent graft with Captivia delivery system to the US market. In 2018, Medtronic received CE mark approval for the Valiant Navion thoracic stent graft system.[2] The Navion device had acceptable safe profiles with a low 30-day perioperative mortality of 2.3% and secondary procedures at 2.3%. Type Ia endoleaks at 1.2% at 1-month imaging follow-up. The Valiant thoracic stent graft is essentially a tube graft composed of polyester graft fabric that is scaffolded by nitinol wires sewn on the outside of the graft, together with nonabsorbable sutures. There is no longitudinal backbone metal support, allowing the advantage of the graft to conform to tortuous patient anatomy. There are several configurations of the graft available, giving a physician the ability to choose between proximal and distal bare-spring extension fixation as well as tapered grafts to accommodate size discrepancies. In the case of large flow lumen, large aneurysms in the descending thoracic distal fixation should be considered. The Valiant offers distal strut configuration for fixation and can be augmented with APTUS fixation systems to prevent device migration in the dynamic thoracic aorta.

Radiopaque markers are embedded into the graft to allow precision deployment at the proximal and distal fabric lines. There are four markers shaped as a figure 8, which delineate the proximal fabric edge. In the midgraft there is a single figure 8 marker showing the minimum amount of overlap needed to treat the longer aortic segments.

The Captiva delivery system is designed for the proximal bare-metal stent thoracic pieces. It allows recapturing and repositioning the stent graft in the event of malpositioned deployment. The deployment system for the closed web stent graft components does not allow recapturing because of the lack of front end bare-metal stent pieces. This ability to recapture the proximal seal zone can be advantageous for precise deployment in zone 0–1 settings.

The indications for use for the Valiant thoracic stent graft with the Captiva delivery system is to repair fusiform aneurysms, saccular aneurysms, and penetrating ulcers of the descending thoracic aorta in patients with appropriate anatomy, including: iliac–femoral vessels compatible with vascular access techniques, devices and accessories, nonaneurysmal aortic diameter ranging from 18 to 42 mm (44 mm for traumatic dissections), and nonaneurysmal aortic proximal and distal neck lengths >20 mm.

Unique to this graft, it does not require a separate sheath and can be barebacked into the patient for lower profile access arteries. The outer diameter of the device (24 French) is on a par with being the lowest available on the market up to 2017. When barebacked, the device has its own hydrophilic lining, allowing ease of delivery and less tissue trauma.

In terms of the safety profile of the device, Conrad et al.[3] demonstrated the 5-year safety data showing a 94.8% freedom from aneurysm-related death, 89% sac showing no growth or shrinking aneurysm, no loss of stent graft integrity, no migration and loss of patency. In terms of endoleaks, Type I endoleaks as an aggregate of the data showed a rate of 7.2% and Type II endoleaks with a rate of 10.7%.

DEVICE INSERTION AND DEPLOYMENT

The delivery and deployment of the Valiant Captiva system can be tailored to the operator's preferences. Based on operator experience, the case will start with obtaining bilateral common femoral artery access. This can be done percutaneously with US guided access and preclosure technique, with the deployment of two Proglide sutures or by an open cutdown. On the contralateral side, a 5-French sheath is placed for a marking flush catheter placed in the proximal aorta and used for an angiogram. On the ipsilateral side, a double curve Lunderquist wire is placed near the aortic root. The wire is delivered through a catheter after systemic heparinization. The device is then mounted on the wire and barebacked into the aorta. A thoracic aortic angiogram is then performed to map the anatomy.

Once the origins of the vessels are marked, the device is positioned. A technical point of note is that during deployment, the Lunderquist wire should have some inward pressure applied to allow the wire to create good outer aortic wall opposition. This allows the device to deploy primarily along the outer curve precisely with relation to the arch vessels and effective seal zone.

To ensure precise deployment at the proximal landing zone, there is benefit to dampening the cardiac impulse. This can be achieved in a variety of mechanisms including pharmacological manipulation, temporary rapid cardiac pacing, or with preload reduction via IVC transient balloon occlusion.

An uncommon event occurs when the thoracic aneurysm is so large that the outer curve of the aneurysm affects the wire bias and deployment of the graft. The physician should then deploy a maximum of two stent pieces so that the Captiva constraining mechanism can allow repositioning of the graft if it becomes displaced by the vacuum of the aneurysm's size.

A point of consideration: if multiple pieces are to be used, the device should be placed in a separate sheath to allow bloodless exchanges.

The clinician at this point has a choice between rapid and slow deployment. Slow deployment is accomplished by turning the large blue handle on the device while keeping the gray (graft) portion secure to prevent any graft migration. If using the Captiva product with bare-metal fixation, the proximal portion of the graft is still partially constrained. A rapid deployment is accomplished by pressing the trigger on the blue handle and dragging the blue away from the fixed gray portion of the deployment system. If Captiva fixation is used, a secondary constraining mechanism is in place that needs to be turned and pulled off to release the bare-metal proximal fixation. Once deployed, the delivery system can be pulled into the abdominal aorta and, depending on the aortic pathology being treated, the final angiogram can be performed with or without the pigtail being repositioned in the proximal aorta. If repositioning is done, the catheter should be straightened with a wire before repositioning so as not to drag on the graft. It is a relatively rare occurrence that the graft will require balloon angioplasty, but if a Type I endoleak occurs, gentle angioplasty should be the first maneuver. If the graft is placed for dissection, oversizing should be minimized and angioplasty is not recommended. During removal of the large sheath, the anesthesiologist should be made aware and communication about blood pressure drop should be noted in case the iliac artery has an iatrogenic pathology. Closure is then completed as per routine.

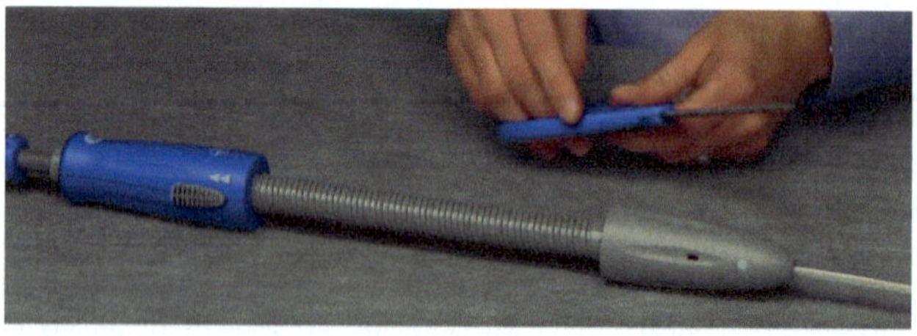

Fig. 23.1

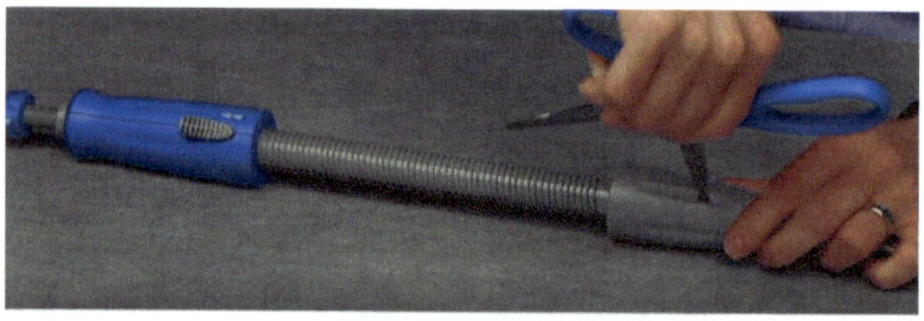

Fig. 23.2

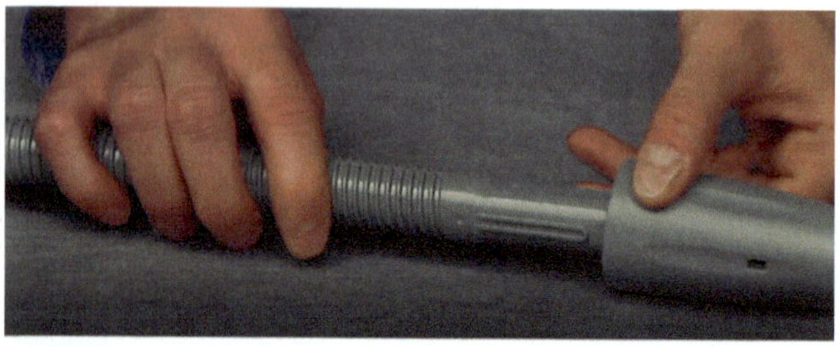

Fig. 23.3

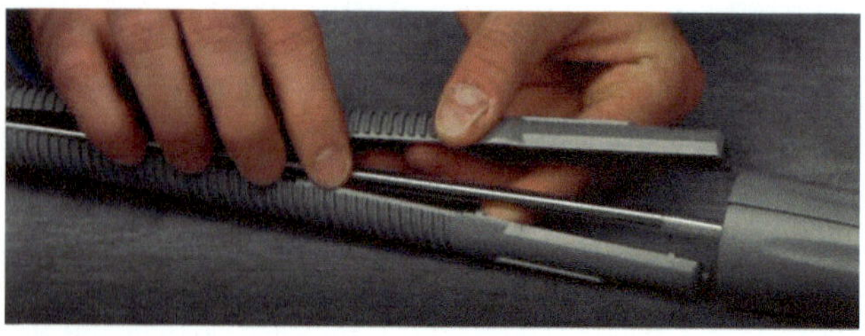

Fig. 23.4

BAILOUT TECHNIQUES

In the event of graft cover severance, which leads to the graft not deploying, the physician will need to disassemble the delivery system manually. The first step is to retract the blue slider all the way back. Take a hemostat and locate the manual disassemble ports on the gray portion of the graft. Push in the ports until a loud pop is heard; this will need to be done on both sides. Step three is to stabilize the delivery

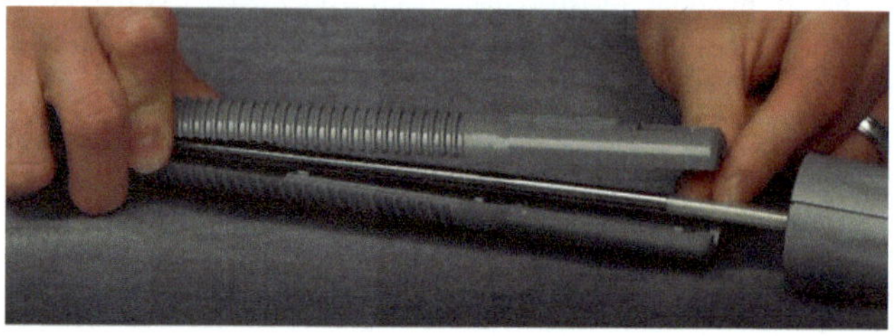

Fig. 23.5

Fr	SG Size (mm)	Covered Length (mm)* 60	100	175	225
18 Fr	20		X		
	22		X	X	
	25		X	X	
20 Fr	28		X	X	
	31		X	X	X
	34	X	X	X	X
	37	X	X	X	X
22 Fr	40	X	X	X	X
	43	X	X	X	X
	46	X	X	X	X

Fig. 23.6

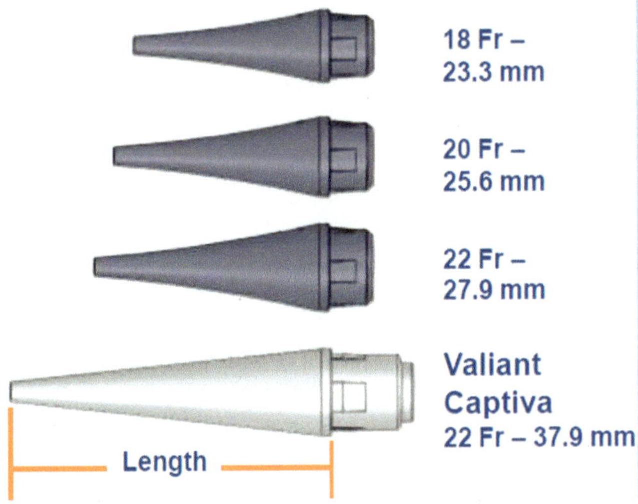

Fig. 23.7

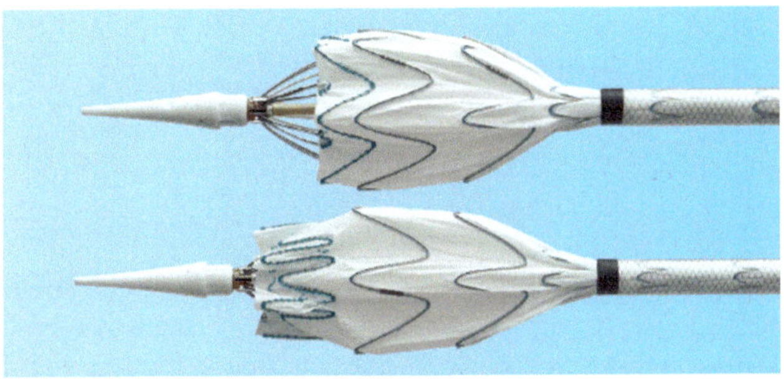

Fig. 23.8

system and to advance the front grip forward. Doing so allows the screw gear to be separated in halves. This exposes the graft cover severance from the main delivery system. Then using hemostat, the graft cover can be pulled back while fixating the graft. This is depicted in Figs. 23.1–23.5.

If an inadvertent subclavian artery coverage occurs, this problem can be handled in a variety of fashions. Angiography may demonstrate adequate flow from vertebral artery filling of the subclavian artery; if this is the case, observation may be warranted. If the arm appears profoundly ischemic, there are two different bailout techniques depending on the anatomy. The first is coming from the arm and using a laser to fenestrate the graft and sealing with a flared covered stent. The second bailout technique is to come from the arm and pass a wire either proximally or distally depending on the anatomy and snorkel or periscope an additional stent graft to maintain patency. Open bailout options include a carotid-to-subclavian bypass for revascularization.

THE VALIANT NAVION

The Valiant Navion is the next generation thoracic stent graft in the Medtronic product line. It offers a lower profile delivery system down to 18 French, with 22 French as the maximum. The device offers a wider range of aortic anatomy, with increased lengths, smaller diameter, and tapers in the figures listed. The taper tip on the Navion was shortened approximately 1 cm compared with the Captiva to allow better tracking through complex anatomy. The working length on the Navion was increased 10 cm to a total distance of 93 cm, with matching lengthening of the hydrophilic coating for deliverability.[4] The shaft handle also received ergonomic upgrades for operator ease-of-use. There are two major configurations available: the FreeFlow and CoveredSeal with tip capture depicted in Figs. 23.6–23.8, providing the choice of additional fixation versus atraumatic placement.

CONCLUSION

Medtronic's thoracic stent graft has historically good safety profiles and with the recent release of the Valiant Navion the clinical application in narrowed and tortuous access vessels can be broadened.

REFERENCES

1. Wang GJ, Jackson BM, Foley PJ, et al. National trends in admissions, repair, and mortality for thoracic aortic aneurysm and type B dissection in the National Inpatient Sample. *J Vasc Surg*. 2018;67(6):1649–1658.
2. Endovascular Today. Medtronic Receives CE Mark Approval for the Valiant Navion Thoracic Stent Graft System. Available at https://evtoday.com/news/medtronic-receives-ce-mark-approval-for-the-valiant-navion-thoracic-stent-graft-system.
3. Conrad MF, Tuchek J, Freezor R, Bavaria J, White R, Fairman R. Results of the VALOR II trial of the Medtronic Valiant Thoracic Stent Graft. *J Vasc Surg*. 2017;66(2):335–342.
4. US Valiant Navion brochure. Available at https://europe.medtronic.com/content/dam/medtronic-com/products/cardiovascular/aortic-stent-graft-products/valiant-navion/documents/us-valiant-navion-brochure.pdf.

24

Complications and Lessons Learned From Global Use of the Streamliner Multilayer Flow Modulator (SMFM) Device

Sherif Sultan, MCh, MD, FRCS, FACS, PhD, Edel P. Kavanagh, MSc, PhD, Ashwini D'Souza, MSc, Yogesh Acharya, MD, MSc, FAcadMEd, AFAMEE and Niamh Hynes, MD, MMSc, ChM, FRSCI, FEBVS

INTRODUCTION

Over the last two decades, endovascular aortic repair (EVAR) has become the preferred treatment with regard to aortic pathologies and is an alternative treatment for patients who do not qualify for open surgery.[1] Although EVAR has been shown to have significantly fewer complications when compared with open surgery, it is associated with complications that can lead to severe morbidity or even mortality.[2] Complication rates after EVAR are as high as 30%, with a 2%–3% rate of late complications requiring intervention.[3] From this, the Streamliner Multilayer Flow Modulator (SMFM; Cardiatis, Isnes, Belgium) technology has evolved. However, many studies involving the SMFM device have described patients who have developed complications, often fatal, after treatment.

The SMFM is an endovascular bare-metal stent for use in aortic, peripheral, visceral, and intracranial aneurysms. Its design comprises multiple interlocked layers of cobalt-alloy metal wire, braided together to create a mesh. Unlike conventional aortic endografts, the SMFM uses the innate physiological response of the human body to remodel the aneurysm sac, rather than excluding it from the circulation, which is the current traditional method. The design permits blood flow to perfuse through the mesh. In this way, it preserves collateral branches, negating the need for surgical branches or fenestrations. Flow within the device is modulated and decreases over time within the surrounding aortic aneurysm sac, theoretically leading to gradual thrombosis of the sac.

When the SMFM technology was first introduced, the Conformité Européenne (CE) labeling was granted without proper compulsion to inform and to train physicians in the new technology. Surgeons used the technology according to their judgment and discretion on a compassionate and trial-and-error basis. As with all new technologies in ill-informed hands, the consequences were disastrous. When the SMFM was first launched, preliminary instructions for use (IFU) were issued to guide physicians' understanding and correct use of the flow modulator technology. Nonetheless, various studies have shown that not all physicians adhered to these instructions, continuing to treat on a compassionate basis patients who were not eligible for other forms of surgery.[4] This, coupled with the surprising lack of awareness of the evolving IFU, has resulted in mortality and unnecessary complications for patients who were already suffering from significant comorbidities.

The SMFM was a relatively new technology, which received CE marking in 2010. Its introduction has been fraught with complication, not only because of its unconventional nature, but also because of lack or ardent operator knowledge, as discussed. This chapter aims to identify the complications in relation to the SMFM, discuss probable causes for these complications, and suggest ways these complications can be avoided in the future.

The Global Registry

The SMFM was a disruptive technology, representing a new concept in the management of aortic disease. The mode of action of this device is completely different from that of conventional aortic devices, which caused much skepticism among the vascular community worldwide. Negative clinical outcomes have forced a more thorough analysis of this new device, and the team at the MFM Global Registry has been undertaking this investigative task. The aim of the Registry is to collect data from surgeons and interventionalists around the world who have used this device, to treat thoracoabdominal aortic pathologies. The experienced team then objectively analyzes the clinical outcomes and engages in biomedical testing of the device. The Registry has, to date, published more than 20 articles on the SMFM and presented its results in over 40 national and international presentations.

SURGICAL TECHNIQUE

Preoperative computed tomography angiography (CTA) with contrast should be carried out to assess aortic vessel and aneurysm/dissection size, including any angulation, proximal/distal landing zones, and femoral access. Accurate measurements are crucial in SMFM size selection and should be assessed using EndoSize virtual deployment software (Therenva SAS, Rennes, France). This software predicts the behavior of the stent through the vessel center-line and anticipates possible foreshortening.

Aneurysm Repair Technique

In aneurysm repair, especially thoracoabdominal, coverage of visceral and spinal branches is inevitable, which is a major downfall of currently available commercial endografts. The SMFM can be deployed across these vessels, without fear of compromised perfusion. This is because of its specific mesh design, which allows flow through the device.

> **TIP 24-1**
>
> The SMFM can cover visceral arteries because of its mesh design.

Preoperatively, the common femoral artery (CFA) is exposed using standard methods. Landing zones, previously identified on CTA, are visualized using intraoperative fluoroscopy. The appropriately sized SMFM (oversized by 25%–30%) is then introduced through a 20-French introducer sheath.

> **TIP 24-2**
>
> The diameter of SMFM should be 25%–30% of the diameter of the target vessel.

> **TIP 24-3**
>
> Visceral vessels to be covered by the SMFM should be surveyed for stenosis, thrombus, or calcification preoperatively.

> **TIP 24-4**
>
> When deploying multiple SMFM, overlap should be 6 cm, with 8 cm recommended in regions of high tortuosity.

An overlapping region of 6 cm between devices is recommended, with 8 cm in areas of tortuosity. In addition, the SMFM should be deployed at a rate of 1 cm/min to enhance aortic wall apposition and further prevent foreshortening, in a method known as "endoquilting." Endoquilting allows accurate conformability to the aortic wall during deployment. All guidewires and delivery sheaths should then be removed and wound closure carried out using standard methods.

If the proximal or distal ends of the SMFM are to be molded, it is recommended that the UnBalloon (LeMaitre, Massachusetts), a mesh-type balloon, be used, because the SMFM wires will inevitably rupture a conventional balloon.

Dissection Repair Technique

The SMFM size should be selected similar to the methods described. In aortic dissection, visceral branches may arise from the false lumen. In these cases, the operator should use a process known as endovascular scissoring (Fig. 24.1). Two 12 × 60 mm balloons should be advanced into both the true and false lumens and concomitantly inflated at the level of the aortic bifurcation. These should then be pulled caudally to cut the septum. Alternatively, a 12-French sheath with two superstiff wires, one in each of the true and false lumens, can be used to divide the septum. The ultimate aim of dividing the septum between the true and false lumens is to equalize the pressure between them.

Where all side branches arise from the true lumen, a 4-French pigtail catheter is used to access the true lumen through an advanced torsion technique. Approximately 2–3 mL of 50% diluted dye should be simultaneously injected to visualize the catheter up to the coronary sinus. Impedance of the catheter at this time should denote entry of the catheter into the false lumen. Where the SMFM is deployed over the aortic arch (for example in a Stanford Type A dissection), the initial 10 cm should be deployed in 20 seconds, during rapid pacing or adenosine-induced cardiac arrest. Endoquilting should then be used for the remainder of the deployment. Similarly, an UnBalloon should be used to inflate the SMFM where necessary. Analogous to the previous technique, all guidewires and delivery sheaths should then be removed and wound closure carried out using standard methods.

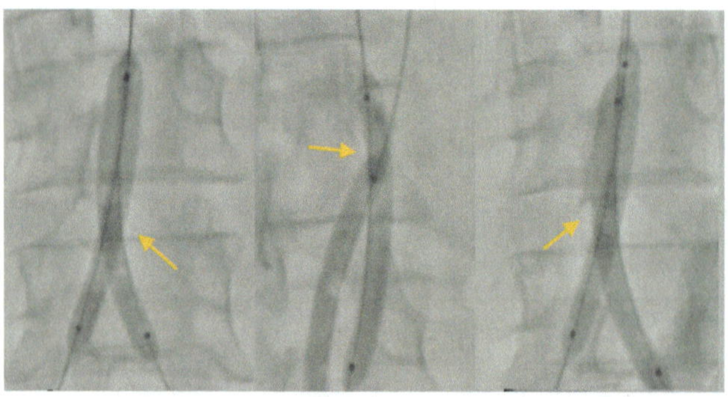

Fig. 24.1 Endovascular Scissoring. Two 12 × 60 mm balloons *(yellow arrows)* are inflated in the true and false lumina, used to cut the septum and equalize the lumen pressures.

SMFM COMPLICATIONS

In preceding years, there has been a slow but nonetheless encouraging learning curve among physicians with regard to the usage of the multilayer technology. This is a direct reflection of the quantity and quality of published literature. So far, there have been a handful of studies and reviews of patient cases from registries, which have shed light on the practical application of the SMFM in patient populations. These studies have included patients who have had complications after implantation of the SMFM and, as will be evident, these are largely a result of noncompliance with the available IFU.

Preoperative Planning and Complications

The Global Registry has previously documented 38 cases in which the SMFM was implanted outside of IFU in patients for treatment of thoracoabdominal aortic aneurysms (TAAA) or Stanford Type B aortic dissection.[4] In all of these cases, zero technical success was achieved, although there were no incidents of death, paraplegia, stroke or renovisceral compromise during the initial hospital stay. Thirteen patients had chronic Stanford Type B dissection with aneurysm dilatation of more than 6 cm. There were also 4 saccular and 6 mycotic aneurysms along with 15 primary TAAA. There was failure to land the device in the normal aorta in 31 (81.6%) cases with 12 inadequate stent overlaps and 11 cases where a smaller SMFM was deployed inside a larger one. Suboptimal sizing of two or more devices relative to each other and to the patient anatomy led to Failure Mode II, which is equivalent to an endoleak Type III, i.e., a leak between overlapping stents.

Ten patients suffered aneurysm ruptures and 23 had previous open or thoracic endovascular repair (TEVAR). Five of the nine cases resulted in a failure mode I (Type I endoleak), in which an undersized device was used. There were eight visceral branch complications. In total, 14 secondary endovascular interventions were required in 11 patients for endoleak or device foreshortening. In those with Stanford Type B dissection, no false lumen was completely thrombosed in the dissecting aneurysms. Follow-up at 10.0 ± 6.9 months showed that all-cause mortality was 89.5%, of which 27 (71.1%) were aneurysm-related deaths. Overall survival, freedom from aneurysm related death, and rupture-free survival estimates were 17.5%, 25.0%, and 31.5%, respectively, at 18 months.

A number of technical failures were recorded in this cohort, such as foreshortening, migration, device collapse, and device undersizing. The authors have reviewed the current manufacturer's IFU and made recommendations for their revision, based on their experience.[5]

Aneurysm Size

The authors have found that in patients with large diameter aneurysms, greater than 6.5 cm, the aneurysm fails to remodel over time, when compared with those with smaller diameters. Lack of aortic remodeling is thought to be caused by adventitial elastolysis, where the structural integrity of the artery wall is lost because of reduction of adventitial elastin. This begins in the aortic wall, restricting remodeling of the aneurysmal sac, which in these cases is larger in diameter (Fig. 24.2). Additionally, a computational study by the authors[6] of six aneurysmal aortic cases found that one patient treated for a TAAA had an extensive aneurysm length. This in turn generated a large volume of flow that could not be modulated by the SMFM devices. This observation led to the conclusion that the SMFM device has no benefit if the sac volume exceeds 400 mL.[5,6] Therefore, to avoid potentially fatal complications, the authors now recommend against using the SMFM in patients with aneurysmal disease of diameter greater than 6.5 cm and/or volume greater than 400 mL.[5,6]

WARNING 24-1

The SMFM is not recommended in aneurysm >6.5 cm maximum aneurysm diameter.

WARNING 24-2

The SMFM is not recommended in TAAA >20 cm maximum aneurysm length.

WARNING 24-3

The SMFM is not recommended in aneurysms with >400 mL total aneurysm volume.

Infectious Aneurysms

Based on current IFU, it is contraindicated to implant the SMFM in mycotic/infectious aneurysms because the infection drastically increases postoperative complications. Interestingly, previous studies have illustrated the successful use of the SMFM in patients with infection. Benjelloun et al.[7] reported the case of a 16-year-old girl treated 4 years previously for a ruptured AAA of tuberculous origin. Three SMFM stents were successively implanted despite being contraindicated in infectious aneurysms. Flis et al.[8] described their experience with treating a primary infected juxtarenal aortic aneurysm with the SMFM. Follow-up imaging showed persistent aneurysm shrinkage of the sac until complete regression to a normal aortic configuration was seen at 1 year.

Reijnen et al.[9] reported their successful treatment of an infected 56-mm saccular aneurysm of the aorta, located at the level of the superior mesenteric artery (SMA), with both renal arteries located within the aneurysm. At 18-month follow-up, the aneurysm was stable and mostly thrombosed, with adequate perfusion of the side branches and no signs of persistent infection.

However, the authors disagree regarding placing the SMFM in any patient with evidence of infection, based on experience with patients with multiple recurrent aortic aneurysms, which subsequently resulted in fatal aneurysm rupture (Fig. 24.3).

Landing Zones

WARNING 24-4

Proximal and distal landing zones should be nonaneurysmal normal aortic wall for a length of at least 20 mm.

The authors recommend, for prevention of endoleak and other complications, deployment within nonaneurysmal native aortic landing zones of at least 20 mm. This will ensure there is adequate radial force to allow self-fixation of the stent against the proximal and distal vessel walls. Since there is a potential for foreshortening during deployment of the SMFM because of its braided design, if the landing zone is selected too far distally, the proximal target zone might not be completely covered (Fig. 24.4). This may lead to failure mode I (Type I endoleak) and to sac rupture when the device cannot properly manipulate the flow. When the SMFM is well placed with good wall apposition in appropriately selected patients, the device laminates blood flow uniformly in parallel layers, allowing regeneration of the endothelium by reduction of peak wall shear stress and slowing of flow into the sac, hence laying down of an organized thrombus.[10]

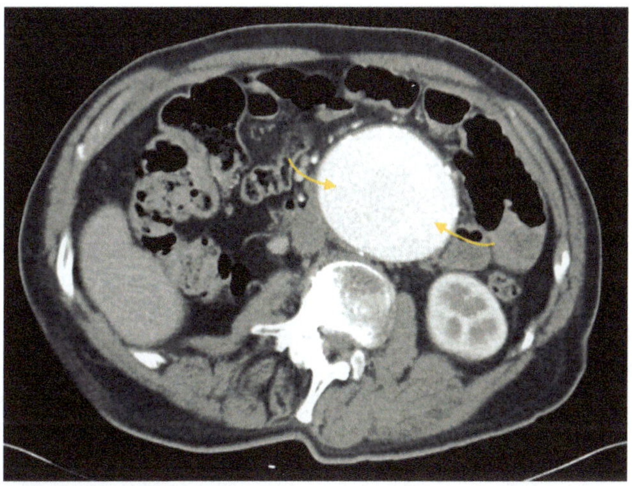

Fig. 24.2 **JuxtaRenal Aneurysm.** Octogenarian male patient with a 7.7-cm juxtarenal aneurysm *(yellow arrows)*, which subsequently ruptured at 48 months post Streamliner Multilayer Flow Modulator implantation.

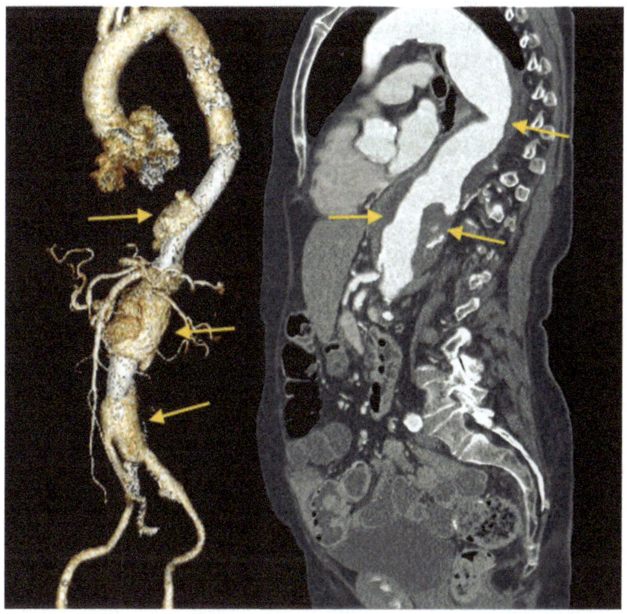

Fig. 24.3 **Infectious Aneurysm.** A 77-year-old male patient with multiple recurrent aortic aneurysms (*yellow arrows*), which subsequently ruptured at 18 months post Streamliner Multilayer Flow Modulator implantation.

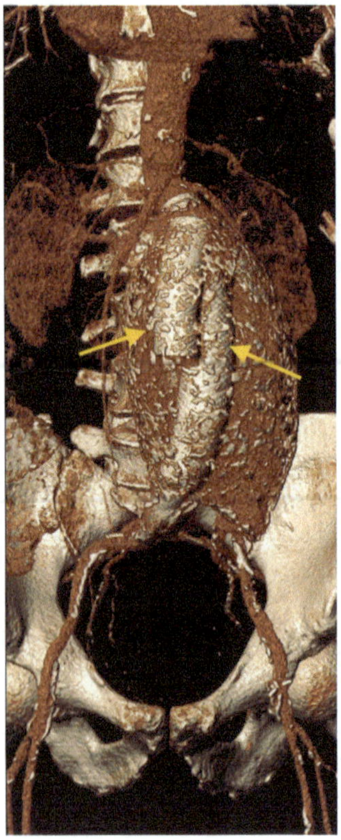

Fig. 24.4 Inadequate Landing Zones. The proximal Streamliner Multilayer Flow Modulator device *(arrow)* was landed distally in the aneurysm sac, while the distal device was landed proximally *(arrow)* in the aneurysm sac.

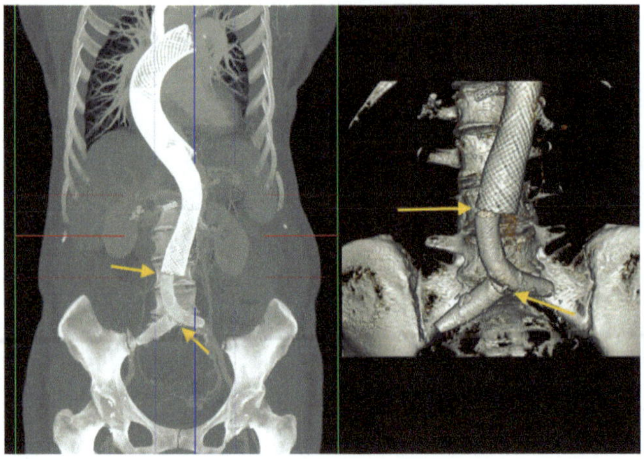

Fig. 24.5 Inadequate Overlap of Streamliner Multilayer Flow Modulator (SMFM) Devices. Lack of minimal overlap between the distal portion of an aortic SMFM device *(arrow)* and bilateral iliac SMFM devices *(arrow)*, resulting in subsequent dislocation.

The authors highlighted previously that correct device placement induced aneurysm flow streamlining, which reduced the dynamic pressure by 23%–66%, and incorrect placements promoted failure mode I (Type I endoleak), with 58% and 16% dynamic pressure increases and aneurysm volume expansion up to 23%.[6]

Perioperative Complications

Inadequate Overlap

In cases that require multiple SMFM devices to cover adequately the aortic pathology to be treated, the smaller diameter SMFM should be implanted first, followed by deployment of a larger SMFM, inside the first device. This engages the radial force of the device, keeping the smaller device open, thus avoiding increased peak wall shear stresses (PWSS) and vortices that could lead to rupture. This was assessed computationally and results highlighted that overlapped devices improved distal perfusion by increasing arch branch outflows from 5% to 24% (Fig. 24.5).[6] The authors recommend using an overlap of 6 cm when deploying multiple SMFM devices. In areas of high tortuosity, an overlap of 8 cm between devices is recommended.

Device Malexpansion

Sultan and Hynes[11] published 1-year results of the MFM in the management of the TAAA and Stanford Type B dissections. In this study, one patient (1 of 55 patients) who had a Crawford Type III TAAA experienced technical failure because the distal portion of the most caudal SMFM did not fully expand. Three attempts at balloon dilating the stent failed where the balloon burst at nominal pressure. Further intervention was decided against, and at 3 months CTA showed the stent had intrinsically expanded (Fig. 24.6). To avoid malexpansion and subsequent balloon rupture in an attempt to inflate the SMFM, the authors recommend that the UnBalloon (LeMaitre, Massachusetts) be used. The operator should also use the technique of endoquilting, which will allow the SMFM to deploy slowly and accurately, encouraging apposition to the wall and preventing collapse. Operators must also be cognizant of vessel tortuosity. In areas of high tortuosity, the SMFM should be deployed slowly, to allow it to conform to the specific curvature of the wall.

Device Foreshortening

Device foreshortening most often occurs during the perioperative phase of deployment of the SMFM. Fig. 24.5 shows an example of foreshortening and dislocation of the proximal SMFM limbs from the main aortic SMFM body. A previous study by Ferrero et al.[12] reported a case of foreshortening in a TAAA patient treated with five SMFM devices. During the procedure, three SMFM devices were deployed from the origin of the left subclavian artery to the aortic bifurcation. However, stent foreshortening occurred with loss of both central overlapping regions. A fourth device was deployed but again foreshortened and dislocated. A fifth device was deployed to cover the dislocated regions. It was reported that this patient died of an aortic arch rupture on postoperative day 5.

To combat foreshortening during deployment, the SMFM should be deployed at a slow rate to increase contact between the device and the aortic wall. Deployment should be steady, gradual, and constant, with forward traction, to avoid foreshortening and boost device placement. Adequate deployment should be evaluated at the end of the procedure using completion angiography. Additionally, a CT scan or magnetic resonance imaging (MRI) should be conducted before patient discharge to check for accurate deployment of the SMFM and possible endoleak.

WARNING 24-5

The SMFM should be deployed slowly to encourage device-to-wall interaction and to prevent foreshortening.

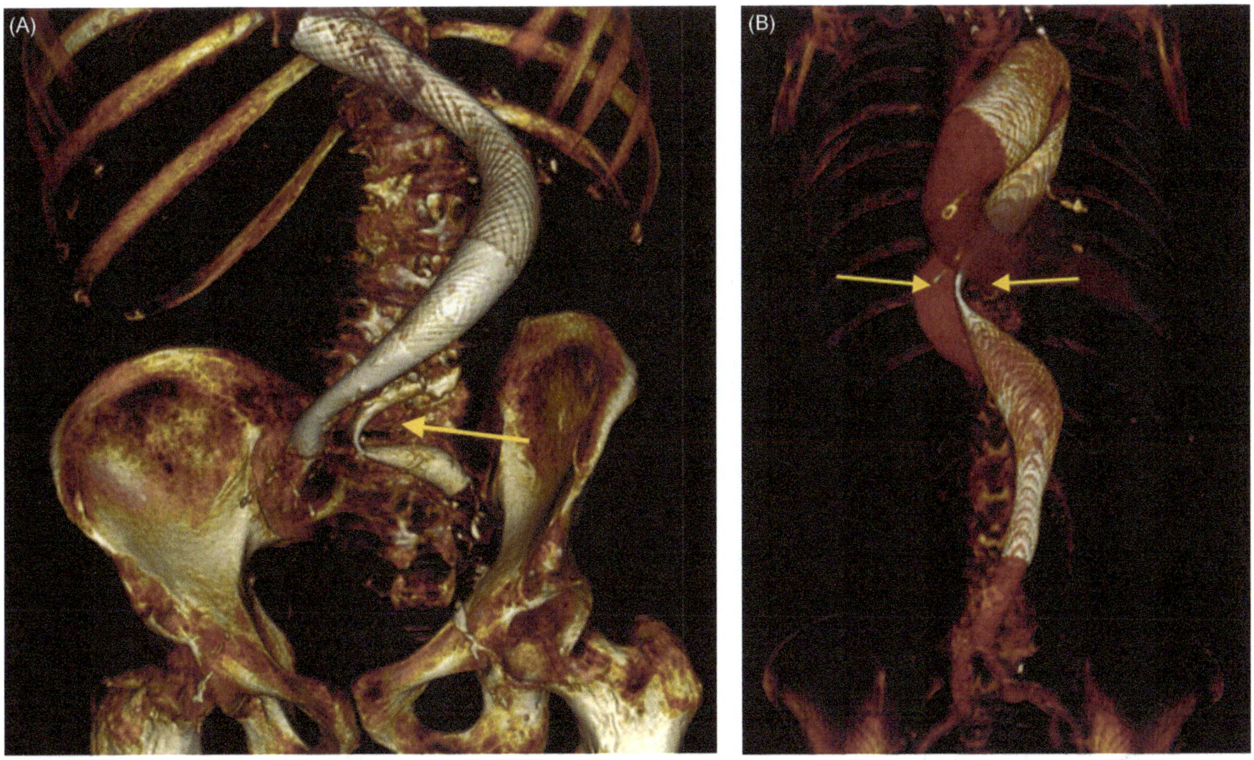

Fig. 24.6 SMFM Malexpansion. (A) Left iliac Streamliner Multilayer Flow Modulator (SMFM) device collapse *(arrow)* in a patient with a juxtarenal aneurysm. (B) A patient with ascending and descending aortic aneurysms, treated with three SMFM, with the second deployed SMFM suffering collapse *(arrows)*.

Postoperative Complications

Device Migration, Dislocation, and Collapse

SMFM device migration, dislocation, and collapse can occur in the postoperative setting. Degree of migration is defined as a movement of the device ≥10 mm relative to the anatomical landmarks designated during the procedure. Lack of correct overlap during deployment can result in subsequent migration of an SMFM (Fig. 24.5). Similarly, inadequate oversizing between multiple devices can lead to a lack of radial force and result in device dislocation or collapse as shown in Figs. 24.6 and 24.7. Lowe et al.[13] implanted the SMFM in 14 patients and reported dislocation of the devices in 4 patients, including dislocation of the main body in the abdominal aorta and in the descending thoracic aorta. To avoid these complications, preoperative planning is vital, such as choosing landing zones in the normal aorta, which should extend beyond 20 mm in both the proximal and distal portions. Choice of SMFM size is also crucial and should be 25%–30% greater than the diameter of the target vessel to ensure good radial force and prevent migration and subsequent dislocation and collapse of the SMFM.

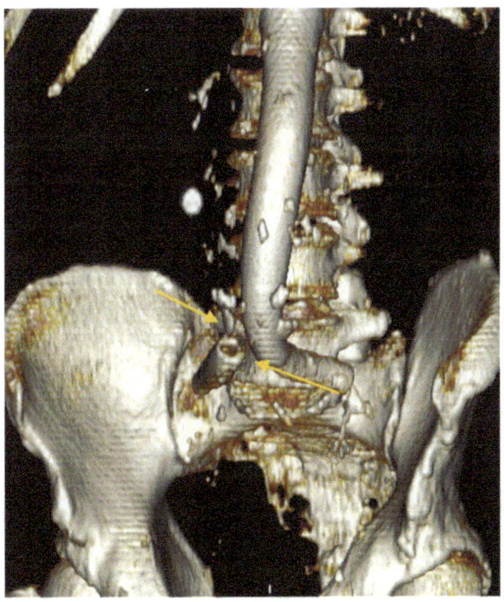

Fig. 24.7 Device Dislocation. Dislocation of the right common iliac artery Streamliner Multilayer Flow Modulator (SMFM) device from the main SMFM aortic body device *(arrows)* at 1-month postimplantation.

Stent Occlusion

Stent occlusion (Fig. 24.8) may also result from inadequate landing zones (for example, in the aneurysm sac; Fig. 24.4), device collapse (Fig. 24.6A), or device dislocation (Fig. 24.7). Ruffino and Rabbia[14] reported six stents that were occluded (11.1%). One was a common iliac artery occlusion at 24 hours in a thrombophilic patient who then underwent surgical aortoiliac bypass. Henry et al.[15] reported their use of the SMFM for treatment of peripheral, visceral, and aortic aneurysms and formulated initial guidelines for the use of SMFM. Nine (10%) devices were reported as occluded, with most occlusions resulting from preexisting conditions. Patency was restored in five occluded SMFM, and four occluded SMFM were asymptomatic and were not treated. All covered side branches were patent except in a patient with thrombophilia who also had an occluded SMFM.

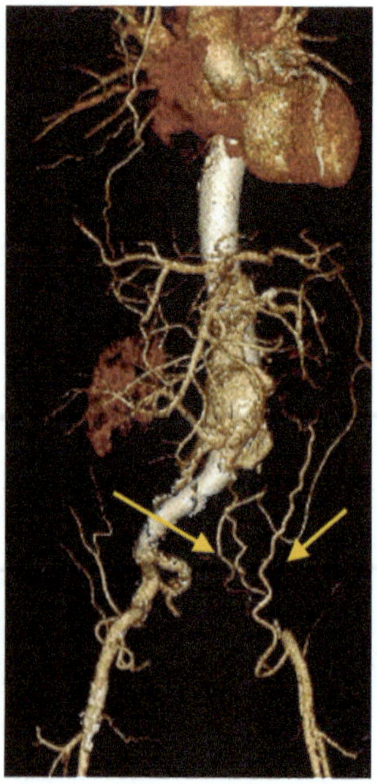

Fig. 24.8 **Streamliner Multilayer Flow Modulator (SMFM) Occlusion.** Left iliac SMFM occlusion *(arrows)* postoperatively, resulting from undersizing, in a patient with bilateral iliac aneurysmal disease.

Vaislic et al.[16] reported 1-year outcomes from the STRATO trial, which involved using the SMFM in repairing TAAA. One patient with two occluded visceral branches underwent successful surgical reintervention. Occlusions were detected in two covered visceral branches (the celiac trunk and SMA with splenic and mesenteric infarction) in one patient 14 days after procedure. This patient was not administered postprocedure dual antiplatelet therapy but was receiving aspirin. The patient underwent successful surgical thrombectomy and bypass of both visceral branches. At 12 months, the celiac trunk and the SMA were patent through the grafts.

Preoperative planning is of utmost importance with regard to stent occlusion. The operator must be aware of any preexisting stenosis or calcification that may exist in visceral arteries. Preoperative CTA is necessary to visualize any partial or full occlusion, and the authors recommend that these be dealt with in advance of SMFM implantation. The authors also recommend that patients receive postoperative clopidogrel (75 mg/day) to reduce the risk of thrombosis and occlusion.

> **TIP 24-5**
>
> Postoperative clopidogrel 75 mg/day should be continued for at least 12 weeks.

Endoleak

When utilizing the SMFM, the terminology "Failure Mode" has been used regarding endoleak formation. Failure Mode I, which is equivalent to an endoleak Type I, is defined as a leak between the proximal stent and the aortic wall (Type Ia) or between the distal stent and the aortic wall (Type Ib). Failure Mode II is equivalent to a Type III endoleak, which is a leak between overlapping stents.

Ruffino and Rabbia[14] reported two cases of stent foreshortening that led to failure mode II at 3 months where the patients suffered from a popliteal aneurysm and internal iliac artery aneurysm, respectively. They both underwent deployment of another SMFM with recovery in device continuity because of inadequate overlap of the stents. They concluded that there has to be a minimum overlap of 3 cm between the stents.

Balderi et al.[17] reported a visceral aneurysm that developed an endoleak from which the splenic and left gastric arteries originated. No reintervention was performed considering the aneurysmal sac's stability at 2-year follow-up. They deemed that stent-graft rigidity and size of delivery systems can preclude placement in distal or tortuous vessels. They had also reached the conclusion, previously, that these devices can cover arising vessels, thus leading to splenic, hepatic, or gastroduodenal infarction, and cannot be used in short or wide-necked vessels.

In a study by Vaislic et al.,[16] endoleaks were identified in five patients (three attachment site and two at device overlap), four of whom underwent reintervention (three additional SMFMs and one stent graft implanted). At 12 months, aneurysms were not thrombosed because of persistent endoleak in two patients. The only death occurred at 11 months in a patient with atrial fibrillation who had experienced a stroke during reintervention for a Failure Mode II at 3 months. Endoleaks (three Failure Mode I and two Failure Mode II) requiring correction were identified in 5 (22%) of the 23 patients, and all were determined to be a result of technical issues. The three Failure Mode I endoleaks were induced by device misplacement (one in a graft in the aortic arch; another in a stenosed area at the top of a gothic aortic arch, and the third within a previously implanted graft), which contributed to incomplete SMFM opening in each case. One of the Failure Mode II endoleaks was caused by placement of a small-diameter SMFM into a larger MFM. In the other case, there was insufficient overlapping of two MFM devices. Reintervention with implantation of one or more additional SMFM devices was performed before 12-month follow-up in one of these cases and after 12-month follow-up in another. One Failure Mode I endoleak was managed by combining stent-graft implantation and left subclavian artery exclusion. Reintervention was declined by the remaining patient with endoleak, who died 18 months after MFM implantation.

The issues described are avoidable if the SMFM intervention is diligently planned preoperatively and deployed with great care. Current, as well as new, recommendations for IFU illustrate that abundant technical guidance is available with regards to device size, number of stents used, device overlap distance, and minimum healthy attachment site requirements.[5]

Aneurysm Rupture

Henry et al.[15] witnessed two aneurysm ruptures for contraindicated use (ruptured aneurysm; mycotic aneurysm). There was one late rupture caused by Failure Mode I. Out of 47 patients, 13.3% experienced endoleaks. Ferrero et al.[12] published a case report on the aortic aneurysm rupture that occurred after the use of the SMFM in a 76-year-old female. The autopsy revealed a 6-cm tear of the aortic arch wall with a visible left hemothorax and that the SMFM overlapping zone was too rigid to accommodate the degree of aortic arch angulation, leading to rupture. Lowe et al.[13] reported deaths, which included four confirmed ruptures, one presumed rupture, and one confirmed dissection with rupture. Examination of these cases alluded to technical failures, such as undersizing and inadequate overlap between devices.

Rupture is also thought to occur in larger diameter aneurysms (>6.5 cm) as a result of adventitial elastolysis (Fig. 24.2), as discussed earlier. Aortic remodeling that allows organized thrombosis and sac shrinkage cannot occur. Examination of previous cases showed that in many of these, the chosen devices were not oversizing appropriately (4%–8%) and had short regions of overlap (3–5 cm). This in turn resulted in incidents of foreshortening, endoleak, and fatal clinical consequences.

EVIDENCE-BASED RECOMMENDATIONS

The Global Registry has conducted a number of reviews, meta-analyses, and computational studies that investigate clinical outcomes as a result of isolating patient cohorts treated outside of IFU from those treated under the IFU. Results illustrated that there are clearly limitations to the SMFM that must be respected when using this technology.

Instructions for Use

The results from a meta-analysis conducted by Hynes et al. of 15 articles,[18] presenting 171 patients, showed that technical success was achieved in 131 cases (76.6%). Among the remaining 40, which were failures, 38 occurred among the cases that were performed outside of SMFM IFU, 10 of whom presented with aortic rupture. Within the IFU subgroup, aneurysm-related survival at 1 year was 93.3% ± 2.79%, which is in sharp contrast to the 38% ± 9% for patients treated outside the IFU. At 18 months, aneurysm-related survival rates remained the same as within the IFU subgroup (93.3% ± 7.64%), whereas the survival estimate fell to 25.6% ± 9.01% for those treated outside the IFU.

Stefanov et al. performed a technically rigorous computational analysis, which provided several important insights that warrant emphasis. Improved flow dynamics were observed when devices were deployed under the IFU.[6] In patients with treatment outside the IFU, mainly as a result of stent foreshortening during positioning, less favorable flow dynamics were observed. Furthermore, in those patients with treatment outside the IFU, aneurysm volume expansion of nearly 25% was seen.[6]

This emphasizes the fact that not adhering to the IFU will most definitely lead to morbidity and even mortality among patients, and those who continue to use the SMFM outside the guidelines are at risk of being negligent toward their patients. It is the treating physicians' responsibility to research the SMFM thoroughly before use and follow the guidelines available in order to achieve the best outcome for their patients.

New Recommendations for IFU

The authors continue to emphasize application of IFU and provide recommendations for the revision of the indications and contraindications for SMFM use.[5] It is now recommended that the diameter of SMFM should be sized to 25%–30% of the diameter of the target vessel and, prior to implantation, a CTA scan must be performed for sizing analysis. This should not be done more than 3 months before procedure. When it is necessary to cover aortic branches such as the left subclavian artery, left common carotid artery, brachiocephalic artery, renal arteries, celiac trunk, and superior mesenteric arteries, the physician should make sure that there is no stenosis, thrombus, or calcification on the preoperative CTA. If the above are detected, we recommend angioplasty and/or stenting of the branch 2 to 4 weeks before the SMFM deployment.

When overlapping devices with different diameters, the smaller diameter device must be deployed first and then the larger diameter should be placed to overlap within the smaller diameter SMFM. To minimize Failure Modes I and II, it is recommended not to have SMFMs overlapping in curved areas. Six centimeters is the minimum recommended overlap, with 8 cm recommended in severe tortuosity of the aorta. During deployment, the SMFM must be in contact with at least one side of the wall, and the device must be deployed using endoquilting. This deployment technique involves a firm, slow, and sustained release mechanism with forward traction, avoids SMFM foreshortening, and maximizes device alignment along the aortic wall. A further precaution must be taken in the form of a postoperative CTA scan or MRI before patient discharge to check for Failure Mode I or II and to treat it promptly.

In addition to the current contraindications for use, the authors recommend against implanting the SMFM in its current state of development in any patients with TAAA. The device should not be deployed in patients with any evidence of infection associated with previously inserted open repair grafts or endografts.[5] The presence of infection from previous open repair will present a hostile environment to the SMFM.[13] The SMFM should not be implanted in patients with a history of myeloproliferative disorders or coagulation problems. The total systemic burden on the patient is thought too great because of platelet consumption during initial thrombosis of the aneurysm sac. The authors now recommend against implantation of the SMFM in patients with a life expectancy of less than 12 months.[5]

CONCLUSION

Several studies showed that the use of the SMFM is associated with an early low incidence of complications, including stroke, paraplegia, and aneurysm rupture. In addition, these studies demonstrated acceptable rates of aneurysm-related survival and visceral branch patency when carried out within the parameters of the IFU, whereas undesirable outcomes have been reported when the SMFM is used outside the IFU. Longer follow-up demonstrated that this technology requires extensive research and development before applying in TAAA patients, but it can be safely used in chronic symptomatic Type B dissection.[19,20] Initially, the SMFM was distributed to the vascular community without dedicated operator knowledge, leading to incorrect and inappropriate use of the device. Early cases invariably included patients with multiple comorbidities and those with no other treatment options. Some of these patients eventually died from preexisting causes. However, these deaths were perpetually linked with poor SMFM clinical outcomes. With poor operator knowledge and inappropriate use outside of IFU, poor clinical outcomes have inevitably resulted.

Despite the mixed evidence in the literature, the authors have reached a consensus that the SMFM, when used within their IFU for symptomatic Type B dissection, represents a valuable option in patients who are deemed to be high risk and are not suitable for open surgery. However, until an advanced dedicated stent is developed, its use in aortic aneurysm cannot be recommended. The flow modulator technology is a promising option in endovascular surgery, and this technological advancement can improve in the future, providing the limitations and IFU of the device are appreciated. Additionally, there is a need to conduct further studies including randomized control trials to explore this emerging technology further.

REFERENCES

1. Sethi RK, Henry AJ, Hevelone ND, et al. Impact of hospital market competition on endovascular aneurysm repair adoption and outcomes. *J Vasc Surg.* 2013;58:596–606.
2. Maleux G, Koolen M, Heye S. Complications after endovascular aneurysm repair. *Sem Intervent Radiol.* 2009;26:3–9.
3. Picel AC, Kansal N. Essentials of endovascular abdominal aortic aneurysm repair imaging: postprocedure surveillance and complications. *Am J Roentgenol.* 2014;203:W358–W372.

4. Sultan S, Hynes N, Sultan M, et al. When not to implant the multilayer flow modulator: lessons learned from application outside the indications for use in patients with thoracoabdominal pathologies. *J Endovasc Ther.* 2014;21:96–112.
5. Sultan S, Kavanagh EP, Costache V, et al. Streamliner Multilayer Flow Modulator for thoracoabdominal aortic pathologies: recommendations for revision of indications and contraindications for use. *Vascular Disease Management.* 2017;14:E90–E99.
6. Stefanov F, Morris L, Elhelali A, et al. Insights from complex aortic surgery with a Streamliner device for aortic arch repair (STAR). *J Thorac Cardiovasc Surg.* 2016;152:1309–1318.
7. Benjelloun A, Henry M, Ghannam A, et al. Endovascular treatment of a tuberculous thoracoabdominal aneurysm with the multilayer stent. *J Endovasc Ther.* 2012;19:115–120.
8. Flis V, Matela J, Breznik S, et al. Treatment of primary infected juxtarenal aortic aneurysm with the Multilayer stent. *J Vasc Endovasc Surg.* 2013;47:561–565.
9. Reijnen MM, van Sterkenburg SM. Treatment of a salmonella-induced rapidly expanding aortic pseudoaneurysm involving the visceral arteries using the Cardiatis Multilayer stent. *J Vasc Surg.* 2014;60:1056–1058.
10. Sultan S, Sultan M, Hynes N. Early mid-term results of the first 103 cases of multilayer flow modulator stent done under indication for use in the management of thoracoabdominal aortic pathology from the independent global MFM registry. *J Cardiovasc Surg (Torino).* 2014;55:21–32.
11. Sultan S, Hynes N. One-year results of the multilayer flow modulator stent in the management of thoracoabdominal aortic aneurysms and Type B dissections. *J Endovasc Ther.* 2013;20:266–377.
12. Ferrero E, Gibello L, Ferri M, et al. Aortic arch rupture after multiple Multilayer stent treatment of a thoracoabdominal aneurysm. *J Vasc Surg.* 2014;60:1348–1352.
13. Lowe C, Worthington A, Serracino-Inglott F, et al. Multi-layer flow-modulating stents for thoraco-abdominal and peri-renal aneurysms: the UK pilot study. *Eur J Vasc Endovasc Surg.* 2016;51:225–231.
14. Ruffino MA, Rabbia C. Endovascular repair of peripheral and visceral aneurysms with cardiatis Multilayer Flow Modulator: one-year results from the Italian Multicentre Registry. *J Endovasc Ther.* 2012;19:599–610.
15. Henry M, Benjelloun A, Wheatley G. The multilayer flow modulator stent for the treatment of arterial aneurysms. *J Cardiovasc Surg (Torino).* 2013;54:763–783.
16. Vaislic CD, Fabiani JN, Chocron S, et al. One-year outcomes following repair of thoracoabdominal aneurysms with the multilayer flow modulator report from the STRATO trail. *J Endovasc Ther.* 2014;21:85–95.
17. Balderi A, Antonietti A, Pedrazzini F, et al. Treatment of visceral aneurysm using multilayer flow modulator stent: two-year follow-up results in five consecutive patients. *Cardiovasc Intervent Radiol.* 2013;36:1256–1261.
18. Hynes N, Sultan S, Elhelali A, et al. Systematic review and patient-level metaanalysis of the Streamliner Multilayer Flow Modulator in the management of complex thoracoabdominal aortic pathology. *J Endovasc Ther.* 2016;23:501–512.
19. Sultan S, Kavanagh EP, Stefanov F, et al. Global MFM Collaborators. Endovascular management of chronic symptomatic aortic dissection with the Streamliner Multilayer Flow Modulator: twelve-month outcomes from the global registry. *J Vasc Surg.* 2017;65(4):940–950.
20. Stefanov F, Sultan S, Morris L, et al. Computational fluid analysis of symptomatic chronic type B aortic dissections managed with the Streamliner Multilayer Flow Modulator. *J Vasc Surg.* 2017;65(4):951–963.

Transcatheter Aortic Valve Replacement

Daniel M. Shivapour, MD, Samir R. Kapadia, MD and Amar Krishnaswamy, MD

TRANSCATHETER AORTIC VALVE REPLACEMENT

Introduction

Aortic stenosis (AS) affects morbidity and mortality as populations continue to age. Recent studies have estimated the prevalence of calcific AS between 2% and 4% among adults over 65 years of age and, for many years, there were limited or no treatment options for certain subsets of patients.[1] In the absence of intervention, once symptoms develop, severe aortic stenosis is associated with a median survival of 1–2 years.[2]

Surgical aortic valve replacement (SAVR) has been the gold standard therapy for severe symptomatic AS and remains important for selected patients.[3] However, at least 30% of patients do not undergo SAVR because of comorbidities and other risk factors believed to place them at prohibitive surgical risk, such as advanced age, prior cardiac surgeries, severe lung disease, frailty, and other significant medical and anatomic considerations.[4] Balloon aortic valvuloplasty (BAV) can increase valve area and offer short-term symptomatic improvement to inoperable patients, but studies have shown a high rate of restenosis and no improvement in survival without definitive valve replacement.[5] To address the unmet need, transcatheter aortic valve replacement (TAVR) was developed.

Cribier and colleagues performed the first TAVR in a human in 2002.[6] Several trials followed and established the safety and efficacy of TAVR.[7–10] The US Food and Drug Administration (FDA) approved TAVR for use in inoperable patients in 2011.[11] TAVR quickly became an established treatment option for a variety of subgroups, including those at high and intermediate risk from surgery, and continues to demonstrate excellent safety and outcomes.

This chapter provides an overview of indications, patient selection, identification, and management of important comorbidities, contraindications, procedural technique and considerations, peri-operative management, and the indication and management of complications of TAVR. We will focus primarily on the transfemoral implantation of two device products currently available in the United States at the time of writing: the balloon-expandable Edwards Sapien XT and S3 valves (Edwards Life Sciences Inc., Irvine, California) and the self-expanding Medtronic CoreValve and Evolute-R valves (Medtronic Inc., Minneapolis, Minnesota).

INDICATIONS AND PATIENT SELECTION

The cornerstone of avoiding complications is appropriate patient selection. This is done with collaborative multidisciplinary evaluation using a "heart team" approach. Each patient is assessed by cardiac surgeons and interventional cardiologists. In some programs, cardiac imaging specialists analyze multimodality imaging to determine anatomic feasibility and valve sizing, while others involve vascular surgeons in screening to determine access options. The key is that each program must critically self-evaluate to ensure that all needs are met to provide appropriate clinical and anatomic evaluation. It is important to understand and to account for specific preferences, goals, expectations, or limitations each individual may have to determine the best treatment strategy.

The diagnosis of severe aortic stenosis can be ascertained by following multidisciplinary consensus guidelines for valvular heart disease.[3] Patients should be symptomatic from their valve disease with at least New York Heart Association (NYHA) Functional Class II symptoms or greater. For high-risk patients with severe aortic stenosis or insufficiency resulting from bioprosthetic valve degeneration, "valve-in-valve" TAVR is approved.

Surgical risk should be assessed by cardiac surgeons and include review of cardiovascular and noncardiovascular comorbid conditions. Clinical decision aids, including the Society of Thoracic Surgeons predicted risk of mortality (STS-PROM) calculator and the European System for Cardiac Operative Risk Evaluation (Logistic EuroSCORE) assist with quantitative risk assessment. It is widely recognized that not all important conditions are included in the risk calculators and that these factors must be considered on a patient-by-patient basis. Factors known to increase substantially the risk of SAVR and/or limit rehabilitation potential following traditional surgery include prior cardiac surgeries/sternotomies, chest wall deformities, prior chest wall radiation, porcelain aorta, prior coronary artery bypass grafting with anatomy lying in unsafe proximity to the chest wall, severe lung disease, cirrhosis, or significant frailty.[12]

The PARTNER IA trial[7] demonstrated an absolute 20% relative risk reduction in mortality with TAVR in comparison with medical therapy. Patients at low surgical risk in the PARTNER-3 and CoreValve low-risk trials were recently demonstrated to have better outcomes with TAVR than surgical AVR when anatomically appropriate.[13,14]

The preferred approach for TAVR is the common femoral artery (transfemoral [TF]). As device profiles and equipment have continued to improve, approximately 90% of patients are able to undergo TF TAVR safely. In patients with acceptable renal function, iliofemoral anatomy and aortic valve annular sizing can both be quickly and reliably assessed using contrast-enhanced computed tomography (CT) scan. Important factors to consider when evaluating patients for iliofemoral suitability of TF TAVR include the minimal luminal diameter (MLD), amount and distribution of calcification, and tortuosity of the iliofemoral vessels, because these can identify patients at high risk of peripheral vascular complications.[15] While the iliofemoral dimensions required are dependent on the type and size of valve chosen, most patients with an iliofemoral MLD of 5.5–6.0 mm are able to accommodate the necessary sheath(s) for TF TAVR. In patients with significant iliofemoral calcification or tortuosity, a larger MLD may be necessary and care should be taken with sheath insertion, valve advancement, and post-TAVR sheath withdrawal, because these patients may be at risk of iliac artery avulsion. For patients whose renal function does not allow contrast CT assessment, other strategies for assessment include noncontrast CT, angiography using minimal contrast dye, or intravascular ultrasound (IVUS) assessment in the catheterization laboratory.

Chest CT images should be gated to cardiac cycle to allow the most accurate sizing of the aortic annulus. The annulus is assessed either manually or using software packages that facilitate semi-automated three-dimensional (3D) reconstruction of CT images. Sizing performed by CT has been shown to be more precise and accurate than measurements using standard echocardiography.[16] Careful assessment of the coronary sinus and aortic root dimensions, calcium distribution in the left ventricular outflow tract, and the height of the coronary ostia from the annular plane are important in selecting the optimal valve size and type. Other strategies for annular assessment include cardiac MRI or echocardiographic modalities (e.g., 3D TEE). It is important to understand the differences in measurements produced by these different modalities, as valve undersizing is an important risk factor for TAVR complications, such as paravalvular regurgitation.

MANAGEMENT OF IMPORTANT COMORBIDITIES PRIOR TO TAVR

It is essential that patients being considered for AVR undergo coronary angiography to assess for obstructive disease. During SAVR, patients with CAD can undergo surgical revascularization (CABG) at the time of their valve replacement. For patients undergoing TAVR, the timing and approach to percutaneous coronary intervention (PCI) for revascularization remains an area of active clinical investigation.

Carotid artery disease is also prevalent in patients with severe AS and must be considered and assessed.

CONTRA-INDICATIONS FOR TAVR

TAVR is not appropriate for patients with severely limited life expectancy as a result of factors outside their AS, clear medical futility, or severe/incapacitating dementia. TAVR is not currently approved for isolated native-valve aortic regurgitation (AR), although this is under investigation. Cardiac surgery can often provide more complete and definitive treatment for patients with other concurrent valve disease not amenable to current transcatheter therapies, patients with concomitant aortopathy, or severe coronary artery disease not amenable to percutaneous coronary intervention (PCI). Additionally, patients whose valve annulus is either too small or too large for currently available transcatheter devices may not be candidates for TAVR.

PROCEDURAL CONSIDERATIONS, EQUIPMENT, AND TECHNIQUE FOR TAVR

Optimal TAVR outcomes are obtained from a multidisciplinary approach with interventional cardiologists, cardiac surgeons, anesthesiologists, nurses, and other support staff working collaboratively. There may be institutional variability in personnel, equipment, and facilities used. In our institution, TF TAVR is most often performed in a minimally invasive fashion, using a fully percutaneous approach with local anesthetic and conscious sedation in a "hybrid" suite. Although rarely required, full surgical preparation of every patient is performed in the event that conversion to an open surgical procedure is necessary.[17]

Preparation and attention to detail when obtaining access is of the highest importance in TF TAVR to mitigate the risk of access site complications (Chapter 1). The common femoral artery should be accessed just above the bifurcation of the profunda and superficial femoral arteries and below the inferior epigastric artery with a micropuncture system under imaging, with verification of location by angiography prior to upsizing. Prior to the insertion of the delivery sheath for the TAVR valve, preclosure of the site can be performed using a variety of devices, such as the Perclose Proglide or ProStar XL devices (Abbott Vascular, Santa Clara, California).

The current Edwards and Medtronic valve series have different sheath sizes. The Edwards SAPIEN-3 is inserted via a 14-French expandable sheath (the 29-mm valve is placed via a 16-French sheath). The Medtronic CoreValve Evolut-R can either be placed using the "in-line" 14-French sheath or through a separate 18-French sheath. The Evolut-Pro utilizes either the in-line 16-French sheath or a separate 20-French sheath. Iliofemoral sizing/access requirements for the SAPIEN-3 and Evolut-R are similar and valve choice is often based on operator preference and aortic root characteristics. The Evolut-Pro requires a larger iliofemoral system.

Additional access is required for placement of a temporary transvenous pacemaker and pigtail catheter to be placed in the noncoronary cusp, to perform aortic root angiography, and to assist in valve positioning. These sheaths can either be placed ipsilateral or contralateral to the delivery sheath. The pigtail catheter can be inserted from a radial artery site; however, it is more difficult to complete endovascular interventions rapidly in the event of an iliofemoral vascular complication and may occupy the access site needed for a cerebrovascular embolic protection device. Some sites routinely place pacemaker wire via the internal jugular (IJ) approach. For patients who already have a permanent pacemaker, the venous sheath can be omitted and rapid pacing for valve deployment performed using a device programmer and the patient's own pacemaker. For patients at high risk of requiring a permanent pacemaker after the procedure (i.e., using a self-expanding valve), we prefer to place an active fixation lead from the right IJ, which can more easily be left in place after the TAVR procedure.

Because cerebrovascular events are one of the most feared complications, we routinely perform our TAVR procedures using cerebral embolic protection (CEP). Currently, the Sentinel device (Claret Medical, Santa Rosa, California) is the only FDA-approved CEP system available in the United States. It consists of one basket in the innominate artery and one basket in the left common carotid artery to capture debris embolized during valvuloplasty and/or valve deployment that are later collapsed and removed at the conclusion of the procedure. The pivotal trial demonstrated a strong trend toward reduced periprocedural cerebrovascular events, and a recent meta-analysis demonstrated that cerebral embolic protection during TAVR was associated with a statistically significant reduction in the primary endpoint of death or stroke.[18,19] Importantly, there were no device-related complications in this trial. It is important that operators are experienced in radial access, radial catheterization, and atraumatic entry to the great vessels when attempting to use this device.

Once vascular access has been obtained and the temporary pacemaker secured, intravenous heparin is given for an activating clotting time (ACT) of 250–300 seconds. The TAVR delivery sheath is inserted over a stiff wire, such as the Lunderquist (Cook Medical, Bloomington, Indiana). Next, the aortic valve is crossed using a catheter and guidewire. In our practice, this is most commonly performed using an

Amplatz Left-1 (AL-1) catheter and a 0.035″ straight-tip guidewire; however, other preformed catheters (e.g., Judkins Right) or specialty wires (e.g., Glidewire [Terumo Medical, Somerset, New Jersey]) can be utilized. It is important to avoid crossing through the mitral subvalvular apparatus, and pass catheters and stiff guidewires slowly into the ventricle to avoid perforation.

Once access to the left ventricle is secured, hemodynamic assessment is performed to assess simultaneous LV and aortic pressure measurements for valve gradient as well as end-diastolic pressures. The catheter can then be used to exchange for a preformed stiff guidewire. For balloon-expandable valves, we prefer the 0.035″ Amplatz Extra-stiff (Cook Medical, Bloomington, Indiana) with a curve at the end of the wire for placement in the LV apex. For self-expanding valves, we routinely utilize the Confida wire (Medtronic, Minneapolis, Minnesota).

An important consideration for optimal valve positioning is to align correctly the inferior margins of the left, right, and noncoronary aortic cusps in a coplanar view. A number of methodologies have been described to aid in finding the best fluoroscopic projections to visualize the annular plane,[20] and the preprocedural CT images can assist; however, we find that a right anterior oblique (RAO) caudal angulation optimized for valve co-axiality is helpful in the majority of patients, to understand the positioning of the valve at the level of the noncoronary sinus (the "lowest" of the three). In current practice, balloon aortic valvuloplasty (BAV) is performed with decreasing frequency prior to balloon-expandable valve placement and rarely for self-expanding valve placement.

The valve is then advanced into position coaxial to the aortic annulus, confirmed using angiography via the pigtail catheter in the noncoronary cusp. Self-expanding valves are placed by unsheathing the device, beginning in the LV outflow tract and continuing until it is completely deployed with the top of the scaffold in the ascending aorta. Rapid right ventricular (RV) pacing is not always required when placing a self-expanding valve, but temporary pacing at a rate of 100–120 beats per minute (bpm) can be used to reduce cardiac output and minimize migration while the valve is unsheathed. For balloon-expandable valves, rapid RV pacing at a rate of 180–220 bpm is required prior to inflation of the device. This temporarily arrests the heart and allows precise placement. Rapid pacing is continued until the valve balloon is completely deflated to prevent the balloon from being ejected from the annulus and inadvertently dislodging the valve. While balloon-expandable valves cannot be repositioned once deployed, current self-expanding valves have the ability to be recaptured/retrieved and repositioned prior to full deployment and release.

Following valve deployment, attention is turned to evaluating the positioning and function of the valve through a combination of aortic root angiography, hemodynamic assessment, and echocardiographic evaluation. Even when not well visualized by echocardiogram, the presence of aortic regurgitation (AR) is suggested by the absence of a dicrotic notch, wide pulse pressure, low aortic diastolic pressures, and elevated LV end-diastolic pressures. The presence of moderate or severe AR has been correlated with poor outcomes after TAVR and interventions to address this (e.g., postdilation of the valve, placement of a second valve in a "valve-in-valve" fashion, percutaneous paravalvular leak closure, etc.) should be considered.[21]

Once the valve has been successfully deployed and no further interventions are anticipated, equipment is removed and hemostasis achieved. The TAVR delivery sheath should always be removed over a wire to maintain vascular access in the event of failure of the predeployed sutures and/or vascular injury. The other arterial access site can be used to perform completion angiography and to exclude occult bleeding stenosis or dissections. Protamine can be given in the absence of contra-indications.

ALTERNATIVES TO TRANSFEMORAL ACCESS

For patients who do not have adequate iliofemoral anatomy, alternative approaches have been developed. Transcatheter valves have been implanted safely following direct surgical access to the thoracic cavity through either a mini-thoracotomy exposing the left ventricular apex (transapical) or direct access to the aorta via a mini-sternotomy (transaortic). In contrast to SAVR, neither of these approaches requires placing the patient on full cardiopulmonary bypass. In more recent years, access has been obtained in the subclavian artery, axillary artery, carotid artery, or via antegrade transseptal or retrograde transcaval–transaortic approach via the femoral veins.[22–27]

PERIOPERATIVE MANAGEMENT AND ADJUNCTIVE THERAPIES

Standard practice at our institution is to monitor patients in the postanesthesia recovery unit overnight. Hospital management is focused on early mobilization and monitoring for vascular and conduction system complications.

Routine antibiotic prophylaxis is recommended for all patients undergoing TAVR to reduce the risk of wound infection and endocarditis.[12] The optimal antithrombotic regimen following TAVR remains unknown. Current guidelines and FDA labeling reflect the protocols used in the initial randomized clinical trials, lifelong low-dose aspirin and 3–6 months of dual antiplatelet therapy (DAPT) with clopidogrel. For patients with a separate indication for therapeutic anticoagulation (e.g., atrial fibrillation, hypercoagulable disorders, etc.), practice varies and may include a short period of "triple therapy" with aspirin, clopidogrel, and anticoagulation or may omit clopidogrel and treat with just low-dose aspirin and anticoagulant. Trials are currently underway to determine whether empiric anticoagulation may be beneficial for valve and clinical outcomes after TAVR.[28]

COMPLICATIONS OF TAVR

The incidence of major complications associated with TAVR continues to decrease. The Valve Academic Research Consortium (VARC-2) has standardized the definitions for important peri- and postprocedural complications and has allowed greater consistency of use.[12] A summary of the notable periprocedural complications after TAVR, their risk factors, and management are summarized in Table 25.1.

Stroke

Stroke is a rare complication that can be devastating. The majority of peri-procedural strokes following TAVR are thought to be embolic, from liberation of calcified debris from the aortic valve annulus and/or aortic arch. Less commonly, patients may suffer strokes from hypotension and global hypoperfusion, which may follow other hemodynamic complications discussed later. The earliest TAVR trials suggested stroke rates may be slightly higher following TAVR compared with SAVR. Subsequent trials and meta-analyses demonstrated either no difference or significantly lower stroke rate with TAVR.[29,30]

Cerebral embolic protection devices represent a modality to reduce the risk of neurovascular complications. Nevertheless, the risk of stroke is never completely mitigated. It is imperative that neurologic

TABLE 25.1 **Complications of TAVR.**

Complication	Risk factors	Prevention	Management
Stroke	• Valve implantation • Post-TAVR atrial fibrillation • Prior cerebrovascular events, old age, female, diabetes, hypertension, prior cardiac surgeries	• Appropriate antithrombotic therapy during and after the procedure • Cerebral embolic protection devices • Minimize unnecessary equipment manipulations in the aortic root and arch	• Immediate neurologic assessment • Emergent cerebrovascular imaging • Possible acute neuro-intervention • Neurology and Neuro-interventional team consultation
Vascular access site complications	• Small, tortuous, or calcified iliofemoral vessels (especially circumferential calcification)	• Careful review of imaging prior to the procedure to identify the optimal access route • Meticulous femoral access techniques with confirmation of placement prior to large-bore sheath insertion • Preclosure of the arteriotomy prior to large-bore sheath insertion • Routine angiography of the access site following sheath removal and hemostasis	• Rapid recognition and prompt endovascular or surgical repair as indicated • Ready availability of endovascular devices in the hybrid suite
Arrhythmias and conduction system disorders	• Pre-existing conduction system disease (particularly right bundle branch block) • Use of self-expanding valves • Highly calcified aortic annulus • Low valve implantation in the left ventricular outflow tract • Valve oversizing	• Proper device sizing and positioning • Consider active-fixation temporary pacemaker placement for high-risk patients and/or those receiving self-expanding valves	• Permanent pacemaker implantation when indicated
Aortic regurgitation and paravalvular leak	• Valve undersizing • Device malpositioning at deployment • Severely calcified or asymmetric annulus	• Proper device sizing and positioning (3D reconstructions from CT or MRI preferred)	• Postdilation • Placement of a second valve • Paravalvular leak closure
Annular rupture and cardiac tamponade	• Valve oversizing • Severely calcified annulus with extension into left ventricular outflow tract • Aggressive postdilation	• Proper device sizing and positioning • Consider self-expanding devices and/or limit postdilation in patients with a severely calcified annulus	• Rapid recognition and prompt pericardiocentesis and/or emergency surgical repair when indicated
Valve malpositioning or embolization	• Valve undersizing • Device malpositioning at deployment • Failure of rapid ventricular pacing during placement of a balloon-expandable valve	• Proper device sizing using 3D imaging • Appropriate valve positioning using proper annulus orientation and aortic root angiography • Importance of maintaining proper pacing wire capture during valve deployment • Slow/methodical inflation of the balloon-expandable valve to allow subtle movement if needed	• Surgical retrieval is required for ventricular embolization • Aortic deployment or surgical removal for distal embolization • Placement of a second valve (valve-in-valve) when indicated for valves which remain in the annulus but are placed too high or too low

assessment is undertaken immediately after the procedure and at routine intervals thereafter. Conscious sedation allows expeditious diagnosis of procedural stroke. For patients with acute neurologic change, rapid CT scan along with involvement of the neuro-interventional team is indicated (Fig. 25.1).

Atrial fibrillation following TAVR has been associated with late neurologic events, and patients with AF should be managed with therapeutic anticoagulation. For patients who are not candidates for anticoagulation, percutaneous left atrial appendage occlusion (LAAO) can be considered. The WATCH TAVR trial randomizing patients to TAVR with or without concomitant WATCHMAN LAAO is currently enrolling.[31] Fig. 25.2 summarizes considerations to mitigate stroke risk in patients undergoing TAVR.

Vascular Complications

Complications at the vascular access site remain the most common procedure-related adverse event. Common risk factors include heavily calcified or tortuous arteries with borderline luminal diameter. Periprocedural vascular issues range in severity from minor access site

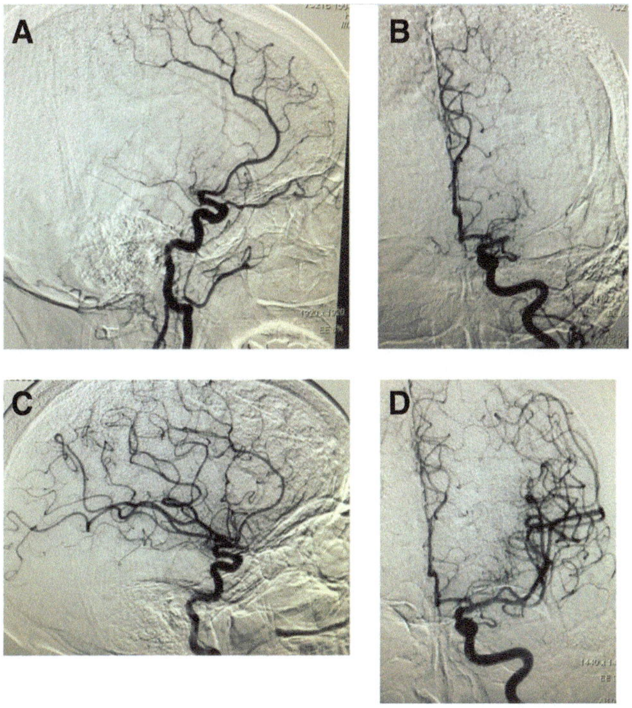

Fig. 25.1 Representative neurologic images from a periprocedural stroke following TAVR. (A) and (B) show representative images from a cerebral angiogram demonstrating middle cerebral artery (MCA) occlusion in a patient following TAVR. (C) and (D) illustrate normal MCA flow after the patient successfully underwent neuro-intervention with thrombectomy.

bleeding (managed expectantly after applying manual pressure) to significant dissections, ruptures, and/or stenosis that require urgent or emergent endovascular repair. For this reason, operators performing TAVR should have experience with peripheral procedures or have immediate access to on-site peripheral vascular specialists.

We routinely place a 5-French common femoral artery (CFA) sheath a few centimeters distal to the TAVR delivery sheath to allow placement of the pigtail catheter in the aortic root as long as the iliofemoral diameter is adequate. Once the delivery sheath is removed, we perform iliofemoral angiography via this sheath. In the event of a vascular complication, intervention is accomplished through the sheath (upsizing as necessary). For patients whose iliofemoral arteries are only large enough for the TAVR delivery sheath, the second arterial access is placed at the contralateral CFA, and angiography after closure of the TAVR access site is accomplished using a 5-French IMA catheter. If intervention is required, we use either a coronary guidewire system or advance a routine peripheral sheath "up-and-over". In cases of CFA stenosis resulting from closure devices or dissection requiring intervention, balloon angioplasty alone is often sufficient. Occasionally, stent placement may be necessary. For large perforations, covered stent placement is usually required, especially if it occurs within the iliac artery. Fig. 25.3 depicts various endovascular procedures to address access site complications in TAVR patients.

It is rare that a vascular complication occurring in the iliofemoral system cannot be addressed using endovascular techniques. However, very rarely, perforation can occur in the aorta, either when advancing the sheath or as the valve is pushed through the sheath. It is therefore wise to have either experience in endovascular aorta grafting (EVAR) or rapid access to vascular surgery.

Arrhythmia

Arrhythmias and high-grade conduction system disease can occur after TAVR and may result in the need for permanent pacemaker (PPM) placement. Studies to date have not shown an association with adverse short- or long-term clinical outcomes after TAVR among those patients who require PPM implantation, although there is some concern regarding the degree of LV function improvement in those patients with LV dysfunction.[32] This is probably as a result of mechanical compression of His bundle fibers as they course through the septal wall of the left ventricular outflow tract (LVOT). Because of its anatomic location, the left bundle is particularly susceptible to this compression and, as a result, patients with a pre-existing right bundle branch block (RBBB) prior to TAVR are at the highest risk of requiring PPM implantation following TAVR. Other anatomic risk factors include a heavily calcified annulus, lower implantation of the valve into the LVOT, and significantly oversizing the prosthesis.[31]

Although the rate of pacemaker use has improved with newer generation self-expanding valves, there is still a substantially higher incidence of requiring a PPM for self-expanding valves compared with balloon-expandable devices. Additionally, while patients requiring a PPM following balloon-expandable valve placement more commonly manifest conduction system defects immediately during the procedure, patients receiving self-expanding devices may manifest in the day or two following implantation. Therefore, it is our practice to place an active-fixation pacemaker lead in all patients receiving a self-expanding TAVR valve and keep this in place for 48–72 hours following the procedure or until discharge.

Aortic Regurgitation

The degree of aortic regurgitation (AR) following TAVR has been correlated with poor outcomes and can be either valvular or paravalvular leak (PVL), or paravalvular aortic regurgitation (PAR). Valvular AR, in a correctly-sized device, is rare. If there is concern for over-expansion of the device resulting in central valvular AR (as may follow aggressive postdilation of a valve), placement of a second valve in a valve-in-valve fashion may be required.

Paravalvular leak is noted significantly more frequently in patients who undergo TAVR rather than SAVR, and newer generation TAVR devices have been modified to address this concern specifically with the addition of skirts on the outside of the valve frame to improve the seal between the valve and what is often a heavily-calcified, asymmetric annulus. Common causes of PVL are heavy and/or asymmetric annular calcification and device undersizing or malpositioning (Fig. 25.4). When significant PVL is identified, postdilation of the valve can sometimes create a tighter seal and reduce the degree of PVL. Other options include percutaneous closure of the defect with vascular plugs or, particularly in cases resulting from device undersizing or malpositioning, placement of a second valve in a valve-in-valve fashion.

Cardiac Trauma

Cardiac tamponade and annular rupture are rare but devastating complications associated with high morbidity and mortality. Etiologies include perforation of the right ventricle from the temporary transvenous pacing wire, perforation of the left ventricle by guidewires, catheters, or the leading edge of the TAVR delivery

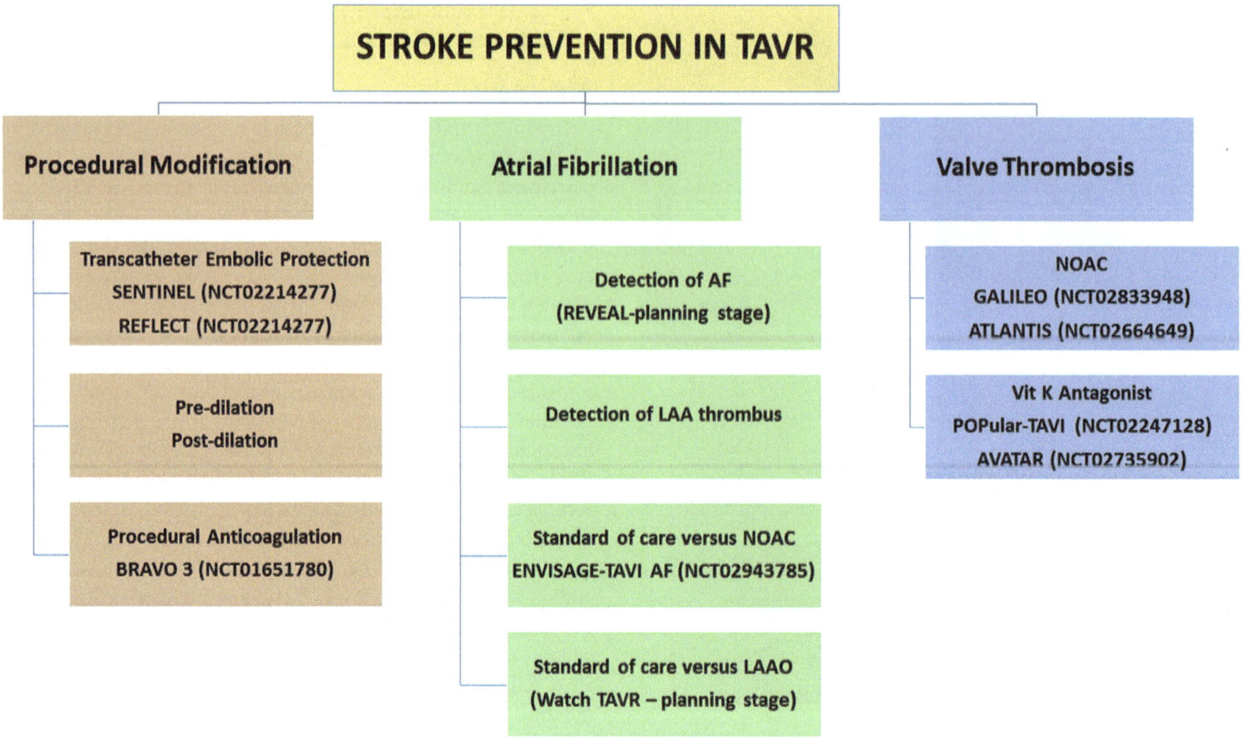

Fig. 25.2 Considerations to mitigate stroke risk with TAVR. AF: atrial fibrillation; LAA: left atrial appendage; NOAC: novel oral anticoagulants; TAVR: transcatheter aortic valve replacement (Reproduced from Kapadia SR, Krishnaswamy A, Tuzcu EM. Atrial fibrillation and transcatheter aortic valve replacement: implications of pre-procedural identification of left atrial appendage thrombus for stroke prevention. *JACC Cardiovasc Interv.* 2017; 10(2):185–187.)

apparatus, or from rupture of the aortic valve annulus after deployment. The key is early recognition and intervention. If emergency echocardiography demonstrates a pericardial effusion, the next step should be to assess the aortic root. If there is no obvious root pathology, perforation is likely. Immediate reversal of anticoagulation is recommended with transfusion of platelets or factors. If the effusion continues to accumulate, emergent pericardiocentesis and drain placement should be performed. Watchful waiting in the operating room is reasonable if the patient remains hemodynamically stable. If this is not successful, consideration should be given to surgical exploration with pericardial patch repair. As long as the patient is stable, we tend not to convert to general anesthesia unless the decision is made for surgical exploration.

Annular rupture is more commonly reported in procedures using balloon-expandable than self-expanding valves and can occur at the supra-annular, intra-annular, or sub-annular levels (or at multiple levels). It can occur following predeployment valvuloplasty (if performed), valve deployment, or postdilation. Risk factors include heavy calcification extending into the LVOT and valve oversizing of >20%.[33] Annular rupture can range in presentation from asymptomatic/contained defects to those that cause the rapid development of hemopericardium and fulminant hemodynamic collapse. Survival is substantially different between these two groups; a small series demonstrated that all patients with contained rupture survived, while the uncontained group had 75% in-hospital mortality.[33]

In situations of annular rupture, emergent echocardiography usually demonstrates hematoma formation at the aortic root. Our approach is to convert the patient immediately to general anesthesia and place a transesophageal echocardiogram probe. This allows real-time observation of the root and provides clear imaging to localize and to demonstrate the extent of the pathology. Aortic root angiography (usually used to assess aortic regurgitation) may also provide evidence of annular rupture. Similar to LV/RV perforation cases, the first steps are reversal of anticoagulation and performance of pericardiocentesis and pericardial drain placement. If the rupture is contained, this conservative management is often adequate (Fig. 25.5). We maintain endotracheal intubation for the first 24 hours with repeat TEE and extubation if stable. If the rupture appears to be extending, or pericardial drainage continues at a significant rate, conversion to open surgery with root repair and surgical AVR may be the only hope for survival.

Valve Leaflet Thrombosis

Aortic valves are susceptible to formation of thrombus on their leaflets. Many patients with mild or moderate leaflet thrombosis are asymptomatic and diagnosis is made on routine CT scan that demonstrates hypoattenuated leaflet thickening (HALT). This has been studied in RESOLVE (assessment of transcatheter and surgical aortic bioprosthetic valve thrombosis and its treatment with anticoagulation) and SAVORY (subclinical aortic valve bioprosthesis thrombosis assessed with four-dimensional CT) registries. These studies demonstrated HALT among 106 of 890 (13%) patients who had undergone TAVR at a median of 83 days.[34] Patients treated with therapeutic anticoagulation after TAVR had a lower incidence of HALT than patients receiving antiplatelet therapy, and all patients who were given anticoagulation after CT findings (36 of 36) resolved their pathology in approximately 6 weeks. Four of eight patients who discontinued anticoagulation had recurrence of reduced leaflet motion (median 164 days).

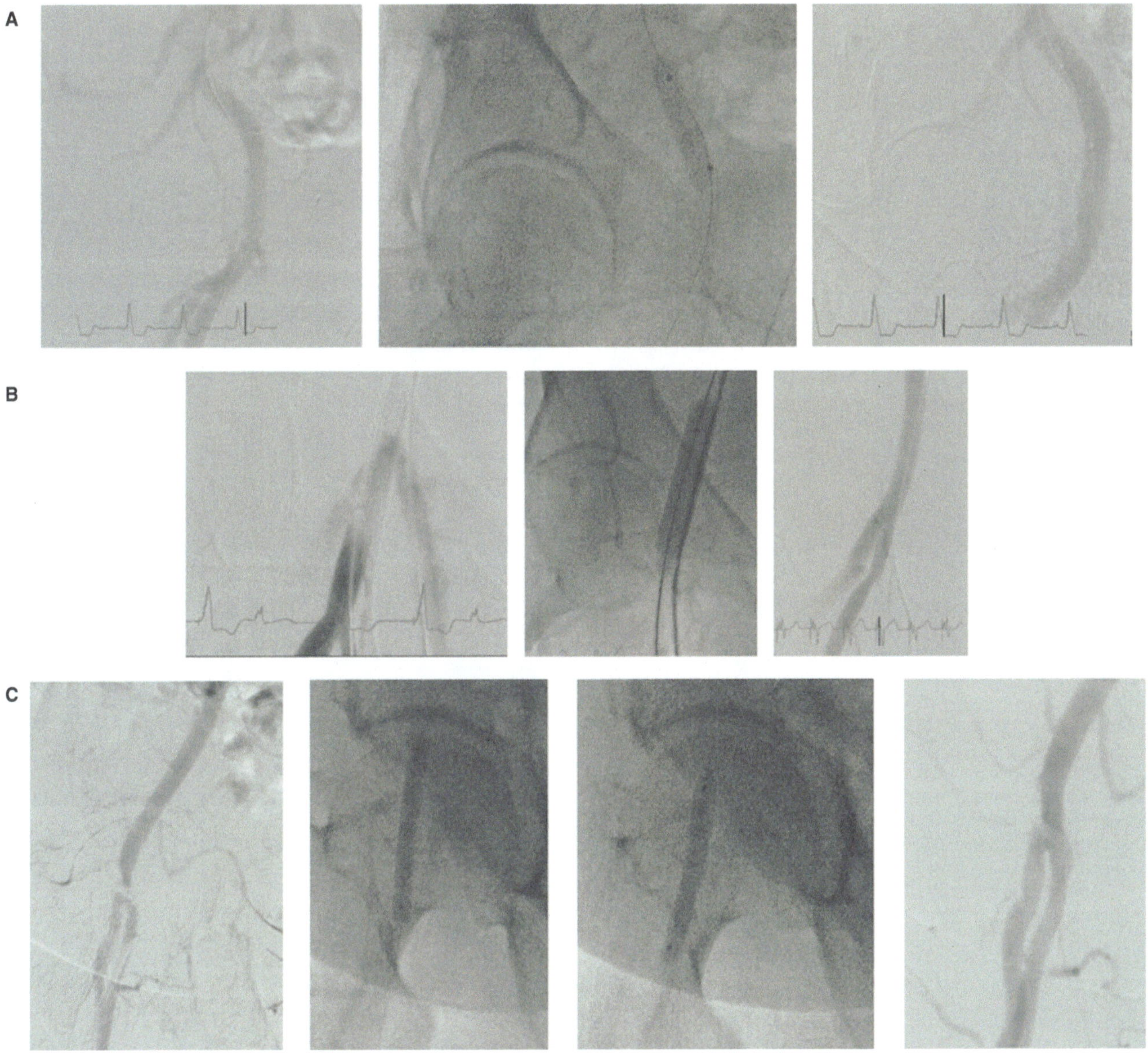

Fig. 25.3 Representative images of endovascular procedures to address access site complications in patients undergoing TAVR. (A) Management of a small, focal perforation. The *left image* illustrates contrast extravasation from the distal right common femoral artery (CFA). The *middle image* demonstrates balloon occlusion, which was performed with a prolonged inflation just proximal to the lesion to stop flow but before the intimal disruption to avoid further exacerbating the arterial injury. The *right image* shows the completion angiogram with no residual stenosis or contrast extravasation. (B) Management of a larger perforation requiring covered stent placement. The *left image* illustrates contrast extravasation from the distal right CFA. The *middle image* demonstrates balloon postdilation immediately following deployment of a self-expanding covered stent to the distal right CFA. The *right image* shows the completion angiogram with no residual stenosis or contrast extravasation. (C) Management of a focal stenosis in the right distal CFA involving the origin of the right superficial femoral (SFA) and profunda arteries. The *second image* shows balloon inflation from the distal CFA into the SFA and the *third image* shows balloon inflation from the distal CFA into the profunda. The *far right image* shows the completion angiogram with no residual obstructive stenosis, dissection, or contrast extravasation and no stenting was required.

Current data suggest there may be a higher risk of transient ischemic attack (TIA) and lower valve durability in patients who experience leaflet thrombosis. The approach to patients with HALT without clinical manifestation is unclear. Further study is underway with trials such as GALILEO to compare treatment with antiplatelet therapy versus rivaroxaban after TAVR.[28] Rates of HALT are lower with surgical bioprostheses, yet TAVR has equivalent or superior outcomes in comparison with SAVR among inoperable, intermediate and high surgical risk patients.

CONCLUSIONS

TAVR is an effective and established therapy for patients with severe, symptomatic aortic stenosis and has excellent results as an alternative to SAVR for a variety of patient subgroups. Considerable efforts are underway to improve existing valve designs to allow lower profiles and smaller peripheral access requirements. A multidisciplinary heart team collaboration is key to the success of any TAVR program and plays a vital role in identifying the best treatment approach for a given patient.

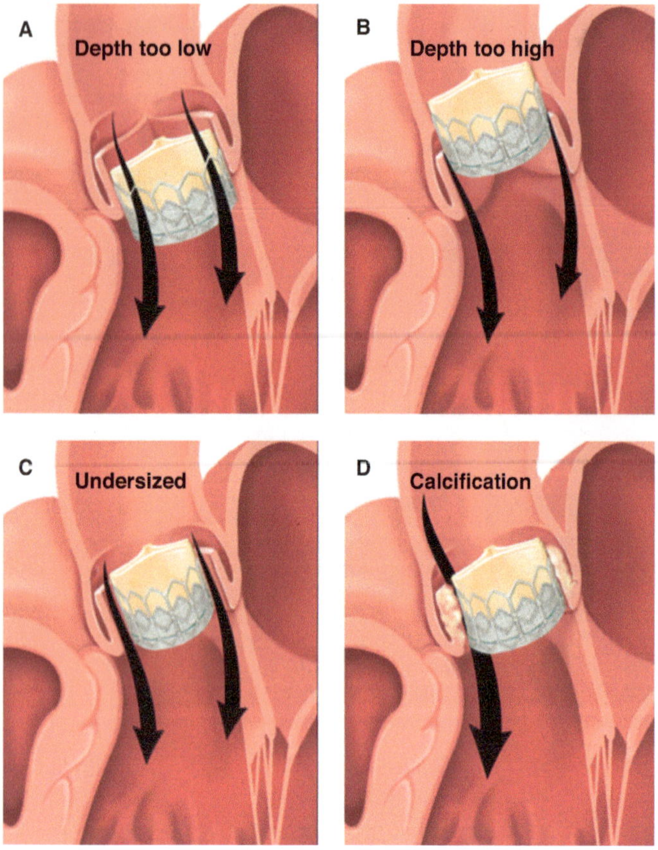

Fig. 25.4 Representative images of the various mechanisms of paravalvular leak in patients undergoing TAVR. (A) Paravalvular leak (PVL) resulting from a valve placed too deep into the left ventricular outflow tract; (B) PVL resulting from a valve placed too high into the aorta; (C) An undersized valve; (D) Focal PVL at the site of focal/asymmetric calcification in the annulus and left ventricular outflow tract (LVOT).

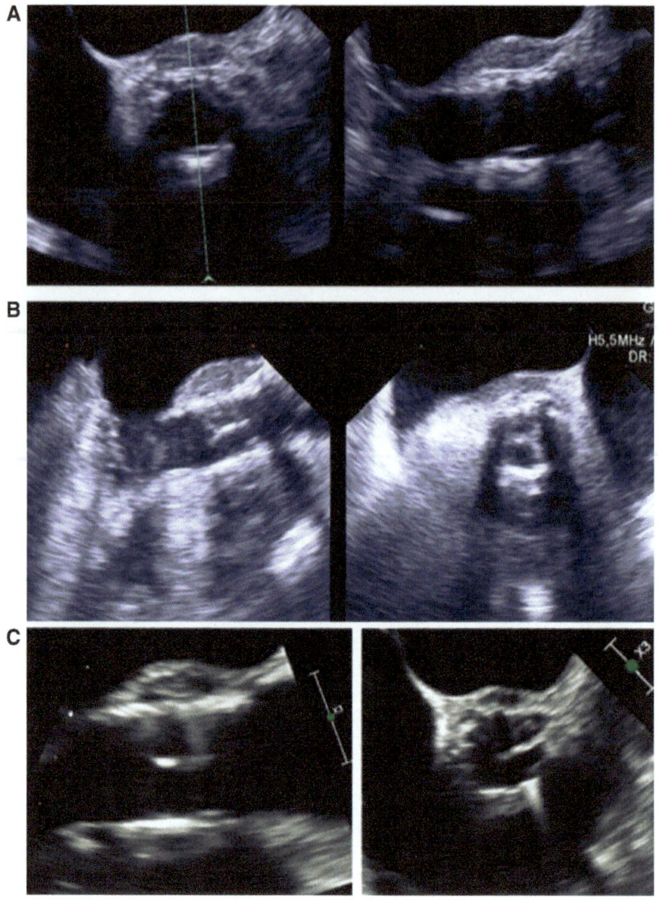

Fig. 25.5 Representative images from a patient with an aortic root hematoma treated conservatively following TAVR. (A) Representative transesophageal echocardiogram (TEE) images of an acute aortic root hematoma observed immediately following TAVR; (B) TEE images obtained after 20 minutes of observation, showing stable findings; (C) TEE images obtained on the day of discharge 8 days later showing resolution of the hematoma.

REFERENCES

1. Freeman RV, Otto CM. Spectrum of calcific aortic valve disease: pathogenesis, disease progression, and treatment strategies. *Circulation.* 2005;111(24):3316–3326.
2. Sarin RK, et al. Combined supravalvular aortic and pulmonary artery stenosis. *Angiology.* 1968;19(5):293–298.
3. Nishimura RA, et al. 2014 AHA/ACC guideline for the management of patients with valvular heart disease: a report of the American College of Cardiology/American Heart Association Task Force on Practice Guidelines. *J Thorac Cardiovasc Surg.* 2014;148(1):e1–e132.
4. Iung B, et al. Decision-making in elderly patients with severe aortic stenosis: why are so many denied surgery? *Eur Heart J.* 2005; 26(24):2714–2720.
5. Kapadia SR, et al. 5-year outcomes of transcatheter aortic valve replacement compared with standard treatment for patients with inoperable aortic stenosis (PARTNER 1): a randomised controlled trial. *Lancet.* 2015; 385(9986):2485–2491.
6. Cribier A, et al. Percutaneous transcatheter implantation of an aortic valve prosthesis for calcific aortic stenosis: first human case description. *Circulation.* 2002;106(24):3006–3008.
7. Leon MB, et al. Transcatheter aortic-valve implantation for aortic stenosis in patients who cannot undergo surgery. *N Engl J Med.* 2010;363(17): 1597–1607.
8. Adams DH, et al. Transcatheter aortic-valve replacement with a self-expanding prosthesis. *N Engl J Med.* 2014;370(19):1790–1798.
9. Popma JJ, et al. Transcatheter aortic valve replacement using a self-expanding bioprosthesis in patients with severe aortic stenosis at extreme risk for surgery. *J Am Coll Cardiol.* 2014;63(19):1972–1981.
10. Smith CR, et al. Transcatheter versus surgical aortic-valve replacement in high-risk patients. *N Engl J Med.* 2011;364(23):2187–2198.
11. Barbash IM, Waksman R. Overview of the 2011 Food and Drug Administration Circulatory System Devices Panel of the Medical Devices Advisory Committee Meeting on the Edwards SAPIEN transcatheter heart valve. *Circulation.* 2012;125(3):550–555.
12. Holmes DR Jr, et al. ACCF/AATS/SCAI/STS expert consensus document on transcatheter aortic valve replacement. *J Am Coll Cardiol.* 2012; 59(13):1200–1254.
13. Mack MJ, et al. Transcatheter aortic-valve replacement with a balloon-expandable valve in low-risk patients. *N Engl J Med.* 2019.
14. Popma JJ, et al. Transcatheter aortic-valve replacement with a self-expanding valve in low-risk patients. *N Engl J Med.* 2019.

15. Krishnaswamy A, et al. Predicting vascular complications during transfemoral transcatheter aortic valve replacement using computed tomography: a novel area-based index. *Catheter Cardiovasc Interv.* 2014;84(5):844–851.
16. O'Brien B, et al. Integration of 3D imaging data in the assessment of aortic stenosis: impact on classification of disease severity. *Circ Cardiovasc Imaging.* 2011;4(5):566–573.
17. Roselli EE, et al. Emergency use of cardiopulmonary bypass in complicated transcatheter aortic valve replacement: importance of a heart team approach. *J Thorac Cardiovasc Surg.* 2014;148(4):1413–1416.
18. Kapadia SR, et al. Protection against cerebral embolism during transcatheter aortic valve replacement. *J Am Coll Cardiol.* 2017;69(4):367–377.
19. Giustino G, et al. Cerebral embolic protection during TAVR: a clinical event meta-analysis. *J Am Coll Cardiol.* 2017;69(4):465–466.
20. Kasel AM, et al. Fluoroscopy-guided aortic root imaging for TAVR: "follow the right cusp" rule. *JACC Cardiovasc Imaging.* 2013;6(2):274–275.
21. Jones BM, et al. Prognostic significance of mild aortic regurgitation in predicting mortality after transcatheter aortic valve replacement. *J Thorac Cardiovasc Surg.* 2016;152(3):783–790.
22. Bruschi G, et al. Alternative approaches for trans-catheter self-expanding aortic bioprosthetic valves implantation: single-center experience. *Eur J Cardiothorac Surg.* 2011;39(6):e151–e158.
23. Al Kindi AH, et al. Alternative access options for transcatheter aortic valve replacement in patients with no conventional access and chest pathology. *J Thorac Cardiovasc Surg.* 2014;147(2):644–651.
24. Thourani VH, et al. High-risk patients with inoperative aortic stenosis: use of transapical, transaortic, and transcarotid techniques. *Ann Thorac Surg.* 2015;99(3):817–823; discussion 823–825.
25. Cohen MG, et al. Transseptal antegrade transcatheter aortic valve replacement for patients with no other access approach - a contemporary experience. *Catheter Cardiovasc Interv.* 2013;82(6):987–993.
26. Chi Lam SC, Bertog S, Sievert H. Transseptal strategy in retrograde transcatheter valve-in-valve implantation for failed surgical aortic bioprosthesis. *Catheter Cardiovasc Interv.* 2014;83(5):817–821.
27. Greenbaum AB, et al. Caval-aortic access to allow transcatheter aortic valve replacement in otherwise ineligible patients: initial human experience. *J Am Coll Cardiol.* 2014;63(25 Pt A):2795–2804.
28. Kapadia SR, Krishnaswamy A, Tuzcu EM. Atrial fibrillation and transcatheter aortic valve replacement: implications of pre-procedural identification of left atrial appendage thrombus for stroke prevention. *JACC Cardiovasc Interv.* 2017;10(2):185–187.
29. Leon MB, et al. Transcatheter or surgical aortic-valve replacement in intermediate-risk patients. *N Engl J Med.* 2016;374(17):1609–1620.
30. Thourani VH, et al. Transcatheter aortic valve replacement versus surgical valve replacement in intermediate-risk patients: a propensity score analysis. *Lancet.* 2016;387(10034):2218–2225.
31. Houthuizen P, et al. Occurrence, fate and consequences of ventricular conduction abnormalities after transcatheter aortic valve implantation. *EuroIntervention.* 2014;9(10):1142–1150.
32. Kapadia SR, Wazni O, Krishnaswamy A. Pacemaker implantation after TAVR. *JACC Cardiovasc Imaging.* 2017;10(10 Pt A):1148–1150.
33. Barbanti M, et al. Anatomical and procedural features associated with aortic root rupture during balloon-expandable transcatheter aortic valve replacement. *Circulation.* 2013;128(3):244–253.
34. Chakravarty T, et al. Subclinical leaflet thrombosis in surgical and transcatheter bioprosthetic aortic valves: an observational study. *Lancet.* 2017;389(10087):2383–2392.

26

Complications in the Endovascular Management of Aortic Dissection

Albeir Y. Mousa, MD, FACS, DFSVS, CWS, MBA, MPH, RPVI and Shadi Abu-Halimah, MD, FACS

INTRODUCTION

Since its inception in 1992, thoracic endovascular aortic repair (TEVAR) was introduced as an alternative treatment option to conventional open surgery for patients with complicated Type B aortic dissection (TBAD), i.e., end-organ malperfusion, refractory hypertension or hypotension, and unrelenting pain.[1] TEVAR is also now considered for treatment of dissections with aneurysmal degeneration with aortic diameter >55 mm or increased aortic diameter of >4 mm/year.[2]

TEVAR VERSUS OPEN SURGERY

TEVAR has been shown to have significantly improved 30-day survival for TAA (84%–95% versus 70%) in contrast to open repair.[3] When studying TBAD specifically, the registry of acute aortic dissection (IRAD) recommended TEVAR be the first line of treatment for patients with complicated TBAD.[3] This report also indicated significant remodeling in favor of TEVAR (expansion of true lumen and regression of false lumen) especially when the stented segment continues to the visceral vessels, directly related to a decrease in the incidence of aortic wall degeneration, with subsequent decrease in likelihood of developing of aneurysms. Likewise, the findings of the VIRTUE study[4] reinforced that aortic remodeling after TEVAR is a continuous process. Accordingly, many respected authorities suggest early endovascular intervention. Also, the recently published Acute Dissection: Stent Graft or Best Medical Therapy (ADSORB) trial[5] found that TEVAR markedly facilitates aortic remodeling compared with medical therapy alone[6], potentially conferring a survival advantage as shown by the INSTEAD trial in 2009 and INSTEAD XL in 2013.[7–10]

TEVAR PROCEDURE

All procedures should be performed in a hybrid suite. Depending on the patient's comorbidities, the surgeon's experience with TEVARs, and the institutional ancillary staff, such procedures can be performed under local anesthesia with MAC sedation or sometimes under general anesthesia. Spinal cord drainage is not typically performed for emergency patients, while selective use in elective cases may be warranted, depending on the planned length of coverage. CTA evaluation is critical to aid in access site determination, with preference to the nondissected vessel if present for direct access to the true lumen. Access can be either surgical or percutaneous, as is standard for large access procedures. Initial access to the true lumen can be obtained with glide wire, Rosen wire, or glide catheter supported by the wire, with the catheter leading, to decrease the chance of dissection with a wire in the false lumen (Fig. 26.1). The wire/catheter is assessed to be in the true lumen by using intravascular ultrasound (IVUS), transesophageal echocardiography (TEE), or a combination of the two, to characterize the extent and the size of the dissection entry point. Then a marked 5-French pigtail is advanced to the aortic arch with image intensifier at 30–40 LAO (left anterior oblique) angle, while an arch angiogram with 20–30 mL Visipaque (GE Health care) is performed. Arch vessels are identified and confirmed with IVUS/TEE (note: marking the monitor or using overlay or road mapping will help proper placement of the stent). Our practice is to keep mean blood pressure around 65–75 mmHg to prevent the windsock effect and to facilitate appropriate placement of the stent. The wire is exchanged for a double curve Landerquist (Cook Medical, Bloomington, Indiana) super stiff wire. The double curve wire enables the stent graft to conform to the outer aortic curvature. An appropriate sized stent graft (i.e., 10% oversized) can be advanced through the true lumen and provide adequate coverage of the dissection entry point (see Fig. 26.2A,B). Further oversizing can be problematic with dissections, especially chronic dissections. The 2-cm landing zone required for aneurysmal dissections is less important, as migration after TEVAR for TBAD is not seen; however, it is critical to cover the entry tear completely. If there is a need to cover arch vessels, assessment of the vertebral flow should be done to minimize stroke risk further (SVS TEVAR guidelines). In order to preserve the cervical vessels, open debranching via carotid–subclavian bypass or parallel graft technique may be considered. In this instance, cannulation of subclavian or left carotid is performed retrograde fashion, and a covered stent (maximum 10% oversizing) is deployed, with the proximal end 4–5 mm proximal to the TEVAR into the aortic arch. Deployment of the thoracic stent graft is first, with sheaths already in place and snorkels/chimneys performed simultaneously. Ballooning of the stent graft, especially in the proximal sealing zone, should be avoided to decrease the risk of retrograde dissection.

If parallel grafts are used, it is important to measure correctly for graft size, using the equation area $= \pi r^2$ to calculate the surface area of chimney stent, stent graft, and native aortic lumen surface area.[11–13]

Although the TEVAR procedure may sound simple, the timing of the procedure, peri-operative management, planning, and managing the potential complications all require a multidisciplinary team of vascular surgeon, cardiac surgeon, intensivist, neurologist, cardiovascular anesthesiologist, and well-trained ancillary staff to recognize and to manage complications. This can be accomplished by creating an Aortic Center of Excellence that manages referrals, facilitates admissions, and places protocols for such pathology.

COMPLICATIONS THAT MAY BE ENCOUNTERED INTRAOPERATIVELY

1. Retrograde dissection: This is the most dreaded intraoperative complication and is directly related to graft oversizing >20 mm.

The incidence in TBAD is 3% compared with 1% in degenerative aortic pathology. The proximal landing zone does not impact this issue and currently used stent configurations do not appear to increase risk, as did some older devices. Some experts suggest using grafts with no proximal hooks or grafts with large aggressive bare-metal stents in the proximal sealing zone to decrease the chance of retrograde dissection. Newer stent generations have no bare-metal parts or short parallel ones and no hooks. Use of TEE can be critical in identifying any proximal dissection after TEVAR completion.

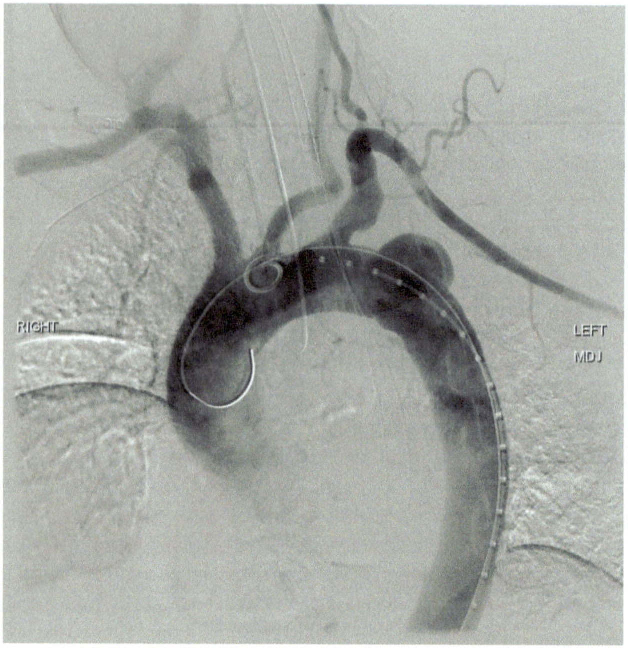

Fig. 26.1 Arch angiogram showing aneurysmal degeneration with TBAD. Note the double curve Landerquist (Cook Medical, Bloomington, Indiana) wire within the true lumen against the aortic valve.

2. Stent maldeployment: Proximal or distal migration resulting from missing the appropriate landing zone can happen. Using a device that the surgeon has experience with decreases that chance. Some devices need more rapid deployment, and others need slow controlled deployment. Some devices offer controlled staged deployment but care must be taken with distal migration. Rigorous control of hypertension and conforming the stent graft to the aortic-outer wall by maintaining forward pressure on Landerquest wire also decrease the risk of maldeployment.
3. Overlooking a large distal fenestration could lead to perfusion of the false lumen, with more chance of distal aortic degeneration, aneurysmal growth, and possible rupture; therefore, meticulous examination of all fenestration between true and false lumina is recommended.
4. Aortic rupture is extremely rare but may occur, especially with patients with connective tissue disease (CTD). In this scenario, emergency aortic occluding balloon and open surgical repair will likely be needed. All patients with known CTD with TBAD should be considered for open repair if judged medically fit.

TECHNICAL RECOMMENDATIONS FOR TEVAR

1. The clinician needs to have clear characterization of true and false lumina.
2. It is imperative to achieve coverage of the proximal entry tear that is usually located at or distal to the left subclavian artery (Fig. 26.3). Strive to have a healthy looking proximal landing zone, even if coverage of the origin of left subclavian is necessary.
3. Strict control of blood pressure.
4. If dissection starts distal to left subclavian artery, cannulation of LSC with a flush catheter may help to guide accurate placement of the stent graft. Double curve Lunderquist Superstiff wire (Cook Medical, Bloomington, Indiana), against the outer border of the aortic arch helps facilitate conforming of the stent graft to the outer aortic curve.
5. Deploy stent graft according to manufacturer instructions. Always make sure to get rid of any tension forward or backward on the deployment because this can cause the graft to jump.
6. Judicious use of heparin after introducing the access sheath.

A

B

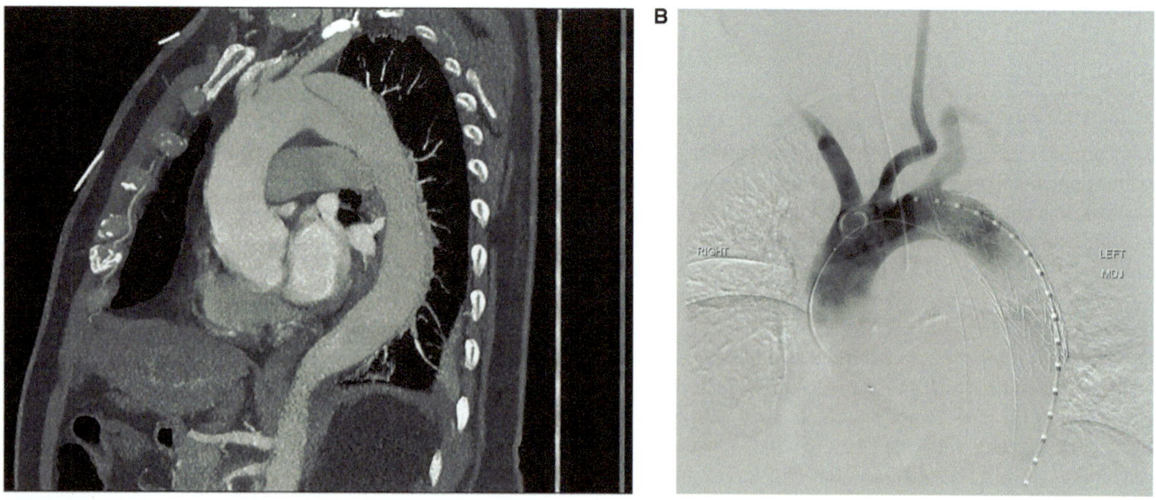

Fig. 26.2 (A) Sagittal view of CT angiogram, showing TBAD with large fenestration just distal to left subclavian artery. (B) Completion angiogram post TEVAR deployment, demonstrating coverage of fenestration just distal to left subclavian artery.

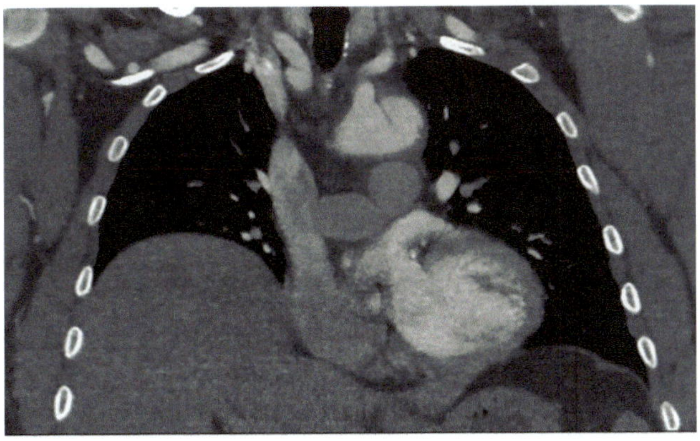

Fig. 26.3 Arch angiogram demonstrating a large proximal entry tear located distal to left subclavian artery.

7. Oversizing: It is best to use 10% oversizing for complicated dissection and 20% for uncomplicated dissection.[6]
8. Evaluate height of bird beak by measuring the gap between the proximal end of the stent graft and the inner curvature of the aortic arch on sagittal multiplanar reformations of CTA images.
9. Follow-up CT scan(s) are needed for surveillance on distal aortic degeneration and possible aneurysmal diseases.
10. Spinal drain: Preoperative drainage of cerebrospinal fluid is considered only for patients at high risk, those with previous aortic surgery, or in whom a long-segment stent graft is planned.
11. Distal entry tears increase the occurrence of aortic events and inhibit aortic remodeling but do not have a significantly negative effect on late survival. Repairing all entry increases the chance of spinal cord ischemia.[14]

PREOPERATIVE CAROTID–LEFT-SUBCLAVIAN BYPASS

Preoperative carotid–left-subclavian bypass is controversial.[15] The Society for Vascular Surgery (SVS)[16] recommends graded carotid subclavian bypass as grade 2C, which is low. The European Association for Cardiothoracic Surgery[17] strongly recommended prophylactic revascularization in selected cases. Still, there is no level 1 evidence to support the procedure. In our practice we perform preoperative LSCA revascularization in elective and non-urgent cases. In emergency cases, no revascularizations are performed, although utilizing snorkel techniques or in situ fenestrations can be helpful.

TEVAR AND COMPLICATED TBAD (CTBAD)

The classic use of TEVAR is in cases of CTBAD. Several prospective trials found decreased 30-day mortality with TEVAR in CTBAD to be 5% to 16%[16,18] compared with 30% after open surgical interventions in the original International Registry of Acute Aortic Dissection (IRAD) report.[3] Such results have paved the road for TEVAR to be considered as front-line therapy for anatomically suitable patients with CTBAD.[6,15,19] Aortic remodeling after TEVAR in CTBAD and a decrease in distal aortic degeneration with subsequent lower prevalence of aneurysmal disease are also noted. These findings open the debate in terms of utilizing TEVAR in uncomplicated TBAD (UCTBAD). Weng et al.[20] reported that the incidence of new entry tear at the distal margin of the stent graft reached 27%, with 30% needing reintervention for complicated distal SINE (stent graft induced new entry). However, a high incidence of SINE has also recently been reported in patients with chronic aortic dissection.[21] Some experts suggest oversizing the distal portion of the stent graft to shut down the false lumen as much as possible.

TEVAR AND UCTBAD

UCTBAD is not a totally benign pathology. Multiple studies have shown delayed aortic complications including development of aneurysmal disease or rupture in up to 25% of patients.[19,20,22]

MULTICHANNELED AORTIC DISSECTION (MCAD)

The incidence of MCAD varies from 5% to 9%.[23] This technical challenge stems from the difficulty to stay within the true lumen. Ando et al.[24,25] noted three-channeled AD in 7.3% in patients with CTBAD who underwent surgical treatment, and the incidence was higher, up to 60%, in patients with Marfan syndrome. However, Sueyoshi et al. found no significant differences between MCAD and double channel aortic dissection in terms of clinical characteristics, including the presence of Marfan syndrome.[26]

PREDICTORS OF PROGRESSION OF AORTIC REMODELING AFTER TEVAR

Several studies have suggested that saccular formation of false lumen, number of intimal tears, large entry tears (≥10 mm), location of the primary entry tear, and configuration of the false lumen may influence the aortic growth rate during the follow-up period.[4,5]

CONCLUSION

TEVAR for TBAD is feasible, safe, and associated with lower perioperative morbidity and mortality than open repair, but it has some significant complications and risks that differ from standard TEVAR for thoracic aneurysm repair. It is a very challenging procedure and requires great attention to detail for each case. Multiple factors need to be considered, including careful characterization of the entry point, relation to arch vessels, distal re-entry, and relation to visceral vessels. Ensuring true lumen location of the stent graft is of utmost importance, in addition to avoiding inappropriate oversizing. In addition, patients' hemodynamics must be closely monitored and controlled.

REFERENCES

1. Walker PJ, Dake MD, Mitchell RS, Miller DC. The use of endovascular techniques for the treatment of complications of aortic dissection. *J Vasc Surg*. 1993;18(6):1042–1051.
2. Lombardi JV, Cambria RP, Nienaber CA, et al. Prospective multicenter clinical trial (STABLE) on the endovascular treatment of complicated type B aortic dissection using a composite device design. *J Vasc Surg*. 2012;55(3):629–640. e2.
3. Fattori R, Montgomery D, Lovato L, et al. Survival after endovascular therapy in patients with type B aortic dissection: a report from the International Registry of Acute Aortic Dissection (IRAD). *JACC Cardiovasc Interv*. 2013;6(8):876–882.
4. Investigators VR. Mid-term outcomes and aortic remodelling after thoracic endovascular repair for acute, subacute, and chronic aortic dissection: the VIRTUE Registry. *Eur J Vasc Endovasc Surg*. 2014;48(4):363–371.
5. Brunkwall J, Kasprzak P, Verhoeven E, et al. Endovascular repair of acute uncomplicated aortic type B dissection promotes aortic remodelling: 1 year results of the ADSORB trial. *Eur J Vasc Endovasc Surg*. 2014;48(3): 285–291.

6. Zhu T, Si Y, Fang Y, et al. Early outcomes of the conformable stent graft for acute complicated and uncomplicated type B aortic dissection. *J Vasc Surg.* 2017;66(6):1644–1652.
7. Nienaber CA. Influence and critique of the INSTEAD Trial (TEVAR versus medical treatment for uncomplicated type B aortic dissection). *Semin Vasc Surg.* 2011;24(3):167–171.
8. Nienaber CA, Rousseau H, Eggebrecht H, et al. Randomized comparison of strategies for type B aortic dissection: the INvestigation of STEnt Grafts in Aortic Dissection (INSTEAD) trial. *Circulation.* 2009;120(25): 2519–2528.
9. Kwolek CJ, Watkins MT. The INvestigation of STEnt Grafts in Aortic Dissection (INSTEAD) trial: the need for ongoing analysis. *Circulation.* 2009;120(25):2513–2514.
10. Nienaber CA, Kische S, Rousseau H, et al. Endovascular repair of type B aortic dissection: long-term results of the randomized investigation of stent grafts in aortic dissection trial. *Circ Cardiovasc Interv.* 2013;6(4): 407–416.
11. Ding X, Hu S, Jiang J. Endovascular Repair with Periscope Technique for Aortic Dissection with an Aberrant Right Subclavian Artery. *Ann Vasc Surg.* 2017;45(264):e9–e13.
12. Trellopoulos G, Georgakarakos E, Pelekas D, Papachristodoulou A, Argyriou C, Georgiadis GS. Chimney and periscope technique for emergent treatment of spontaneous aortic rupture. *Ann Vasc Surg.* 2014; 28(5):1324–1328.
13. Krankenberg H, Bader R, Sixt S, et al. Endovascular repair of ascending aortic aneurysm by transapical approach and periscope technique. *J Endovasc Ther.* 2013;20(1):13–17.
14. Zhu C, Huang B, Zhao J, et al. Influence of distal entry tears in acute type B aortic dissection after thoracic endovascular aortic repair. *J Vasc Surg.* 2017;66(2):375–385.
15. White RA, Miller DC, Criado FJ, et al. Report on the results of thoracic endovascular aortic repair for acute, complicated, type B aortic dissection at 30 days and 1 year from a multidisciplinary subcommittee of the Society for Vascular Surgery Outcomes Committee. *J Vasc Surg.* 2011;53(4):1082–1090.
16. Matsumura JS, Lee WA, Mitchell RS, et al. The Society for Vascular Surgery Practice Guidelines: management of the left subclavian artery with thoracic endovascular aortic repair. *J Vasc Surg.* 2009;50(5): 1155–1158.
17. Wojciechowski J, Znaniecki L, Bury K, Rogowski J. Thoracic endovascular aortic repair with left subclavian artery coverage without prophylactic revascularisation-early and midterm results. *Langenbecks Arch Surg.* 2014;399(5):619–627.
18. Makaroun MS, Dillavou ED, Kee ST, et al. Endovascular treatment of thoracic aortic aneurysms: results of the phase II multicenter trial of the GORE TAG thoracic endoprosthesis. *J Vasc Surg.* 2005;41(1):1–9.
19. Zhu T, Si Y, Fang Y, et al. Early outcomes of the conformable stent graft for acute complicated and uncomplicated type B aortic dissection. *J Vasc Surg.* 2017.
20. Weng SH, Weng CF, Chen WY, et al. Reintervention for distal stent graft-induced new entry after endovascular repair with a stainless steel-based device in aortic dissection. *J Vasc Surg.* 2013;57(1):64–71.
21. Jang H, Kim MD, Kim GM, et al. Risk factors for stent graft-induced new entry after thoracic endovascular aortic repair for Stanford type B aortic dissection. *J Vasc Surg.* 2017;65(3):676–685.
22. Akin I, Kische S, Rehders TC, Ince H, Nienaber CA. Thoracic endovascular stent-graft therapy in aortic dissection. *Curr Opin Cardiol.* 2010;25(6): 552–559.
23. Guo B, Hou K, Guo D, et al. Outcomes of thoracic endovascular repair for type B aortic dissection with multichanneled morphology. *J Vasc Surg.* 2017.
24. Ando M, Okita Y, Tagusari O, Kitamura S, Matsuo H. Surgery in three-channeled aortic dissection. A 31-patient review. *Jpn J Thorac Cardiovasc Surg.* 2000;48(6):339–343.
25. Ando M, Okita Y, Tagusari O, Morota T, Kitamura S. Three-channeled aortic dissection in Marfan syndrome. *Cardiovasc Surg.* 2000;8(2): 153–158.
26. Guo B, Hou K, Guo D, et al. Outcomes of thoracic endovascular repair for type B aortic dissection with multichanneled morphology. *J Vasc Surg.* 2017;66(4):1007–1017.

27

Complications of Endovascular Septal Fenestration in the Management of Patients With Aortic Dissection

Quirine L. Eijkenboom, BS and Michael D. Dake, MD, FSIR, FCIRSE

INTRODUCTION

Endovascular fenestration is used to manage complicated aortic dissection in a manner analogous to open surgical septectomy. The intent to create a large communication between the aortic true and false lumina providing free interluminal flow and equalization of pressure differentials. The technique depends on the clinical situation. The two most commonly reported include endovascular balloon septectomy and longitudinal guidewire-mediated septectomy.

Balloon fenestration of the dissection septum is most frequently performed in acute dissection complicated by branch vessel ischemia. The purpose is to create a hole or tear within the septum separating the true and false lumina. This produces a more balanced admixture of blood flow in the aortic lumina and functionally reduces or relieves malperfusion of tissue beds supplied by branch arteries originating from a previously compromised aortic lumen.

Guidewire-mediated longitudinal septal fenestration is typically used in cases of chronic dissection associated with false lumen aneurysm formation within the thoracic and/or abdominal aorta. In the setting of chronic dissection, branch vessel malperfusion is rarely critical, and the role of fenestration therefore has another focus. In selected patients at high risk of open aneurysm repair, endograft placement may offer an alternative therapy. However, the presence of the dissection prevents the graft from obtaining an adequate seal and graft expansion. Consequently, a Type I endoleak commonly occurs.

The intent of a longitudinal fenestration is to divide the septum and to create a uniluminal segment including an appropriate transaortic diameter neck suitable for endograft anchoring around the entire outer circumference of the aorta across both lumina. Now, with the endograft channeling all the blood flow, the aneurysm sac is isolated, thus mitigating the risk of progressive aneurysm enlargement.

FENESTRATION AND ACUTE AORTIC DISSECTION

Branch vessel malperfusion, caused by acute aortic dissection, is a potentially life-threatening condition if untreated. Mechanisms of branch vessel obstruction secondary to aortic dissection are classified as static, dynamic, or a combination of both. Static involvement is caused by direct extension of the dissection process and the aortic septum into a branch artery resulting in mechanical obstruction. If associated with evidence of critical ischemia, static branch vessel compromise is typically treated by placement of stents within the true lumen of the affected branch.

Dynamic obstruction is caused by prolapse of the dissection septum over branch vessel origins. In cases of acute dissection complicated by dynamic branch vessel malperfusion, compromised flow to critical abdominal and/or leg arteries is frequently a result of false lumen compression of the aortic true lumen (true lumen collapse) that supplies these ischemic branches. When aortic true lumen obliteration exists, there is typically an imbalance in flow and pressure within the two aortic lumina. Often there is a very large primary intimal entry tear, and the resultant false lumen in-flow is frequently greater than its outflow capacity. Consequently, the aortic false lumen diastolic blood pressure is commonly greater than that in the aortic true lumen. In this clinical situation, placement of an aortic stent graft in the true lumen over the primary entry tear results in a dramatic decrease in false lumen in-flow and an almost instantaneous relief of aortic true lumen compromise and the ischemia involving branch arteries originating from it. This is the standard current therapy for so-called "dynamic branch vessel involvement." However, in cases with unfavorable or unsuitable anatomy for endograft placement or when the appropriate device is unavailable, endovascular septal fenestration is an option. The procedure is performed within the infrarenal aorta where a balloon is inflated across the septum to create a hole or tear. In the setting of acute dissection, this tear is predictably a linear transverse rent in the lamella oriented perpendicular to the longitudinal course of the aorta. The immediate result is a decrease in the resistance to false lumen outflow, increasing flow from the false lumen. This effectively decompresses the aortic false lumen and relieves the upstream compromise affecting branch vessels originating from the true lumen.

The technique is dependent on successfully transgressing the septum—usually from the diminutive, narrowed aortic true lumen to the much larger, dominant false lumen—using a 21-gauge needle directed through a curved, relatively rigid cannula or guide catheter oriented perpendicular to the lamella.[1,2] Correlation between live fluoroscopy and preprocedural computed tomography (CT) imaging helps to orient the guiding cannula so that it is pointed in the direction of the mid septum. Real-time intravascular ultrasound imaging is invaluable in confirming direction of the needle puncture. Once the needle is advanced 4 mm to 6 mm to cross the septum, a 0.014″ or 0.018″ guidewire is advanced until it is well proximal to the level of septal transgression. A 4-French or 5-French catheter is advanced over the needle and guidewire. After their removal, an injection of contrast media is used to confirm successful crossing. A 0.035″ guidewire is then introduced and the catheter and guiding cannula are removed.

A series of sequentially larger diameter angioplasty balloons are then inflated across the septum. After reaching a diameter of 20–24 mm, aortography is performed to confirm the adequacy of the new communication and the flow to previously compromised branch vessels originating from the aortic true lumen. In most cases, balloon septectomy to the range of diameters previously detailed is sufficient to relieve critical compromise of aortic true lumen branches. This may be difficult to determine definitively intraprocedurally and may require close monitoring of symptoms, blood chemistry studies, and peripheral hemodynamics as appropriate in the immediate postprocedural period before a final determination of whether the fenestration was successful in reversing branch ischemia.

The salutary effect in terms of true lumen enlargement on CT imaging following balloon fenestration is never as dramatic anatomically as that observed following aortic stent graft placement of the primary entry tear, but physiologically, an improvement in true lumen flow is usually evident when the aortic fenestration is performed distal to the involved branches as opposed to more proximally in the distal thoracic segment. A balloon fenestration proximal to the involved abdominal branches should be avoided because it acts as a secondary entry tear and may exaggerate the imbalance in flow between the lumina and do little to alleviate aortic true lumen obliteration in the abdomen.

If the clinical outcome is deemed inadequate, supplemental revision may be undertaken. This may involve placement of a large self-expanding noncovered metallic stent across the fenestration, such as a baffle, guiding flow proximal in the aortic false lumen to distally in the true lumen via the existing fenestration. A large 20–24 mm diameter Wallstent (Boston Scientific Inc., Watertown, Massachusetts) that is between 40 mm and 80 mm long is frequently selected to serve as a frame to buttress open the fenestration and improve the desired hemodynamic effect.

Alternatively, the balloon fenestration may be extended or a new communication created longitudinally using a guidewire-mediated septectomy. This procedure is more commonly used in chronic dissections to create a segmental uniluminal channel. This technique is described later. Both methods are usually successful in reversing symptoms in the majority of acute dissection patients unresponsive to balloon septectomy alone.

In a study by Park et al.,[3] 16 patients received aortic fenestration and/or branch stenting as treatment; 30-day mortality was 8.3% and branch vessel malperfusion improved in 90%, although there was also expansion of the outer aortic diameter at 1-year follow-up.

In a study by Midulla et al.,[4] 35 patients with aortic dissections were treated with endovascular fenestration. All were technically successful, with 26 patients requiring additional stenting; 30-day mortality was 34%, 8 of 23 survivors suffered from ischemic complications, and all patients had a patent false lumen.

Complications

Serious adverse events related to balloon fenestration are relatively uncommon and tend to be associated with the steps performed prior to the actual balloon inflation. Inadvertent injury to access vessels or the distal aorta during insertion and advancement of the guiding cannula or sheath, which needs to be somewhat rigid to allow accurate directional orientation for needle passage across the flap, is a risk. Similarly, attempts at a needle transgression of the septum from one aortic lumen to the other may be inaccurate with puncture through the outer wall of the aorta into surrounding tissues, the inferior vena cava, or ureter. Depending on the needle size and subsequent passage of any catheters or larger devices, lack of recognition of the unanticipated transaortic tract may lead to bleeding, vessel rupture, arteriovenous fistula, or ureteral laceration. Any of these complications may prove catastrophic and require keen awareness that an unexpected problem exists and prompt attention to treating it appropriately. One way to mitigate a serious adverse event is to use a small-gauge needle, such as a 21-gauge Chiba needle for the septal puncture rather than a larger 18- or 19-gauge needle. Alternately, TourGuide deflectable sheaths may be used in combination with re-entry catheters/devices with intravascular ultrasound to cross the septum more accurately and to avoid puncture extrinsic to the aorta. Although the fenestration should be placed infrarenally, going too low frequently leads to the lack of a successful procedure for restoration of perfusion to the viscera.

Another risk of this procedure exists when thrombus is present at the level of fenestration. This more frequently involves the presence of clot within the false lumen, but it may also exist in the true lumen. The risk of distal embolization may occur from endovascular device manipulation within any partially thrombosed vessel. This is still quite rare. This procedure is relatively safe with concerns usually more related to whether the septectomy has provided clinically successful and complete reversal of branch vessel obstruction and tissue malperfusion.

If the operation is inadequate and extension of the fenestration or its buttressing with a stent as described earlier is undertaken, these techniques become more complicated with additional steps that may be associated with more serious adverse effects. The complications associated with longitudinal guidewire-mediated fenestration will be described later in the chapter, but creation of a baffle using a large self-expanding stent to buttress the septectomy may have unique related risks.

The main risk is the possibility of branch vessel narrowing or obstruction resulting from the presence of the aortic stent overlying its origin. Although a bare, noncovered stent is used, it may have to be placed with a portion of the device within the true lumen of the visceral segment of the abdominal aorta. Depending on its precise position within the aortic true channel, it may abut or cross true lumen branches that may be impaired at their origin. If this is observed, placement of a branch vessel ostial stent delivered through and expanded across the overlying struts of the self-expanding aortic stent is an effective treatment.

In all cases, vigilant postfenestration imaging surveillance at regular intervals is necessary to check for disease progression. In general, the main risk in chronic dissection is false lumen aneurysm formation, but following fenestration there is ongoing risk of branch vessel compromise as its morphology evolves. One example of late recurrent branch vessel ischemia following balloon fenestration was reported by Williams et al.[5] Two months after percutaneous transfemoral fenestration in a Type III aortic dissection, subacute mesenteric ischemia was diagnosed. Continued expansion of the false lumen required aortic resection and graft replacement of the distal thoracic and abdominal aorta.

FENESTRATION AND CHRONIC AORTIC DISSECTION

False lumen thrombosis is traditionally regarded as a measure of success in thoracic endovascular aortic repair (TEVAR) for acute Type B aortic dissection. However, residual distal septal communications and patent intercostal and lumbar arteries may still provide perfusion and tension to the false lumen, leading to progressive expansion. The effect of this phenomenon on subsequent false lumen aneurysm formation is difficult to predict, but in many cases, complete healing of the aorta is unlikely to be achieved.[6]

A patent false lumen is considered a predictor for late death caused by false lumen rupture and for retreatment of the descending aorta to manage progressive false lumen enlargement.[7] In addition, patients with acute Type B aortic dissection who have a partially thrombosed aortic false lumen exhibit a significantly higher annual growth rate when compared with patients having a patent or completely thrombosed false lumen. Consequently, patients with partial thrombosis require more intense follow-up imaging surveillance and may benefit from prophylactic intervention to avoid false lumen aneurysm formation and rupture.[8]

Treating chronic Type B aortic dissection with TEVAR has several unique concerns. The proximal stent graft landing zone is often compromised because of proximity to arch vessels and lack of a healthy distal neck. In most post-TEVAR cases, the false lumen in the abdominal aorta is not completely excluded, with patency maintained by residual fenestrations distal to the stent graft that perfuse the thoracic false lumen in a retrograde fashion. In this situation, the lower thoracic aortic false lumen remains pressurized and, as a result, is at risk of progressive expansion.

In chronic Type B dissection with false lumen aneurysm, the presence of a septum dividing the aorta into two lumina within proximal and/or distal potential neck segments, in anatomy otherwise suitable for endograft aneurysm exclusion, represents a challenge for endovascular management. In this setting, guidewire-mediated septectomy with longitudinal cutting of the dissection septum may be a useful adjunct to endograft placement by providing a suitable landing zone to anchor and to seal the device.

The rationale for endovascular longitudinal septectomy is to create a uniluminal neck segment either in the distal thoracic aorta to facilitate isolation of a thoracic false lumen aneurysm (proximal device placement in a usual landing zone) or in the infrarenal aorta to create a suitable proximal landing zone to anchor a standard EVAR device to treat an abdominal aneurysm. The restoration of a single channel proximal and/or distal to an aneurysm provides a neck segment that allows circumferential sealing of an endograft against the outer wall of the aorta without an intervening dissection lamella.

The existence of two flow channels in dissection is often associated with pressure and flow discrepancies that cause progressive false lumen dilation and aneurysm formation. Longitudinal septal cutting divides the aortic lamella and has been shown to equalize the flow and pressure in the true and false lumina while it creates a uniluminal channel more amenable to (T)EVAR.

The procedure starts by obtaining bilateral common femoral access, although occasionally it is possible to perform through unilateral groin access. Catheters are introduced into both lumina, guided by CT imaging, arteriography, and/or intravascular ultrasound to identify the orientation of the two channels in the iliofemoral conduit arteries, to detail the termination of the dissection process, and to pinpoint existing natural fenestrations in the septum. Once access is obtained, the septum is punctured at the desired level with a needle directed by a guiding cannula in a manner identical to that described previously. In most cases the puncture is made with the needle advanced from the smaller aortic true lumen across the septum toward a larger false lumen. Once successful passage is confirmed, a guidewire is introduced into the false lumen and snared. The snare and guidewire are then withdrawn and exteriorized such that the wire forms a loop from the aortic true lumen, across the lamella and out of the false lumen. The exact location of the needle puncture to initiate balloon or guidewire septectomy is variable and based on the specific anatomic configuration and orientation of the septum and the related clinical symptoms found in each individual case of dissection.

With both ends of the guidewire outside the patient, the access sheaths in the groins are positioned close (3–5 cm) below the wire segment transgressing the septum to provide support for the fenestration maneuver. Two techniques for initiating the next step of septal division have been described. One involves applying simple downward traction on the ends of the guidewire to create a cleavage tear in the lamella. Once the "break-in" rent is made, the guidewire is pulled distally like a cheese wire to extend the rip in the septum.

Alternatively, the guidewire-mediated fenestration may be initiated by pulling the guidewire back and forth in a sawing motion, like a Gigli wire saw. Once the initial cut is established the sawing motion is continued with a downward force to continue the septal division inferiorly to the desired distal location. Irrespective of the technique used, the starting point of the fenestration must be well proximal (4–7 cm) to the intended landing zone of the proximal margin of an EVAR device. This also applies to creating a suitable distal landing zone for TEVAR isolation of thoracic false lumen aneurysm where a generously long longitudinal fenestration is necessary both proximal and distal to the intended distal aspect of the endograft to facilitate its full expansion and to ensure a circumferential seal to prevent endoleak.

After the septum is longitudinally divided like a curtain, the procedure is completed with standard (T)EVAR graft placement with anchoring of the device within uniluminal neck segment(s). There is no consensus regarding the relative superiority of the techniques in the setting of chronic aortic dissection. There has never been a direct comparison reported. Our experience suggests that less downward traction force is required when a back-and-forth sawing motion is applied during guidewire-mediated longitudinal fenestration.

Several reports in the medical literature have described the technique of guidewire-mediated longitudinal septal fenestration.[9–13] Those who report the procedure performed in conjunction with standard endograft placement to manage a false lumen aneurysm associated with aortic dissection stress the importance of preprocedural planning to ensure that the proposed landing zone created after septotomy is dimensionally suitable with a transaortic diameter within the treatment range of available devices. In cases where the resultant diameter of the uniluminal neck after fenestration is too large, other options are preferred.

Complications

Arterial tortuosity and variations in septal tissue composition (fibrosis, calcification), dimensions (thickness), and adjacent luminal properties (mural thrombus) may reduce the effectiveness of guidewire-mediated fenestration and influence the risks of the procedure. Unstable arterial ulcerations, dense plaque, and luminal thrombus may result in an increased risk of peripheral embolization during the procedure.[11] Indeed, longitudinal guidewire septotomy irrespective of these variables is associated with potential complications.

There is a risk of aortic wall damage or rupture during the procedure distinct from an incidence of endoleaks (Types Ia and Ib) caused by incomplete sealing following endograft placement with persistent aneurysm perfusion, growth, and rupture. Intraprocedural aortic rupture has not been reported in the literature, but it remains a key concern.

Clearly, the technique of guidewire-mediated septotomy is not precisely controllable in terms of constraining the longitudinal course of lamella tearing, which may result in obstruction of branch arteries. Prolapsing septal segments following guidewire fenestration may cause malperfusion by covering branch vessel origins, resulting in ischemia involving the viscera, kidneys, spinal cord, or lower extremities. Similarly, it is possible that sheared septal tissue may actually prolapse into branch vessel ostia and compromise flow or that a septal flap may narrow an aortic lumen (true or false) proximal to a branch that it supplies.

Fortunately, with prompt recognition, these untoward events may be amenable to endovascular rescue using stents or stent grafts placed within the aorta and/or affected branch. Malperfusion of arteries branching from the aorta may also result from a shift in false lumen thrombus during either guidewire fenestration or as a consequence of stent graft placement. We have experience with one case of renal artery obstruction (Fig. 27.1) where this may be the responsible mechanism. To decrease the risk of inadvertent ischemia, consideration should be given to obtaining wire access to the lowest renal prior to septotomy, to allow for parallel graft rescue should prolapse of the septum occur.

In addition, there are isolated case reports of patients with long-standing intestinal hypoperfusion caused by chronic aortic true lumen

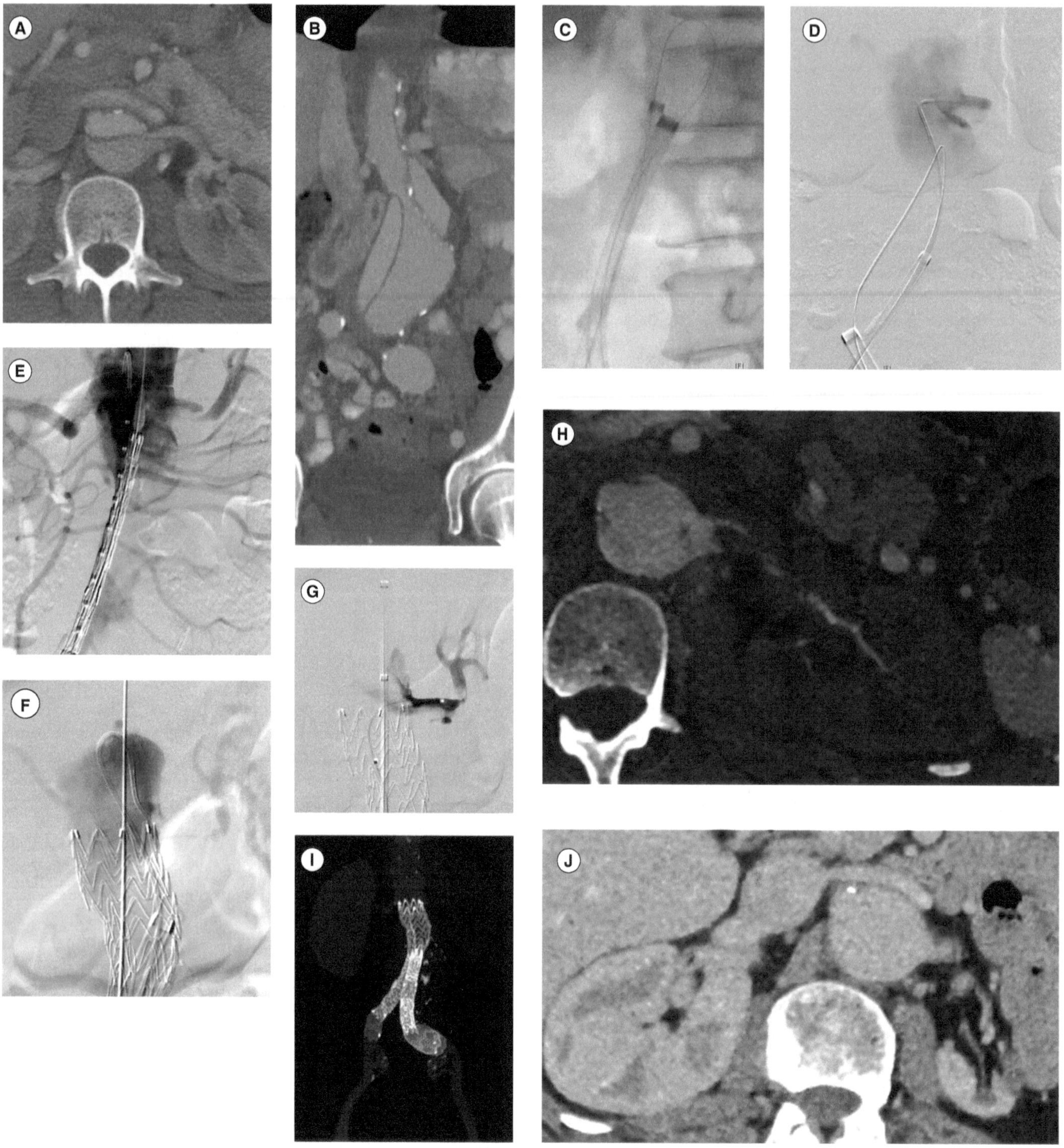

Fig. 27.1 A 60-year-old man with chronic Type B aortic dissection status post stent graft placement in thoracic aorta and enlarging abdominal aortic aneurysm treated with guidewire septectomy and abdominal endograft complicated by left renal artery occlusion. (A) Axial computed tomography (CT) image preseptectomy shows dissection septum extending directly into left renal artery. (B) Coronal reconstruction of CT data set preseptectomy shows complex aortic dissection with associated infrarenal abdominal aortic aneurysm. Transaortic diameter at the level of the renal arteries is 33 mm. (C) Fluoroscopic image after establishing 0.018″ guidewire loop across the dissection septum at the level of the celiac trunk. Two angiographic sheaths, one in the true lumen and one in the false, are positioned for support just below the loop. (D) Abdominal aortogram performed immediately after guidewire septectomy displays filling of the true and false aortic lumina with proximal opacification of the dissected left renal artery, but no distal flow. (E) Aortogram performed with aortic stent graft positioned immediately below the renal arteries before deployment. Both aortic lumina are opacified, as are the right renal artery of the false lumen and the dissected left renal artery, now with distal flow. (F) Aortogram post stent graft deployment without filling of the left renal artery. (G) Post-balloon angioplasty of the left renal artery, flow is restored, albeit poor, to the left kidney. (H) Axial CT reconstruction through the left renal artery shows a diminutive nearly occluded lumen with only a faint nephrogram indicating a lack of perfusion 3 days after the procedure. (I) Shaded-surface display of CT data set performed 3 days after the procedure shows thrombosed aneurysm sac after septectomy and endograft placement, patent right renal artery, and grossly asymmetric nephrograms associated with near occlusion of left renal artery. (J) Delayed postintravenous contrast axial image from CT performed 10 months after the procedure shows markedly decreased left renal size, scant left kidney perfusion, and markedly delayed nephrogram.

collapse who, upon fenestration, experienced reperfusion-related shock that led to intra-operative death.[11]

Another risk involves folding or collapsing of the septum rather than the desired cutting of the lamella. This could result in septal tissue collapse like accordion pleats into an obstructing mass below the fenestration causing peripheral ischemia.[4] In most cases, as long as guidewire access into the more proximal aorta is maintained, resulting stenosis and occlusions of the terminal aorta and/or iliac arteries can be successfully managed depending on the scenario by placement of stents or, alternatively, stent grafts using a tube graft, an aorto-unilateral or a bifurcated endograft to buttress open a lumen or lumina.

CONCLUSION

Percutaneous septal fenestration is a valuable technique to include in our endovascular armamentarium to manage highly selected cases of complicated acute and chronic aortic dissection. Although not required frequently, it is an option that should be considered when standard treatments to manage branch vessel malperfusion in acute dissection or false lumen aneurysm in chronic cases are not anatomically feasible or too high risk. Fortuitously, based on what is reported, most of the known complications of septal fenestration are amenable to successful endovascular treatment without the need for open surgical correction.

REFERENCES

1. Hartnell GG, Gates J. Aortic fenestration: a why, when, and how-to guide. *Radiographics.* 2005;25:175–189.
2. Wuest W, Goltz J, Ritter C, Yildirim C, Hahn D, Kickuth R. Fenestration of aortic dissection using a fluoroscopy-based needle re-entry catheter system. *Cardiovasc Interv Radiol.* 2011;34:S44–S47.
3. Park K, Do Y, Kim S, et al. Endovascular treatment of acute complicated aortic dissection: long-term follow-up of clinical outcomes and CT findings. *J Vasc Interv Radiol.* 2009;20:334–341.
4. Midulla M, Renaud A, Martinelli T, et al. Endovascular fenestration in aortic dissection with acute malperfusion syndrome: immediate and late follow-up. *J Thorac Cardiovasc Surg.* 2011;142:66–72.
5. Williams DM, Brothers TE, Messina LM. Relief of mesenteric ischemia in type III aortic dissection with percutaneous fenestration of the aortic septum. *Radiology.* 1990;174:450–452.
6. Qing KX, Yiu WK, Cheng SW. A morphologic study of chronic type B aortic dissection and aneurysms after thoracic endovascular stent grafting. *J Vasc Surg.* 2012;55:1268–1275.
7. Fattouch K, Sampognaro R, Navarra E, et al. Long-term results after repair of type A acute aortic dissection according to false lumen patency. *Ann Thorac Surg.* 2009;88:1244–1250.
8. Trimarchi S, Tolenaar JL, Jonker FH, et al. Importance of false lumen thrombosis in type B aortic dissection prognosis. *J Thorac Cardiovasc Surg.* 2013;145:S208–S212.
9. Tashiro J, Baqai A, Goldstein LJ, Salsamendi JT, Taubman M, Rey J. "Cheese wire" fenestration of a chronic aortic dissection flap for endovascular repair of a contained aneurysm rupture. *J Vasc Surg.* 2014;60:497–499.
10. Ullery BW, Chandra V, Dake M, Lee JT. Cheese wire fenestration of a chronic juxtarenal dissection flap to facilitate proximal neck fixation during EVAR. *Ann Vasc Surg.* 2015;29(124):e1–e5.
11. Kos S, Gürke L, Jacob AL. A novel fenestration technique for abdominal aortic dissection membranes using a combination of a needle re-entry catheter and the "cheese-wire" technique. *Cardiovasc Interv Radiol.* 2011;34:1296–1302.
12. Watkinson AF. A novel "cheese wire" technique for stent positioning following difficult iliac artery subintimal dissection and aortic re-entry. *Cardiovasc Interv Radiol.* 2009;32:781–784.
13. Gissler MC, Lee JT, Chandra V, Dake MD. Percutaneous septectomy in chronic dissection with AAA creates uniluminal neck for EVAR. *Cardiovasc Interv Radiol.* 2017;40:1522–1528.

28

Renal and Mesenteric Aneurysms

Jared T. Feyko, DO and Luke Marone, MD, DFSVS

INTRODUCTION

Aneurysms of the mesenteric circulation are a rare but potentially fatal pathology. Therefore, a thorough understanding of the natural history and treatment options available is critical to the vascular surgeon potentially faced with treating this entity. Successful treatment with standard open surgical techniques was first described in the 1950s. Since that time, a major paradigm shift toward endovascular treatment has occurred not unlike many vascular pathologies we commonly encounter. Furthermore, the quality of cross-sectional imaging has improved dramatically, which has led to more frequent incidental detection of mesenteric aneurysms. At the same time, technologic advances have made an increasing number of devices available for the treatment of mesenteric aneurysms. This chapter will cover the epidemiology of mesenteric aneurysm including incidence and standard treatment indications. We will focus primarily on contemporary endovascular treatment techniques, descriptions of currently available devices, and how to avoid common complications.

BACKGROUND

Visceral artery aneurysms are defined as aneurysms involving the celiac artery, superior mesenteric artery, inferior mesenteric artery, or any branch of these arteries. Renal artery aneurysms are classified separately and discussed in the following section. Estimates of the true incidence of visceral artery aneurysms vary from as low as 0.1% to 2 % in adults. The proportionate distribution of visceral aneurysms is more clearly understood than the overall incidence and is as follows: 60% splenic artery, 20% hepatic artery, 5.5% superior mesenteric artery, 4% celiac artery, 4% gastric artery, jejunal, ilial, and colic arteries 3%, pancreaticoduodenal artery 2%, gastroduodenal artery 1.5%, and inferior mesenteric artery <1%. The traditional definition of aneurysms applies with aneurysm defined as 1.5 times the diameter of the normal nondilated vessel. Visceral aneurysms include a large proportion of degenerative fusiform aneurysms, pseudoaneurysms, and saccular aneurysms. Underlying etiologies are varied as well and include, atherosclerosis, medial degeneration, collagen vascular disease, fibromuscular dysplasia, infectious etiologies, inflammatory etiologies, vasculitis, iatrogenic injury, and trauma. In previous decades it was more common for mesenteric aneurysms to present ruptured, with associated mortality as high as 70%. Exact rates of mesenteric aneurysm rupture are still not well established, but with improved imaging quality more incidental nonrupture aneurysms are being discovered.[1]

Congruent with the global trend in vascular surgery there is a shift towards endovascular treatment of mesenteric aneurysms as a first line option. This is secondary to advances in technology and an increasing array of devices available to practitioners. Standard open surgical techniques can certainly still be applied to intact or ruptured mesenteric aneurysms, but retrospective data have demonstrated equivalent survival between open and endovascular treatment for intact aneurysms and decreased morbidity with endovascular repair. Additionally, in the ruptured cohort endovascular treatment was shown to have significantly lower postoperative mortality (7.4% versus 28.6%).[2] Therefore, the trend toward treatment with endovascular techniques is likely to continue. This chapter will describe available methods for each anatomic location, as well as generally accepted indications.

INDICATIONS

Treatment indications vary by anatomic location. For splenic aneurysms, indications are diameter greater than 2 cm, symptomatic, ruptured, pseudoaneurysm, pregnancy, child-bearing age, orthotopic liver transplant, and portal hypertension. Hepatic artery aneurysms are the next most common mesenteric aneurysm and treatment indications are ruptured, symptomatic, pseudoaneurysm, multiple aneurysms, polyarteritis nodosa, other inflammatory conditions, and size greater than 2 cm. Superior mesenteric aneurysms are less common, but all SMA aneurysms should be repaired in appropriate surgical candidates. Similarly, all celiac artery aneurysms, gastric, gastroepiploic, pancreaticoduodenal, gastroduodenal, inferior mesenteric, jejunal, ileal, and colic artery aneurysms should be repaired unless the patient is deemed too high risk with respect to comorbidities. Finally, mesenteric venous aneurysms can generally be safely observed unless they become symptomatic.[1]

ENDOVASCULAR TREATMENT OPTIONS

Regardless of the treatment technique used, the therapeutic goal is the exclusion of the aneurysm from systemic circulation, thereby eliminating rupture risk or symptoms if present. A variety of embolic materials can be utilized either to exclude the aneurysm from circulation or to be placed directly in the aneurysm sac to induce thrombosis. The materials available are various types of coils, liquid embolic agents (such as glue or thrombin), and vascular plugs. Coils are the most commonly used and are a permanent agent that can be made of either stainless steel or platinum. Coils are available in an array of lengths, diameters, and shapes. Coils are also available in a fibered variety with increased thrombogenicity. Additionally, coils are classified by delivery mechanism into pushable (where they are advanced precisely to the desired location by advancing a wire behind the coil), injectable (where the coil is advanced quickly by injecting fluid through the catheter in a burst), or detachable (where the coils are connected to a guidewire that must be disconnected prior to final placement, adding an element of precision and safety). The profile of coils ranges from 0.035″ for large and medium sized vessels to 0.018″ microcoils that can be advanced through a microcatheter into small vessels with sizes available as small as 2 mm. Pushable coils include the Nestor and Tornado coils (Cook Medical, Bloomington, IN), which are available in both 0.035″ and 0.018″ sizes. Interlock coils (Boston Scientific, Marlborough, MA) are of the detachable variety and also come in both 0.035″ and 0.018″ sizes. Our preferred microcatheters include the Renegade (Boston Scientific, Marlborough, MA) Highflow and the Direxion. Coils may be used in one of several different techniques. Sac packing is a frequently used technique that refers to the aneurysm itself and only the aneurysm being filled with coils, thereby inducing thrombosis. This technique is useful for pseudoaneurysms where preservation of the end artery is needed, leading to thrombosis of only the pseudoaneurysm and not any other segment of the parent vessel. This can be technically challenging to perform, and the sac packing technique can be used in conjunction with a bare-metal stent covering the neck of the aneurysm, with the coils deployed through a microcatheter placed between the interstices of the stent. This technique is referred to as stent-assisted coiling and has the advantage of preventing coils from being inadvertently placed outside the desired area. It is useful for wide-necked aneurysms where sac packing may otherwise lead to nontarget vessel embolization. A similar technique is referred to as balloon remodeling, originally described for the treatment of intracerebral aneurysms. In this technique, a compliant angioplasty balloon the size of the parent vessel is deployed and the pseudoaneurysm is cannulated with a microcatheter between the balloon and the vessel wall. When performing this technique, we place the microcatheter in the aneurysm prior to balloon inflation, yet have the balloon catheter in place prior to cannulation with the microcatheter. We recommend inflation to no more than 4 atm and use of an 8-French sheath, minimum. For the 0.035″ platform and 6-French sheath for the 0.018″ platform. Additionally, we recommend weight-based anticoagulation with heparin. With the balloon in place, coils are deployed in the aneurysm and the balloon is deflated once the sac is filled with coils. This provides the same benefit as the stent-assisted coiling technique but permits use of a temporary balloon occlusion rather than permanently deploying a stent. The coils should be 20%–30% greater than the diameter of the artery. The potential complications of coil embolization are nontarget embolization in which coils end up in a non-desired location. Rupture of the pseudoaneurysm during vigorous coil deployment may also occur, as may failure of the aneurysm to thrombose. The latter is particularly true in patients with abnormal coagulation parameters. Embolization may also be achieved with other agents such as glues (N-butyl cyanoacrylate), which form a cast when coming in contact with blood. When using this type of glue, a hydrophilic microcatheter should be used to decrease the rate of polymerization in the catheter. Additionally, lyophilized thrombin can be used, which triggers the coagulation cascade and results in the formation of a fibrin plug in the desired location. N-butyl cyanoacrylate may result in polymerization within the catheter, which must be flushed with 5% dextrose before and after administration and both agents may also result in nontarget embolization. Additionally, if the glue occludes the catheter, access will be lost and will need to be the vessel reselected. It is therefore common to utilize the balloon remodeling technique with these agents. Vascular plugs such as the Amplatzer (St. Jude Medical, Minnesota) is an additional option. It is a three-dimensional nitinol mesh, which is well suited to occlude the vessel leading to the aneurysmal segment. They are attached to a delivery device, which must be unscrewed after deployment in the proper location. The plugs should be oversized (30%–50%) and are a good option for medium-sized vessels. They are highly effective and precise in their deployment mechanism. More recently, the MVP Micro Vascular Plug System (Medtronic, Bloomington, Minnesota) has become available, allowing exclusion of small and medium diameter vessels using a 5-French catheter. Vascular plugs or coils may also be used with the so-called "sandwich technique". In this technique the vessel proximal and distal to the aneurysmal segment is occluded with either plugs or coils rather than simply filling the sac itself. This technique is effective but must be limited to situations where occlusion of the parent vessel will not cause significant clinical sequelae. This technique is especially successful in the treatment of large splenic artery aneurysms.

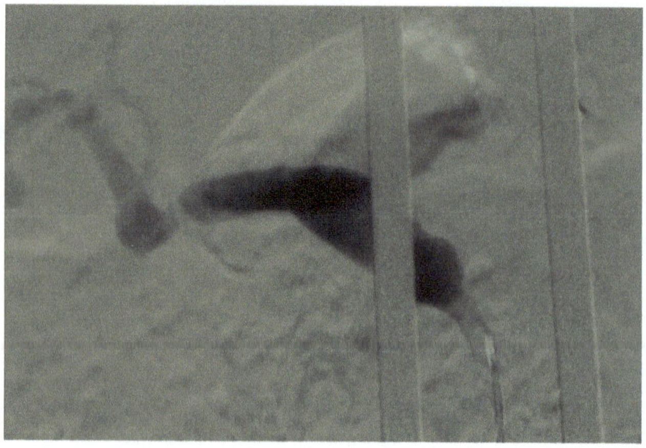

Fig. 28.1 A 2.6-cm common hepatic artery aneurysm.

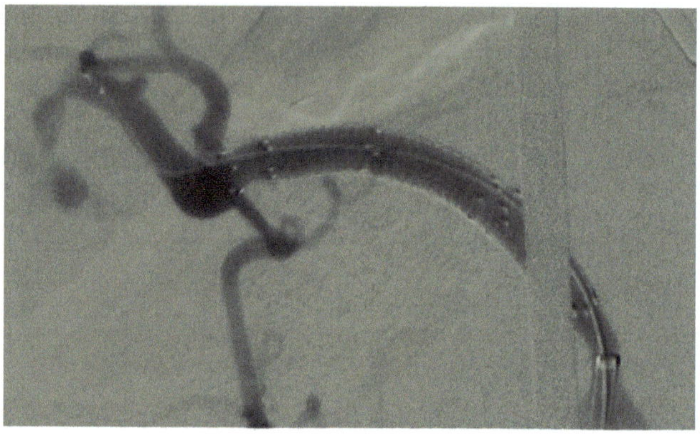

Fig. 28.2 Common hepatic artery aneurysm after treatment with covered stent.

Covered stents are also an option in the treatment of mesenteric aneurysms. This technique involves placement of a stent graft across the aneurysm in the parent vessel, excluding the aneurysm from circulation, but preserving the patency of the vessel. This requires the use of a longer sheath and advancement into the mesenteric artery for support in delivering the covered stent. It is recommended to have at least 1 cm proximal and distal to the aneurysm to achieve an adequate seal. Self-expanding and balloon-expandable varieties are available depending on the anatomic location. Covered stents come in sizes as small as 5 mm and require a minimum sheath size of 6 French. Therefore, this technique can work well in some of the larger mesenteric aneurysms but is not an option for smaller branch vessel aneurysms (Fig. 28.1 and Fig. 28.2).[3]

ENDOVASCULAR TREATMENT TECHNIQUES

Interventions are most commonly performed via common femoral access. Brachial access is another option, but as with any intervention there is a higher incidence of access-related complications as well as sheath size limitations. We advocate femoral access whenever feasible, with brachial access being a good option for mesenteric vessels with a steep take-off angle from the aorta. Use of a steerable guide catheter such as the IMA (Cordis, Santa Clara, CA) guiding catheter or the JR5 (Cordis, Santa Clara, CA) guiding catheter helps reduce the need for brachial access. After percutaneous access is obtained, the patient is systemically heparinized. Standard diagnostic arteriograms are performed, including

AP and lateral aortograms, as well as selective mesenteric arteriograms depending on the location of the aneurysm to confirm the location, determine size, and collateral circulation. The target vessel is selected and a sheath (6 French for 0.035″ coils and 5 French for 0.018″ coils) is advanced over a stiff wire such as Rosen (Cook Medical, Bloomington, IN), Supracore (Abbott, Abbott Park, IL), or MagicTorque (Boston Scientific, Marlborogh, MA) to secure access to the origin of the mesenteric vessel. Through this sheath a guidewire is used to select the aneurysm and an appropriate size selective catheter is used to gain access to the aneurysm. If simple sac packing technique is used, this set-up can be used to advance appropriately sized coils, using a wire into the aneurysm until it is sufficiently packed (Fig. 28.3 and Fig. 28.4). If a simple sac packing technique is to be used with microcoils, a telescoping method can be used with a microcatheter advanced into the aneurysm through a standard size selective catheter and coils can be delivered by either advancing with a wire or saline injection. Detachable coils can be delivered using the same set-up, with the added step of confirming adequate placement prior to detaching the coil from the delivery device. Thrombin or N-butyl cyanoacrylate can also be delivered via this set-up. Additional steps should be taken to dilute the material with ethiodized oil appropriately so that it does not set-up too early, and the catheter must be flushed with 5% dextrose before and after each infusion to prevent occlusion. The sac packing technique works well with narrow-neck aneurysms, but for wide-necked aneurysms the stent-supported coil embolization technique or balloon-remodeling technique can aid safe coil delivery. In this approach the bare-metal stent is deployed first across the aneurysm origin. A selective microcatheter is then used from a separate access or through the original support sheath to cannulate the aneurysm sac through the stent interstices and coils are deployed in the usual fashion. The balloon remodeling technique is performed similarly, but the aneurysm sac is cannulated prior to advancing the balloon across the aneurysm neck and then inflated prior to delivery of coils or glue (6-French sheath for 0.018″ platform and microcatheter and 8-French sheath for 0.035″ platform). After coiling or glue delivery is complete, the balloon is deflated and removed. Coiling, using the sandwich technique as opposed to sac packing, is effective for occluding the parent vessel when it is not necessary to preserve its patency. In this technique the catheter is first placed distal to the origin of the aneurysm, coils are delivered to occlude the distal segment fully, then the catheter is withdrawn proximal to the aneurysm, and additional coils are placed to occlude the proximal segment. It should also be noted that any significant branches coming directly off the aneurysm should also be embolized prior to the sandwich technique. The sandwich technique can be performed using vascular plugs proximally and distally or a combination of coils and plugs. Lastly, covered stent placement can be performed after sheath access to the proximal mesenteric vessel is secured. This requires larger sheaths and greater sheath purchase to be able to deliver the stent and is therefore limited to the treatment of more proximal mesenteric aneurysms. Covered stents should be 10%–20% oversized in order to achieve adequate seal.[4]

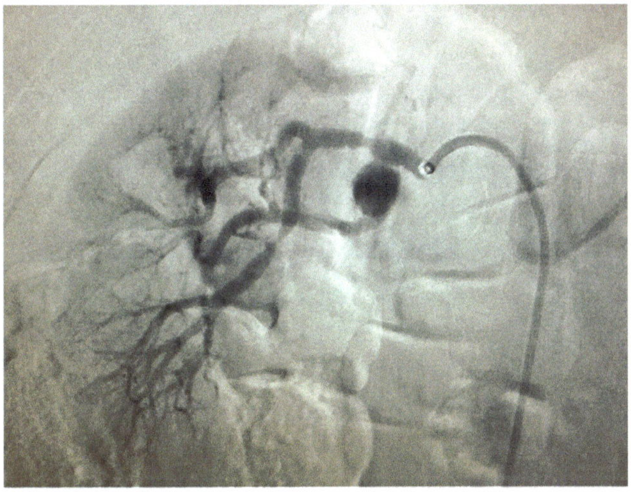

Fig. 28.3 Pretreatment renal artery aneurysm.

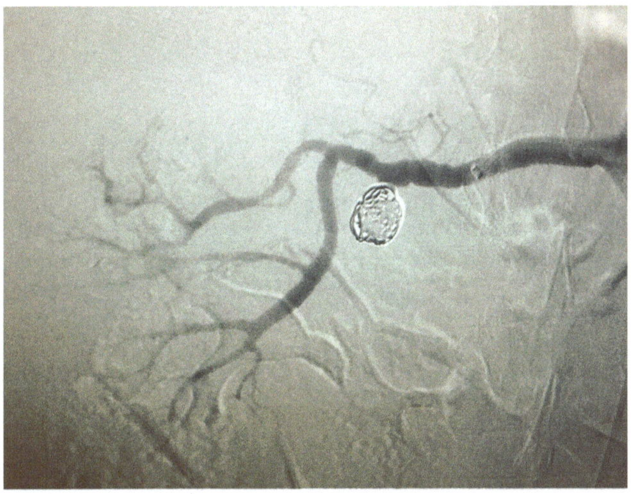

Fig. 28.4 Coil embolization of renal artery aneurysm with sacrifice of Renal Parenchyma.

RENAL ANEURYSMS

Background

Renal artery aneurysms are rarely encountered, but they are an important pathology with which to be familiar. The incidence of renal artery aneurysm is estimated to be 0.7%–0.9%. Renal aneurysms may be degenerative, pseudoaneurysms, dissecting, intrarenal, or extrarenal. The majority of true aneurysms are extrarenal (90%) and occur at the primary or secondary bifurcation. They are infrequently confined to the main renal artery, which complicates treatment. The majority of true renal aneurysms are saccular (75%) and occur at the primary renal artery bifurcation. Fusiform renal aneurysms are less common, usually less than 2 cm in diameter, and typically involve only the main renal artery distal to a significant stenosis. Renal aneurysms may be associated with medial fibroplasia or may be pseudoaneurysms secondary to trauma or iatrogenic injury. Renal artery aneurysm rupture is rare and indications for intervention are rupture, symptoms, pseudoaneurysm, pregnancy, and size greater than 2 cm.[5]

Treatment

Treatment for renal aneurysms follow many of the same decisions for treatment as visceral aneurysms. Open techniques are well established and have good results. However, when feasible the trend is for endovascular repair because of the decreased morbidity. Specific treatment techniques are similar to those endovascular treatment options available for mesenteric aneurysms. These include various embolizing agents, vascular plugs, and covered stents. As previously mentioned, these aneurysms most commonly occur at distal branch points. This complicates treatment, making covered stent placement often unfeasible without compromising perfusion to a segment of the kidney.

Embolization is still technically feasible for many of these aneurysms, utilizing the array of agents and techniques previously described. In contrast to visceral aneurysms, a portion of the renal parenchyma may be sacrificed if preservation is not feasible. Additionally, in the scenario of a nonviable kidney the entire circulation to the kidney may be sacrificed to prevent ongoing hemorrhage. Intrarenal aneurysms are rare but deserve mention. These aneurysm can be coiled but may result in partial parenchymal loss and even require partial nephrectomy.

Complications/Troubleshooting

Complications are infrequent and are often related to inappropriate initi al procedure planning. The most frequent complications include access site thrombosis and or iatrogenic femoral pseudoaneurysm, nontarget vessel inadvertent embolization, vessel/aneurysm rupture, and vessel dissection. These are discussed in more detail in other chapters.

Upon identification of the target vessel we support the use of a tri-axial sheath/catheter configuration to allow for maximal support for coil delivery and or other embolic adjuncts mentioned previously in the chapter. Tri-axial mesenteric vessel purchase allows for more accurate device placement and increased stability. These features not only help in the avoidance of complication but they also assist in the management of complications should they occur. The tri-axial system consists of a 5- or 6-French sheath, a telescoped glide type catheter, and a secondarily telescoped microcatheter (for coil/embolic agent delivery). This configuration enables the delivery of embolic agents in a controlled manner even through highly tortuous vessels. In cases where stent graft placement is considered, a standard sheath placement with adequate purchase of the target vessel is recommended over a high support wire (Rosen [Cook Medical, Bloomington, IN], Supracore [Abbott, Abbott Park, IL]). Additionally, vessel purchase and stability is critical when utilizing the balloon remodeling technique and the stent-assisted coiling technique for wide-neck aneurysms. When inadvertent coil placement occurs, the proceduralist can easily snare the coil for removal. When vessel rupture is identified, a stent graft can be placed or the vessel can be occluded distal and proximal to the rupture site to avoid further hemorrhage, and anticoagulation should be reversed. The balloon should be re-inflated across the perforation and materials gathered expeditiously. If rupture occurs, with only 5-French access there exists risk of loss of wire to upsize to a larger sheath should this situation occur and the rupture should be definitively managed with coil embolization. Finally, if dissection is identified and noted to be flow-limiting, a self-expanding nitinol stent can be placed to restore normal flow and eliminate the area of vessel injury. In short, appropriate preprocedure planning, choice of equipment and target vessel stability are critical in the avoidance of and the treatment of potential iatrogenic issues.

REFERENCES

1. Lakin R, Kashyap V. Splanchic Artery Aneurysms. In: Cronenwett J, Johnston KW, eds. *Rutherford's Vascular Surgery*. 8th ed. Philadelphia: Saunders; 2014:2220–2235.
2. Shukla A, Eid R, Fish L, et al. Contemporary outcomes of intact and ruptured visceral artery aneurysms. *Journal of Vascular Surgery*. 2015; 61:1442–1448.
3. Madhusudhan K, Venkatesh H, Gamanagatti S, et al. Interventional Radiology in the Management of Visceral Artery Pseudoaneurysms: A Review of Techniques and Embolic Materials. *Korean Journal of Radiology*. 2016;17(3):351–363.
4. Hemp J, Sabri S. Endovascular Management of Visceral Arterial Aneurysms. *Techniques in Vascular and Interventional Radiology*. 2015;18:14–23.
5. Calligaro K, Dougherty M. Renovascular Disease: Aneurysms and Arteriovenous Fistulae. In: Cronenwett J, Johnston KW, eds. *Rutherford's Vascular Surgery*. 8th ed. Philadelphia: Saunders; 2014:2326–2344.

29

Mesenteric Embolization: Solid Organ, Pelvic Trauma, and GI Bleeding

Dolly Thakkar Doshi, MD, FVIR and Michael D. Dake, MD, FSIR, FCIRSE

INTRODUCTION

The common goal of catheter-based embolization procedures is to cease the flow of blood mechanically in a particular vessel or vascular territory using either a temporary or permanent agent. In the history of interventional radiology, embolization has an established key role as a frequently used, clinically valuable, and widely applicable endovascular procedure. This is partly a result of its elegance and simplicity as a minimally invasive technique capable of achieving impressive life-saving results.

Untreated or unapparent arterial hemorrhage constitutes one of the most preventable causes of death in abdominal and pelvic trauma.[1] Recent advances in noninvasive imaging and interventional angiography have enabled earlier identification of critical arterial hemorrhage to facilitate prompt and precise endovascular treatments that yield improved outcomes compared with historical results from past decades. Now it is not only identified early, but also treated promptly and with great precision.

Technological advances of computed tomography (CT), CT angiography (CTA), have indispensably replaced the conventional diagnostic angiography to evaluate the cause and pinpoint the site of vascular injury. Currently, laparotomy has been replaced from the first line of management for hemodynamically stable patients, because CTA and nonoperative management have shown favorable benefits. Arterial embolization is now an irreplaceable component of primary resuscitation, more so with further breakthroughs in endovascular techniques.[2–5]

The key for successful embolization lies in mastering a thorough knowledge of the available equipment/materials and applying it appropriately. (Fig. 29.1 lists the various embolization materials available currently.)

In this chapter, we present the necessary inventory currently used for delivery of different embolization materials, the relevant tricks of the trade for their optimal use and tips to avoid adverse effects. Most importantly, we shall discuss how to recover once a mistake or complication occurs during the course of an embolization procedure.

PARTICLE EMBOLIZATION (GELFOAM AND POLYVINYL ALCOHOL)

Procedure Recommendations: The Dos and Don'ts

Ideally, it is best to prepare a separate embolization table distinct from the standard procedural set-up for catheters, guidewires, etc., with two distinct bowls of saline and contrast. Use small syringes (<5 mL) for embolization and specifically mark them as "embolization" or "particles". After selective catheterization, always ensure optimal catheter positioning prior to embolization by performing a test injection of contrast to assess the potential for reflux of embolic material into nontarget areas.

Magnify the field of view to focus on the target region, collimate the borders, and under constant fluoroscopic guidance begin to slowly inject particles in a series of small puff-like injections, using the same pressure for each. Commonly, particles and Gelfoam have a tendency to aggregate and to form a clump at the junction of the tip of the syringe and the hub of the catheter. This may form a plug and result in catheter occlusion. Plug formation can be prevented by flushing the catheter after each syringe of particles injected to ensure a purged or clean catheter that is free from any residual embolization material. The key to this technique is to continue flushing normal saline until the operator no longer visualizes the opacified agent and there is free flow of saline with minimal injection force.

Occasionally, operators may encounter sudden and/or increased resistance during embolization. In this situation, a common mistake is to forcefully flush large volumes of saline with increasingly higher pressure in a vigorous attempt to clear the blocked catheter. This forceful maneuver may lead to an explosive and uncontrolled dislodgement of embolization agent into nontarget area(s) as the obstruction is relieved. Encountering such resistance is common, and it can be better addressed by injecting small aliquots of saline using a 1-mL syringe.

It is important to remember that as embolization with particles or Gelfoam progresses, the speed and dynamics of vascular flow change. Peripheral flow in distal small vessels becomes progressively stagnant, and further embolization can lead to reflux into nontarget vessels, proximal to the catheter tip. Approaching the end of the embolization process, it is critical to recognize that the catheter system is still full of the embolization agent and large puffs of contrast or saline, even during catheter withdrawal, can cause accidental nontarget embolization of other organs.

Special care should be taken while performing postembolization arteriography to avoid any inadvertent use of embolization syringes, because residual particles can transiently adhere to the wall and/or hubs of syringes. Similarly, it is a good precautionary practice following embolization to aspirate and to discard one syringe of blood before performing a completion arteriogram.

Temporary Agent—Gelfoam—Properties and Uses

Gelfoam is a water-soluble, readily available, temporary embolic agent supplied as a powder or pad that can be easily prepared for transcatheter use. Postembolization, it is completely absorbed by the body with an arterial vascular recanalization time of 2–3 weeks.[6] Gelfoam is available in powder form with a particle size of 40 to 60 μm, which is preferable for distal capillary-level embolization. Alternatively, a slurry of Gelfoam is prepared by scrapping the sponge in a bowl of contrast or chopping out 1- to 2-mm cubes with scissors from a larger pad and then mixing

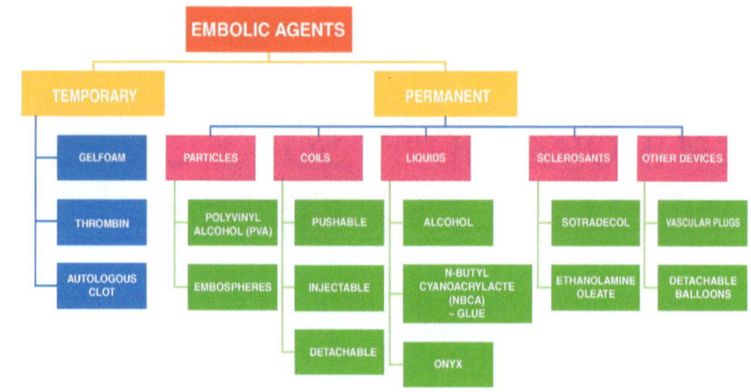

Fig. 29.1 Various embolization materials.

them with contrast to attain a size variation of 500 and 2000 μm. A microcatheter with a relatively large lumen of 0.027–0.028″ is generally recommended for delivery of the agent is this form.

A single large piece or "torpedo" of Gelfoam can be used for proximal embolization, but difficult catheter loading and catheter occlusion are potential disadvantages, especially when using catheters with an internal diameter of less than 0.035″. The most distinctive characteristic of Gelfoam is its rapid absorbability by macrophages, thus restoring vascular patency in a relatively short timeframe of a few days to weeks.[7]

Semipermanent Agents: Properties and Uses

The most commonly used embolic particles include polyvinyl alcohol (PVA), tris-acryl gelatin microspheres (TAGM), and hydrogel particles. These work on the same principle as Gelfoam, with the main difference being the uniformity of particle size and the property to cause permanent or semipermanent vessel occlusion. They can lead to occlusion either by mechanical obstruction or by clinging to the vessel wall and inciting an inflammatory response. It is not uncommon during embolization to develop a conglomerate or clustered mixture of particles within the catheter hub that impedes further injection. This can be avoided by preparing the agent with the use of a ≥50% contrast mix with saline and constant agitation of the injection syringes with frequent resuspension of particles. Of note, over-diluting contrast with too much saline will make fluoroscopic visualization more difficult, especially in obese patients or when motion artefacts are encountered.

- PVA particles (Contour SE Boston Scientific, Natick, Massachusetts) are uniformly-sized particles available in calibrated vials of specific size ranges, with the smallest spanning from 100 to 300 μm and the largest from 900 to 1200 μm.
- TAGM spheres or Embospheres (Biosphere Medical, Rockland, Massachusetts) are uniformly spherical-shaped spheres produced from acrylic polymer matrix impregnated with porcine gelatin and coated with a hydrophilic surface, which prevents aggregation.
- Bead block microspheres (Biocompatibles, distributed by Terumo, Somerset, New Jersey) are made of biocompatible microporous PVA hydrogel and behave more like the TAGM particles than PVA particles. They exhibit good flexibility and compressibility, which facilitates smooth injection and allows them to be tightly packed as they are capable of undergoing 20% to 30% deformation.
- Embozene microspheres (CeloNova Biosciences, Newnan, Georgia) are highly compressible hydrogel spheres coated with Polyzene to provide a lubricious outer covering. These newer agents are color-coded and available in relatively narrow size distributions, with an average diameter range of 50 μm within each size offering. They are available over a wide range of diameters starting at 40, 100, 250, 400 μm up to the largest size of 900 μm.
- QuadraSpheres (Biosphere Medical, Rockland, Massachusetts) are polyvinyl alcohol sodium acrylate spheres that feature the distinct property of size expansion when the spheres contact blood, nonionic contrast, or saline. They have an expansion capacity of up to four times their original dry state nominal diameter within a short span of about 10 minutes, resulting in increased surface area. This enables tighter packing between spheres and facilitates near-total luminal occlusion. At present, these are predominantly used for drug delivery in hepatocellular carcinoma and uterine fibroids.

Postembolization Complications

Multiple studies have described an increased complication rate of rebleeding following Gelfoam embolization of traumatic abdominal and pelvic hemorrhage, despite arteriographic documentation of hemostasis upon completion of the procedure.[7–11] Alternatively, the opposite effect can occur with overly aggressive embolization when a Gelfoam slurry occludes an entire segment of a mesenteric vessel and prevents any re-entry of blood through proximal or distal collateral pathways leading to target organ infarction.[12,13] Additionally, on occasion it is possible for aerobic organisms to multiply in the retained air bubbles, with promoted infection and abscess formation.[14] This complication is typically managed by administration of appropriate antibiotic therapy.

COIL EMBOLIZATION

Procedure Recommendations: The Dos and Don'ts

The first step begins with choosing the desired diameter of the wire element composing the coil and a compatible catheter system. The selection is based on a number of factors including size and location of vessel at the site of coil deposition, but paying special attention to correctly matching the chosen coil with a delivery catheter is critical to prevent complications, such as getting a coil stuck within the catheter. Standard coils require a 0.035″ or 0.038″ inner diameter catheter lumen while microcoils require anywhere from a 0.010″, 0.014″, 0.018″, to a 0.021″ microcatheter lumen for deployment.

It is always standard policy to use an end-hole catheter rather than a catheter with side holes, because a coil may wedge a side hole and prevent advancement beyond the catheter tip. Of note, coils will not deploy through side holes.

Difficult coil delivery, failed deployment, or deployment in an unwanted area can occur when a mismatched delivery catheter is used with a sufficiently oversized luminal diameter for the selected coil platform diameter. As a result, the wire or pusher used to advance the coil can override the proximal end of the coil, resulting in jamming within the oversized catheter lumen. In cases when such an inadvertent event occurs and a coil becomes stuck in the catheter, it is always best to withdraw the "coil in catheter" system together and re-engage with an appropriate fresh catheter via an introducer sheath. As a rule, angiographic introducer sheaths should always be used in embolization procedures to maintain arterial access to the branch with smaller catheters to the site for embolization, in the event of an untoward event, such as a partial or failed coil deployment. This avoids loss of access site and wasted time.

It is crucial to size the vessel correctly at the point where the coil is to be placed. Coils should be sized according to the vessel size. Soft coils can be oversized by 20%–30%, but stiff coils allow less than 1 mm of oversizing, otherwise they tend to remain elongated in a sinusoidal form once deployed. A very large or oversized coil can kick back the catheter during deployment, whereas a coil that is too small and undersized will fly off and migrate distally.

Upon loading a coil into the delivery catheter, it is necessary to ensure an end-to-end snug approximation of the catheter hub with the coil-loading cartridge to avoid inadvertent premature coil deployment in the catheter hub that typically causes catheter occlusion and coil damage. It is important to use coil pushers that are specifically provided for delivery of compatible microcoils through recommended microcatheters. Another commonly encountered problem is recoil of the catheter during coil deployment that results in unintended nontarget deployment. The potential for this may be assessed using the wire test method. This simply involves advancing a few centimeters of the guidewire or pusher selected for coil advancement and watching for push-back of the catheter tip. If no tip displacement is observed, it suggests a stable catheter position that will support accurate coil placement. If a kick-back of the catheter tip is noted during the wire test, it is a good idea to obtain a more stable catheter position by advancing distally or by switching to a co-axial catheter system to insure precise deployment accuracy and the support to obtain dense packing of coils, if desired. If the coil is still kicking back the parent system, use a firm grip to hold the system in place and use a stiffer wire pusher for deployment. If the problem persists, the key lies in using a shorter and smaller coil to resolve the issue. If catheter stability is questionable in critical areas where pinpoint accuracy is essential, detachable coils can be used to assure accurate deployment.

The complication of recanalization of previously coiled vessels can be prevented by creating a compact packing or nesting of coils. This can be achieved by using the scaffold technique or the anchor technique. In the scaffold technique, a large stiff coil is placed initially, followed by a dense packing with softer coils within the larger framing coil. The anchor technique involves placing the initial segment of a coil in a small branch vessel to provide good anchorage to the coil and a foundation to secure subsequent coils to form a dense coil nest. Usually it takes less than 5 minutes to attain complete thrombosis once a tight coil mass has been created. Sometimes, operators are concerned when persistent flow is observed through the embolized vessel immediately after coil placement, but predictably with patience and time, a focal coil pack will induce thrombosis and vessel occlusion within a few minutes.

Experience and expertise are necessary for deploying coils that are pushed effectively and without mishap, as they cannot be withdrawn or repositioned easily like detachable coils. If these coils migrate or are misplaced, it may be necessary to retrieve them promptly using a snare or similar retrieval device. If inadvertently a coil is partially left inside the catheter with the most of its length already deployed, then, as an initial maneuver, the coil–catheter combination can be pushed forward as a system to try to re-engage the target site and complete deployment. Detachable coil systems are ideal for controlled release of coils and for accurate embolization in complex anatomical situations. These coils are designed to address the concerns associated with coils that can be pushed and to enable testing coil formations and placement accuracy within the target site prior to release. Although considerably more expensive than coils that can be pushed, detachable coil systems provide interventionalists with the confidence of knowing that a coil may be tested, retrieved, and retested as many times as necessary in order to achieve the desired configuration, and only then is a commitment to deployment made.

Postembolization Complications

The most commonly encountered complication of coil embolization for abdominal/pelvic hemorrhage is rebleeding secondary to coil migration. Distal migration of a coil, for example, in cases of splenic artery embolization, may also be complicated by resultant ischemia, infarction, and infection. This is decreased by the correct sizing of coils. Occasionally, if unresponsive to antibiotic administration, this can necessitate splenectomy.[15–19]

LIQUID EMBOLIZATION AGENTS

Absolute alcohol or other sclerosing agents are not used in mesenteric embolization because they result in tissue necrosis. Successful embolization of abdominal or pelvic hemorrhage, irrespective of a patient's coagulation status, can be achieved by using N-butyl cyanoacrylate or glue (Trufill NBCA, Cordis Neurovascular, Fremont, California) or ethylene vinyl alcohol copolymer or Onyx (Medtronic Inc., Minneapolis, Minnesota).

N-butyl cyanoacrylate or glue is a fast-acting, life-saving, effective, and safe embolic material with multiple benefits.[20] It is mixed with an iodized oil such as lipiodol in varying rations of 1:1 to 1:3 depending on the viscosity desired to account most effectively for the blood flow and position of the catheter tip relative to the intended site of vessel occlusion.[21] When in contact with blood, it undergoes fast polymerization and leads to complete hemostasis. Catheter occlusion is a challenge that many interventionalists face during their first few experiences with glue embolization. The risk of this complication can be mitigated by using a meticulous technique and by following basic guidelines such as careful flushing of all catheter system components with 5% dextrose solution prior to glue injection to prevent premature polymerization of NBCA in the catheter.

Ethylene vinyl alcohol copolymer (EVOH) or Onyx is a nonadhesive liquid embolic agent dissolved in dimethyl sulfoxide (DMSO) and suspended in micronized tantalum powder to provide contrast for better fluoroscopic visualization. The kit contains a 1.5-mL vial of Onyx, 1.5-mL vial of DMSO, and three 1-mL Onyx delivery syringes. A DMSO compatible delivery microcatheter is required (Marathon, Rebar, or Ultraflow HPC catheters) to gain access to the embolization site.[22] Two forms of Onyx are available: Onyx 18 and Onyx 34. Onyx 18 is less viscous and is therefore capable of traveling more distally from the catheter tip to an intended site of occlusion.

Slow injection under fluoroscopic control through a microcatheter is required to allow maximum control during the infusion. Unlike glue, it does not have adhesive properties when in contact with arterial walls but instead relies upon filling up the lumen to achieve its effect. Following embolization, it does not adhere to the vascular endothelium and thus, as opposed to glue, reflux along the catheter during injection does not cause permanent adhesion of the catheter to the vessel.

If a long segment of microcatheter is within a tortuous artery leading to the embolization site, it could make catheter removal difficult. This situation results as a consequence of mechanical trapping rather than adhesion of the catheter, and slow gradual traction is the key to safe microcatheter withdrawal. If further difficulties exist with withdrawal, use of a wire in the catheter is also advised to decrease the risk of avulsion.[23] Occasionally vasospasm occurs as a result of overuse of DMSO to prepare the microcatheter preliminarily and purge its lumen.[24] It is always best to inject only the volume of DMSO calibrated to match the specified dead space of the microcatheter lumen. This is performed in a slow, controlled manner, never to exceed a maximum dose of 200 mg/kg. The injection rate should not exceed 0.3 mL/min. Vigilance is always needed throughout the course of Onyx embolization to avoid its passage into nontarget areas.

High cost and the need for comprehensive expertise in handling complications related to the flow of liquid embolic agents into nontarget areas are the major limitations restricting more widespread use of glue and onyx for embolization.[25]

OCCLUSION DEVICES

Amplatz vascular plugs (AVPs) are thrombogenic occlusion devices, consisting of bare-metal nitinol mesh configurations, typically oversized by 30%–50% of the luminal diameter when placed at the desired site of occlusion. After placing a guiding sheath or catheter at the target location, these plugs are easily deployed by unsheathing and then releasing a screw attachment mechanism. One notable advantage is that they can be resheathed if not in an ideal position after initial unsheathing, and then redeployed and simply detached by counterclockwise rotation of the delivery cable once in the preferred position. These devices are recommended for the occlusion of appropriate medium and larger vessels, such as renal or splenic arteries, where standard coils would pose the risk of accidental misplacement, unwanted migration, or ineffective embolization.[26] Although a plug is much more expensive than a coil, its use as a solitary embolization device has made it handy and a favored choice for instantaneous use when compared with the cost and relative inefficiency of deploying multiple coils. One major challenge to the application of vascular plugs in cases of hemorrhage is the inability to navigate a relatively stiff device through tortuous vasculature to the desired site of embolization. These vascular plugs are available in various shapes and a wide variety of sizes to suit a range of vascular anatomies.

MVP Microvascular Plug System (Medtronic Inc, Bloomington, Minnesota) is a thrombogenic occlusion device that can be advanced using a 5-French catheter. Similar to the Amplatzer plug, these are more expensive than coils and can be used for similar applications.

Covered stents, unlike other embolization agents, maintain the flow pathway while providing hemostasis when there has been a traumatic injury to a relatively large (>5 mm diameter), straight, nonbranched proximal arterial segment. Their use has already been established in hepatic, splenic, renal, and iliac arteries to effectively manage traumatic hemorrhage, pseudoaneurysm, and fistula and iatrogenic traumatic injuries in the abdomen and pelvis.[27–29]

Standard complications associated with the use of a metal stent, such as kinking, deformation, dislodgement, and occlusion, can all occur. In addition, it is critical to choose appropriate anatomy when considering a covered stent to avoid graft occlusion of vital uninvolved side branches.

CONCLUSION

Various embolization agents such as coils, Gelfoam pledgets, liquid embolics, vascular plugs, or a combination of these can be selected to endovascularly treat most causes of mesenteric hemorrhage, traumatic solid organ injury and pelvic bleeding. These agents provide good proximal occlusion effectively and may also be used in sandwich technique, typically in regions of potential collateralization, to secure a successful outcome.[6] As an extremely versatile endovascular procedure, the benefits of transcatheter embolization techniques are well-established.

Unfortunately, with the variety of applications and innovations in embolization comes a wide range of potential complications that are difficult to summarize and easily classify. A strong foundation in arterial anatomy, good knowledge of angiographic techniques, access to a wide variety of the available embolic agents, and sound procedural judgment are all important prerequisites to ensure interventionalists are optimally prepared to face the various challenges that occur during embolization of abdominal/pelvic bleeding, to avoid the recognized complications, and to manage any untoward outcomes thus limiting clinical harm.

REFERENCES

1. Zealley IA, Chakraverty S. The role of interventional radiology in trauma. *BMJ*. 2010;340:c497.
2. Velmahos GC, Toutouzas KG, Vassiliu P, et al. A prospective study on the safety and efficacy of angiographic embolization for pelvic and visceral injuries. *J Trauma*. 2002;53:303–308.
3. Nijhof HW, Willemssen FE, Jukema GN. Transcatheter arterial embolization in a hemodynamically unstable patient with grade IV blunt liver injury: is nonsurgical management an option? *Emerg Radiol*. 2006;12:111–115.
4. Tanizaki S, Maeda S, Hayashi H, et al. Early embolization without external fixation in pelvic trauma. *Am J Emerg Med*. 2011;30:342–346.
5. Monnin V, Sengel C, Thony F, et al. Place of arterial embolization in severe blunt hepatic trauma: a multidisciplinary approach. *Cardiovasc Intervent Radiol*. 2008;31:875–882.
6. Konez O. Medscape Reference. Vascular Lesion Embolization Imaging 2011. Available at http://emedicine.medscape.com/article/419614-overview.
7. Franco F, Monaco D, Volpi A, Marcato C, Larini P, Rossi C. The role of arterial embolization in blunt splenic injury. *Radiol Med*. 2011;116:454–465.
8. Liu PP, Lee WC, Cheng YF, et al. Use of splenic artery embolization as an adjunct to nonsurgical management of blunt splenic injury. *J Trauma*. 2004;56:768–773.
9. Smith HE, Biffl WL, Majercik SD, Jednacz J, Lambiase R, Cioffi WG. Splenic artery embolization: have we gone too far? *J Trauma*. 2006;61:541–546.
10. Jander HP, Russinovich NA. Transcatheter gelfoam embolization in abdominal, retroperitoneal, and pelvic hemorrhage. *Radiology*. 1980;136:337–344.
11. Omert LA, Salyer D, Dunham CM, Porter J, Silva A, Protetch J. Implications of the "contrast blush" finding on computed tomographic scan of the spleen in trauma. *J Trauma*. 2001;51:272–278.
12. Wu SC, Chow KC, Lee KH, Tung CC, Yang AD, Lo CJ. Early selective angioembolization improves success of nonoperative management of blunt splenic injury. *Am Surgeon*. 2007;73:897–902.
13. Sclafani SJ, Shaftan GW, Scalea TM, et al. Nonoperative salvage of computed tomography—diagnosed splenic injuries: utilization of angiography for triage and embolization for hemostasis. *J Trauma*. 1995;39:818–827.
14. Abada HT, Golzarian J. Gelatine sponge particles: handling characteristics for endovascular use. *Tech Vasc Interv Radiol*. 2007;10:257–260.
15. Dasgupta N, Matsumoto AH, Arslan B, Turba UC, Sabri S, Angle JF. Embolization therapy for traumatic splenic lacerations. *Cardiovasc Intervent Radiol*. 2012;35:795–806.
16. Ekeh AP, Khalaf S, Ilyas S, Kauffman S, Walusimbi M, McCarthy MC. Complications arising from splenic artery embolization: a review of an 11-year experience. *Am J Surg*. 2013;205:250–254.
17. Haan JM, Biffl W, Knudson MM, et al. Splenic embolization revisited: a multicenter review. *J Trauma*. 2004;56:542–547.
18. Ekeh AP, McCarthy MC, Woods RJ, Haley E. Complications arising from splenic embolization after blunt splenic trauma. *Am J Surg*. 2005;189:335–339.
19. Bessoud B, Duchosal MA, Siegrist CA, et al. Proximal splenic artery embolization for blunt splenic injury: clinical, immunologic, and ultrasound-Doppler follow-up. *J Trauma*. 2007;62:1481–1486.
20. Jae HJ, Chung JW, Jung AY, Lee W, Park JH. Transcatheter arterial embolization of nonvariceal upper gastrointestinal bleeding with N-butyl cyanoacrylate. *Korean J Radiol*. 2007;8(1):48–56.
21. Parildar M, Oran I, Memis A. Embolization of visceral pseudoaneurysms with platinum coils and N-butyl cyanoacrylate. *Abdom Imaging*. 2003; 28(1):36–40.

22. Simon SD, Reig AS, Archer KJ, Mericle RA. Biomechanical attributes of microcatheters used in liquid embolization of intracranial aneurysms. *J Neurointerv Surg.* 2012;4:211–214.
23. Walcott BP, Gerrard JL, Nogueira RG, Nahed BV, Terry AR, Ogilvy CS. Microsurgical retrieval of an endovascular microcatheter trapped during Onyx embolization of a cerebral arteriovenous malformation. *J Neurointerv Surg.* 2011;3:77–79.
24. Lv X, Li Y, Jiang C, Wu Z. The incidence of trigeminocardiac reflex in endovascular treatment of dural arteriovenous fistula with Onyx. *Interv Neuroradiol.* 2010;16:59–63.
25. Mavili E, Donmez H, Ozcan N, Akcali Y. Endovascular treatment of lower limb penetrating arterial traumas. *Cardiovasc Intervent Radiol.* 2007;30:1124–1129.
26. Widlus DM, Moeslein FM, Richard HM III. Evaluation of the Amplatzer vascular plug for proximal splenic artery embolization. *J Vasc Interv Radiol.* 2008;19:652–656.
27. Burdick TR, Hoffer EK, Kooy T, et al. Which arteries are expendable? The practice and pitfalls of embolization throughout the body. *Semin Intervent Radiol.* 2008;25:191–203.
28. Parodi JC, Schönholz C, Ferreira LM, Bergan J. Endovascular stent-graft treatment of traumatic arterial lesions. *Ann Vasc Surg.* 1999;13:121–129.
29. Piffaretti G, Tozzi M, Lomazzi C, et al. Endovascular treatment for traumatic injuries of the peripheral arteries following blunt trauma. *Injury.* 2007;38:1091–1097.

30

Complications in Angioplasty and Stenting of Mesenteric and Renal Artery Disease

Tiziano Tallarita, MD, Emanuel R. Tenorio, MD, PhD, Jussi M. Kärkkäinen, MD, PhD and Gustavo S. Oderich, MD

INTRODUCTION

Chronic mesenteric ischemia (CMI) is a relatively uncommon disorder, accounting for <1 per 100,000 hospital admissions in the United States. Prophylactic revascularization is not recommended in patients with either renal or mesenteric artery disease. Treatment is indicated in select patients who present with symptoms of chronic mesenteric ischemia, such as intestinal angina, weight loss, and fear of eating. This occurs because of the after-meal pain associated with the condition. The combination of angioplasty and stenting has become the first line of treatment and is associated with lower mortality and morbidity compared with open surgical reconstruction. Open surgical reconstruction is currently relegated to patients who are not candidates or fail endovascular therapy and those with recalcitrant, recurrent in-stent stenosis, or occlusion.[1] The aim of this chapter is to summarize the most common intraprocedural and postoperative complications of mesenteric angioplasty and stenting for mesenteric and renal artery disease.

MESENTERIC ANGIOPLASTY AND STENTING

Selection of open versus endovascular approach is based on careful review of preprocedure computed tomography angiography and clinical risk. The superior mesenteric artery (SMA) is the primary target for revascularization and, as such, the anatomy of the SMA is the most important determinant of choice of therapy. The ideal lesion for angioplasty and stenting is a short, focal stenosis or occlusion with minimal to moderate calcification or thrombus, but interventions can be indicated in patients with more complex lesions. Celiac axis angioplasty and stenting carries a higher risk of restenosis[2] and should not be performed if there is active compression by the median arcuate ligament, unless this has been surgically released. Intraprocedural complications may occur more frequently with severely calcified lesions and occlusions.[3]

INTRAOPERATIVE COMPLICATIONS

Despite the minimally invasive approach, mesenteric angioplasty and stent placement carry a risk of significant morbidity. The rate of intraoperative complications is poorly reported in the literature.[4–7] Our group reported intraoperative complications in 18% of the patients[8], including residual stenosis in 9%, stent dislodgement or dissection in 5% each, and vessel occlusion, perforation, or mesenteric hematoma in <1%–2%. Distal embolization occurs in 8% of patients treated by SMA stenting without embolic protection, with higher rates among patients with subacute symptoms, occlusion, long lesions (>30 mm), and severe calcification. Finally, access-related complications range between 3% and 16%.[3]

Access-Related Complications

Brachial approach offers excellent access in patients with acute angles at the vessel origin, occlusions, or long lesions. Nevertheless, brachial punctures are more prone to access-related complications, including potentially disabling neuropraxia of the median nerve from developing hematoma.[3]

Branch Perforation and Mesenteric Hematoma

Branch perforations may result from inadvertent catheter manipulations or excessive guidewire advancement into small branches. Therefore, the guidewire should ideally be placed in the main trunk of the SMA and should be visualized at all times (Fig. 30.1).

Dissections and Thrombosis

Problems such as dissections (Fig. 30.2) may also occur with small or larger profile devices. Excessive catheter and guidewire manipulation, fragile vessel wall or excessive dilatation, or oversizing of the stent can all cause dissection. Dissections occur more frequently adjacent to the distal edge of the stent, but also distally or within side branches. It is important to maintain guidewire access, which facilitates management. If the origin and extension of dissection is unclear, intravascular ultrasound helps identify the entry and end-point. Treatment can be done by distal extension using self-expandable stent (Fig. 30.2), avoiding dilatation. If guidewire access has been lost, management can be difficult. If the dissection is flow-limiting, regaining access to the true lumen can be attempted and then stenting can be continued. However, if the main trunk is occluded and guidewire access cannot be achieved, open surgical revision is necessary (Fig. 30.3). In these cases, proximal control can be obtained by balloon inflation, the dissection flap is excised and the arteriotomy is closed over a patch (Fig. 30.3). Less frequently, bypass may be necessary.

Stent Dislodgement, Fracture, and Compression

The incidence of stent dislodgement has been reported up to 8% in the past[8] with hand-mounted stents but is now rare; dislodgement can also be caused by incorrect measurement of the target diameter and stent downsizing. This complication can occur with covered stents (stent slippage) or in patients with recalcitrant lesions that are prone to "watermelon seed" the stent (Fig. 30.4) during deployment. It is critical to maintain guidewire access. The stent can be locked with a balloon and relocated into a normal arterial segment within the mesenteric or iliac arteries. Finally, the SMA lesion can be restented. If access has been lost, the stent can be compressed against the arterial by placement of a second stent.

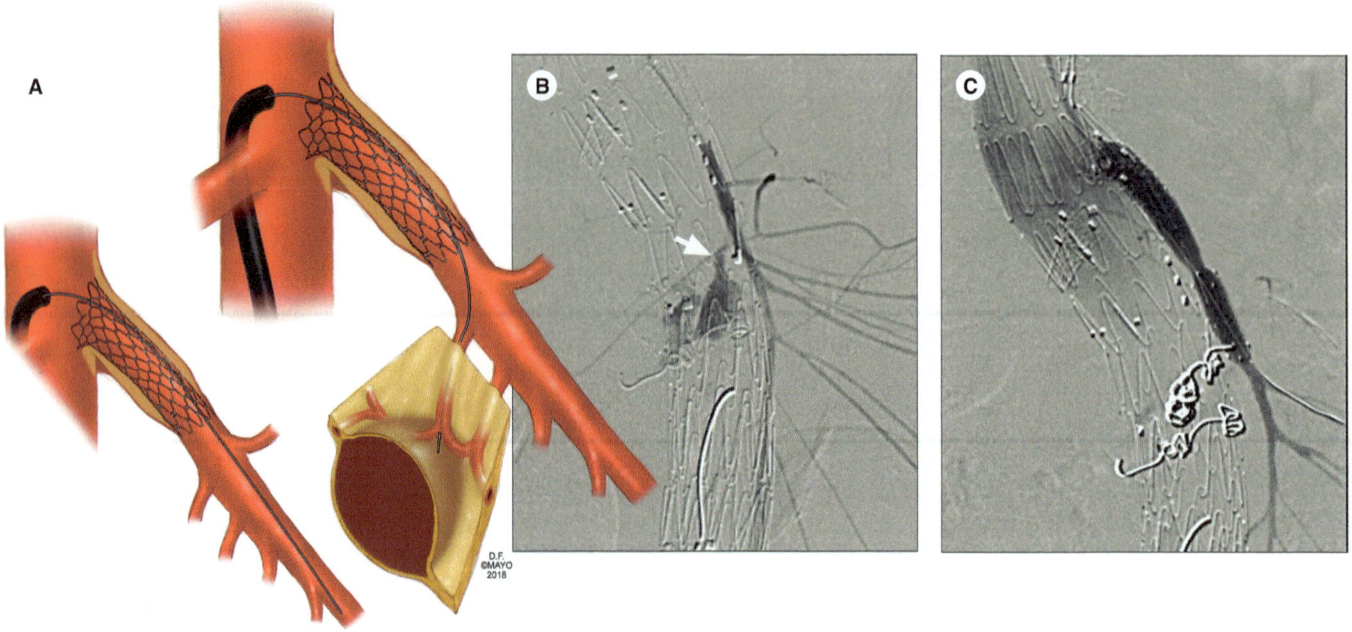

Fig. 30.1 (A) Jejunal branch perforation during superior mesenteric artery (SMA) angioplasty and stenting. (B) Angiography of the SMA showing contrast extravasation of a jejunal branch *(white arrow)*. (C) Angiography of the SMA showing no contrast extravasation after selective embolization using 0.038″ coils and angioplasty with covered stent of the branch origin.

Stent fracture is an uncommon cause of recurrent stenosis or occlusion (Fig. 30.5); stent fractures have been well documented in other areas and are more prevalent in arteries that cross flexion points, such as the popliteal artery. Flow-limiting stent fractures can often be addressed endovascularly.

Stent compression or in-folding can be seen in patients treated by fenestrated endografts, or when the delivery system of the aortic device compresses the leaflets of a balloon expandable stent (Figs. 30.6 and 30.7). Reballooning the stent or overlap address the issue.

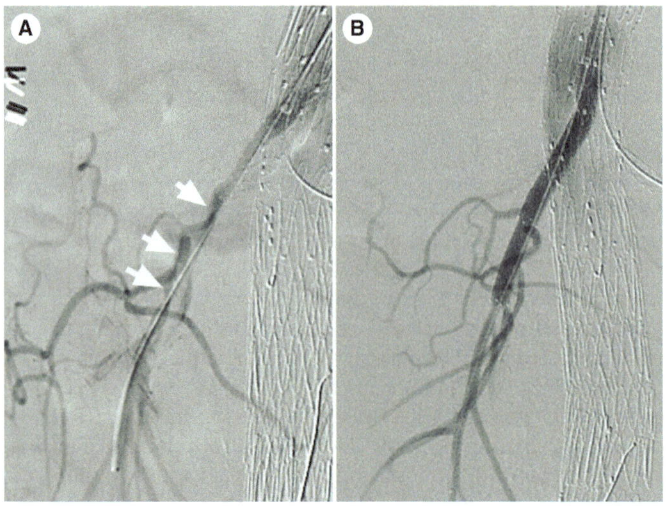

Fig. 30.2 (A) Angiography showing dissection of the middle third of the superior mesenteric artery *(white arrows)* during fenestrated-branched endovascular repair. (B) Angioplasty was performed with self-expandable stent with resolution of the dissection.

Embolization

Endovascular interventions carry a relatively low risk of visceral vessels embolization. However, the embolic event can result in life-threatening complications or permanent disability. Use of a filter may decrease the incidence of distal emboli, especially in long stenosis or occluded lesions, but does not completely eliminate the risk of it. Embolization can still occur during filter retrieval or formation of debris beyond the embolic protection device (EPD) as a result of stagnant flow or inadequate systemic heparinization. Acute emboli may be treated using plasminogen activator (t-PA), catheter aspiration, intra-arterial nitroglycerin, angioplasty and stenting at the location of the embolization, and retrieval of the embolic material using an EPD or over-the-wire embolectomy (Fig. 30.8). In case of persistent emboli, continuous catheter-directed thrombolysis is considered with multiple checks up to 5 days. However, prolongation of thrombolytic therapy increases the risk of hemorrhagic complications.

Postoperative Medical Complications

The most common medical complications include acute kidney injury in 2% to 8%, acute bowel ischemia in 1% to 7%, gastrointestinal bleeding in 1% to 5%, cardiac events in 1% to 7%, and respiratory complications in 1% to 7%. Mortality is usually related to cardiac events, gastrointestinal bleeding and bowel ischemia. The latter is typically associated with intraprocedural complications such as distal embolization, thrombosis, or dissection.

We recommend admitting patients for observation overnight. Worsening abdominal pain after the procedure is unusual and warrants evaluation to rule out thrombosis, embolization, or a mesenteric

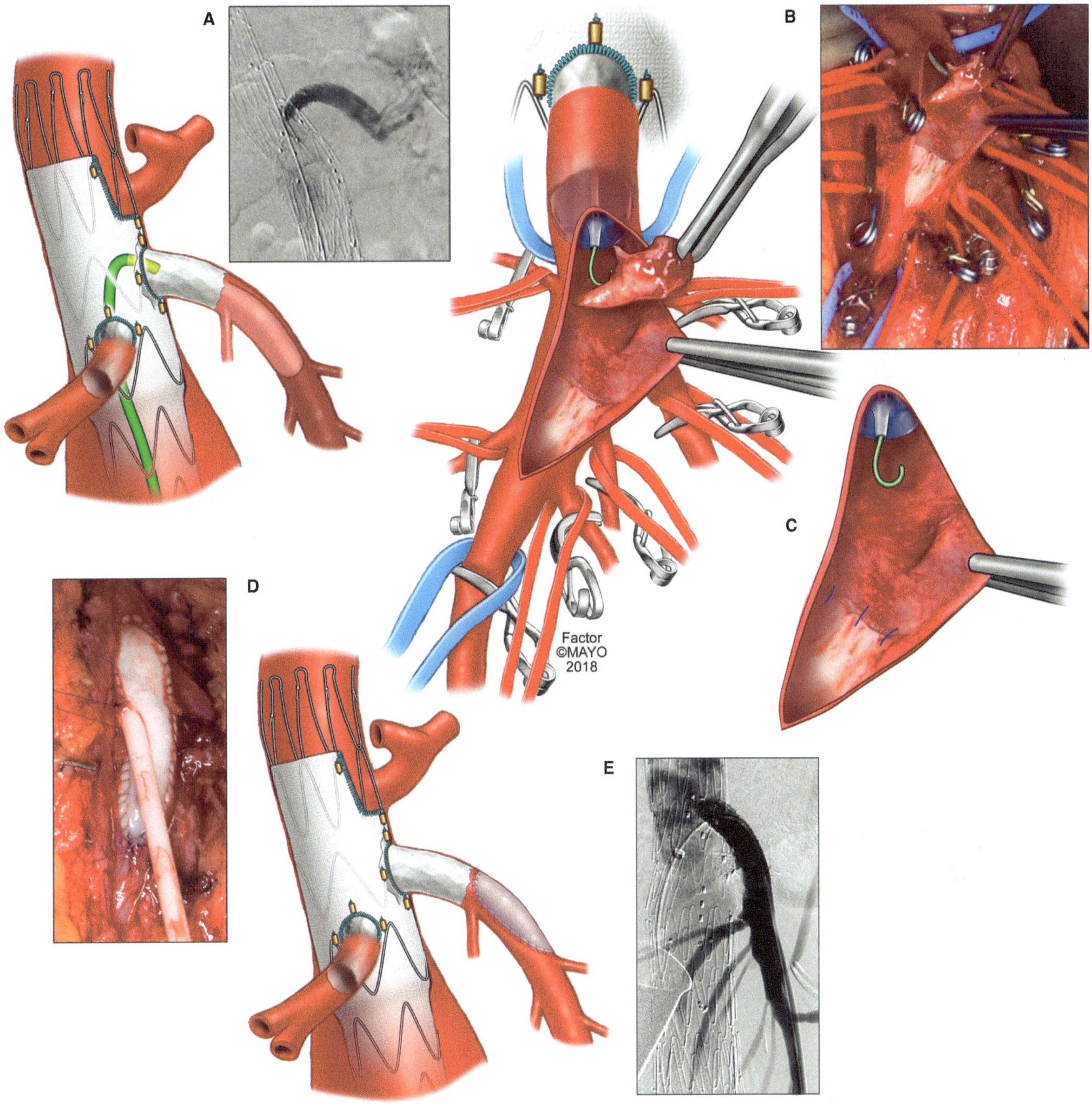

Fig. 30.3 (A) Dissection with occlusion of the mid-distal third of the superior mesenteric artery (SMA) during fenestrated-branched endovascular aortic repair. (B) The SMA was surgically exposed via midline laparotomy, and multiple jejunal side branches were controlled with silastic vessel loops. (C) Longitudinal arteriotomy was performed, with removal of the dissection flap and fixation of the distal intima with 5-0 proline. (D) Angioplasty with bovine pericardial path and retrograde mesenteric stent was performed. (E) Angiography showing patent stent with resolution of prior SMA dissection.

hematoma from jejunal branch perforation. Patients are allowed to resume a regular diet within 6 to 8 hours. Antiplatelet therapy is typically started prior to the intervention with acetylsalicylic acid and continued indefinitely thereafter. Clopidogrel is started the day of the intervention, with a loading dose of 300 mg, and continued for 6 to 8 weeks as a dual antiplatelet agent or indefinitely if a covered stent is used. A duplex ultrasound scan prior to discharge or within the first few days after the procedure serves as a baseline for future comparison. Follow-up includes clinical examination and duplex ultrasound every 6 months during the first year and annually thereafter.

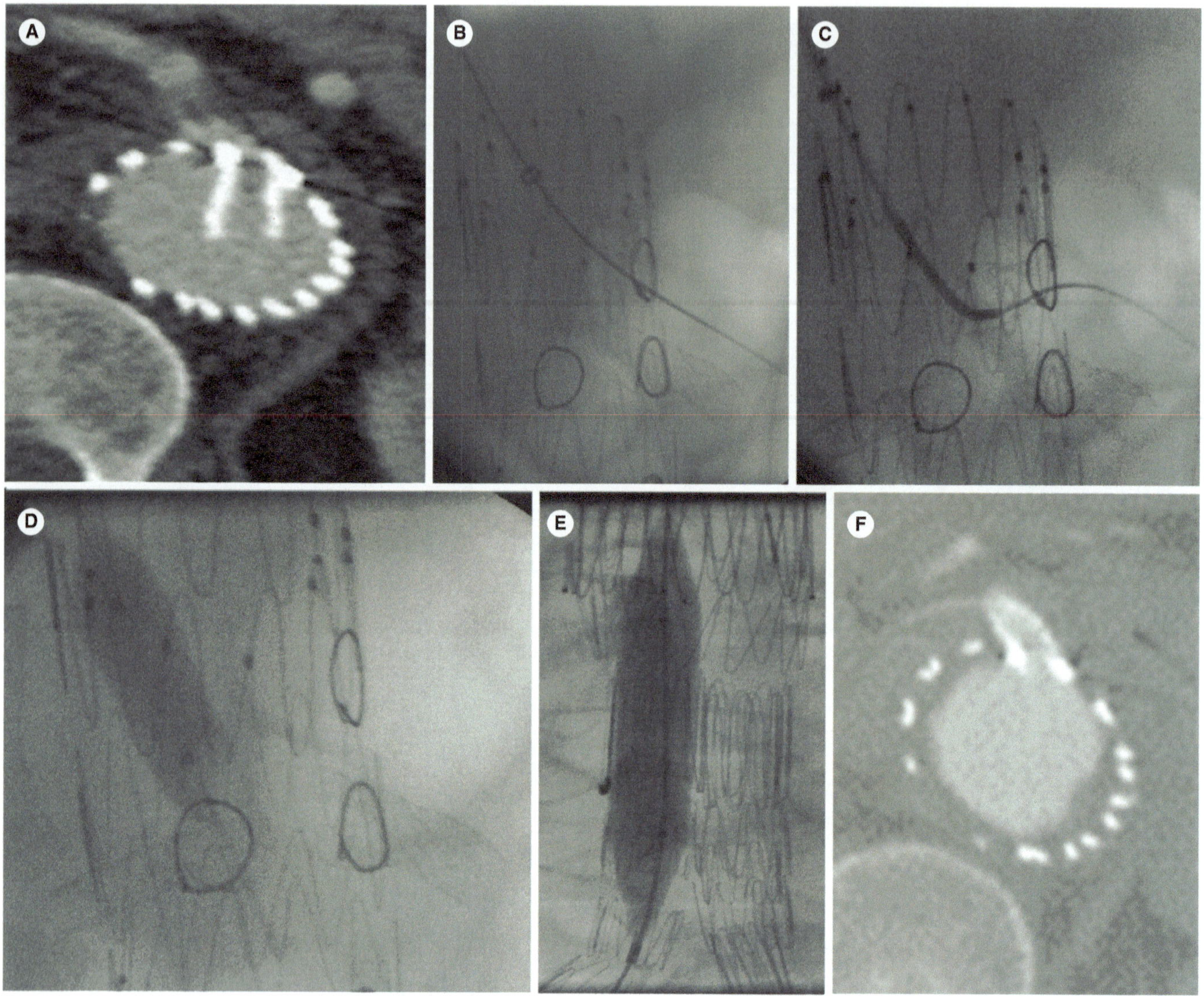

Fig. 30.4 (A) Migration of the celiac stent graft after fenestrated-branched endovascular aortic repair. (B and C) Using a 5-French Kumpe catheter, the celiac stent was selectively catheterized. The Amplatz wire was advanced to the hepatic artery. The stent graft was attached to the celiac artery by only 2 or 3 mm and was almost completely out of the fenestration. (D) A 10-mm balloon was successfully inflated and, with minimal manipulation, the stent graft promptly came out of the celiac artery. (E) This was then carefully moved downward toward the right iliac limb. (E) The balloon-expandable stent was then able to enter the right iliac limb fully and was inflated to 12 mm. (F) Finally, celiac artery re-angioplasty with covered stent was performed.

RENAL ARTERY ANGIOPLASTY AND STENTING

Development of endovascular techniques led to an explosion in renal artery interventions, often with poorly defined indications. It is important that vascular interventionists understand the rationale for disease management and which endovascular techniques should be applied to revascularize renal artery lesions when indicated.

Percutaneous femoral artery access is used in most patients. Brachial or radial artery approach may be needed in select patients with difficult renal artery lesions, particularly if there is caudal angulation or severe aortoiliac occlusive disease.[9–11] The authors prefer using a guide catheter with single or two-wire ("no touch") technique and low profile, rapid exchange system. Predilatation is generally not required and may be associated with microembolization of plaque fragments to the renal parenchyma. The stent should not be oversized and should be positioned across the lesion, with 1 to 3 mm projecting into the aorta for ostial lesions.

INTRAOPERATIVE COMPLICATIONS

Technical success is most commonly defined as residual stenosis of less than 30%, with no evidence of flow-limiting dissection, perforation or branch vessel compromise. A meta-analysis of primary renal artery stenting by Isles[18] and associates documented a technical success rate of 96% to 100%. The most common cause of technical failure is the inability to traverse the lesion with a guidewire in 2% to 5% of patients or inadequate dilatation or coverage of the lesion.[12] The use of stents has resulted in increased technical success (>95%) and improved patency rates when compared with balloon angioplasty alone. Complication rates are low in most reports but can reach up to 36%.

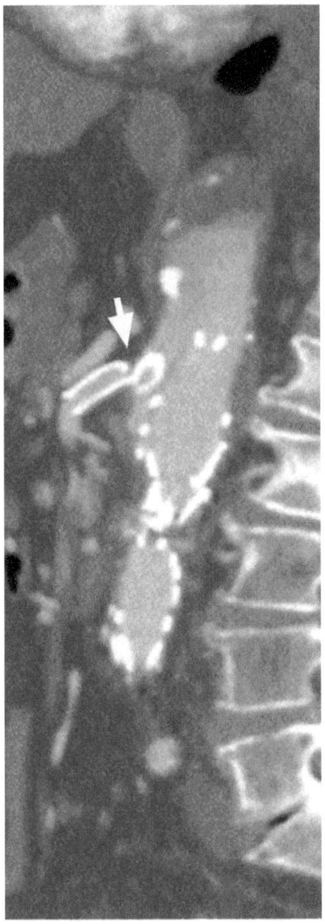

Fig. 30.5 Angiography showing a fracture of the superior mesenteric artery stent *(white arrow)*.

Access-Related Complications

The most common complications are access site hematoma or pseudoaneurysm in approximately 5% of patients. Use of ultrasound during access, avoidance of severely calcified vessels or anterior wall plaque, as well as appropriate reversal of systemic heparinization helps minimize risk. In patients with brachial access, surgical exposure decreases risk of complications because of the higher risk of hematoma and neuropraxia with percutaneous approach.

Perforation and Parenchymal Hematoma

Iatrogenic renal artery or parenchyma perforation (Fig. 30.9) is a well-known complication during endovascular treatment of renal artery stenosis. The risk seems to increase when a high-grade stenosis or occlusion is encountered. In case of tight stenosis or occlusion, a soft-tip hydrophilic guidewire can facilitate crossing the lesion. Hydrophilic tipped-wires may inadvertently perforate small branches if not used with caution. Therefore, we recommend exchanging the wire for a braided 0.014–0.018″ wire as soon as the lesion is crossed and to avoid positioning the wire too deep in the renal branches. Smaller wires in particular can easily perforate the renal capsule, leading to a large perirenal hematoma. Stable, nonexpanding subcapsular, perirenal, or pararenal hematoma can be observed. Covered stents are reserved for perforations of the main trunk; in the case of more distal perforation, embolization of small distal branches can be accomplished with microcoils, preserving as much as possible of the renal parenchyma. Immediate hypotension seen in the case of branch perforation is usually a result of a vasovagal response rather than massive blood loss. Intravascular fluids should be administered. Severe bradycardia and hypotension may be treated with atropine (0.5 mg) if necessary.

Dissections and Thrombosis

Dissection is most common during catheterization of the renal arteries (Fig. 30.10), although it can also result from aggressive angioplasty or stent insertion. It tends to occur more commonly with high-grade or heavily calcified lesions. Non-flow-limiting dissections may be observed, but flow-limiting lesions should be treated by distal extension of the stent. If an unsuccessful endovascular attempt has been made, surgery should be considered if the patient cannot afford to lose the kidney (i.e., single kidney).

Renal artery stent thrombosis is an unfortunate complication that often leads to the loss of the kidney. Unrecognized renal artery dissection can lead to thrombosis. Early detection is key to increase the chance of salvaging the kidney. Thrombosis may be treated by t-PA, mechanical thrombectomy, or stenting. Early stent thrombosis is often a result of technical problems, such as persistent stenosis, dissection, or stent compression.

Stent Dislodgement

Stent dislodgement was more commonly seen with hand-mounted stents and is rare with premounted stents. Precise vessel diameter measurement and better control of stent deployment with gentle "pull-traction" maneuver of the wire and sheath can help in avoiding them.

Embolization

The incidence of symptomatic renal artery embolization varied from 1% to 8%, with renal artery occlusion rates ranging between 0.8% and 2.5%. Embolization of aortic debris can occur during complex endovascular aortic repair (Fig. 30.11). The use of curved-tip catheter can facilitate cannulation of the renal artery but, at the same time, carries intrinsic risk of athero-embolic complications. The "no touch technique" overcomes this issue by using a buddy 0.035″ wire in the aorta and avoiding the tip of the catheter coming in contact with the ostium of the vessel or the suprarenal aorta itself. Modification of this technique with an over-the-wire balloon or microcatheter has also been described. Filter devices can be considered, but they are not commonly used for renal arteries. The filter device needs to traverse the lesion first and this may cause thrombo-embolism.

Postoperative Medical Problems

Large retrospective series (>100 patients) have shown that early mortality and morbidity are 0%–3.7% and 2%–17%, respectively.[11] Davies et al.[10] analyzed 592 renal artery interventions and found that 186 kidneys (31%) suffered >5% loss of total parenchyma, resulting in lower Estimated Glomerular Filtration rate (eGFR) compared with those that did not have parenchyma loss. The procedure-related complication rate did not differ significantly for these two groups, although patients who had renal parenchyma loss did experience more complications (21% versus 16%).

In several randomized trials[13,14], the two most important endpoints of blood pressure control and stabilization or improvement of renal function, for which renal stenting is usually performed, were not statistically better than the control medical group. However, many methodological issues have been attributed to these results, in particular poor patient selection.

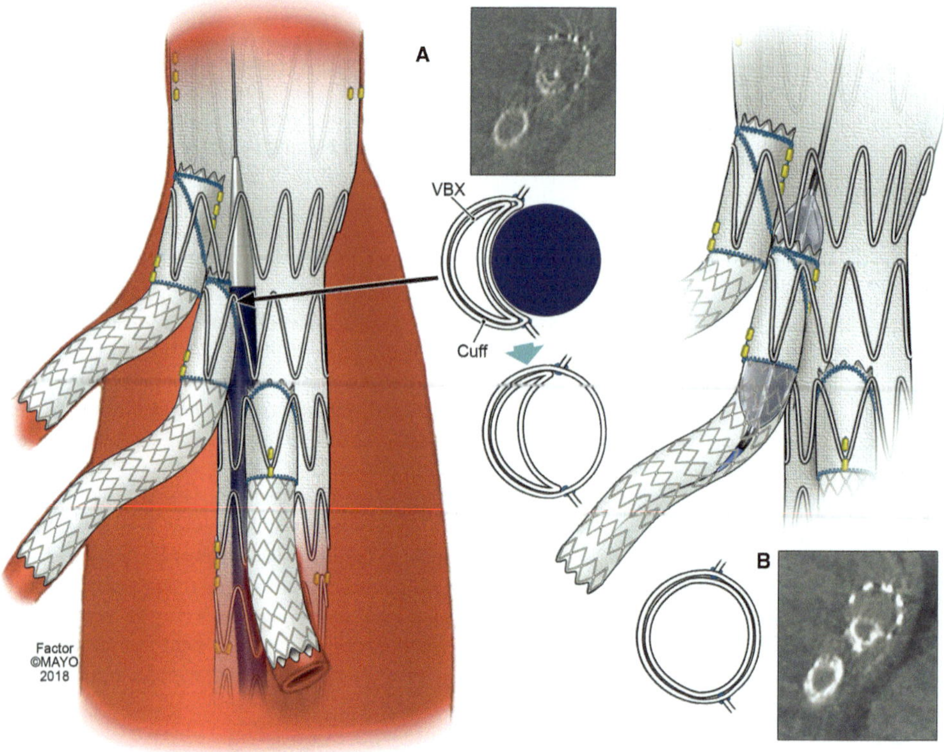

Fig. 30.6 (A) Compression of the superior mesenteric artery (SMA) stent caused by the advancement of a thoracic stent graft in a patient with prior fenestrated-branched endovascular aortic repair. (B) After balloon angioplasty the SMA stent was patent and fully expanded.

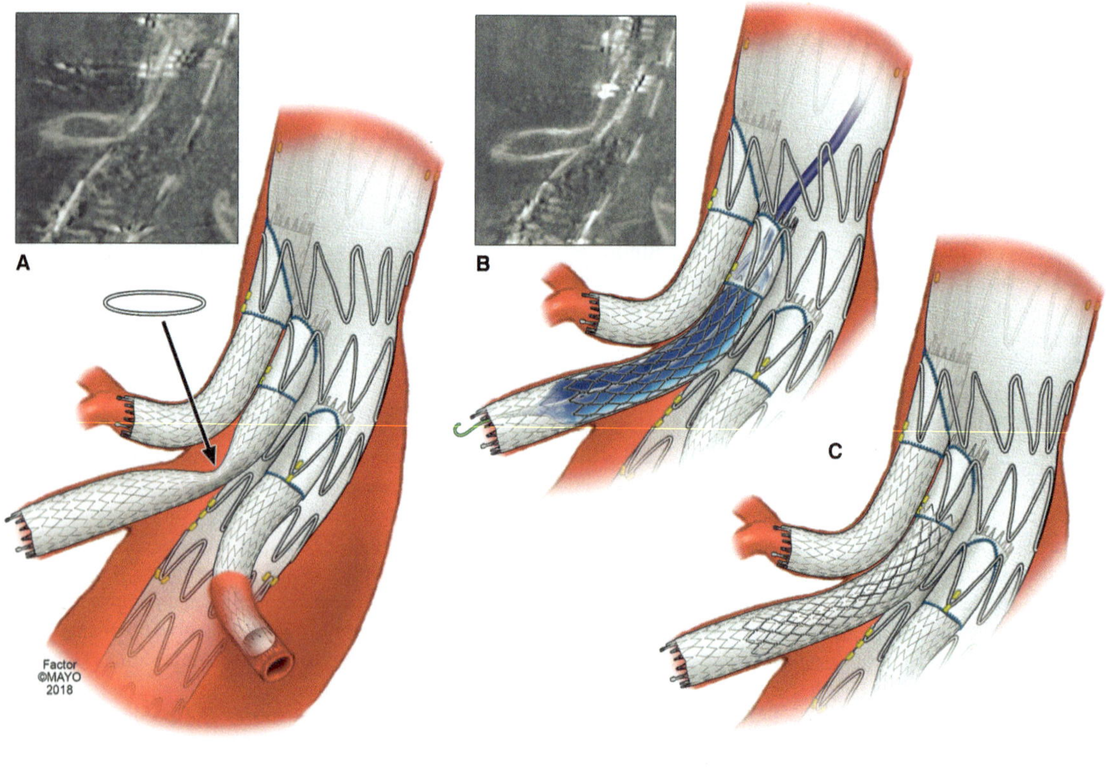

Fig. 30.7 (A) Compression of the superior mesenteric artery (SMA) stent during fenestrated-branched endovascular aortic repair. (B) Performed adjuvant angioplasty with self-expandable stent. (C) Illustration showing the stent of SMA patent and fully expanded.

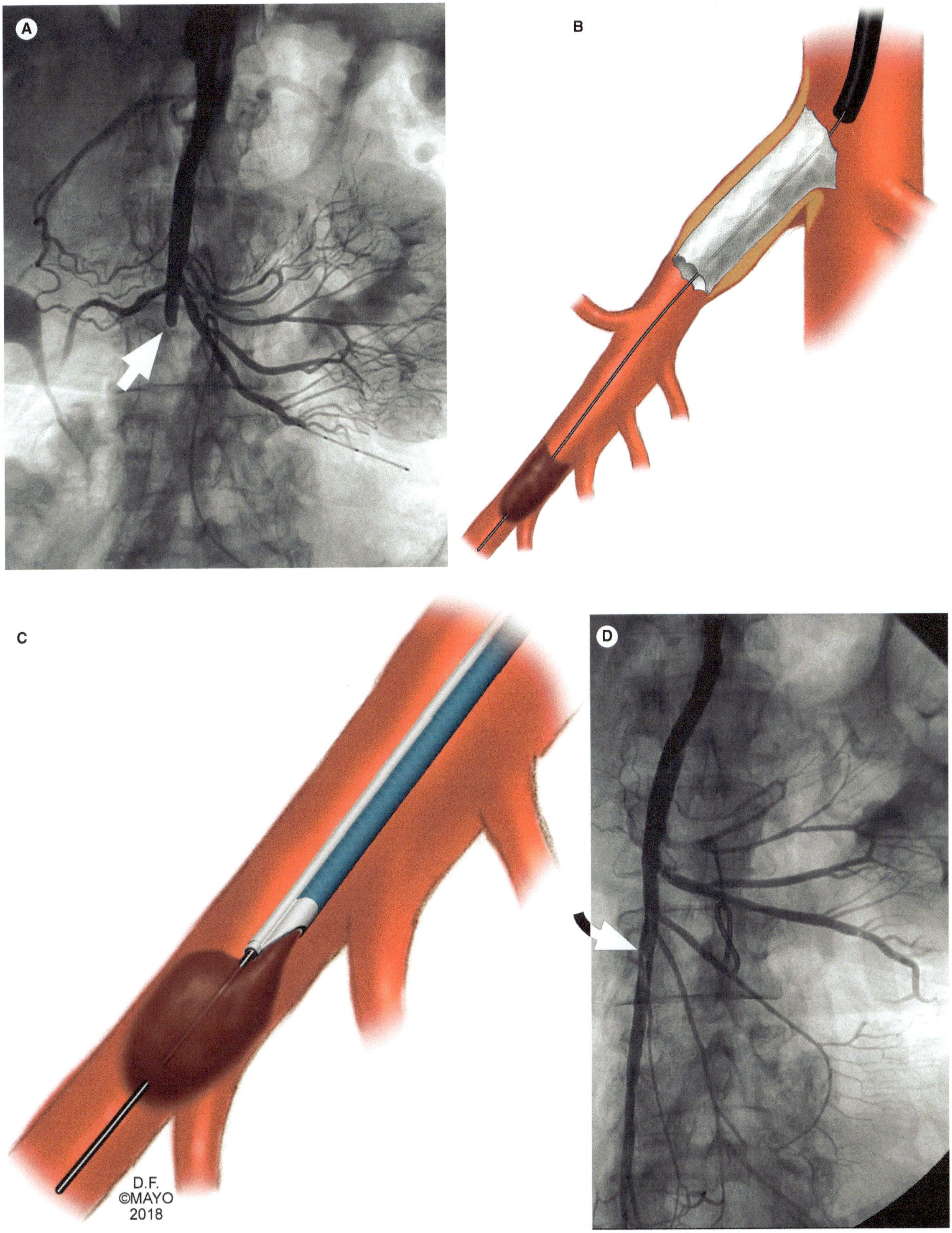

Fig. 30.8 (A and B) Successful recanalization of an occluded superior mesenteric artery (SMA) was complicated by distal embolization *(white arrow)*, which was (C) successfully salvaged by catheter-directed thrombolysis and aspiration with an Export aspiration catheter (Medtronic, Minneapolis, Minnesota) over a 0.014″ wire. (D) Completion angiography showed widely patent SMA with a small, non–flow-limiting dissection flap *(white arrow)*.

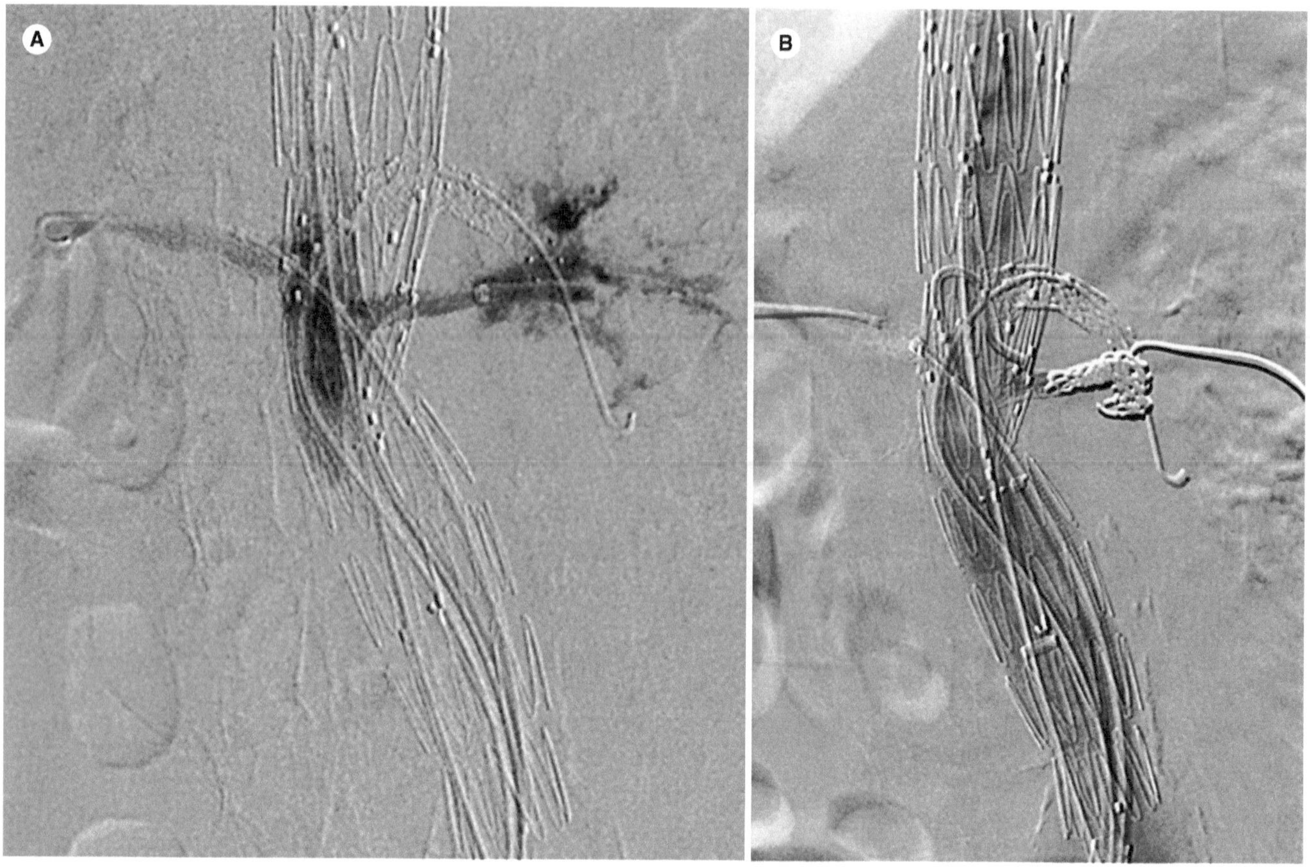

Fig. 30.9 (A) Angiography showing perforation of the left renal artery during fenestrated-branched endovascular aortic repair. (B) Performed embolization using 0.038″ coils to control bleeding.

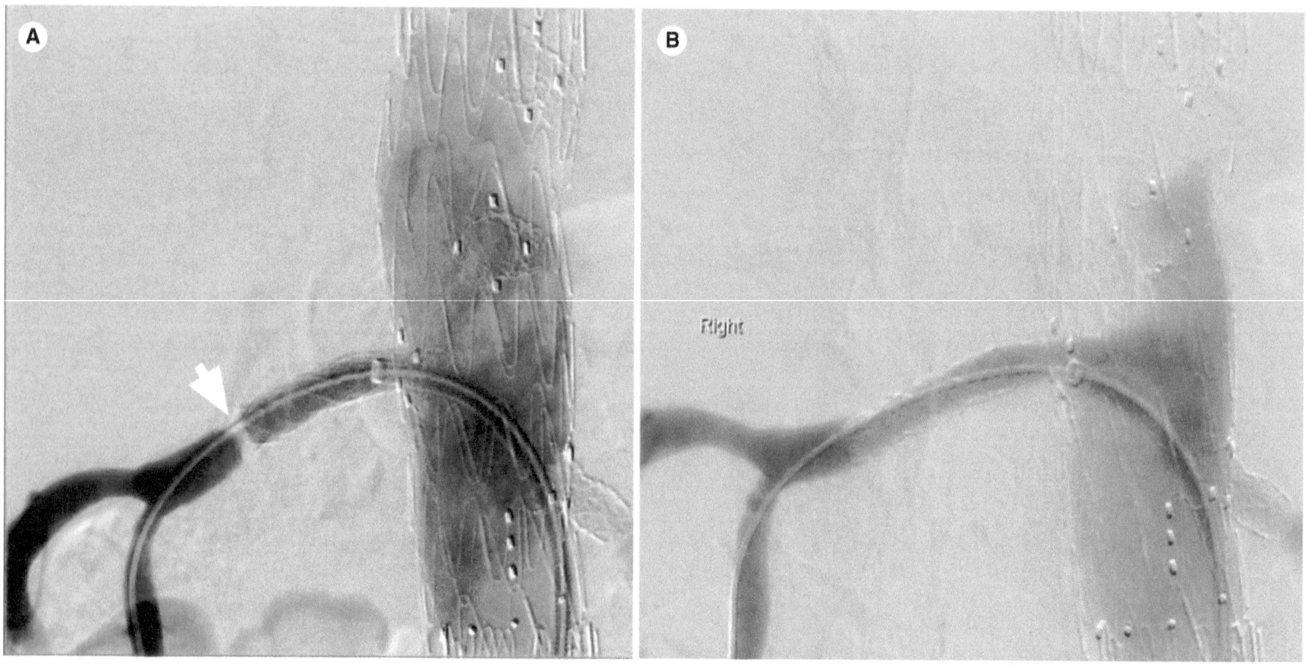

Fig. 30.10 (A) Angiography showing neo-intimal hyperplasia with important stenosis in the distal portion of the right renal stent *(white arrow)*. (B) Complete resolution of stenosis after angioplasty with covered stent.

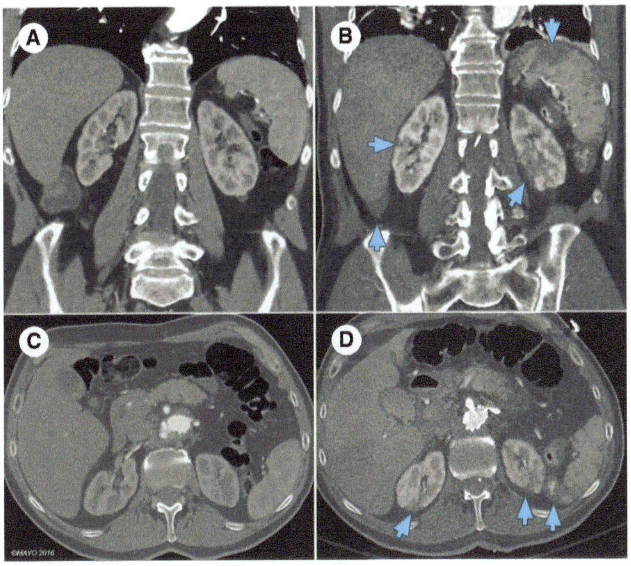

Fig. 30.11 Coronal and axial images of the (A and C) preoperative and (B and D) early postoperative computed tomography angiograms (CTAs). The *arrows* depict infarction areas in the liver, kidneys (bilateral), and spleen. (Used with permission of Mayo Foundation for Medical Education and Research. All rights reserved.)

Patients are allowed to resume a regular diet within 6 to 8 hours. Hemoglobin and creatinine are checked on the first day postoperatively. Worsening flank pain may warrant an urgent ultrasound to check for stent patency and rule out capsular or perirenal hematoma. Antiplatelet therapy is typically started prior to the intervention with acetylsalicylic acid and continued indefinitely thereafter. Clopidogrel is started the day of the intervention with a loading dose of 300 mg and continued for 6 to 8 weeks as a dual antiplatelet agent or indefinitely if a covered stent is used. A duplex ultrasound scan prior to discharge or within the first few days after the procedure serves as a baseline for future comparison. Follow-up includes clinical examination and duplex ultrasound every 6 months during the first year and annually thereafter.

Branch Instability After Fenestrated-Branched Endovascular Aortic Repair

The term branch instability was coined in 2015 by Mastracci et al.[15] to describe any branch-related death, rupture, or complication that triggered a re-intervention. Oderich et al.[16] analyzed 496 target vessels and found no difference in branch instability for fenestrations (93%) versus directional branches (92%), although there was a trend toward lower freedom from branch instability for renal (89%) compared with mesenteric arteries (93%). Mastracci et al.[15] reported freedom from branch instability of 94% at 1 year and 84% at 5 years, which compares favorably with our rate of 93% at 1 year. In a European multicenter study, among 23 renal artery adverse events, 9 (39%) were occlusions and 4 (17%) were stenosis, and the left renal artery was the most frequent involved. Restenting was performed in all four stenoses. Finally, Greenberg et al.[17] reported 4 and 2 cases of in-stent stenosis or occlusion among 57 patients followed at 2 years; of these cases, 5 required re-stenting in a multicenter trial of fenestrated endograft repair for juxtarenal abdominal aortic aneurysms.

CONCLUSIONS

Endovascular treatment, whenever feasible, has become the first choice of treatment for both mesenteric and renal artery atherosclerotic disease, because it has lower morbidity and mortality when compared with open surgery. Careful evaluation of symptoms is key because there are no specific symptoms to diagnose mesenteric or renal stenosis; good judgment and extensive pre-operative evaluation will help in defining the best interventional strategy for each patient (i.e., femoral versus brachial approach) and to lower intra-operative complication. All symptomatic lesions need to be treated and, in expert hands, peri-operative complications can be low. Whenever a complication happens, this can be life-threatening, as in the case of mesenteric embolism. Prompt recognition is mandatory and may reduce dismal outcome.

REFERENCES

1. Patel VI, Conrad MF, Kwolek CJ, LaMuraglia GM, Chung TK, Cambria RP. Renal artery revascularization: outcomes stratified by indication for intervention. *J Vasc Surg.* 2009;49(6):1480–1489.
2. Malgor RD, Oderich GS, McKusick MA, et al. Results of single- and two-vessel mesenteric artery stents for chronic mesenteric ischemia. *Ann Vasc Surg.* 2010;24(8):1094–1101.
3. Oderich GS, Tallarita T, Gloviczki P, et al. Mesenteric artery complications during angioplasty and stent placement for atherosclerotic chronic mesenteric ischemia. *J Vasc Surg.* 2012;55(4):1063–1071.
4. Aburahma AF, Campbell JE, Stone PA, et al. Perioperative and late clinical outcomes of percutaneous transluminal stentings of the celiac and superior mesenteric arteries over the past decade. *J Vasc Surg.* 2013;57(4):1052–1061.
5. Dias NV, Acosta S, Resch T, et al. Mid-term outcome of endovascular revascularization for chronic mesenteric ischaemia. *Brit J Surg.* 2010;97(2):195–201.
6. Oderich GS, Erdoes LS, Lesar C, et al. Comparison of covered stents versus bare metal stents for treatment of chronic atherosclerotic mesenteric arterial disease. *J Vasc Surg.* 2013;58(5):1316–1323.
7. Sarac TP, Altinel O, Kashyap V, et al. Endovascular treatment of stenotic and occluded visceral arteries for chronic mesenteric ischemia. *J Vasc Surg.* 2008;47(3):485–491.
8. Oderich GS, Malgor RD, Ricotta JJ, 2nd. Open and endovascular revascularization for chronic mesenteric ischemia: tabular review of the literature. *Ann Vasc Surg.* 2009;23(5):700–712.
9. Burket MW, Cooper CJ, Kennedy DJ, et al. Renal artery angioplasty and stent placement: predictors of a favorable outcome. *Am Heart J.* 2000;139(1 Pt 1):64–71.
10. Davies MG, Saad WE, Bismuth J, Naoum JJ, Peden EK, Lumsden AB. Renal parenchymal preservation after percutaneous renal angioplasty and stenting. *J Vasc Surg.* 2010;51(5):1222–1229; discussion 9.
11. Kashyap VS, Sepulveda RN, Bena JF, et al. The management of renal artery atherosclerosis for renal salvage: does stenting help? *J Vasc Surg.* 2007;45(1):101–108; discussion 8–9.
12. Leertouwer TC, Gussenhoven EJ, Bosch JL, et al. Stent placement for renal arterial stenosis: where do we stand? A meta-analysis. *Radiology.* 2000;216(1):78–85.
13. van Jaarsveld BC, Krijnen P, Pieterman H, et al. The effect of balloon angioplasty on hypertension in atherosclerotic renal-artery stenosis. Dutch Renal Artery Stenosis Intervention Cooperative Study Group. *N Engl J Med.* 2000;342(14):1007–1014.
14. Cooper CJ, Murphy TP, Cutlip DE, et al. Stenting and medical therapy for atherosclerotic renal-artery stenosis. *N Engl J Med.* 2014;370(1):13–22.
15. Mastracci TM, Greenberg RK, Eagleton MJ, Hernandez AV. Durability of branches in branched and fenestrated endografts. *J Vasc Surg.* 2013; 57(4):926–933.
16. Oderich GS, Ribeiro M, Hofer J, et al. Prospective, nonrandomized study to evaluate endovascular repair of pararenal and thoracoabdominal aortic aneurysms using fenestrated-branched endografts based on supraceliac sealing zones. *J Vasc Surg.* 2017;65(5):1249–1259.e10.
17. Greenberg RK, Sternbergh WC, 3rd. Makaroun M, et al.; Fenestrated Investigators. Intermediate results of a United States multicenter trial of fenestrated endograft repair for juxtarenal abdominal aortic aneurysms. *J Vasc Surg.* 2009;50(4):730–737.
18. Isles, et al. QJM. 1999;92(3):159–67.

31

Thrombolysis in Acute Limb Ischemia

Catherine C. Go, MD, Efthymios D. Avgerinos, MD, PhD, MSc and Rabih A. Chaer, MD, MSc

INTRODUCTION

Acute limb ischemia (ALI) arguably presents one of the most challenging problems that vascular surgeons face. The diagnosis is often clinical, but the etiology and appropriate treatment strategy are not always straightforward. A missed or delayed diagnosis can have grave consequences, such as limb loss or even death. Its estimated incidence is 1.5 cases per 10,000 people annually.[1] Each patient's physical examination will vary based on etiology, time of insult, and level of occlusion. This may range from asymptomatic to profound ischemia, depending on the presence of collateral flow (Table 31.1). As a general rule, the severity of the ischemia typically determines the urgency and type of revascularization. While open surgery remains the gold standard, over the past couple decades, endovascular interventions have expanded and may eventually dominate the field. The purpose of this chapter is to describe the role, indications, and outcomes of endovascular interventions in patients presenting with lower extremity acute limb ischemia, primarily focusing on complications and strategies to avoid them.

ACUTE LIMB ISCHEMIA TREATMENT ALTERNATIVES

The mainstay of treatment for ALI is expeditious prevention of clot propagation and reversal of ischemia. Anticoagulation is paramount and should be started immediately to prevent secondary thrombosis. Common practice is a bolus of 100 units/kg of unfractionated heparin (UFH) following by an infusion of 18 units/kg/h.

Class II and class III ischemia require immediate intervention, and patients should be transferred to a hospital with the full gamut of vascular options. Historically, class IIB ischemia is a criterion for open surgical intervention because it can restore perfusion more rapidly than traditional catheter-directed therapy (CDT). However, new studies suggest that advances in endovascular therapy, such as high-dose/accelerated CDT or pharmacomechanical thrombolysis (PMT), may offer times comparable to reperfusion as surgical therapy, which will be discussed later.[2,3] (See Fig. 31.1 for the recommended ALI treatment algorithm.)

BOX 31.1

Computed tomography angiograms (CTA) may aid in a diagnosis and operative planning, but it is based on physician preference. It is our preference to reserve CTA for patients with diminished femoral pulses, complicated surgical history, or multiple bypasses.

Surgery versus Catheter Intervention

The debate between surgical revascularization and endovascular thrombolysis has been ongoing since the 1990s, with two randomized control trials (RCTs) serving as the foundation. Post hoc analysis of one of the RCTs—the Surgery versus Thrombolysis for Ischemia of the Lower Extremity (STILE) trial—concluded that in patients with symptoms of ischemia of 14 days or less had better amputation-free survival at 6 months with thrombolysis over surgery. In the Thrombolysis or Peripheral Arterial Surgery (TOPAS) trial, the rates of limb salvage and death were comparable. In both trials, the rates of hemorrhage and complications were higher in the thrombolysis groups.[4,5] Despite no clear superiority in 30-day limb salvage or mortality, surgery continues to be performed 3–5 times more often than CDT, based on European and United States national registry data, and are likely secondary to the feared complications that will be discussed later in this chapter.[6]

University of Pittsburgh Medical Center (UPMC) Experience

It is our practice to take most patients with aortoiliac and femoral occlusions for open thromboembolectomy. Postintervention angiogram is on a physician preference basis, but generally if back bleeding is poor, or there are concerns for advanced peripheral arterial disease, or there are no distal doppler signals, angiography is obtained. At this point, chronic disease can be treated either with endovascular means or open surgery, or if distal embolization is evident, a 2–4 mg bolus of recombinant-tPA (rtPA) can be used to lyse some of the occluded outflow. If the result remains unsatisfactory, however, popliteal or pedal cutdowns may be necessary.

The benefit of surgical intervention is expeditious revascularization, but the rapidity of reperfusion needs to be weighed against the complications seen with open surgery and the inability to clear smaller outflow vessels. In our experience, which is summarized in a 2015 retrospective review of open surgery versus endovascular therapy for ALI, 326 acute limbs (classes I–III ischemia) underwent open surgery with 87%–91% technical success, which was significantly higher than CDT or PMT. However, there was no difference in amputation rates and, compared with patients who were managed with endovascular techniques, surgical patients had significantly higher 30-day and 1-year mortality, wound infection, rethrombosis, fasciotomy, return to the OR, postoperative renal failure, and new hemodialysis rates. Additionally, their lengths of stay were also extended by an average of 3 days.[7]

Catheter-Directed Lysis

The principle behind CDT is the dissolution of clots to uncover the underlying lesion that caused thrombosis. Additionally, it offers the advantage of lysing both large and small arteries, potentially providing better run-off. The likelihood of successful reperfusion with CDT increases when the occlusion is less than 14 days old, the thrombus is easily crossed by a wire, the graft being lysed has been patent for at least 1 year, and if a culprit lesion is found and can be treated (Fig. 31.2). In fact, one study reported a 2-year native vessel patency rate after lysis of 79% if a lesion was found and treated versus 9.8% if no lesion was found.[3]

TABLE 31.1 **Rutherford classification of severity, signs, and symptoms of acute limb ischemia.**

		SYMPTOMS/FINDINGS		DOPPLER SIGNALS	
Category	**Description/prognosis**	**Sensory**	**Motor**	**Arterial**	**Venous**
I. Viable	Not immediately	None	None	Audible	Audible
II. Threatened					
a. Marginally	Salvageable if promptly treated	Minimal	None	Inaudible	Audible
b. Immediately	Salvageable with immediate revascularization	Rest pain	Mild	Inaudible	Audible
III. Irreversible	Major tissue loss or permanent nerve damage	Anesthetic	Paralysis	Inaudible	Inaudible

From Earnshaw JJ. Acute Ischemia. In: Cronenwett JL, Johnston KW, et al. *Rutherford's Vascular Surgery*, 8th ed. Philadelphia: Saunders; 2014:2518–2543.

The authors' practice is to access the contralateral femoral artery with a single puncture in a retrograde fashion, typically under ultrasound guidance in order to minimize the likelihood of puncture site hematomas. Diagnostic images are obtained to evaluate the extent of thrombosis and the quality of the outflow. After the extent of thrombosis is defined, a 4- or 5-French Cragg-McNamara (Covidien, Mansfield, Massachusetts) multi-side-hole catheter is embedded in the thrombus. If the clot extends into the tibial vessels, a ProStream (Covidien, Mansfield, Massachusetts) infusion wire is used in a coaxial manner (Fig. 31.3). Although there is controversy over the dose and rate of thrombolytic delivery, the author uses a 2–4-mg bolus of rtPA followed by an infusion rate of 0.25–1.00 mg/h through each catheter. UFH at 500 units/h is infused through the sheath to prevent pericatheter thrombosis. Follow-up angiography is performed 6–12 hours later. During the follow-up angiogram, depending on the rate of clot clearance, the operator may opt to continue lysis by repositioning the catheters or finalize the procedure by ballooning or stenting uncovered lesions as needed.

While infusion catheters are in place and lytic agents are actively being administered, ICU management is commonly advocated. Continuous monitoring of vitals and neurologic status are essential. Any change in neurologic exam or sudden headache should be treated like a hemorrhagic stroke until ruled out by CT scan. The ICU can also provide hourly access site surveillance to ensure no growing hematomas and to perform regular neurovascular checks to evaluate the progress of lysis. Controversy exists on whether laboratory monitoring is essential.[3] It is the authors' practice to check hemoglobin and fibrinogen levels every 6 hours and to titrate the infusion rate with precipitous drops in fibrinogen. If levels decrease by 50%, the infusion rate is generally halved. At fibrinogen levels below 100 mg/dL, the infusion rate is decreased to 0.25 mg/h or paused entirely.

Patients are routinely kept on either clear liquid diets or no food at all. They are maintained on bedrest while the femoral sheath is in place, with the leg kept straight to decrease risk of puncture site hematoma. A Foley catheter can be utilized, which will also help with urine output monitoring.

Intravenous hydration while restoring flow to an acutely ischemic limb is essential. Reperfusion of the ischemic limb leads to release of acidic metabolites and myoglobin and can lead to metabolic derangement and/or renal failure. Patient education is also tantamount. Patients undergoing CDT should be informed that their pain may wax and wane with microembolization and then subsequent lysis of emboli. If PMT is used, tea-colored urine may result from red blood cell lysis. This is especially true with the AngioJet device discussed in the following section.

Pharmacomechanical Thrombectomy

One of the limitations of CDT is the time to reperfusion may not be rapid enough to prevent irreversible neuromuscular injury. This is precisely why Rutherford IIB ischemic patients generally undergo open surgery rather than lysis. However, since the advent of CDT, innovation has introduced endovascular mechanical clot removal devices that can be considered in conjunction with pharmacologic thrombolytics to accelerate clot dissolution and, in turn, decrease the dose of lytic agent given. Below are the three most widely used catheters for PMT in ALI.

AngioJet

The AngioJet Thrombectomy System (Boston Scientific, Maple Grove, Minnesota) is a rheolytic device that produces high-pressure jets of saline to fragment thrombus at the tip of the catheter, which, in turn, creates a relative low-pressure area that acts a suction tip whereby clot particles can be removed from the body. The PEARL Registry (PEripheral use of AngioJet Rheolytic thrombectomy with a variety of catheter Lengths) prospectively enrolled 283 patients with ALI who were treated with the AngioJet with or without CDT. Approximately 26% of patients presented with class I ischemia, 38% with class IIA, and 35% with class IIB. Overall, there was 83% success, defined as not requiring open surgery. Those who underwent PMT completed their surgery in one session, had shorter procedures, and received significantly less thrombolytic agents. Amputation-free survival at 6 and 12 months were 85% and 81%, respectively. Safety outcomes were similar to other PMT studies, with 4.3% of major bleeding requiring transfusion. A caveat to note is that 80% of the patients enrolled in the PEARL registry had symptoms for 7 days or less, which may have contributed to high success rates.[8]

UPMC Experience

Our experience with PMT for ALI is predominantly with the AngioJet catheter for femoral–popliteal thrombus, followed by CDT for residual thrombus. Although some surgeons prefer to use embolic protection devices (EPDs), we generally do not. Instead, the AngioJet is initially used to clear the proximal clot without crossing the distal cap to avoid potential distal embolization. This is done with power pulse mode with 6–12 mg of rtPA in 100–250 mL of normal saline, followed by thrombectomy mode after 15–20 minutes dwell time. The distal cap is

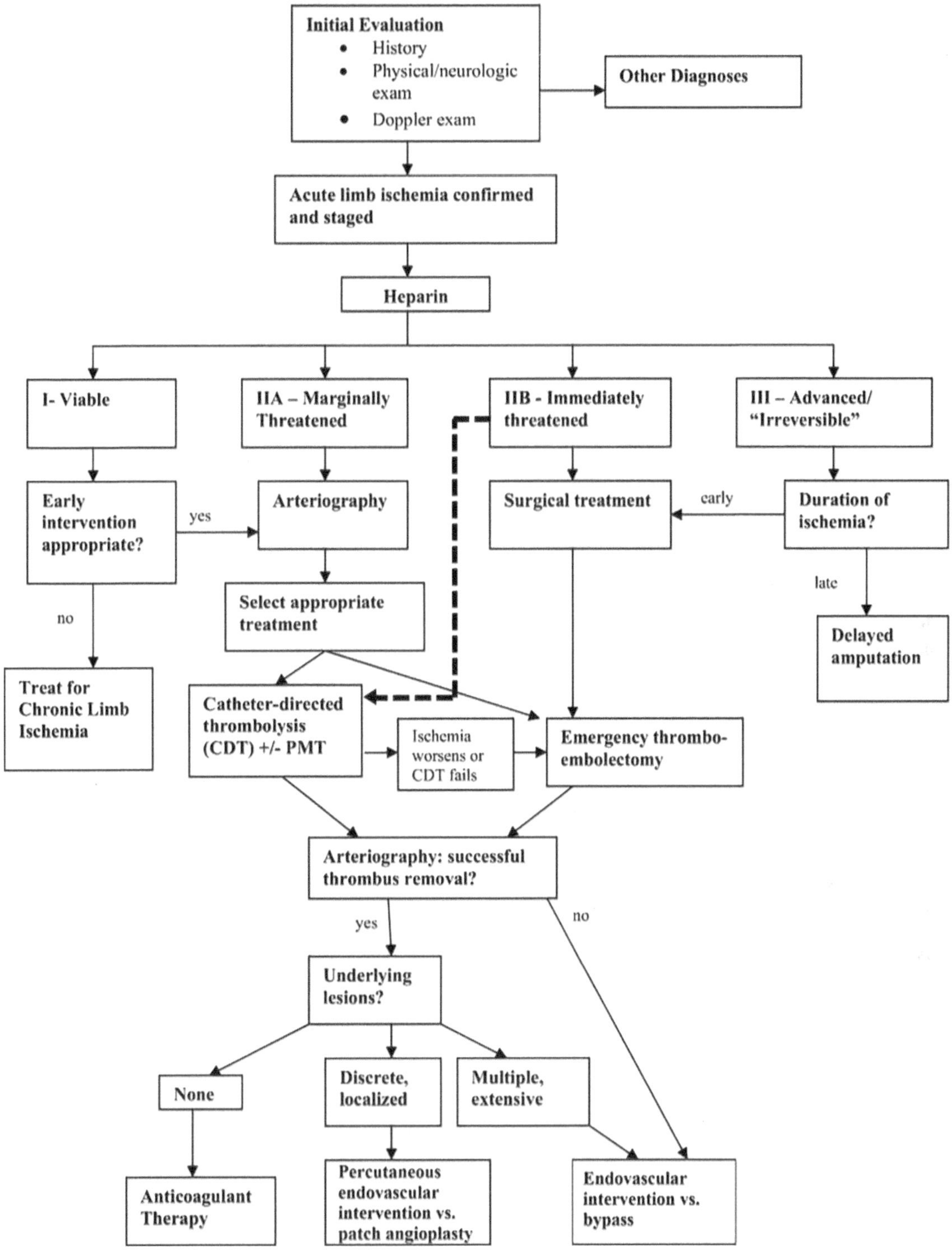

Fig. 31.1 Treatment algorithm for acute limb ischemia separated by Rutherford degree of ischemia. Rutherford class IIB ischemia is classically treated with surgical revascularization, but with the development of advanced endovascular techniques, catheter-directed therapy (CDT) or pharmacomechanical thrombolysis (PMT) may be the treatment option of choice for some surgeons. This is depicted with a *dashed line.*

(Figure adapted from Rutherford RB. Clinical staging of acute limb ischemia as the basis for choice of revascularization method: when and how to intervene. *Sem Vasc Surg* 2009;22(1):5–9.)

crossed after clearance of the proximal thrombus. In our retrospective review of 154 limbs that received CDT versus PMT, there was a significant difference in technical success favoring PMT (90.1% versus 78.3%). Although not statistically significant, more instances of embolization occurred in the PMT group (14% versus 6%). However, there was no difference in duration of lysis, amputation, patency, or mortality at 2 years. With regards to complications, there was a significant difference in rates of access site hematoma, with more occurring in the PMT group. There were also three occurrences of transient acute renal failure in the PMT group and none in the CDT group. This figure did not reach significance. We therefore conclude that PMT offers increased chance of technical success compared with CDT and

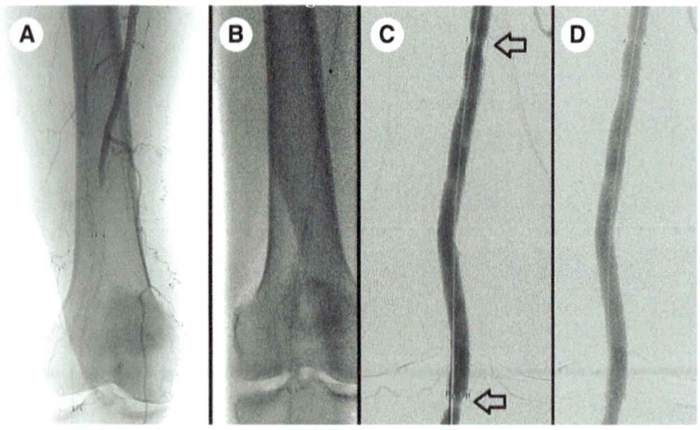

Fig. 31.2 (A) Initial angiogram of a 73-year-old woman with a previous popliteal stent graft for rest pain who presented with ALI and found to have occluded stent. (B) A Cragg-McNamara catheter embedded within the in-stent thrombosis. (C) Culprit lesions uncovered after 12 hours of catheter-directed therapy seen at proximal and distal ends of the stent graft *(arrows).* (D) Completion angiogram after drug-coated balloon angioplasty to both lesions with minimal residual stenosis.

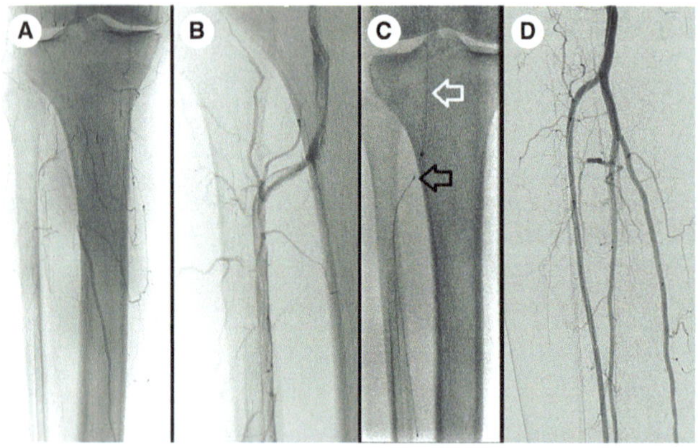

Fig. 31.3 (A) Angiogram of the thrombosed outflow of the same 73-year-old woman with an occluded popliteal stent. (B) Anterior tibial (AT) artery with thrombus. (C) A Cragg-McNamara catheter was placed within the clotted stent *(white arrow)* with a co-axial Pro-Stream wire *(black arrow)* placed into the AT. (D) Completion angiogram after 12 hours of catheter-directed therapy demonstrating 3-vessel outflow without stenosis.

similar clinical and patency outcomes. However, we proceed with caution in patients with renal insufficiency.[9]

Penumbra

The Penumbra/Indigo system (Penumbra, Alameda, California) is an aspiration thrombo-embolectomy catheter available in sizes 3- to 8-French that is vacuum-driven for consistent suction and first became available in 1985 as an alternative to balloon embolectomy (Box 31.2). The PRISM trial was a single-arm, multicenter, retrospective review of 79 patients who underwent endovascular suction thrombectomy as either initial or adjunctive therapy after other revascularization attempts. Standard technique is to place the tip of the catheter at the proximal edge of the thrombus and begin aspiration. Technical success was measured by angiographic assessment using a Thrombolysis in Myocardial Infarction (TIMI) score with 0 meaning no perfusion and 3 meaning complete perfusion. Ninety-nine percent of cases began with a TIMI score of 0–1 and use of the Penumbra thrombectomy catheter improved TIMI grade to 2–3 in 87.2% of patients. There were no long-term outcomes described. Complications included anemia, compartment syndrome, and other medical complications, including renal insufficiency, confusion, and respiratory failure.[10]

> **BOX 31.2**
>
> The varying catheter sizes of the Penumbra allow for versatility. In ALI, the 8-French system is generally used in the aortoiliac, femoral, and popliteal regions. The 5- and 6-French systems are useful in the tibial arteries, while the 3-French system is reserved for the pedal arteries. The powerful negative pressure supplied by the device possibly makes it the most effective in pure occlusions. In the setting of partially restored flow, the system appears simply to aspirate blood.

EndoWave

The EndoWave catheter (EKOS Corporation, Bothell, Washington) uses ultrasound technology to fragment thromboemboli mechanically while also infusing thrombolytics to accelerate clot dissolution. In a small retrospective review that compared 75 patients undergoing PMT with the EndoWave catheter to 27 patients undergoing traditional CDT, there were no statistical significant differences in technical success, limb salvage, and mortality.[11] There were multiple limitations to this study, including a small sample size, use of urokinase for CDT, and exclusion of Rutherford IIB ischemia. Notably, there were more bleeding events in the CDT-only group and a trend toward more embolization in the EKOS group. The DUET trial is a randomized trial comparing ultrasound-assisted thrombolysis and CDT that enrolled 60 patients and showed no difference in technical success, 30-day patency, and mortality.[12]

In addition to PMT techniques described earlier, there are two prospective observational studies from Poland describing high-dose and accelerated CDT that had similar technical success to previously reported CDT rates and did not lead to more bleeding complications. With high-dose/accelerated CDT and PMT devices, the time to perfusion can be shortened, which would allow patients with more advanced ischemia to be candidates for endovascular treatment.[2,13] Although data for use in advanced ischemia are scarce, PMT provides a suitable alternative with equivalent outcomes to CDT, which has long been studied and validated as a treatment for ALI.[3]

Contraindications

The contraindications to CDT and PMT are based on the exclusion criteria used for the randomized control trials and the contraindications used for systemic thrombolysis. These are summarized in Table 31.2. In our institution, patients with a contraindication to lysis are offered open revascularization or PMT with minimal to no use of rtPA.

COMPLICATIONS

Hemorrhagic complications are the feared potential sequelae of lytic therapy. These events can range from access site hematoma to fatal intracranial or systemic bleeding. For these reasons, aggressive monitoring is a necessity while tPA is being infused. Table 31.3 summarizes the anticipated complications.

Major Hemorrhage

Although performed in the 1990s with urokinase, the pivotal randomized control trials comparing lysis and open surgery had similar

TABLE 31.2 **List of contraindications to systemic pharmacologic thrombolysis. As a result of the improved safety profile of catheter-directed lysis, the decision to administer regional tPA is highly dependent on the individual's practice.**

Contraindications to thrombolysis
Absolute contraindications
1. Established cerebrovascular event within previous 2 months (excluding TIA)
2. Active bleeding diathesis
3. Recent gastrointestinal bleeding within previous 10 days
4. Intracranial or spinal surgery within previous 3 months
5. Intracranial trauma within previous 3 months
Relative contraindications
1. Cardiopulmonary resuscitation within previous 10 days
2. Major nonvascular surgery or trauma within previous 10 days
3. Uncontrolled hypertension (systolic >180 mmHg or diastolic >110 mmHg)
4. Puncture of noncompressible vessel
5. Intracranial tumor
6. Recent eye surgery
Minor contraindications
1. Hepatic failure, coagulopathy
2. Bacterial endocarditis
3. Pregnancy
4. Active diabetic proliferative retinopathy

From Norgren L, Hiatt WR, Dormandy JA, et al. Inter-Society Consensus for the Management of Peripheral Arterial Disease (TASC II). *J Vasc Surg.* 2007;45 (Suppl S):S40A–S47A.

outcomes with regard to life-threatening hemorrhage. These events were defined as bleeding that produced hypotension, required transfusion, or intracranial hemorrhage. The thrombolysis group endured significantly more hemorrhagic complications at a rate of 5.6%–12.5% compared with 0.7%–5.5% in the open surgical cohort. Specifically, intracranial hemorrhage occurred in 1.2%–1.6% of patients.[4,14] The only significant predisposing factor for hemorrhagic complications was the use of therapeutic heparin. For this reason, the standard CDT protocols use subtherapeutic systemic heparin during lysis, usually at a rate of 500 units/h infused through the sheath.

In our 2015 study comparing open surgery and endovascular intervention, there were no significant bleeding events in the open surgery group, but systemic bleeding occurred in eight patients (5.2%) in the endovascular group. These were four gastrointestinal bleeds, three retroperitoneal bleeds, and one brainstem hemorrhage. Four of these bleeds were fatal, including the brainstem hemorrhage.[7,9] In a 2017 retrospective study of 689 limbs treated with CDT for ALI, only three patients (0.4%) suffered from intracranial hemorrhage.[5]

In the accelerated and high-dose CDT studies from Poland, in which 138 patients received 40–60 mg rtPA in 2.5–3.5 hours, only one patient suffered hemorrhagic stroke. All other bleeding complications (10%) were not life-threatening, although three hematomas required evacuation. Although more studies are needed to vet these accelerated protocols, there are data that support the use of high-dose

TABLE 31.3 **Summary of most common complications associated with CDT and their incidence.**

Complication	Rate
Major hemorrhage	
Intracranial bleeding	0.4%–1.6%
Systemic, life-threatening bleeding	5%–12%
Minor hemorrhage	
Access site hematoma	5%–10%
Compartment syndrome	1%–3%
Other	
Acute renal failure	1%–5%
Embolism	5%–10%

CDT, Catheter-directed therapy.

rtPA in acute coronary syndrome or pulmonary embolism while maintaining similar safety profiles.[2,13] In the PEARL study, there were five patients (4.3%) with bleeding requiring transfusion, without any intracranial hemorrhage associated with the AngioJet device.[14]

In the event of intracranial or life-threatening hemorrhage, thrombolysis should be terminated immediately. If there is concern for neurologic changes or new headache, a plain CT scan of the head should be obtained and neurosurgical consultation sought. All anticoagulation and antiplatelet therapy should be held until clearance from neurosurgery and resumed based on clinical judgement. Currently, the evidence regarding fibrinogen levels and their predictive value with respect to hemorrhagic complications is unproven.[15]

Minor Hemorrhage

Minor bleeding predominantly refers to access site hematoma and remote bleeding that may lead to compartment syndrome. Hematoma at the site of puncture is the most common bleeding complication associated with CDT and PMT, occurring anywhere from 5% to10% of cases. For this reason, a low threshold to use ultrasound guidance for arterial access is recommended. In the majority of these events, expectant management or manual compression is sufficient. In some instances, patients may require duplex evaluation to rule out pseudoaneurysm. Based on sonographic findings, thrombin injection or primary surgical repair can be pursued.

Compartment Syndrome

Compartment syndrome is a complication associated with ALI treatment. It is not endospecific but can be associated with wire trauma or reperfusion. In fact, it is more commonly seen after open surgical revascularization or PMT. Because of the gradual resolution of ischemia, patients who undergo CDT are less likely to have severe reperfusion swelling. It is recommended, however, that any patient with motor changes (class IIB or class III ischemia) receive prophylactic fasciotomies or be closely monitored for signs and symptoms of compartment syndrome. Occasionally, lytic infusion may lead to bleeding in the affected limb that may lead to mass effect requiring fasciotomy.[3,6] The rate of fasciotomy post-revascularization for ALI is 5.3% in the United States. However, among CDT patients only, the rate of compartment syndrome is roughly 1%–3%, while our experience with the AngioJet revealed a rate of 3.2%.

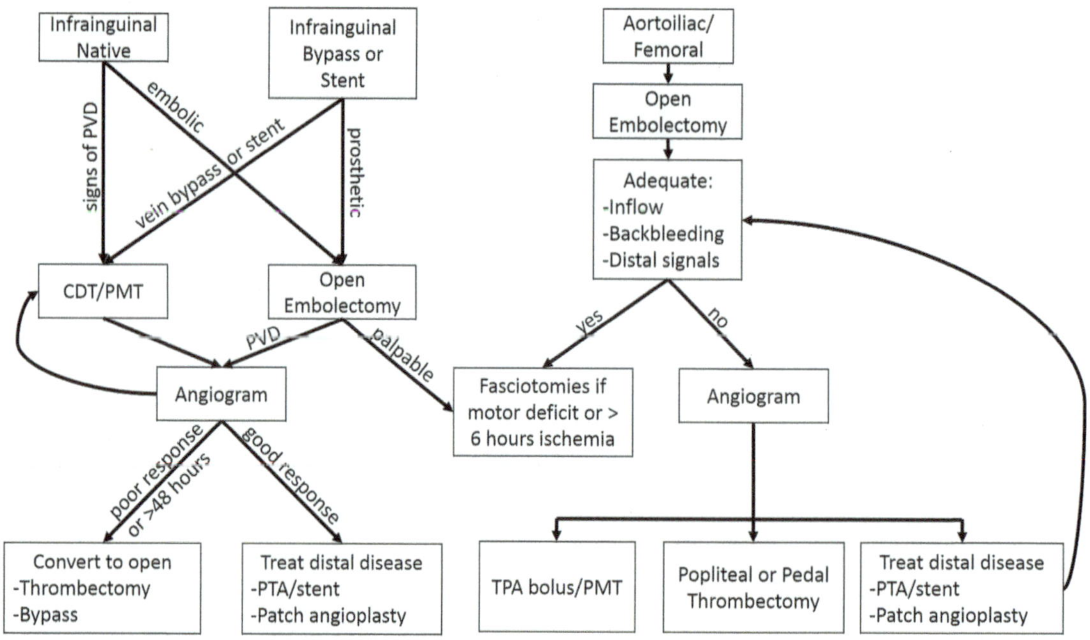

Fig. 31.4 Summary of the University of Pittsburgh Medical Center treatment algorithm for Rutherford Class IIA and IIB. Our preference is to use the AngioJet or Penumbra when using pharmacomechanical thrombosis (PMT) in the lower extremities. CDT, catheter-directed therapy; percutaneous transluminal angioplasty (PTA); peripheral vascular disease (PVD); tissue plasminogen activator (TPA).

The treatment for suspected compartment syndrome is four-compartment fasciotomy. The anterior compartment is most often involved, but a deep posterior compartment syndrome would be the most functionally devastating because of the tibial nerve's course through it.

Renal Failure and Myoglobinuria

Acute renal failure is not uncommon after ALI treatment secondary to myoglobinuria, hemoglobinuria, and iodinated contrast loads. Hemoglobinuria is especially prevalent after PMT secondary to red blood cell lysis. In the case of the AngioJet, renal complications appear to be correlated with run times greater than 5–10 minutes, infusion volumes exceeding 300 mL, and a 10% drop in hematocrit. Myoglobinuria can be seen in up to 20% of patients after open and endo treatment of ALI. With CDT and PMT, acute renal failure occurs in 1%–5% of cases, with new hemodialysis requirements occurring in less than 1% of patients treated.[7,9]

Management includes strict monitoring of urine output and aggressive, but judicious, intravenous hydration. Alkalinization of urine with sodium bicarbonate will prevent the crystallization of myoglobin, the main culprit in causing tubular necrosis. Nephrology consultation may also prove helpful as some patients may require temporary dialysis until recovery of kidney function. Mannitol and plasmapheresis have not shown any benefit.[3,6]

Embolism

Although more common in PMT, distal embolization during CDT is common. Patients often report waxing and waning pain and paresthesia in the affected limb as emboli lodge distally and then dissolve with continued lysis. The patient's Doppler examination may also change, therefore educating the patient and nursing staff is key. If the patient's pain does not improve or worsens over the following hours, angiography with or without surgery may be warranted. At our institution, if there is no improvement of symptoms or angiographic decrease in clot burden, lysis is stopped at 48 hours and other techniques are pursued (Fig. 31.4).

Embolism is seen in 5%–10% of patients undergoing CDT and up to 14% in PMT, with the majority requiring no additional intervention except for continued lytic infusion. Those whose symptoms did not abate with continued lysis required repositioning of catheters, thrombectomy, and occasionally patch angioplasty as discussed in the clinical case in the next section. Some recommend embedding catheters in the thrombus without crossing the distal end of the clot, which functions as natural embolic protection. This advice, however, is anecdotal.[2,6] Some surgeons use embolic protection devices (EPDs) to prevent distal embolization, such as the SpiderFX embolic protection device (Medtronic, Minneapolis, Minnesota). Although more studies are needed, the results appear positive with one study concluding that the use of EPDs during CDT decreased patients' analgesia requirements and lytic infusion duration.[16]

Clinical Case

A 49-year-old woman with a previous history of claudication presented to an outside hospital with acute paresthesia of the right foot. A CT angiogram revealed a focal right superficial femoral artery (SFA) occlusion and distal tibial occlusions. Her ankle brachial index was normal on the left and 0.47 on the right. She was taken for a right popliteal cut-down, successful SFA embolectomy but poor return after tibial embolectomy. Subsequent angiogram showed no improvement in the outflow. She was transferred to UPMC for continued paresthesia. Another angiogram was performed and PMT was attempted with the Penumbra and Export (Medtronic, Minneapolis, Minnesota) catheters and a 2-mg bolus of rtPA. There was no improvement angiographically. A pedal thrombectomy was then performed with a palpable PT at the end of the case with resolution of symptoms (Fig. 31.5).

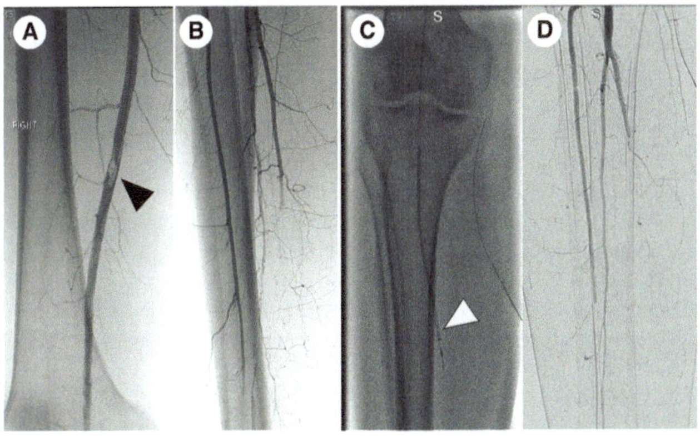

Fig. 31.5 (A) Initial angiogram of superficial femoral artery/popliteal segment with embolus *(black arrow)*. (B) Prior to tibial embolectomy, all three outflow vessels were occluded. (C) Penumbra catheter seen in tibial arteries *(white arrow)*. (D) Minimal improvement seen after pharmacomechanical thrombolysis. Patient subsequently underwent pedal thrombectomy with recanalization of her posterior tibial artery (not shown).

OUTCOMES

Technical Success

Successful revascularization is generally defined as restoration of in-line flow to the foot without need for surgical conversion. CDT achieves success rates of 75%–92% of patients with ALI, which is comparable to open revascularization. Roughly 75%–90% of patients who undergo successful endovascular treatment will need an adjunctive procedure based on etiology of the ischemia. In a large retrospective study in Sweden, 689 limbs were treated with CDT. Technical success was within the range listed here. The rate of adjunctive procedure was 77% for all ischemic limbs except for those caused by emboli (67%, P = 0.002) in the first 30 days.[5]

Modes of failure include ongoing ischemia/inadequate response, bleeding requiring termination, or distal embolization. Factors that portend poor outcomes include end-stage renal disease (ESRD), diabetes, current smoking, and lysis of prosthetic bypass graft. Because of poor success rates and subsequent patency of prosthetic bypass grafts, some recommend de novo bypass grafting rather than thrombolysis as initial therapy. In general, the likelihood of technical success increases with the number of patent pedal outflow vessels.[3,6]

Limb Salvage

As previously discussed, ALI poses a serious limb loss threat with a 30-day amputation rate of 5%–15%. Patients with Rutherford III ischemia and occluded popliteal aneurysms were more likely to have primary amputation. Among Rutherford II ischemic limbs, 30-day amputation rates are comparable between open and endo interventions. Furthermore, above-knee amputation is four times more prevalent than below-knee amputations in ALI contrasted with the even distribution in chronic limb ischemia.[6]

Amputation rates at 6 months to 1 year are in the range of 12%–20%. At 5 years, this increases to 25%. Patients who initially presented with embolic ALI have significantly lower amputation rates in long-term follow-up studies, whereas those who presented with an occluded graft/stent suffer from higher amputation rates (20%–40%). Risk factors that predict limb loss include ESRD, diabetes, cerebrovascular disease, age greater than 65 years, and female sex.[5,17]

Survival

Although the risk of 30-day mortality for patients with ALI has been quoted as high as 26%, the 30-day survival in patients with ALI treated with CDT ranges from 90% to 100%. The most common cause of 30-day death is bleeding complication.

Survival at 1 year and 5 years post-CDT is roughly 80% and 50%, respectively. Although the study at our institution shows a survival benefit in those who underwent endovascular intervention over open surgery at 1 and 2 years, a meta-analysis performed in 2016 showed no significant difference in mortality between the two treatment paradigms at 1, 6, and 12 months. Patients who presented with a thrombosed popliteal aneurysm had significantly better survival at 5 years (83% versus 54%) compared with patients who presented with other etiologies of ALI. The strongest predictors of mortality are ESRD and advanced ischemia. Other predictors include age, preoperative anemia, atrial fibrillation, cerebrovascular disease, ischemic heart disease, and COPD.[1,9]

CONCLUSIONS

Despite the feared complication of intracranial hemorrhage, which occurs in less than 1% of patients undergoing thrombolysis, CDT and PMT present minimally invasive alternatives to open surgery for ALI, with comparable outcomes in terms of technical success and limb loss. With the added benefit of shorter hospital stays, lower rates of compartment syndrome, wound infection, and less complex adjunctive procedures, endovascular techniques continue to gain momentum and popularity. Although at this time, CDT and PMT have for the most part been reserved for less advanced ischemia, their role in more advanced ischemia as demonstrated above may be justified as they can allow expeditious restoration of flow with less embolic complications with the use of an embolic protection device. As more data accumulate and with new endovascular advances and devices in the pipeline, most patients with threatened limbs can be candidates for endovascular therapy.

REFERENCES

1. Enezate TH, Omran J, Mahmud E, et al. Endovascular versus surgical treatment for acute limb ischemia: a systematic review and meta-analysis of clinical trials. *Cardiovasc Diagn Ther.* 2017;7(3):264–271.
2. Lukasiewicz A, Lichota W, Thews M. Outcomes of accelerated catheter-directed thrombolysis in patients with acute arterial thrombosis. *Vasc Med.* 2016;21(5):453–458.
3. Earnshaw JJ. Acute Ischemia. In: Cronenwett JL, Johnston KW, et al. *Rutherford's Vascular Surgery*, 8th ed. Philadelphia: Saunders; 2014:2518–2543.
4. Ouriel K, Veith FJ, Sasahara AA, et al. A comparison of recombinant urokinase with vascular surgery as initial treatment for acute arterial occlusion of the legs. Thrombolysis of Peripheral Arterial Surgery TOPAS) Investigators. *N Engl J Med.* 1998;19:1021–1030.
5. Grip O, Wanhainen A, Acosta S, et al. Long-term outcome after thrombolysis for acute lower limb ischemia. *Eur J Vasc Endovasc Surg.* 2017;53(6):853–861.
6. Norgren L, Hiatt WR, Dormandy JA, et al. Inter-Society Consensus for the Management of Peripheral Arterial Disease (TASC II). *J Vasc Surg.* 2007;45(Suppl S):S40A–S44A.
7. Taha AG, Byrne RM, Avgerinos ED, et al. Comparative effectiveness of endovascular versus surgical revascularization for acute lower extremity ischemia. *J Vasc Surg.* 2015;61:147–154.
8. Leung DA, Blitz LR, Nelson T, et al. Rheolytic pharmacomechanical thrombectomy for the management of acute limb ischemia: results from the PEARL registry. *J Endovasc Ther.* 2015;22(4):546–557.
9. Byrne RM, Taha AG, Avgerinos ED, et al. Contemporary outcomes of endovascular interventions for acute limb ischemia. *J Vasc Surg.* 2014; 59(4):988–995.

10. Saxon RR, Benenati JF, Teigen C, et al. Utility of a power aspiration-based extraction technique as an initial and secondary approach in the treatment in peripheral arterial thromboembolism: results of the multicenter PRISM trial. *J Vasc Interv Radiol.* 2017;S1051-0443(17):1–9.
11. Schernthaner MB, Samuels S, Biegler P, et al. Ultrasound-accelerated versus standard catheter-directed thrombolysis in 102 patients with acute and subacute limb ischemia. *J Vasc Interv Radiol.* 2014;25(8):1149–1156.
12. Schrijver AM, van Leersum M, Fioole B, et al. Dutch randomized trial comparing standard catheter-directed thrombolysis and ultrasound-accelerated thrombolysis for arterial thromboembolic infrainguinal disease (DUET). *J Endovasc Ther.* 2015;22(1):87–95.
13. Falkowski A, Poncyljusz W, Samad RA, et al. Safety and efficacy of ultra-high-dose, short-term thrombolysis with rt-PA for acute lower limb ischemia. *Eur J Vasc Endovasc Surg.* 2013;46:118–123.
14. The STILE Investigators. Results of a prospective randomized trial evaluating surgery versus thrombolysis for ischemia of the lower extremity. *Ann Surg.* 1994;220:251–266.
15. Poorthuis MH, Brand EC, Hazenberg CE, et al. Plasma fibrinogen level as a potential predictor of hemorrhagic complications after catheter-directed thrombolysis for peripheral arterial occlusions. *J Vasc Surg.* 2017;65(5):1519–1527.
16. Irani Z, Oklu R. The use of embolic protection device in lower extremity catheter-directed thrombolysis. *Diagn Interv Imaging.* 2016;97(2):273–275.
17. Schrijver AM, de Vries JP, van den Heuvel DA, et al. Long-term outcomes of catheter-directed thrombolysis for acute lower extremity occlusions of native arteries and prosthetic bypass grafts. *Ann Vasc Surg.* 2016;31:134–142.

32

Aortoiliac Interventions for Occlusive Disease

Mariel Rivero, MD and Hasan H. Dosluoglu, MD, FACS

INTRODUCTION

Endovascular treatment of complex (TASC C and D)[1] lesions of the aortoiliac arteries has been increasingly adopted since the early 2000s, especially after the introduction of stent grafts. Although the primary patency rates are reported to be 60%–86% at 5 years, which is lower than with direct revascularization, secondary patency rates are comparable ranging from 80% to 98%.[2] In the most recent meta-analysis, the 5-year patency rates were reported to be 91% in patients with claudication and 87% in patients with critical limb ischemia.[3] Mortality and morbidity were 3.3% and 8.3%, which is the main reason for adopting minimally invasive alternatives. There are no modern studies comparing direct revascularization with endovascular revascularization in patients with complex aortoiliac occlusive disease in large numbers; however, a few small series have explored this issue. Overall, they have shown that endovascular treatment has inferior primary patency with similar secondary patency rates and lower morbidity and mortality.[4–6]

In contrast to outcomes in the femoropopliteal segment, patency of TASC C and D lesions in the iliac segment has been reported to be comparable with that of TASC A and B lesions.[6–8] In a series of 433 patients who had systematic iliac stenting between 1997 and 2009, with a median follow-up of 72 months, primary patency rates at 5 and 10 years were 83% and 71%, respectively, in the TASC II C/D group and 88% and 83% in the TASC II A/B group ($P = 0.17$).[6] However, the risk of complications (vessel rupture, dissections, loss of branch vessels, early and late occlusions, distal embolization) increased with the complexity of the revascularization. The complication rate was higher in the C/D group (9% versus 3%, $P = 0.014$), with significantly longer procedure times in the above referenced study.[6]

The most important aspect of aortoiliac revascularization is to anticipate and to avoid complications via careful preoperative planning. In addition to obtaining a detailed history and physical examination, any patient with suspected aortoiliac occlusive disease should undergo preoperative imaging, ideally with a computed tomography angiogram. The amount of calcium and clot content within the vessels, the anatomy of the critical vessels, and the anticipated re-entry level are all crucial to planning treatment of these lesions. However, despite appropriate planning, complications will occur and, in that event, timely and appropriate management can minimize adverse outcomes.

PATIENT PREPARATION

Management of aortoiliac disease often requires a combination of both open and endovascular techniques. While many complex lesions can be addressed percutaneously, a significant proportion of patients (up to 20%)[4,9] have bulky common femoral artery disease and will require concomitant femoral endarterectomy. Open access may also be preferred in the setting of acute or subacute occlusion, as it facilitates protection from distal embolization. In addition, antegrade iliac crossing may result in a common femoral dissection, which is typically managed via open repair. If open femoral intervention is either likely or anticipated, the procedure should be performed in a setting appropriate for a hybrid repair.[10]

Crossing aortoiliac lesions can be performed in either a retrograde or antegrade fashion and it is not unusual to need a combination of both approaches. Therefore, the possibility of both brachial and femoral access should be anticipated, and the patient should be prepared accordingly at the beginning of the procedure. Upper extremity access typically requires a sheath at least 90 cm in length. However, longer sheaths and crossing catheters up to 125 cm should be available for taller patients or in the event that a radial approach is preferred. When crossing via a contralateral femoral approach, a deflectable sheath may be necessary to increase support, especially when dealing with a short common iliac stump.

In the rare event that an aortoiliac lesion cannot be crossed, there should be a clear plan for open intervention. If revascularization is urgent, the patient should be prepared for possible femoral–femoral or axillary–femoral bypass at the beginning of the procedure.

CROSSING AND TREATING AORTO-ILIAC LESIONS

There are four main issues to address when planning an endovascular intervention for aortoiliac lesions: (1) antegrade versus retrograde crossing; (2) femoral versus brachial access; (3) re-entry method; (4) stent selection. Of these, the crossing direction is the most important as it will, in many respects, dictate each of the subsequent choices. However, every decision is ultimately predicated on the desire to minimize the risks of vessel perforation, embolization, and occlusion associated with a difficult re-entry.

Crossing Direction and Access Site

Though crossing an aortoiliac lesion can be performed in either a retrograde or an antegrade fashion, our preferred initial approach to most lesions is antegrade. This strategy prevents proximal extension of the re-entry site, which can weaken the aortic wall and lead to either perforation or development of an obstructive flap. In addition, an antegrade approach provides more flexibility in the event that percutaneous re-entry is unsuccessful. Wire retrieval through a femoral cut-down is relatively straightforward and well-tolerated in most patients. For patients with external iliac artery occlusions and a patent internal iliac artery, crossing in an antegrade fashion also minimizes the chance that a dissection will compromise the internal iliac branch.

If the ipsilateral common iliac artery is patent, then we typically start with a contralateral femoral approach. The internal iliac artery is selectively cannulated and the initial wire is exchanged for a support wire (Storq, Cordis, Cardinal Health, Dublin, OH; Bentson, Boston Scientific, Marlborough, MA). A sheath is then placed from the contralateral femoral artery into the distal common iliac artery (CIA) and the occlusion is crossed with a Glidewire-Glidecatheter combination (Glidewire, Glidecath, Terumo, Somerset, NJ). If additional support is desired, then a 0.014″ or

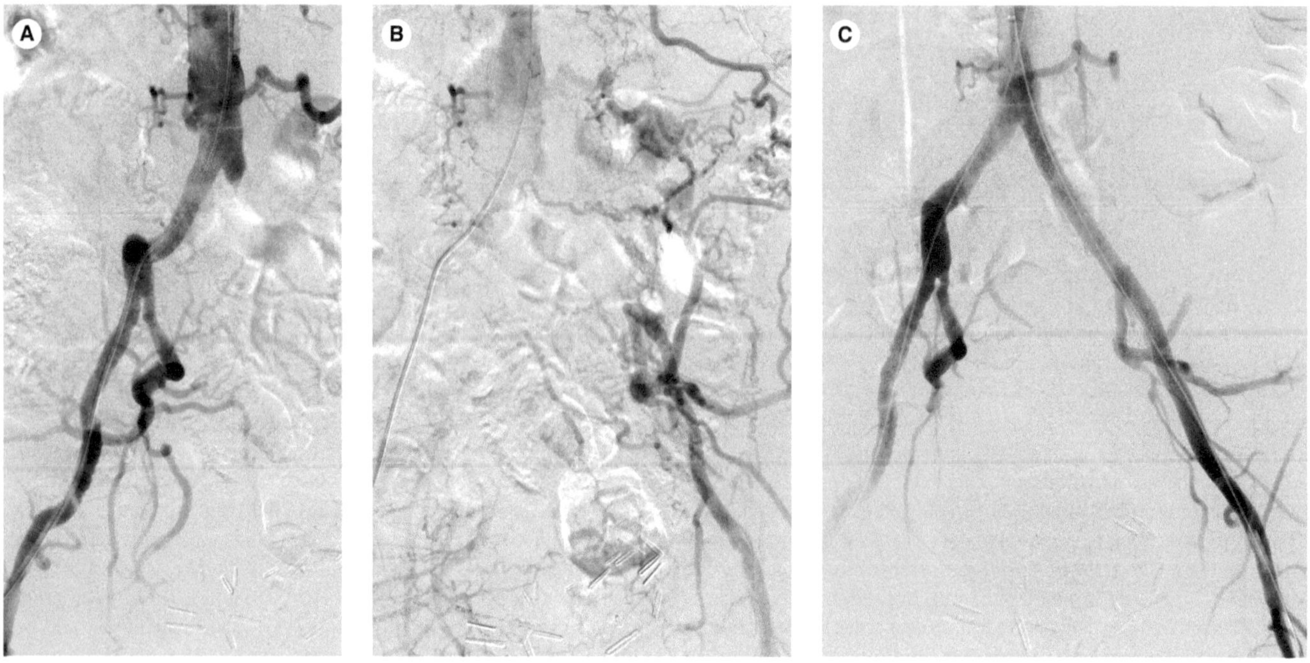

Fig. 32.1 A 62-year-old patient with left leg claudication, with left common iliac artery occlusion, reconstituting above the internal-external iliac bifurcation (A, B). After crossing retrograde from left femoral access, an Atrium stent graft was placed (C).

0.018″ wire can be left in the internal iliac artery for support while a crossing catheter is delivered to the distal CIA in buddy-wire fashion.

While an internal iliac artery occlusion or the presence of a short common iliac stump can make antegrade crossing from the contralateral femoral artery more challenging, it is still our initial approach in most patients. In this situation we begin by probing the common iliac artery with a catheter (our preference is either the Omni flush or the IM catheter) and a stiff straight Glidewire. If the occlusion cannot be entered or the common iliac artery does not provide adequate purchase, a deflectable sheath can be used to support the wire-catheter combination. However, ultimately a brachial approach with a 90-cm sheath (typically 5 French) may be necessary. A brachial approach offers better support for the crossing wire and is our first choice in the setting of a flush iliac occlusion or extensive aortic involvement.

Although we typically prefer antegrade crossing of iliac lesions, there are situations in which retrograde crossing is preferable. In patients with a CIA occlusion and a large, patent internal iliac artery, retrograde crossing via an ipsilateral femoral access should be the preferred initial approach, as it minimizes the chance that the internal iliac artery will be occluded by extension of the dissection plane (Fig. 32.1). Furthermore, an ipsilateral common femoral artery (CFA) access will ultimately be needed when placing a CIA stent; therefore, in cases that do not require stent extension above the aortic bifurcation, this approach allows the entire procedure to be completed via a single puncture. We also consider a retrograde approach when dealing with an isolated external iliac occlusion in combination with an occluded or diminutive internal iliac artery. In this case, there is little risk to the pelvic circulation and a retrograde approach can both simplify the procedure and increase support for the crossing wire/catheter.

Re-Entry Technique and Stent Selection

In severely calcified and chronic lesions, crossing is most likely to be subintimal and the distal re-entry must be carefully managed to limit the extent of the dissection plane and prevent occlusion of critical branch vessels. If the wire does not re-enter the true lumen at or above the CFA when crossing an iliac lesion in an antegrade fashion, the most expedient and safest solution is usually to perform a femoral cut-down, retrieve the wire manually, and then repair the distal aspect of the dissection surgically. A sheath can then be advanced over the wire in a retrograde fashion, while maintaining the wire externalized from the initial femoral or brachial access for support, and the iliac lesion treated via stenting. Our preference for the external iliac artery location is a self-expanding covered stent, because the course of the wire while crossing an occlusion is unpredictable. The guidewire path may be subadventitial and, in our observation, ballooning up the very thin arterial wall may result in external iliac artery rupture, which sometimes occurs in a delayed fashion.

When an iliac lesion is crossed retrograde, the main concern is continuation of the dissection into the aorta such that the re-entry point ends up proximal to the aortic bifurcation. Even in cases in which the crossing seemed easy, it is possible to have a higher re-entry point than suggested by the angiogram and a low threshold should be maintained for using intravascular ultrasound (IVUS) to confirm the course of the crossing wire. We use IVUS routinely when planning to place an iliac stent precisely at or just below the aortic bifurcation. If the re-entry site is above the aortic bifurcation, it may be necessary to raise the bifurcation with kissing stents (Fig. 32.2). Alternatively, a re-entry device (Pioneer or Outback) can be used to re-enter the aorta distally in a more controlled fashion.[11] This is our first choice when our goal is to land an iliac stent precisely at the bifurcation and also in those cases is which the distal aortic wall is known to be very diseased, such that it will resist luminal re-entry. We generally prefer the ultrasound-guided re-entry device (Pioneer) because it allows for direct visualization of the re-entry target and, consequently, reduces the number of attempts to achieve successful re-entry; however, Outback can be used equally effectively (Fig. 32.3). In patients with heavy calcification of the iliac arteries, Outback is preferred because of the superior deliverability of the device to the target. The Pioneer is less sturdy to advance, even after balloon dilatation of the tract.

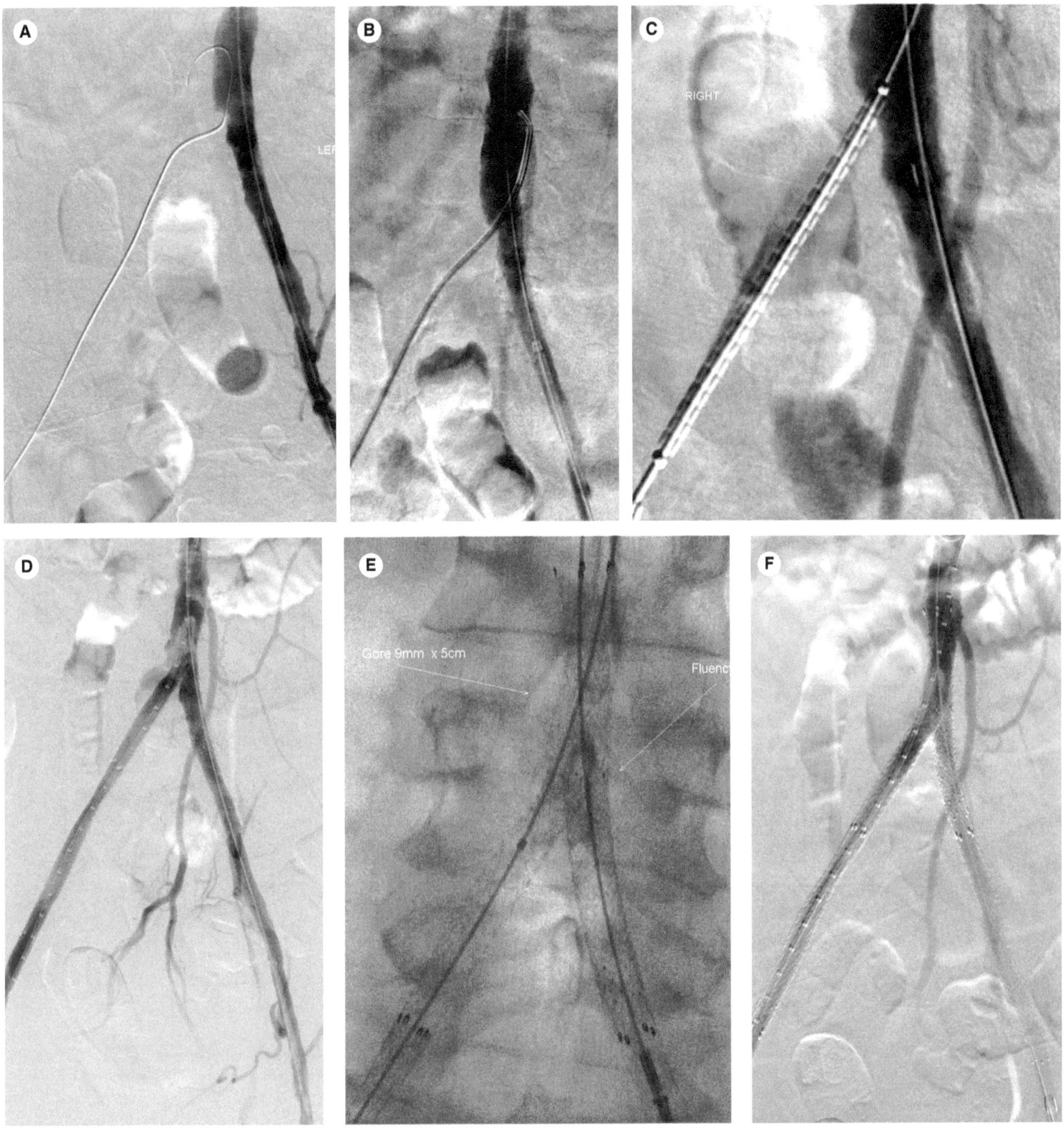

Fig. 32.2 A 54-year-old patient with right leg disabling claudication, right common iliac artery (CIA) and external iliac artery (EIA) occlusion, and bulky right common femoral artery (CFA) disease. After exposure of the right CFA, the iliac occlusion was crossed with stiff Glidewire. Glidewire initially remained subintimal in the aortic wall (A), then entered the aortic lumen seemingly at the distal aorta (B). An Atrium stent graft was placed in the CIA and a Fluency stent graft was placed in the EIA (C). An angiogram showed dissection extending proximally (D), which was addressed by placing two covered stents to the aorta proximal to the dissection (E, F).

Reconstruction of the distal aorta can be performed using double-barrel bare or covered stents or by using the Covered Endovascular Reconstruction of the Aortic Bifurcation (CERAB) technique[12] in which a large, balloon-expandable stent graft is placed in the aorta, with kissing stents extending from the bilateral common iliac arteries up into the aortic stent graft. CERAB was initially described using a 12-mm Atrium stent in the aorta (size not currently available in the United States), which was postdilated up to 16 mm. However, Gore VBX or self-expanding stent grafts (short iliac limb of Gore or Endurant graft) are reasonable alternatives.

Use of bifurcated stent grafts (Endologix) has also been increasingly reported[13,14], not only in patients who have large aneurysms, but also in cases with small aneurysms or those with significant clot layering of the aorta proximal to the occlusion (Fig. 32.4). However, the diameters of the CIA and the external iliac artery (EIA) on one side must allow for passage of a 17-French sheath, for passage of the aortic stent graft. In patients with

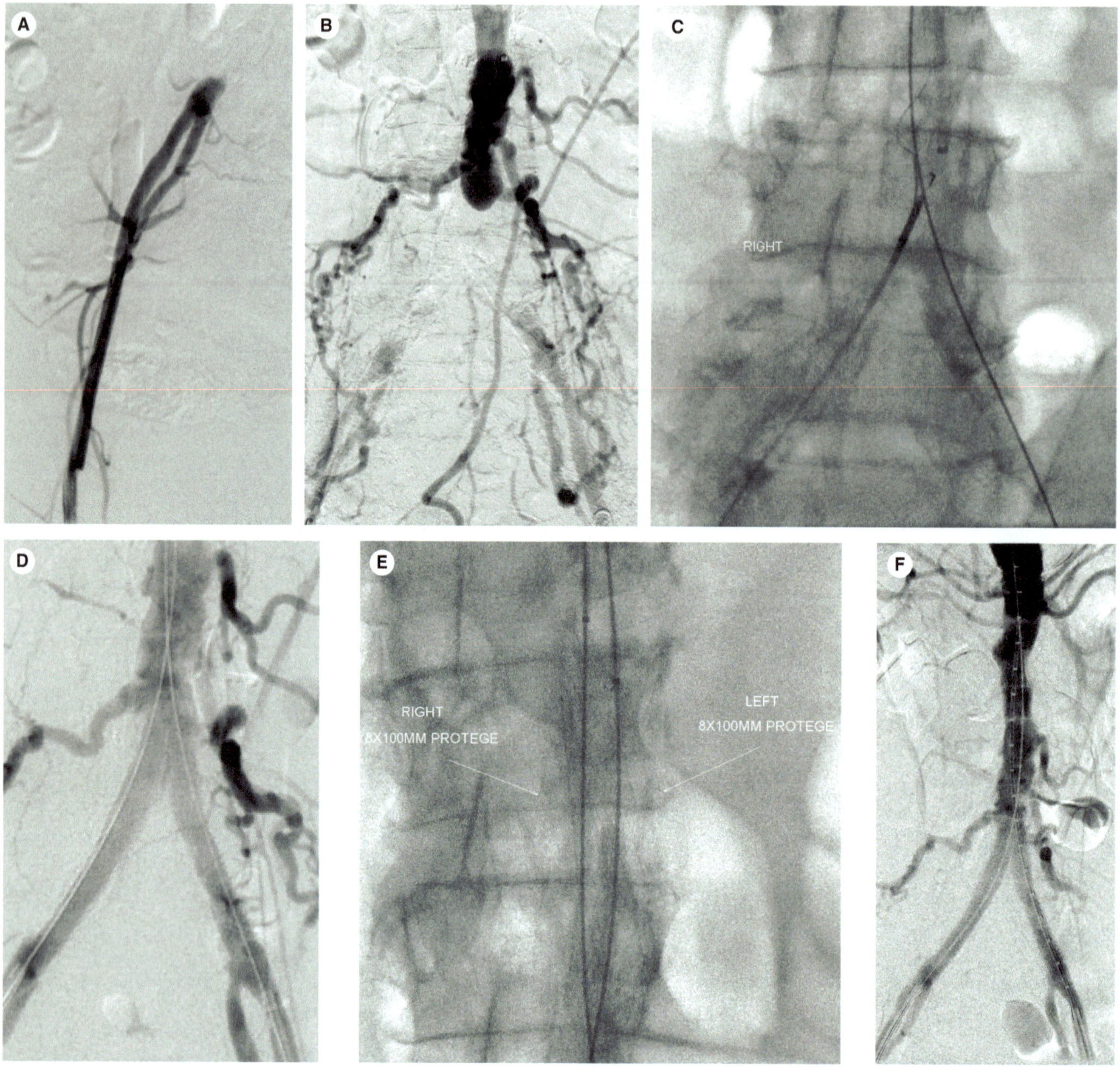

Fig. 32.3 A 78-year-old patient with right toe ulcer and distal aortic occlusion extending to common iliac artery (CIA) (A, B). Transbrachial approach failed to break the cap, therefore Outback was used for re-entry bilaterally and Atrium stent grafts were used in the CIA bilaterally (C, D), extending proximally with self-expending nitinol stents (E, F).

severe calcification of the CIA, a balloon-expandable covered CIA stent may need to be placed to allow passage of the main bifurcated graft.[15] When treating significant bilateral common iliac disease with a bifurcated device, it may be necessary to predilate the contralateral CIA and then advance an 8- or 9-French sheath to the aortic bifurcation. The proximal position of the sheath prevents the contralateral limb from catching on the diseased CIA when the main body is lowered onto the aortic bifurcation. After placement of the bifurcated main body, if there is a need to extend the graft proximally, we typically do not release the contralateral limb before advancing the 17-French sheath proximally. Delaying deployment of the contralateral limb helps to stabilize the main body while advancing the large ipsilateral sheath through narrow iliac vessels. Most patients will also need to have extension of the iliac limbs to the internal–external iliac artery bifurcation, typically using balloon-expandable covered stents (ICast, Atrium Medical Corporation, Merrimack, NH: Viabahn VBX, Gore Medical, Flagstaff, AZ), and in patients with diseased distal CIA and patent internal iliac artery (IIA), bare stents can be used to preserve the IIA and this typically does not result in the loss of the IIA; however, it is important to remember that the IIA may get occluded as a result of plaque shift with placement of the stent. If IIA preservation is important, sizing the balloon by the EIA diameter makes this less likely to occur.

CONCOMITANT FEMORAL ENDARTERECTOMY (HYBRID) PROCEDURES

Femoral endarterectomy (FEA) is necessary in approximately 15%–20% of patients with aortoiliac occlusive disease, most of whom have

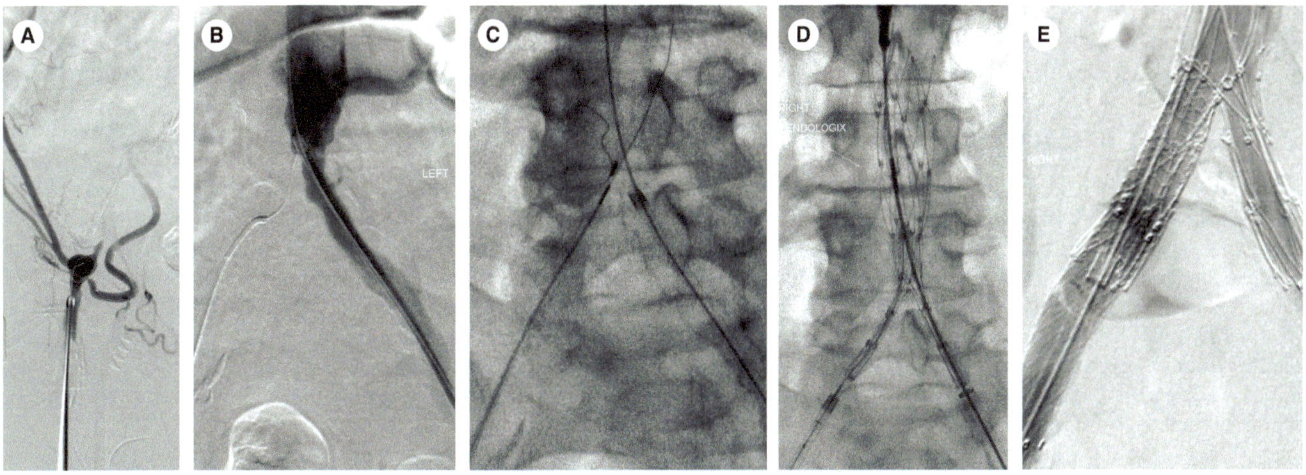

Fig. 32.4 A 66-year-old patient with right disabling claudication was found to have 5.0-cm abdominal aortic aneurysm with occluded right common iliac artery (CIA) and external iliac artery (EIA) (A). A Glidewire was passed in a retrograde fashion (B) and a Pioneer catheter was used for re-entry (C) followed by Endologix placement (D) and relining of CIA and EIA (E).

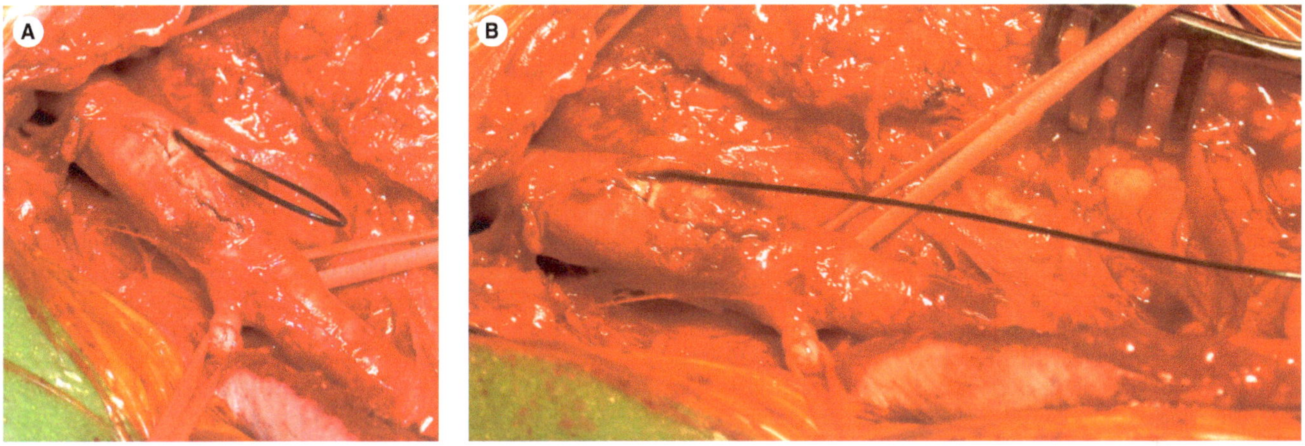

Fig. 32.5 (A, B) Retrieval of Glidewire during arteriotomy.

EIA occlusion or disease with or without concomitant CIA occlusion. When FEA is planned, we expose the CFA before attempting to cross the occlusion. The occlusion is then crossed **before** making the arteriotomy for the endarterectomy (pre-arteriotomy guidewire access, PAGA).[15] This technique ensures preservation of the inflow early in the procedure. The guidewire is positioned across the lesion and maintained throughout the endarterectomy and patching, and then the iliac artery is treated after the patch is completed. Although we typically use Glidewires during crossing, we exchange them for a nonhydrophilic wire as early as possible to minimize the chance that the crossing wire is inadvertently lost or pulled out. The wire can be kept at the anastomotic suture line and hemostasis maintained by cinching the ends of the running suture (our preferred approach), or brought out through the patch, by puncture in the midpatch with introducer needle, and back threading the wire prior to beginning the anastomosis. The iliac vessels are treated with covered stents (our preference is Fluency in those with calcifications or Viabahn in those with soft plaque or organized clot component) because the course of the wire during crossing can be very close to the adventitia, leaving only a thin residual wall. In this setting, a bare-metal stent can cause iliac rupture, which may present immediately or as an iliac pseudoaneurysm during follow-up.

In patients with a diseased, but patent, CFA in whom retrograde crossing is planned, we typically access the exposed CFA with a microwire because it will remain in the small, but patent, lumen as proximally as possible. The access is then upsized as needed to cross the iliac lesions. Once the iliac arteries are crossed and the guidewire is in the aorta, we recommend placing a 7-French or larger sheath across the lesion before starting the endarterectomy to prevent disruption of the thin walled vessel after the endarterectomy. After the continuity of the calcified plaque between the distal EIA and CFA is disrupted by endarterectomy, the interface between the distal EIA and the endarterectomized wall of the CFA is very weak. At that point, any resistance to advancing a sheath across the iliac lesions can cause complete disruption of the interface, which will necessitate a difficult oversewing of the calcified EIA stump (may require 0 prolene with a strong needle) and an extra-anatomic bypass.

If an antegrade crossing is planned, the wire is advanced to the level of the common femoral artery and then retrieved at the time of the arteriotomy.[10] In this case, it is unnecessary to re-enter the true lumen (Fig. 32.5). The wire is maintained externally at both sites during the endarterectomy. If the dissection has continued to the level of the common femoral artery, the re-entry point can be defined surgically after the vessel is open. Once the wire has been retrieved from the arteriotomy, a sheath can be advanced across the iliac occlusion and the endarterectomy and stenting may proceed as described.

MANAGEMENT OF COMPLICATIONS

Despite all planning, complications will occur, and the physician must be prepared to address these in a timely manner because the consequences of delay can be highly morbid or even fatal. A variety of covered stents, snares, wires, catheters, re-entry devices, and ideally IVUS should be available on the shelf. Most complications can be managed endovascularly; however, for non-surgeons performing complex aortoiliac procedures, we highly recommend that they work in an environment where emergency surgical consultation is immediately available. Surgical conversion is more likely to be necessary in patients with severe calcification, bulky CFA disease, and those with subacute occlusions (3–6-month history with easy crossing of occluded arteries). These conditions increase the likelihood of distal embolization and extensive CFA dissection, both of which are easier and safer to manage via open conversion rather than through the use of stent extension, thrombectomy devices, or thrombolysis.

Dissection

Dissection of diseased iliac arteries can occur from the very beginning of a percutaneous procedure, even with placement of a relatively delicate micropuncture wire. All guidewires should be advanced under fluoroscopic guidance and the slightest resistance should prompt the physician to verify the anatomy by placing a catheter and performing a low-pressure dye injection by hand. However, dye should never be injected without blood return, because this can cause air embolization and may extend a dissection when given in high pressures. If a dissection is identified early, a 0.014″ nontraumatic tip guidewire (i.e., All Star, Abbott Laboratories, Chicago, IL) can be advanced from the initial access site and redirected into the true lumen. Once the wire has reached the aorta, it can be gradually upsized to a 0.035″ guidewire using straight, hydrophilic catheters (Quick-Cross, Phillips Healthcare, Andover MA; Seeker, Bard Medical, Franklin Lakes, NJ; Renegade, Boston Scientific, Marlborough, MA) and the case can proceed normally. Since the initial dissection plane is retrograde, it is unlikely to continue expanding; however, as the involved vessels are typically quite diseased, we maintain a low threshold for placing a self-expanding bare-metal stent at the end of the procedure.

If a retrograde dissection is not recognized early and larger wires, catheters, and sheaths are placed, it can rapidly become complicated and difficult to cross. In this situation, crossing antegrade via either a contralateral femoral or brachial access is usually successful. Once the guidewire is beyond the dissection, it can be snared via the ipsilateral femoral access, and then the case can proceed as planned. However, rarely, when the dissection plane has become large, it may be difficult to get an antegrade wire and retrograde snare into the same plane. In this case, a balloon can be inflated within the retrograde dissection plane from the ipsilateral femoral access while a re-entry device (either Outback, Cordis, Cardinal Health, Dublin, OH or Pioneer, Phillips Healthcare, Andover MA) is loaded over the antegrade wire. The balloon then becomes the target for the needle on the re-entry device. Once a connection between the antegrade and retrograde planes is confirmed by puncturing the balloon, a wire can be advanced through the re-entry device and into the retrograde plane. This wire can then either be snared or backed out of the ipsilateral femoral access with the ruptured balloon.

While dissection can be problematic at the beginning of a case, it much more commonly becomes an issue when crossing an occlusion in a subintimal plane. If the dissection plane extends beyond the end of the occlusion, it can result in the loss of critical side branches or, in the case of proximal aortic extension, limit flow through the entire reconstruction. In a patient with retrograde crossing of a CIA occlusion into the aorta and suspected dissection, it is very important to use IVUS to identify the most proximal extent of dissection (aortic re-entry). If the point of re-entry is proximal to the aortic bifurcation, the patient will need stenting of both common iliac arteries, typically with double-barrel bare or covered stents. Unilateral iliac stent placement will cause obstruction of the contralateral common iliac artery. In patients with concomitant aortic clots or aneurysm, in whom a bifurcated monobody (AFX, Endologix Inc, Irvine, CA) device is planned, it may be reasonable to withdraw the wire and either come from the contralateral access and snare the wire in the subintimal plane (rendezvous technique) or, if the re-entry is close to the bifurcation, simply complete the procedure with the understanding that the graft will be sitting higher than the actual bifurcation.

If the desired point of re-entry is within the iliac arteries, extension of the dissection plane may cause occlusion of the hypogastric, deep femoral, or superficial femoral arteries. When the internal iliac artery is occluded during crossing of a CIA lesion, contralateral access and placement of a wire into the IIA can be attempted while maintaining the wire from the ipsilateral femoral artery. Once the IIA is accessed, kissing stents (bare or covered) can be placed into the IIA and EIA to reestablish flow and to tack down the intimal flap (Fig. 32.6).

If the re-entry point is too low in the CFA and noticed early, the wire can be pulled back to the distal EIA near the point of reconstitution and a re-entry device can be used to re-enter at a more proximal level. If there is bulky CFA disease, the dissection can be addressed during the ensuing FEA. However, if a low re-entry is not recognized and the dissection extends to the femoral bifurcation, this will manifest on the completion angiogram with occlusion/narrowing of the deep femoral artery (DFA) or superficial femoral artery (SFA). In this situation, surgical conversion is the safest and most effective solution. The femoral vessels are easily accessible and direct assessment simplifies identification of the relevant planes and placement of tacking sutures.

A completely percutaneous approach to femoral bifurcation salvage may be considered in poor risk patients, although it often proves more technically demanding than open conversion. This strategy typically requires retrograde puncture of the superficial femoral or popliteal artery and then snaring the wire via the contralateral sheath. A second wire can then be positioned in the DFA and the dissection treated via placement of kissing stents. In this situation, IVUS should be considered to define the anatomy better and to confirm the course of the crossing wires.

Arterial Perforation

Arterial perforation can occur during wire manipulation and is typically not an issue when it is recognized immediately and the wire is pulled back. The more clinically significant vessel perforations result either from overdilation or from failure to recognize that a wire passage occurred in a subadventitial, rather than a subintimal, plane with subsequent angioplasty or bare metal stenting of the tract (Fig. 32.7). The most common cause of EIA rupture is oversizing of angioplasty balloons. Consequently, we predilate with a balloon 1 mm smaller (5 or 6 mm) than our estimated final diameter goal and then use the appropriately-sized stent. We also have a very low threshold for using covered stents in the EIA, particularly in those with bulky disease extending to the CFA, because the patency has been shown to be superior, as well as the risk of rupture being eliminated.

Although iliac rupture can sometimes present in a delayed fashion, either as a pseudoaneurysm or a late rupture, the most common presentation is immediate onset of excessive pain and hypotension from massive retroperitoneal bleeding. Once rupture occurs in the iliac

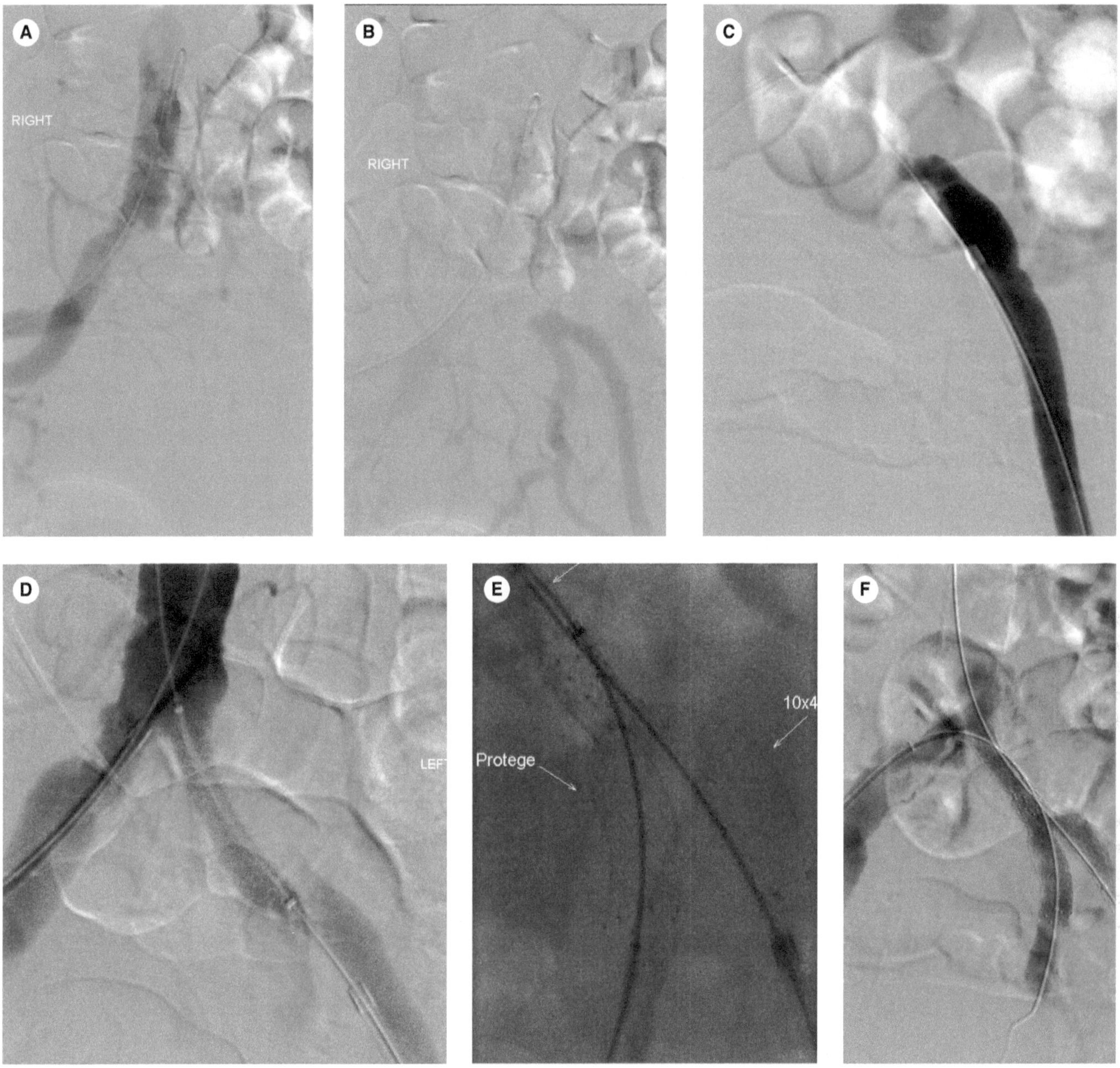

Fig. 32.6 A 70-year-old patient with left foot ulcer with left common iliac artery (CIA) occlusion. Antegrade crossing resulted in loss of left internal iliac artery (IIA) after placing covered stent to left CIA (A–D). The left IIA was accessed via contralateral access while the wire was maintained from left femoral access and kissing stents were placed to IIA and the external iliac artery (E, F).

artery, swift and decisive action is necessary to prevent significant morbidity and mortality. A quick dye injection will allow identification of the rupture site and then a balloon, typically the same balloon that was inflated prior to the rupture, should be introduced to tamponade the vessel, usually at nominal pressures only. It is critical not to panic and not to lose wire access across the lesion. After temporary control has been established, a stent graft and appropriately-sized sheath should be identified. If multiple maneuvers will be necessary, such as upsizing the sheath, consideration should be given to establishing contralateral access and placing an occlusion balloon more proximally in either the CIA or aorta. However, in most cases, a covered stent can be placed expeditiously with rapid control of the rupture, as long as wire control is maintained.

In patients with a perforation close to the internal iliac artery, an initial attempt can be made to place a covered stent right at the take-off of the IIA. However, if bleeding persists, then the IIA should be sacrificed. Complete disruption of the IIA take-off is unusual but can occur when using larger sheaths. In this situation, simple coverage of the IIA may not provide adequate control and open repair may be necessary. In patients with CIA rupture, balloon-expandable covered stents can be used for control. However, if a patient has severe calcification or bulky common iliac disease, we prefer to use covered stents preemptively to avoid this occurrence. It is extremely unlikely to have a perforation at the aortoiliac junction; however, in such cases, expeditious repair is essential. The first attempt at control is typically placement of kissing covered stents in the bilateral common iliac arteries.

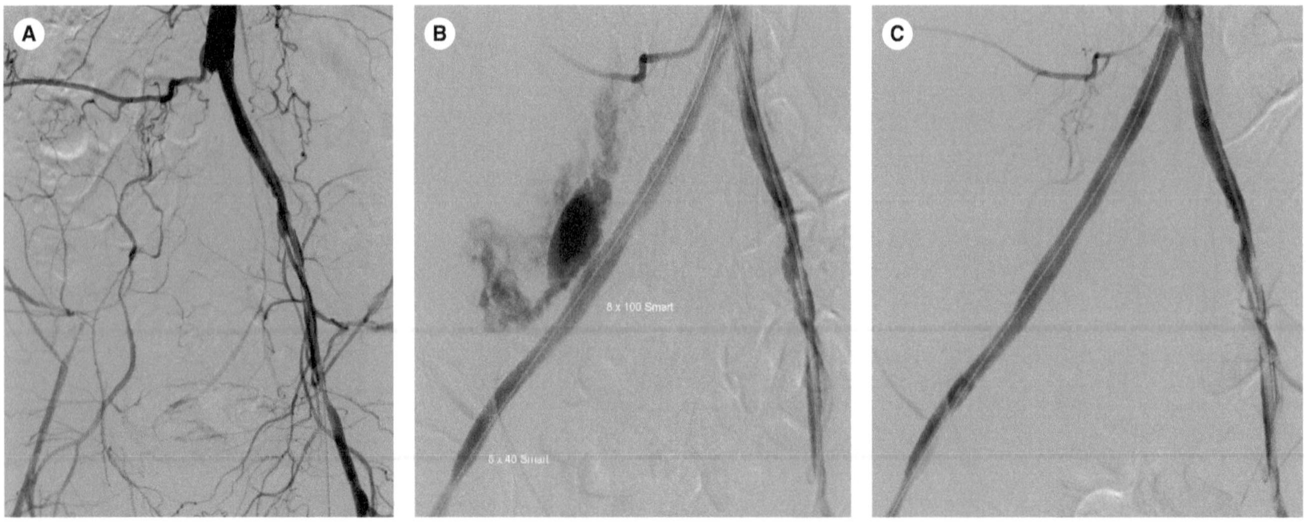

Fig. 32.7 Iliac perforation after self-expanding stent postdilatation (A, B), treated with covered stent placement (C).

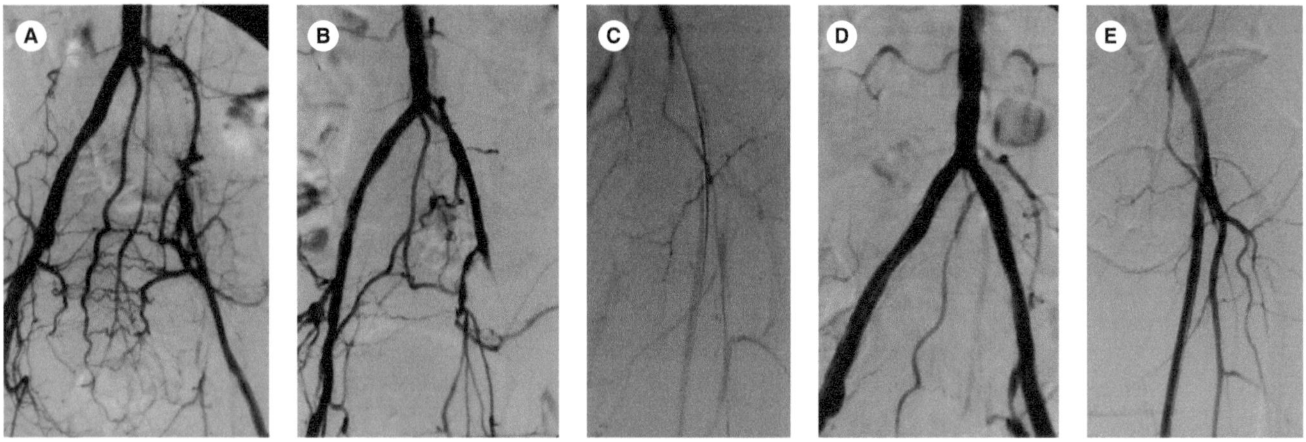

Fig. 32.8 A 67-year-old with 4-month history of left leg claudication. Left common iliac artery occlusion easily crossed and stented, resulting in occlusion of left external iliac artery, with repeat stenting to trap the clot resulting in occlusion of the common femoral artery (A–C). Thrombectomy and thrombolysis successfully cleared all clots (D, E).

However, placement of an aortoiliac stent graft and femorofemoral bypass with or without coil embolization of the CIA may be necessary. The risk of kissing stent grafts in this circumstance is continued bleeding from the gutter between the grafts if the lesion extends to the bifurcation area.

Embolization

Embolization is most likely to occur in patients with either acute or subacute arterial occlusions. This should be considered, prior to intervention, based on the patients' presentation history and the ease of crossing the lesion. In these cases, either femoral cut-down with clamping of the distal branches or thrombolysis should be considered before proceeding with recanalization (balloon angioplasty and stenting). Filter deployment may also be useful once the occlusion has been crossed. However, this often requires placement of either a buddy wire for support or use of two filters (one in the SFA and one in the DFA) with interventions being performed over both wires, all of which is frequently cumbersome and not completely protective. Regardless of the preventative steps taken, it is critical to establish the patency of the run-off vessels at the start of the procedure and also immediately after crossing any occlusions, so that embolization can be recognized and managed in a timely fashion.

In patients with organizing clots, the entire occluded segment may move down distally (toothpasting) (Fig. 32.8). This problem can be addressed using thrombolysis if the leg is not ischemic. However, in patents with large clot embolization, simple exploration and thrombectomy is usually the safest and most efficient option. In the case of small, distal emboli, there are a variety of thrombectomy catheters (suction or mechanical such as Angiojet, Boston Scientific, Marlborough, MA; Indigo, Penumbra Inc, Alameida, CA) that can help to retrieve the clot. However, the devices themselves can cause additional embolization to more distal vessels, even with the use of protective filters. Consequently, adjunctive thrombolysis will still be necessary in many of these cases.

Embolization of renal or mesenteric arteries can occur in patients with juxtarenal aortic occlusions during wire manipulations near the renal arteries. In these cases, the emboli often consist of atherosclerotic debris rather than clot and, as a result, may not respond to thrombolysis. Consequently, we prefer aortobifemoral bypass in good risk patients and extra-anatomic bypass for higher risk patients. Although treatment of juxtarenal occlusions with an aortic stent graft and snorkeling of the renal arteries and SMA has been described[16], the risk of wire manipulation with associated "trashing" is too high and should only be considered in extreme cases.

REFERENCES

1. Norgren L, Hiatt WR, Dormandy JA, et al. Inter-Society Consensus for the Management of Peripheral Arterial Disease (TASC II). *J Vasc Surg.* 2007;45(Suppl S):S5–S67.
2. Jongkind V, Akkersdijk GJ, Yeung KK, et al. Asystematic review of endovascular treatment of extensive aortoiliac occlusive disease. *J Vasc Surg.* 2010;52:1376–1383.
3. de Vries SO, Hunink MG. Results of aortic bifurcation grafts for aortoiliac occlusive disease: a meta-analysis. *J Vasc Surg.* 1997;26:558–569.
4. Kashyap VS, Pavkov ML, Bena JF, et al. The management of severe aortoiliac occlusive disease: endovascular therapy rivals open reconstruction. *J Vasc Surg.* 2008;48:1451–1457.
5. Sachwani GR, Hans SS, Khoury MD, et al. Long-term results of iliac stenting and aortofemoral grafting for iliac artery occlusions. *J Vasc Surg.* 2013;57:1030–1037.
6. Dosluoglu HH, Lall P, Harris LM, et al. Long term durability of endovascular and open revascularization for disabling claudication. *J Vasc Surg.* 2012;56:1478–1479.
7. Ichihashi S, Higashiura W, Itoh H, et al. Longterm outcomes for systematic primary stent placement in complex iliac artery occlusive disease classified according to Trans-Atlantic Inter-Society Consensus (TASC)-II. *J Vasc Surg.* 2011;53:992–999.
8. Koizumi A, Kumakura H, Kanai H, et al. Ten year patency and factors causing restenosis after endovascular treatment of iliac artery lesions. *Circ J.* 2009;73:860–866.
9. Pulli R, Dorigo W, Fargion A, et al. Early and long-term comparison of endovascular treatment of iliac artery occlusions and stenosis. *J Vasc Surg.* 2011;53:92–98.
10. Dosluoglu HH, Harris LM, Cherr GS. Recanalization of concomitant iliac artery and common femoral artery occlusions using an antegrade hybrid (open/endovascular) approach. *Vasc and Endovasc Surg.* 2007;41: 130–134.
11. Jacobs DL, Motaganahalli RL, Cox DE, et al. True lumen re-entry devices facilitate subintimal angioplasty and stenting of total chronic occlusions: initial report. *J Vasc Surg.* 2006;43:1291–1296.
12. Grimme FA, Goverde PC, Verbruggen PJ, Zeebregts CJ, Reijnen MM. Editor's Choice-First Results of the Covered Endovascular Reconstruction of the Aortic Bifurcation (CERAB) Technique for Aortoiliac Occlusive Disease. *Eur J Vasc Endovasc Surg.* 2015;50(5):638–647.
13. Maldonado TS, Westin GG, Jazaeri O, et al. Treatment of Aortoiliac Occlusive Disease with the Endologix AFX Unibody Endograft. *Eur J Vasc Endovasc Surg.* 2016;52(1):64–74.
14. Van Haren RM, Goldstein LJ, Velazquez OC, Karmacharya J, Bornak A. Endovascular treatment of TransAtlantic Inter-Society Consensus D aortoiliac occlusive disease using unibody bifurcated endografts. *J Vasc Surg.* 2017;65(2):398–405.
15. Dosluoglu HH, Cherr GS. Pre-arteriotomy guidewire access (PAGA). A crucial maneuver for securing inflow and/or outflow in patients with bulky iliofemoral occlusive disease undergoing combined (open/endovascular) procedures. *Eur J Vasc Endovasc Surg.* 2006;32:97–100.
16. Bin Jabr A, Sonesson B, Lindblad B, Dias N, Resch T, Malina M. Chimney grafts preserve visceral flow and allow safe stenting of juxtarenal aortic occlusion. *J Vasc Surg.* 2013;57(2):399–405.

33

Complications of Femoropopliteal Interventions for Occlusive Disease

James F. McKinsey, MD, FACS and Reid Ravin, MD

INTRODUCTION

There has been a dramatic change over the past several decades in management of patients with femoropopliteal occlusive disease transitioning from open to minimally invasive endovascular repair. Optimal medical therapy continues to be the first-line therapy for patients with claudication caused by femoropopliteal disease. This includes smoking cessation and cardiovascular risk reduction, including antiplatelet therapy, cholesterol manipulation, exercise therapy, and oral statins.[1] Supervised exercise programs have proven to be efficacious, but they require consistent participation from highly motivated patients. Revascularization may be appropriate in patients with claudication who still have lifestyle altering symptoms despite medical management. Patients with critical limb ischemia (CLI) require intervention to achieve limb salvage. These patients usually have multilevel vascular disease and often require complex procedures.

Currently, in many centers, endovascular management of superficial femoral artery (SFA) and proximal popliteal lesions is the first-line therapy regardless of degree of stenosis, extent of calcification, total plaque occlusion, or length of the lesion.

Plaque etiology and composition impacts on the ability to perform endovascular procedures. Lesions can be composed of smooth muscle cell intimal hyperplasia, calcific lesions, thrombotic material, arterial necrotic core material, and a combination. The plaque constituents also impact procedure success and long-term patency. Studies have shown that the greater extent of calcification, the less the likelihood of immediate and long-term success.[2]

PATIENT EVALUATION

Many medical processes can cause lower extremity symptoms, and a careful history and physical help clarify the potential etiology. If there is concern for peripheral artery disease (PAD), we generally perform noninvasive vascular laboratory studies to evaluate further. We have found that these studies can accurately identify the arterial occlusive lesions and direct intervention. Arterial duplex confirms the location of the lesions and the extent and degree of calcification. If duplex reveals a long segment calcific SFA occlusion and an adequate venous conduit, we schedule the hybrid angiographic suite for diagnostic angiography and potential endovascular or open bypass. Other vascular surgeons and interventionalists have reported added benefit to preintervention CT angiography of the aorta and lower extremities,[3,4] including more sizing of balloons and stents.

ARTERIAL ACCESS

In our institution, all arterial access is performed under ultrasonic guidance. The common femoral artery (CFA) is accessed antegrade or retrograde with micropuncture system. To confirm location and orientation, we pass the inner dilator of the micropuncture sheath into the femoral vessel and perform oblique angiogram, confirming optimal access. The micropuncture sheath with the inner and outer dilators reconnected is reinserted and the system exchanged to a 0.035″ wire and 4–5-French sheath.

Access for femoropopliteal occlusive lesions are routinely performed antegrade or retrograde, with the approach tailored to patient anatomy. Antegrade access is used with patent aortoiliac, CFA, and proximal SFA, and planned intervention in mid-distal SFA, popliteal, or tibial vessels. Antegrade access allows greater "pushability" to traverse arterial total occlusions and control of the wire and catheter torque for selective catheterization of branch vessels. Steep aortic bifurcations and extremely tall patients, where catheter length becomes an issue, are well served by antegrade approach. Possible drawbacks are a higher rate of hematoma and pseudoaneurysm, although this may have abated in more recent series.[5] Antegrade access can be more uncomfortable for the operator, as most endovascular suites are better oriented to facilitate retrograde femoral access. To maintain the usual orientation of controls and not have to work around the head and upper body of the patient, we frequently place a longer sheath into the proximal SFA, using an 0.035″ support wire with approximately 20 cm of sheath externalized. The sheath is then gently curved to the patient's contralateral groin in an approximation of up-and-over position. An occlusive Ioban drape secures this in place. This allows direct access from the more conventional retrograde approach, with added stability.

Similar technique is used for retrograde access. Retrograde access allows visualization of the suprarenal, perivisceral, aortoiliac inflow regions, and bilateral lower extremity arterial run-off vessels. Aortoiliac angulation and calcification can make retrograde access more challenging. Once aortoiliac angiography has been completed, angiography of the contralateral lower extremity is performed. It is critical that angiography be carried out to the level of the foot to have a thorough understanding of the vasculature of the patient. To facilitate higher-quality imaging and decrease contrast load, imaging is performed from the contralateral external iliac artery. If the SFA is patent, the catheter is advanced to the popliteal over a wire and run-off of tibial and pedal vessels performed. If there is SFA occlusion, better visualization of the popliteal and tibial vessels may require a more proximal catheter in the external iliac artery, such that collateralization from the profunda femoral artery (PFA) allows visualization of the popliteal through geniculate vessels. Severe angulation within the aortoiliac segment can make passage of a sheath more challenging. Options for facilitating placement of an up-and-over sheath include positioning a wire within the contralateral distal SFA. If that is unsuccessful, passing a stiffer catheter with a more supportive wire, such as Rosen or Amplatz may facilitate sheath passage. If the sheath will still not pass, we take a long dilator and pass it over the stiffer wire into the contralateral iliac system. With the dilator in place, the shorter sheath can be advanced over the shoulders of the dilator into the contralateral iliac artery. Additionally, by separating the dilator and sheath slightly, it is often possible to "walk" the sheath over steep bifurcations. Finally, if the sheath will not advance, contralateral femoral access can be obtained and a small sheath inserted, snaring the wire. With through-and-through access, the sheath can be advanced into the iliac arteries.

FEMORAL INTERVENTIONS

Once the sheath is in place, characteristics of the plaque determine type of intervention. Characteristics that impact intervention include calcification, location of the plaque relative to branch points, degree of stenosis, presence of previously placed stents, presence or absence of in-stent restenosis, and length of lesion. First, the plaque must be crossed with a guidewire. We usually use a 0.035″ hydrophilic coated wire. Traversing a totally occluded plaque can be challenging but is possible even with long calcific lesions. A central luminal or true lumen crossing is considered by many to be optimal.[6] In order to accomplish this, a supportive catheter is placed through the sheath and brought into close proximity of the total arterial occlusion. The hydrophilic wire gently probes the cap of the occlusion, attempting to find a small microchannel allowing the wire to engage and to advance. Care is taken not to form a loop at this point because of the high probability of a subadventitial dissection. The subadventitial plane is actually misnamed subintimal and is actually a plane between the media and adventitia, similar to the plane encountered when performing carotid endarterectomy.

Once the hydrophilic wire advances, the support catheter is advanced to allow better pushability and control of the wire. The tip of the wire is continually rotated in a circular fashion to attempt to stay in the central luminal plane. If there is significant spiraling of the wire, it is likely the wire is in the subadventitial plane. The wire and catheter are advanced in sequential fashion until the reconstitution point is reached. It is extremely important that the arterial reconstitution point is identified prior to attempting crossing, to prevent the catheter and wire from propagating a dissection flap within the patent vessel rather than re-entering the true lumen. In Fig. 33.1, we demonstrate use of the Crosser for crossing the distal cap of a chronic total occlusion in order to maintain true luminal position. By stopping immediately proximal to the distal cap, a wire can be used to probe to find a re-entry point. Once the wire passes into the true lumen, the catheter should be advanced, the wire removed, and the catheter aspirated to see whether there is a blood return. If there is a blood return, an angiogram should be performed confirming true-lumen re-entry.

It is possible to have blood return even if the catheter is still in a dissection plane. If the proximal aspect of the plaque cannot be engaged or the central luminal plane cannot be re-entered, there are several options. First, especially in long SFA occlusions, the question should be asked whether the patient is a surgical candidate. The patency of long-segment transatlantic inter society consensus classification D (TASC D) lesions endovascular interventions have not been favorable and, when appropriate, surgical bypass is recommended.[7]

If the patient is not a good candidate for bypass, the Bolia technique creates a narrow loop in the hydrophilic wire just proximal to the proximal cap, advancing the wire into the subadventitial plane (subintimal) down to the reconstitution point of the occluded artery and then using a directional catheter to re-enter into true lumen.[8] This technique does create an eccentric dissection plane within the subadventitial plane, which may impact on success and complication rates.

There are devices designed to aid in the traversing of the proximal and distal caps. The Crosser (BD Bard, Franklin Lakes, New Jersey) has

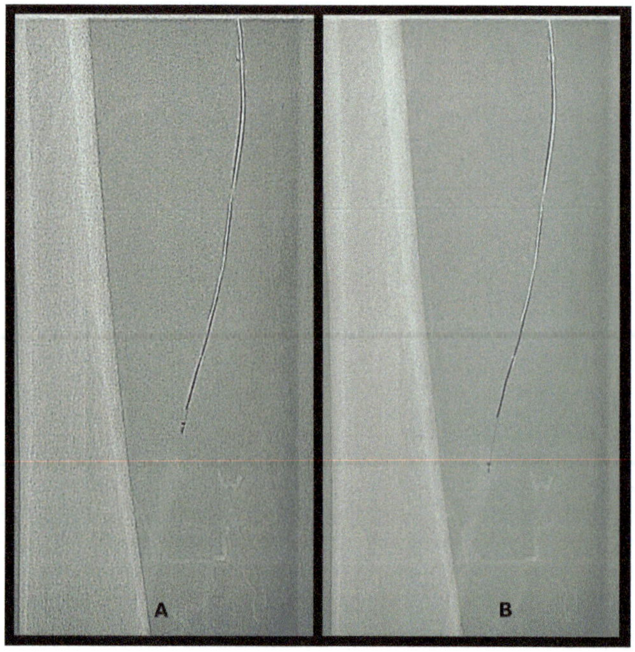

Fig. 33.1 Use of the Crosser for crossing a distal cap of a chronic total occlusion to maintain true luminal position. (A) Crosser brought in contact with cap of occlusion. (B) Crosser activated and crossing lesion.

an indication for proximal plaque traversing. It is placed just proximal to the plaque, activated, and gently brought in contact with the proximal plaque (Fig. 33.1). Using a hydraulic (jackhammer) affect, the device gently probes the proximal cap and attempts to engage into microchannels and is slowly advanced.[9] Traversing the main portion of the plaque is generally fairly straightforward until the distal cap, which can also be somewhat dense. The device is advanced slowly and works to re-enter the true lumen. Care must be taken that the Crosser device does not advance within a subadventitial plane and create a dissection.

The step-by-step technique uses the Spectranetics Excimer laser (Philips Medical, Colorado Springs, Colorado). The laser fiber is brought into close proximity to the proximal plaque, activated, and gently allowed to advance into the proximal cap. Once the proximal cap has been traversed by the laser fiber, the wire is advanced, and allowed to track through the plaque until the distal cap is encountered. The laser may be required to be activated again, traversing through the distal cap. This technique also performs initial laser atherectomy of the underlying plaque.

All of the techniques described are most effective if performed as primary therapy, rather than being attempted once wire and catheter traversal has failed. With attempted wire catheter crossing, channels can be created so that the crossing devices will engage and follow the same path, rather than creating a new path. If the plaque can be traversed through the proximal cap and the main body of the plaque, even in a subadventitial plane, but re-entry cannot be accomplished, a re-entry device can be used.

Several devices are available, and mechanism of action is generally insertion of a curved needle into true lumen from the extraluminal plaque, either using ultrasonic (Pioneer, Philips, Amsterdam, Netherlands) or fluoroscopic guidance (Outback, Cordis, Hialeah, FL). This has been shown to be highly effective for re-entry and can be accomplished after failed wire catheter traversal attempts.[10]

Finally, Spinosa described a retrograde tibial or popliteal access, SAFARI technique.[11] A small sheath or a bareback 0.018″ crossing catheter (our preference) is inserted into distal patent vasculature, usually by ultrasonic guidance, and manipulated proximally through the plaque. Once the wire has traversed the plaque, it is snared from above establishing through-and-through wire access, facilitating endovascular intervention. This is demonstrated in Fig. 33.2, where retrograde peroneal artery access is shown. Additionally, SAFARI techniques can be combined with outback re-entry devices (Fig. 33.3). In that case, an outback catheter is used in conjunction with retrograde puncture and balloon inflation in order to obtain antegrade access into a tibial vessel.

As the profiles of the endovascular devices have decreased, some authors recommend primary retrograde intervention from tibial or popliteal access, without antegrade catheterization.[12,13] In cases of instant restenosis and occlusion, care has to be taken to assure that you stay within the stent and not traverse the interstices. If there is concern, a small balloon can be passed over the crossing wire to confirm that struts have not been traversed. The stent can also be accessed percutaneously under fluoroscopic guidance, and then the 0.035″ wire can be advanced through the stent and captured with a snare for a through-and-through access if unable to cross from above or below (Fig. 33.4).

ENDOVASCULAR TREATMENT OPTIONS

Dr. Charles Dotter initially introduced sequential arterial dilatation using semi-rigid dilators in 1964.[14] In 1979, Dr. Andreas Grüntzig described percutaneously placed balloon angioplasty (PTA), dramatically changing management of coronary artery disease and PAD.[15] Initially POBA (plain old balloon angioplasty) was recommended for short, focal, nonoccluded stenosis, with reasonable results. There was concern for plaque recoil and restenosis, dissection, and vessel perforation. Shillinger reports 1-year patency of POBA at 37% in femoral lesions.[16] To address this, metallic stents were developed.[17] Because of the need for flexibility and mobility in lower extremity, self-expanding stents were developed. Initial stent results were good, with 1-year primary patency approximately 66%.[18] Long-term complications include stent fracture, occlusion or in-stent restenosis, and recurrent symptoms. Short focal stents are more effective than long-segment, entire SFA stenting.[19] Current attempts to improve outcomes of intra-arterial stent placement have included use of medications to inhibit the

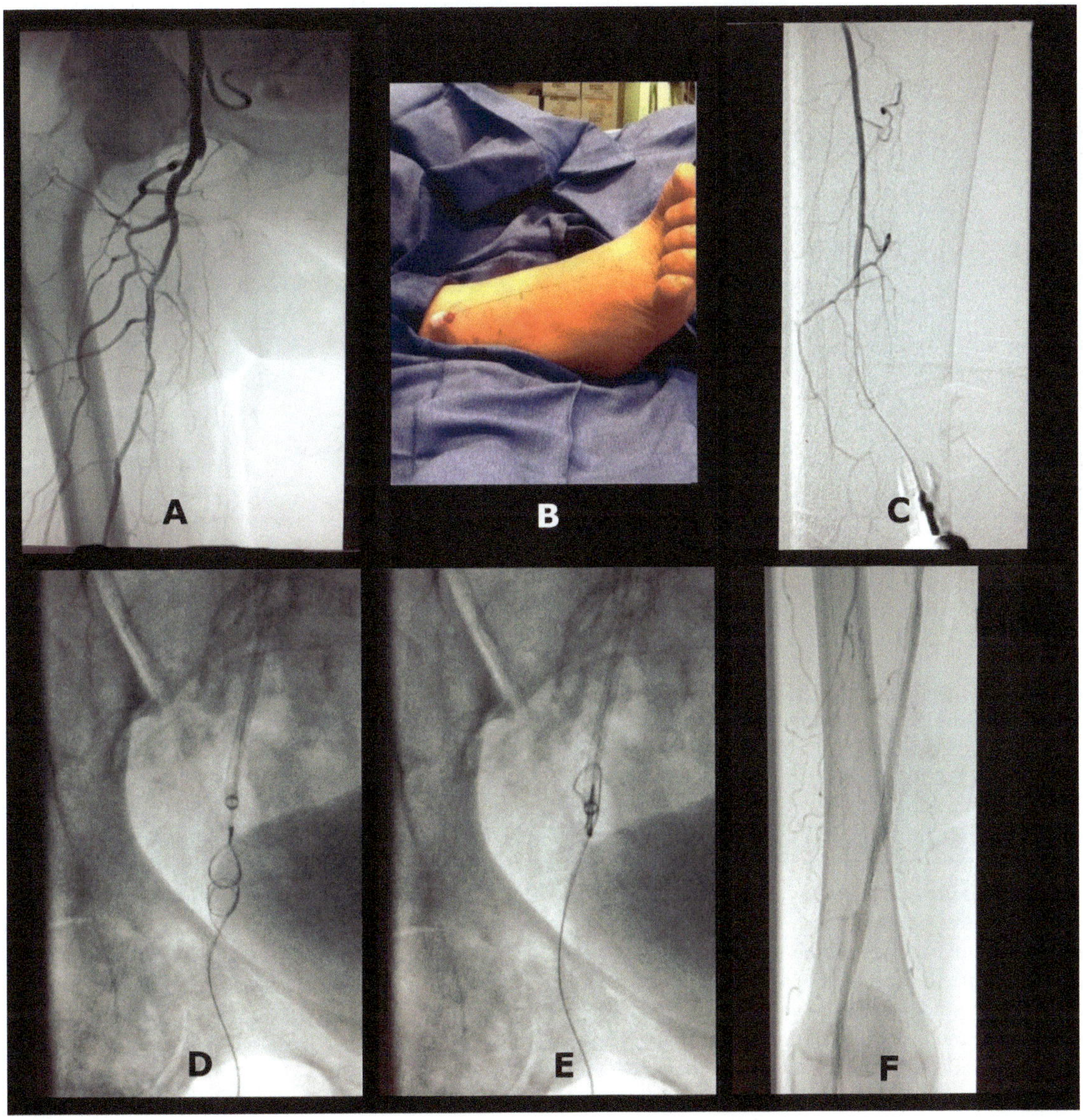

Fig. 33.2 Retrograde peroneal access with snaring for SAFARI technique. (A) Occluded superficial femoral artery (SFA). (B) Peroneal access. (C) Peroneal access. (D) Snaring from up and over. (E) Crossing wire brought in to sheath. (F) Recanalized SFA.

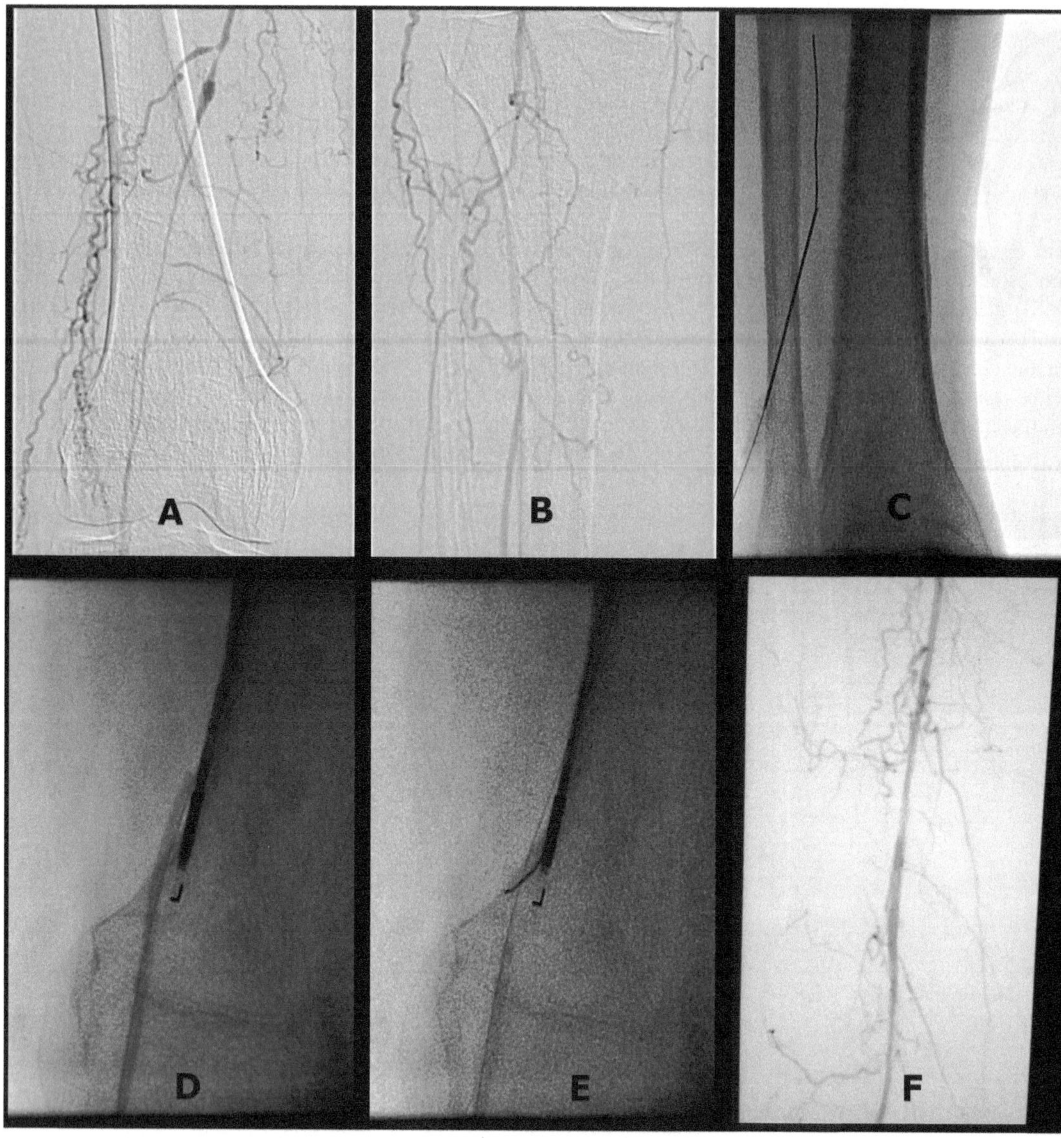

Fig. 33.3 SAFARI technique combined with Outback re-entry device. (A) Occluded popliteal (B) Patent tibial vessels. (C) Peroneal access. (D) Outback lined up for accessing true lumen—marked with wire from below. (E) Outback deployed with wire entering true lumen. (F) Recanalized popliteal artery.

proliferative response resulting in intimal hyperplasia. The Zilver PTX (Cook Medical, Bloomington, IN) drug-eluting stent 5-year data have shown 80% clinical benefit versus 59% for POBA and patency of 66% Zilver PTX versus 43% POBA.[20] Recently, Eluvia Drug Eluting Stent (Boston Scientific, Marlborough, MA) reported primary patency at 1 year of 88%. Our current practice for longer or complex arterial plaques is to use drug-eluding stents, when a stent is indicated, provided that no other antimyeloproliferative therapy is administered simultaneously. We tend to limit use of stents because of concern for long-term complications of stent fracture and the stent itself acting as a mechanical barrier to future therapeutic modalities. Additional antimyeloproliferative therapy is now available using primarily paclitaxel-coated balloons. There are multiple different drug concentrations and crystalline structures available on paclitaxel-coated balloons. A larger crystalline structure has been associated with potential longer duration of drug exposure in the arterial wall in a "depot" mechanism of action. There is concern for possible distal embolization in these larger crystalline coatings. This has not been shown to be clinically significant nor to impact wound healing. Safety-related outcomes, major amputation, and death have been equivalent between POBA and drug-coated balloon (DCB) groups in pivotal trials. The long-term clinical benefits of DCB use are more equivocal over longer follow-up. The LEVANT II trial of the CR Bard drug-coated balloon Lutonix showed significant improvement in primary patency at 12 months (65.2% versus 52.6%, $P = 0.02$). However, this was reduced to a 5.6% improvement in primary patency at 24 months.[21] Results of the Medtronic DCB IN.PACT SFA randomized trial have had more promising durability results, with primary patency advantage remaining at 36 months (69.5% versus 45.1%, $P < 0.001$).[22] The ILLUMENATE pivotal trial for the Stellarex drug-coated balloon, showed similar durable advantage for DCB up to 24 months.[23]

In December 2018, a meta-analysis found an increase in later term all-cause mortality from exposure to paclitaxel.[1] At 2 years, all-cause mortality showed a negative impact, and by 4 to 5 years this was more pronounced. (14.7% versus 8.1% with an odds ratio of 1.93.) This meta-analysis was a compilation of three randomly controlled trials (Zilver-PTX, Thunder and IN.PACT SFA), none of which was powered

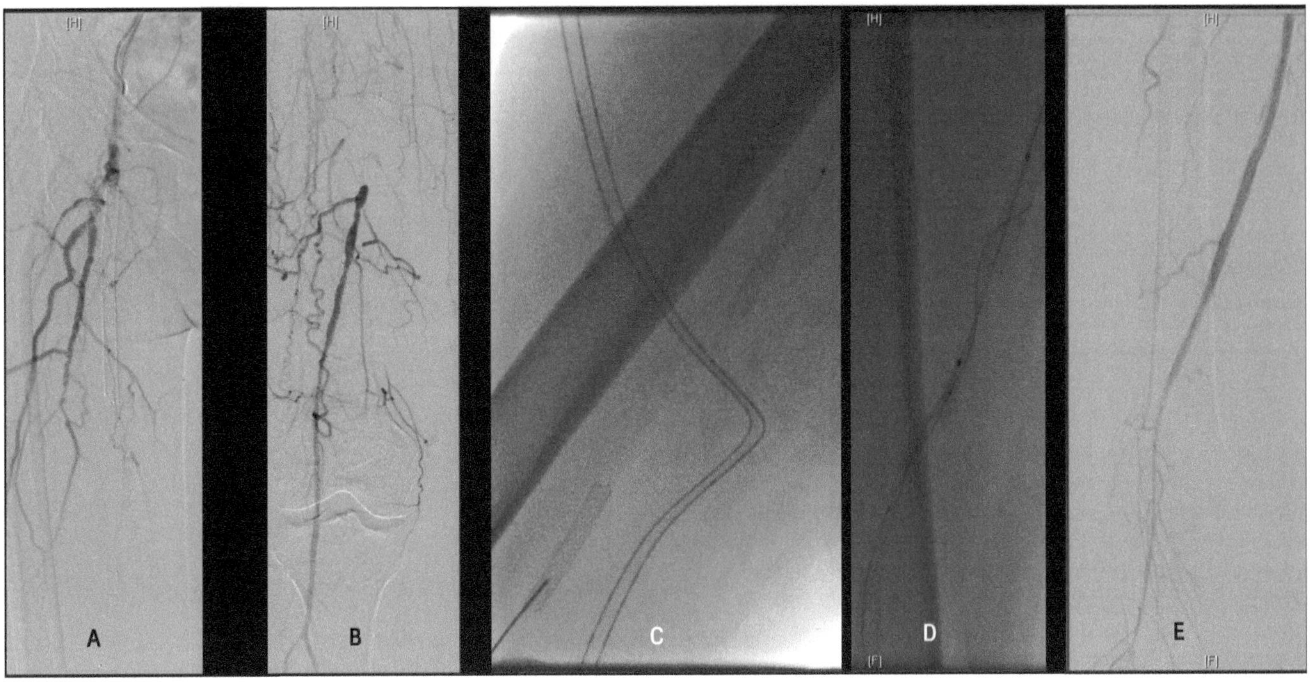

Fig. 33.4 Percutaneous accessing of occluded stent to recanalize occluded SFA. (A) Occluded superficial femoral artery (SFA). (B) Reconstitution of distal SFA. (C) Percutaneous access directly into SFA stent. (D) Snaring percutaneous wire through stent. (E) Recanalized SFA.

to evaluate the impact on all-cause mortality. This has drawn significant attention and discussion by physicians, industry, vascular societies, and regulatory agencies. The US Food and Drug Administration (FDA) initially released a notification of their concern in January 2019. (Paclitaxel in much higher doses has been used in treatment of patients with breast cancer without associated increase in long-term all-cause mortality.) In March and June 2019, the FDA stated that "While analyses are ongoing, preliminary review of this data has identified a potentially concerning signal of increased long-term mortality in study subjects treated with paclitaxel-coated products compared to patients treated with uncoated devices." Their analysis further showed "In total, among this 975 subjects in these three trials, there was an approximately 50% increased risk mortality in subjects treated with the paclitaxel coated devices (20.1% versus 13.4% crude risk of death at five years)." The FDA recommendations are to continue diligent monitoring, to make treatment recommendations, and to include in the informed consent process the potential increase in all-cause long-term mortality with a discussion of risk and benefits for all available PAD treatment options. For some patients who are typically high risk for restenosis, the benefits may outweigh the potential risk of using the paclitaxel-containing products, thereby justifying their use.

Before this analysis, we were fairly liberal with the use of paclitaxel-containing products in all PAD patients. We now tend to use other modalities in patients with claudication. In patients with CLI and long highly calcific lesions or restenotic lesions, we consider use of paclitaxel after a thorough discussion with the patient and include this as part of informed consent.

Polytetrafluoroethylene (PTFE) has been used to cover a self-expanding stent to prevent intimal hyperplasia formation through the interstices. Covered stents are also effective in treatment of complications, including arterial perforation, pseudo-aneurysm formation or shaggy thrombotic lesions. The VIBRANT trial reported that at 3 years, there was no difference in patency of Viabahn covered stent grafts compared with bare-metal stenting, although they did note a 50% stent fracture rate in the bare-metal stents compared with 2.6% in Viabahn.[24] Retrospective series suggest there may be a utility to using Viabahn stents in long-segment chronic total occlusions because patency seems less dependent on lesion length.[25]

Many plaques and recurrent stenoses are mixed consistency, including calcification, smooth muscle cell intimal hyperplasia, thrombus, and necrotic material. As a result of this mixed nature, POBA has been associated with distal embolization and outflow arterial occlusion. In patients with significant risk of thrombus or necrotic material, we advocate the use of mechanical thromboatherectomy in the initial intervention. If the hydrophilic wire easily passes through an occluded vessel, concern for thrombus or necrotic material is significantly increased. Mechanical thrombectomy with aspiration allows removal of this thrombus and necrotic material, as well as initial atherectomy debulking. This allows better visualization and selective endovascular intervention with spot stenting or post mechanical thrombectomy/atherectomy angioplasty. If there is significant thrombus burden within the plaque, distal embolic protection devices are generally utilized in conjunction with therapeutic interventions. Some authors recommend routine use of embolic protection devices in all endovascular interventions.

Angioplasty and stenting do not remove or debulk atherosclerotic lesions but simply disrupt the internal and/or external elastic lamina, allowing the lumen to increase. Atherectomy debulks plaque and removes it. Each of the atherectomy devices has strengths and weaknesses (Table 33.1). The devices are defined by the mechanism in which it debulks and include directional, rotational, orbital, and laser photoablative devices. Directional devices can be used effectively in eccentric and concentric plaques, and typically atheromatous material is stored in the device nosecone, which requires intermittent removal and cleaning. The DEFINITIVE LE study prospectively reviewed 800 patients undergoing directional atherectomy, revealing a 78% primary patency and freedom from reintervention in lesions up to 20 cm in length in SFA, popliteal, and tibial vessels.[26] Embolization rate was 3%, with

TABLE 33.1 Atherectomy devices.

Lesion type	Calcium	Thrombus	Intimal hyperplasia	Mixed plaque
TurboHawk/ HawkOne	+++	+	+++	++++
Turboelite Laser	+	++++	+++	+++
JetStream	++	++++	++++	++
DiamondBack 360 CSI	++++	−	+	++

1.6% requiring intervention. Preliminary results indicate that using directional atherectomy and DCB compared with DCB alone is potentially effective in long or highly calcific lesions. Highly calcific lesions can act as a mechanical barrier to prevent the penetration of the antiproliferative agents to the medial smooth muscle cells. Debulking before DCB treatment could allow better exposure of the underlying smooth muscle cells to the antimyeloproliferative agent. Directional atherectomy can excise calcified lesions but is associated with significant distal embolization, and embolic protection devices should be routinely used. Rotational atherectomy allows aspiration and one-time insertion but are limited in luminal gain. However, the Jetstream atherectomy device (Boston Scientific) increased luminal diameter by approximately 3.4 mm.[27] Rotational atherectomy is effective in removing organized thrombus and atherosclerotic plaque.[28] Orbital atherectomy is effective with short focal calcific lesions and, theoretically, reduces calcified plaque to minuscule particles washed out through the outflow bed. It is not effective with thrombus or intimal hyperplasia. A large registry study found that plaque reduction was most effective in calcified lesions and least in soft, fibrotic lesions. This study included three orbital atherectomy devices manufactured by CSI (St. Paul, Minnesota). On average, lesions achieved a stenosis reduction of 35%–88% prior to angioplasty.[29]

Recently, the FDA approved the PQ Bypass DETOUR trial evaluating the possibility of an endovascular femoropopliteal bypass using the femoral vein as the conduit for covered stent grafts to traverse the SFA occlusion. Retrograde arterial access is obtained from the contralateral femoral artery and a catheter is inserted in the CFA. The femoral vein and the superficial femoral artery above and below the area of occlusions are identified and, through catheter manipulation, a covered stent is passed from the SFA above the area of occlusion to the SFA below using the femoral vein as the conduit for the covered stent graft to traverse. Clinical results are pending.

Lesion location can impact selection of endovascular therapy. Lesions within areas of flexion such as the CFA and popliteal artery have previously been considered "no stent zones," but additional studies have shown that flexible stents can be used in these regions.[30] In non-high risk patients, surgical intervention on the CFA is considered first-line therapy. High-risk patients and patients with hostile groins who are not good surgical candidates are considered for endovascular intervention. Directional atherectomy has been shown to be very effective in debulking femoral lesions with low risk of perforation or embolization (Fig. 33.5).

Lesions at arterial branch points are challenging for angioplasty or stent placement. Angioplasty can result in plaque shift and vessel obstruction. Buddy wires into both vessels and simultaneous kissing balloon angioplasty helps prevent plaque shift and vessel occlusion, which requires a 7-French sheath minimum. Stent deployment can

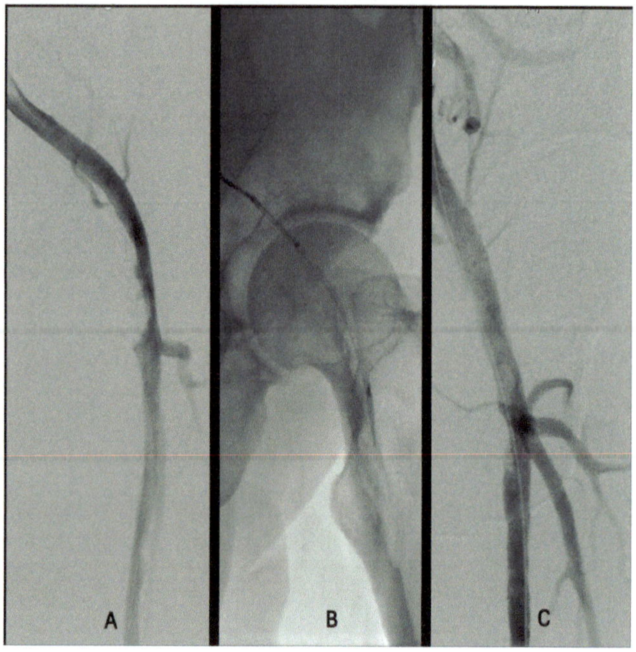

Fig. 33.5 Directional atherectomy for bulky lesion treatment. (A) Bulky common femoral artery (CFA) lesion. (B) Directional atherectomy of CFA lesion. (C) Completion imaging after debulking of CFA.

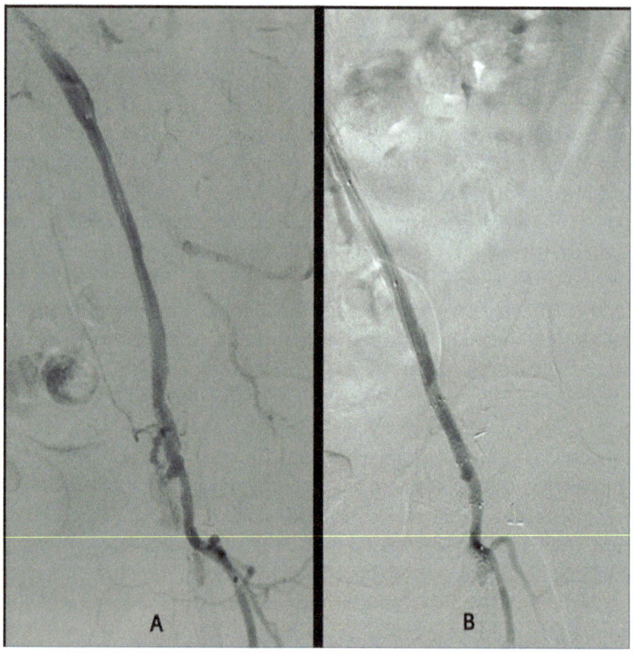

Fig. 33.6 (A) Perforation after endovascular intervention. (B) Stent graft coverage of perforation.

impinge on the orifice of the branch vessel and "jail it" such that further intervention is difficult. In particular, stent positioning and accuracy is required when treating the very proximal SFA to limit impingement on the PFA. Finally, distal SFA and proximal popliteal lesions need to be carefully evaluated to insure that the endovascular intervention does not alter the potential surgical bypass target for distal anastomosis.

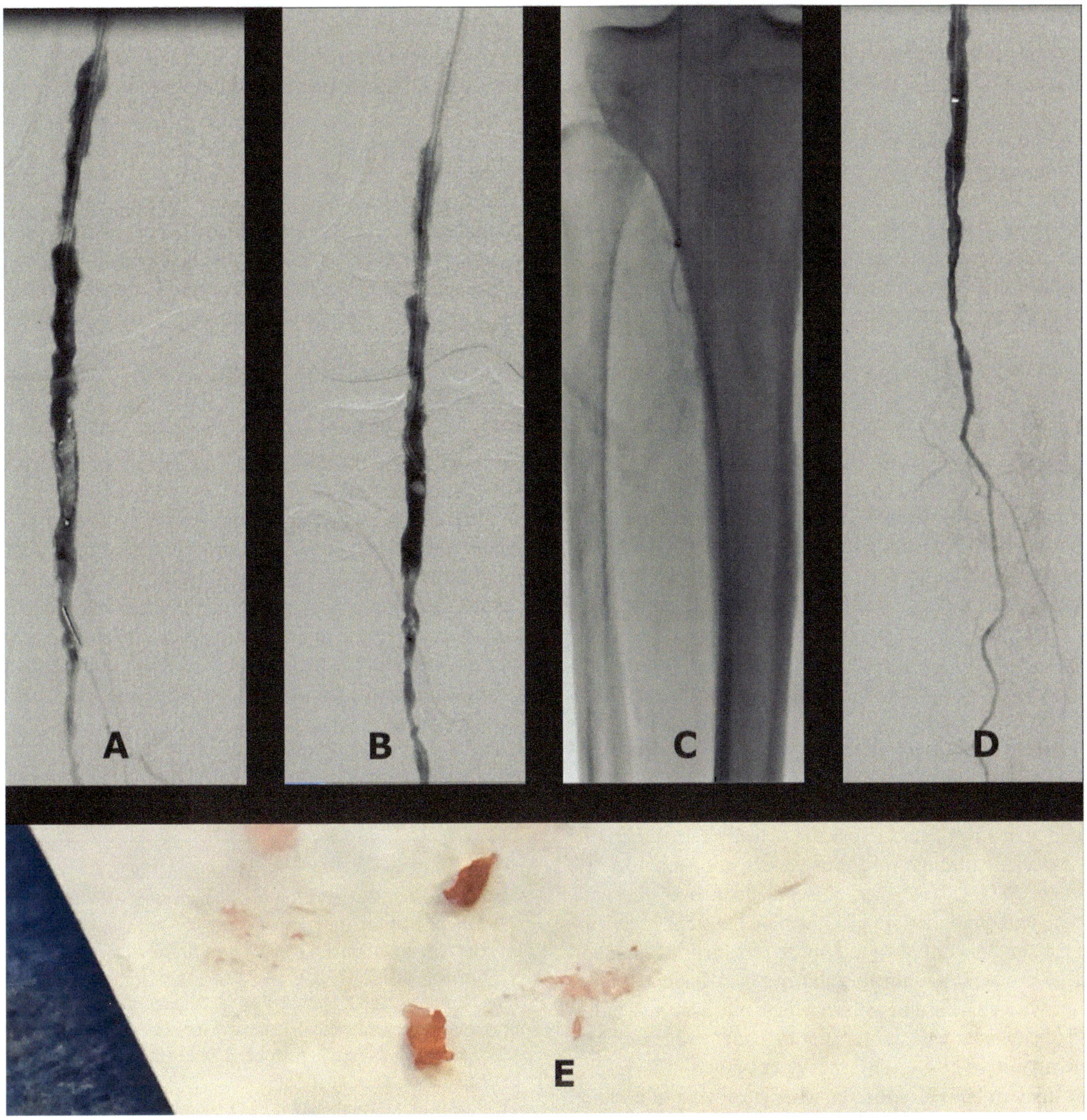

Fig. 33.7 Embolization after endovascular intervention. A 4-French sheath as aspiration catheter. (A) Visible debris trapped in an embolic protection filter. (B) Residual embolic material still in popliteal artery after filter recapture. (C) Aspiration with 4-French aspiration catheter. (D) Completion angiogram.

COMPLICATIONS

Perforation

Arterial perforation can occur with catheter and wire manipulation, balloon angioplasty, stent placement, and atherectomy. Early perforation appears as a blush within the arterial wall but without frank extravasation. Wire or catheter perforation, especially through side branches, can be managed with simple balloon inflation and reversal of anticoagulation. True artery perforation may require embolization with embolic material or coils. Larger vessel perforation will be initially managed with prolonged balloon tamponade with a low-pressure inflation and external pressure if the vessel is accessible. If unresolved, covered stent is used. Highly calcific vessels are more prone to perforation and rupture and more liberal use of covered stents is recommended. Treatment of totally occluded arteries increases risk of rupture (Fig. 33.6).

Dissection

Wire manipulation and catheter advancement can lead to arterial dissection if the hydrophilic wire engages a plaque and creates a subintimal dissection, which then propagates along the arterial wall. Catheter manipulation especially in higher flow regions can create a small tear in the intima, acting as a nidus for propagation of a dissection with arterial forward flow. Percutaneous angioplasty creates a dissection just by the nature of inflating and disrupting the internal elastic lamina in the atherosclerotic plaque, but in most cases, this is non-flow limiting. Non-flow-limiting dissections generally heal without intervention. Flow-limiting dissections can lead to hypoperfusion and thrombosis and should be treated. It is imperative that wire access across the zone be maintained until it is confirmed that a dissection or perforation has not occurred. If wire access is lost, regaining true lumen to true lumen access may be extremely challenging. If this occurs, meticulous technique must be used to try to regain wire position within the true lumen, sometimes requiring retrograde access through the distal vessels. Low-pressure sustained balloon inflation is first-line therapy. If that is unsuccessful, self-expanding stent placement is therapeutic in most cases. In selected cases in which a stent is not desired, we have utilized directional atherectomy to excise the flap, thereby resolving the dissection. In rare cases, especially when wire access is lost, surgical bypass or direct suture repair may be required to restore perfusion.

Embolization

During endovascular intervention, atherosclerotic plaque, thrombus, and rarely catheter tip, stents, or portions of wire can embolize, obstructing arterial perfusion to the limb. If there is high risk of embolization based on heavily calcified lesions or organized thrombus, embolic protection devices should be considered. A properly sized and positioned filter can be invaluable. Even with proper case planning and use of embolic protection, embolization can occur. The size of the embolus and its consistency determine which technique is utilized to extract the embolus. If it is small, catheter-directed aspiration devices or a 4-French long vascular sheath can be used to aspirate. Monorail aspiration catheters are available with a small channel for the wire, allowing maintenance of wire access. Emboli can precipitate thrombosis, and thrombolytic therapy may be needed in conjunction with embolectomy. For this reason, it is critical to maintain adequate anticoagulation after embolization. For calcific emboli, simple POBA of the embolus may embed it into the arterial wall and out of the flow channel, although these pebble-like emboli are notoriously hard to aspirate. New advances in mechanical thrombectomy are available that generate significant negative aspiration force and have an auger at the catheter tip that can break up more organized thrombus, which can then be aspirated. The penumbra device has proved effective in peripheral applications and is now FDA approved.[31] If it is a larger foreign body or plaque, snaring may be required. In Fig. 33.7 we demonstrate use of a 4-French sheath as an aspiration catheter. Finally, if endovascular attempts are ineffective and the limb is ischemic, surgical thrombectomy or bypass should be considered.

Stent embolization can occur in two different scenarios. First, balloon-mounted stents can detach from the delivery catheter during manipulation, especially through torturous vessels, and embolize into the outflow artery. Passing a smaller caliber balloon over the wire, through the stent, and gently inflating can deploy the stent in its current location or it can be withdrawn to a more proximal location and fully deployed. If the stent cannot be captured by a balloon or has embolized off the wire, snaring and withdrawing it into a large sheath is the next option. Occasionally the stent cannot be fully withdrawn into the sheath and may need to be retrieved by cut-down. The second mechanism for stent embolization occurs when deploying in a region that has an hourglass stenosis or changing caliber such that the stent "watermelon seeds" either distally or proximally and geographically misses the treatment area. This is more common in venous stenoses. These stents generally have to be either deployed in their new location if they are balloon-expandable or snared and retrieved if they are self-expanding. Finally, if the stent is undersized, it can embolize distally and have to be deployed at that location. A second properly sized stent is then placed in the intended area. The original embolized stent may need to be snared and retrieved.

In-Stent Restenosis

With increased use of self-expanding stents, there has also been increased incidence of stent related complications. In-stent restenosis from myo-intimal hyperplasia is the leading cause of refigintervention caused by recurrent stenosis. This is very challenging to treat and is a barrier to sustained patency. POBA or drug-coated balloon therapy is the dominant treatment option but has a high recurrence rate.[32] Directional and rotation atherectomy have been attempted but also have a high recurrence rate and directional atherectomy is contraindicated. The EXCITE trial using the Spectranetics Excimer laser to debulk the fibrotic animal hyperplastic tissue within the stent followed by balloon angioplasty was shown to be statistically more efficient compared with POBA.[33] Additionally, stent fracture may occur. If significant fracturing is noted during reintervention, relining with a new stent or a covered stent is optimal. If multiple episodes of restenosis occur, surgical bypass should be considered.

CONCLUSIONS

Femoropopliteal lesions commonly occur in both CLI and intermittent claudication. This area is difficult to treat because lesions tend to be long and the artery is quite dynamic. Open vascular reconstruction is effective and durable, as long as there is reasonable conduit and runoff. The endovascular era has brought many advantages, but there are continued concerns about the long-term durability. Despite the development of several new modalities of treatment, progress has been incremental, and the patency is still measured in months, not years. Reintervention rates are a major cause of concern and it is likely that there will be continued focus on innovation in femoropopliteal occlusive disease treatment.

This chapter serves as an overview of the current state of endovascular intervention in the femoropopliteal segment. Common treatment modalities are summarized and described, along with their failure methods, and common complications are detailed. Given the large number of therapeutic modalities available and the relative paucity of comparative data, there is no single idealized treatment algorithm, and therapies need to be tailored to the patient and their disease pattern.

REFERENCES

1. 2018 ACC/AHA/AACVPR/AAPA/ABC/ACPM/ADA/AGS/APhA/ASPC/NLA/PCNA Guideline on the Management of Blood Cholesterol: A Report of the American College of Cardiology Foundation/American Heart Association Task Force on Clinical Practice Guidelines. *J Am Coll Cardiol.* 2019;73(24):3168–3209.
2. Okuno S, Lida O, Shiraki T, et al. Impact of calcification on clinical outcomes after endovascular therapy for superficial femoral artery disease: Assessment using the peripheral artery calcification scoring system. *J Endovasc Ther.* 2016;23(5):731–737.
3. Kaladji A, Giovannetti M, Pascot R, et al. Preoperative CT-scan-based sizing and in-stent restenosis in peripheral endovascular revascularizations. *Vascular.* 2017;25(5):504–513.
4. Itoga NK, Kim T, Sailer AM, Fleischmann D, Mell MW. Lower extremity computed tomography angiography can help predict technical success of endovascular revascularization in the superficial femoral and popliteal artery. *J Vasc Surg.* 2017;66(3):835–843.
5. Wheatley BJ, Mansour MA, Grossman PM, et al. Complication rates for percutaneous lower extremity arterial antegrade access. *Arch Surg.* 2011;146(4):432–435.
6. Chang Z, Zheng J, Liu Z. Subintimal angioplasty for lower limb arterial chronic total occlusions. *Cochrane Database Syst Rev.* 2016;11:CD009418.
7. Norgren L, Hiatt WR, Dormandy JA, et al., TASC II Working Group. Inter-society consensus for the Management of Peripheral Arterial Disease (TASC II) *J Vasc Surg.* 2007;45(Suppl S):S5–S67.
8. Bolia A, Miles KA, Brennan J, Bell PRF. Percutaneous transluminal angioplasty of occlusion of the SFA by subintimal dissection. *Cardiovasc Interv Radiol.* 1990;357–363.
9. Intraluminal Crossing Via Atherectomy. c2016. Tempe, AZ. [accessed 2019 Jan 20]. https://www.crbard.com/CRBard/media/ProductAssets/BardPeripheralVascularInc/PF10026/en-US/5w8s9x4kanid8o2h9fe8sljvrbl4h6eq.pdf
10. Jacobs DL, Motaganahalli RL, Cox DE, Wittgen CM, Peterson GJ. True lumen re-entry devices facilitate subintimal angioplasty and stent of total chronic occlusions: Initial report. *J Vasc Surg.* 2006;43(6):1291–1296.
11. Spinosa DJ, Harthun NL, Bissonette EA, et al. Subintimal arterial flossing with antegrade-retrograde intervention (SAFARI) for subintimal

recanalization to treat chronic critical limb ischemia. *J Vasc Interv Radiol.* 2005;16(1):37–44.
12. El-Sayed H, Bennett ME, Loh TM, Davies MG. Retrograde pedal access and endovascular revascularization: A safe and effective technique for high-risk patients with complex tibial vessel disease. *Ann Vasc Surg.* 2016;31:91–98.
13. Sanghvi KA, Kusick J, Krathen C. Retrograde tibio-pedal access for revascularization of lower-extremity peripheral artery disease using a 6 Fr slender sheath: The "pedal-first" pilot project. *J Invasive Cardiol.* 2018; 30(9):334–340.
14. Dotter CT, Judkins MP. Transluminal treatment of arteriosclerotic obstruction. Description of a new technic and a preliminary report of its application. *Circulation.* 1964;30:654–670.
15. Gruntzig A, Kumpe DA. Technique of percutaneous trans-luminal angioplasty with the Gruntzig balloon catheter. *Am J Roentgenol.* 1979;132:547–552.
16. Schillinger M, Sabeti S, Loewe C, et al. Balloon angioplasty versus implantation of nitinol stents in the superficial femoral artery. *N Engl J Med.* 2006;354(18):1879–1888.
17. Palmaz JC, Sibbit RR, Reuter SR, Tio FO, Rice WJ. Expandable intraluminal graft: a preliminary study. Work in progress. *Radiology.* 1985;156(1):73–77.
18. Krankenberg H, Schluter M, Steinkamp HJ, et al. Nitinol stent implantation versus percutaneous transluminal angioplasty in the superficial femoral artery lesions up to 10 cm in length, the femoral artery stent trial (FAST). *Circulation.* 2007;116(3):285–292.
19. Conroy RM, Gordon IL, Tobis JM, et al. Angioplasty and stent placement in chronic occlusion of the superficial femoral artery: technique and results. *J Vasc Interv Radiol.* 2000;11(8):1009–1020.
20. Dake MD, Ansel GM, Jaff MR, et al., Zilver PTX Investigators Durable clinical effectiveness with paclitaxel-eluting stents in the femoropopliteal artery: 5-year results of the Zilver PTX randomized trial. *Circulation.* 2016;133 (15):1472–1483.
21. Bard touts 2-year data on Lutonix. June 19, 2015. [accessed 2019 Jan 20]. https://www.massdevice.com/bard-touts-2-year-data-on-lutonix
22. Schneider PA, Laird JR, Tepe G, et al., IN.PACT SFA trial investigators. Treatment Effect of Drug-Coated Balloons is Durable to 3 Years in the Femoropopliteal Arteries: Long-term results of the IN.PACT SFA randomized trial. *Circ Cardiovasc Interv.* 2018;11(1).
23. Zellter T. ILLUMINATE global study. Presented at LINC 2017; January 24–27, 2017; Leipzig, Germany.
24. Geraghty PJ, Mewissen MW, Jaff MR, Ansel GM, VIBRANT Investigators. Three-year results of the VIBRANT trial of VIABAHN endoprosthesis versus bare nitinol stent implantation for complex superficial femoral artery occlusive disease. *J Vasc Surg.* 2013; 58(2):386–395.
25. Saxon RR, Coffman JM, Gooding JM, Ponec DJ. Long-term patency and clinical outcome of the Viabahn stent-graft for femoropopliteal artery obstructions. *J Vasc Interv Radiol.* 2007;18(11):1341–1349.
26. McKinsey JF, Zeller T, Rocha-Singh KJ, Jaff MR, Garcia LA, DEFINITIVE LE Investigators. Lower extremity revascularization using directional atherectomy:12-month prospective results for the DEFINITIVE LE study. *JACC Cardiovasc Interv.* 2014;7(8):923–933.
27. Maehara A, Mintz GS, Shimshak TM, et al. Intravascular ultrasound evaluation of JETSTREAM atherectomy removal of superficial calcium in peripheral arteries. *EuroIntervention.* 2015;11(1):96–103.
28. Kim TH, Chavarria N, Dahal K, Azrin M, Lee J. Jetstream XC device for treatment of long Viabahn stents occlusions in the superficial femoral artery: A report of two cases. *Ann Vasc Dis.* 2017;10(4):441–445.
29. Das T, Mustapha J, Indes J, et al. Technique optimization of orbital atherectomy in calcified peripheral lesions of the lower extremities: The CONFIRM series, a prospective multicenter registry. *Catheter Cardiovasc Interv.* 2014;83(1):115–122.
30. Varcoe RL. Current and evolving strategies for the treatment of atherosclerotic disease of the popliteal artery. *J Cardiovasc Surg.* 2015; 56(1):55–65.
31. Penumbra Indigo System Separator. c2019. [accessed 2019 Jan 20]. https://www.penumbrainc.com/peripheral-device/indigo-system-separator/
32. Ho KJ, Owens CD. Diagnosis, classification, and treatment of femoropopliteal artery in-stent restenosis. *J Vasc Surg.* 2017;65(2):545–557.
33. Dippel EJ, Makam P, Kovach R, et al., EXCITE ISR Investigators Randomized controlled study of excimer laser atherectomy for treatment of femoropopliteal in-stent restenosis: initial results from the EXCITE ISR trial (EXCImer laser randomized controlled study for treatment of femoropopliTEal in-stent restenosis). *JACC Cardiovasc Interv.* 2015; 8(1 pt A):92–101.

34

Complications of Endovascular Repair of Popliteal Artery Aneurysms

Mathew Wooster, MD, Jeffrey B. Edwards, MD and Murray L. Shames, MD, DFSVS, FACS

INTRODUCTION

Popliteal artery aneurysms (PAAs) occur at an incidence of 7.39 per 100,000 people, accounting for 80% of peripheral artery aneurysms.[1] Typically asymptomatic, they are most commonly found incidentally on peripheral arterial disease screening examinations or when screening is based on the known presence of an aortic aneurysm, which confers a 12%–40% chance of popliteal artery aneurysm occurrence.[2] PAAs may occasionally cause symptoms related to compression of surrounding structures (nerve palsy or leg swelling), but more frequently the symptoms are directly correlated with arterial occlusion in the form of emboli (i.e., blue toe syndrome) or acute limb ischemia from aneurysm thrombosis. Repair is recommended for PAAs ≥2 cm maximum diameter or when symptoms are present.[1–4] Consideration should also be given to prophylactic repair for smaller aneurysms without symptoms when there is evidence of significant thrombus burden with prior embolization (poor run-off).

Traditionally, PAAs have been treated with open surgical techniques. Repair options include interposition reconstruction with excision of the aneurysmal segment or bypass with proximal and distal ligation of the aneurysm. Both medial and posterior approaches are well described, with the use of autologous vein preferred, but prosthetic conduits perform relatively well compared with its use in occlusive disease.[2] Elective open surgical repair for PAAs is frequently reported, with greater than 80% cumulative patency at 3 years.[5]

Despite the high patency rates for open repair, endovascular stent grafts provide an alternative to open PAA repair, with a greater number of patients undergoing endovascular repair than ever before. Early reports of endovascular PAA repair utilized the Wallgraft (Boston Scientific, Minneapolis, Minnesota), a self-expanding covered stent based on the Wallstent platform.[1] At the time, it was the only available self-expanding covered stent, but it has limitations given its stainless steel base, which gives it limited flexibility and allows for a fair amount of lengthening and foreshortening depending upon the vessel diameter in which it is deployed. With the introduction of newer nitinol-based endoprosthesis, namely the Gore Viabahn (Gore Medical, Flagstaff, Arizona), came the potential of increased flexibility and easier deployment without the concerns of foreshortening, thus opening the door for more widespread use of the technique.

Endovascular repair of popliteal aneurysms has been reported with patency greater than 70% up to 4 years. Secondary interventions are most common for loss of patency, with in-stent stenosis resulting from kinking or in-folding of grafts.[3] Additional reintervention may be required for extension of aneurysmal disease with subsequent endoleaks.

Evaluation for endovascular versus open repair of popliteal aneurysms is based on a variety of factors, including medical risk for anesthesia, baseline functional capacity, patient lifestyle, vascular anatomic characteristics, and acuity of presentation. In general, emergency repairs are a result of thrombotic events and thus are most frequently treated by open repair in our practice. This is not a mandate, of course, because catheter-directed therapies for management of acute thrombosis are being more frequently used and can allow more expeditious clot removal even for Rutherford IIb patients, but this has been our general experience to date. Patient concerns regarding recovery time from surgery may lead toward endovascular repair for highly functional patients needing to return to work quickly or to help care for loved ones. Similarly, older individuals and those with more medical comorbidities are more likely to be preferred for endovascular repair, but this will be balanced with objective evaluation of endovascular candidacy. Although a near infinite subjective discussion can be had regarding personal or patient preferences for when to perform open versus endovascular repair, a more appropriate first question concerns simple anatomic adequacy for repair, which will be discussed in greater detail later.

Specific Concerns

Recognizing the increased interest in an endovascular first approach to treatment, it is important to realize that there is a particular set of challenges for PAA repair. During preoperative planning, we focus first on the anatomic challenges, including length of the distal seal zone and status of the tibial run-off for assessing candidacy for endovascular repair. The necessary landing zone for adequate seal is not well established for popliteal aneurysms. Most would agree 1–2 cm should be adequate, but this can be a challenge for the distal landing zone in particular. There is great variability in the origin of the anterior tibial artery, with many patients having a high origin, which compromises the length of a distal landing zone. If necessary, the anterior tibial artery can be sacrificed and the length extended to the tibioperoneal trunk for a landing zone. This is not without a cost, of course, because it decreases the run-off from three to two vessels and the tibioperoneal trunk is typically a smaller caliber vessel than the popliteal artery, which makes the size match between the distal and proximal landing zones more challenging.

Run-off scoring is an important data-point when comparing patency of lower extremity interventions for occlusive disease.[4,5] The same is true when treating popliteal aneurysms. Patients with compromised tibial outflow have consistently worse outcomes compared with patients with three-vessel run-off.[5] The outflow may or may not be able to be modified with endovascular techniques, and this must be taken into account when deciding upon open versus endovascular repair. As a general practice, we have not routinely treated tibial occlusive disease pre-emptively with a goal of improving run-off score because the general patency for tibial interventions remains somewhat hindered. This is a consideration that warrants future evaluation because below-the-knee intervention skill sets and tools continue to improve.

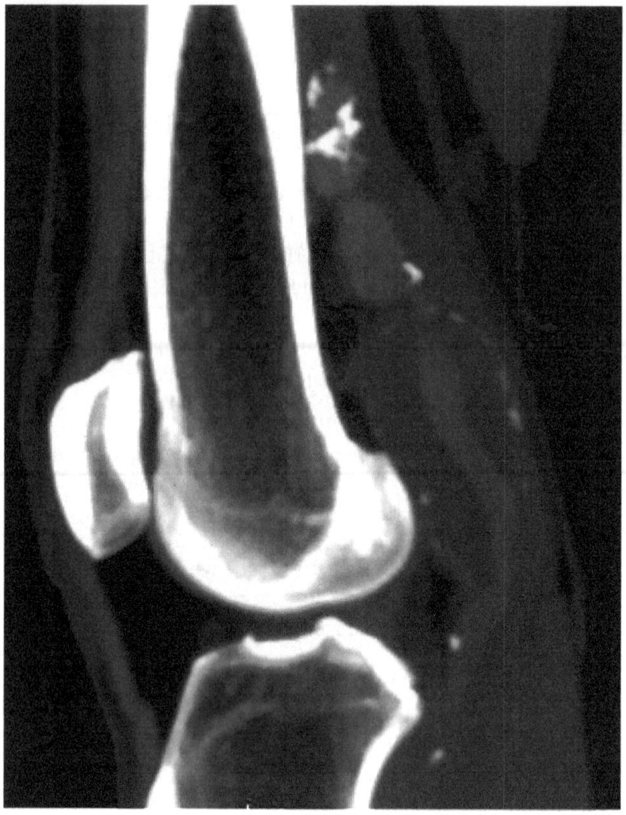

Fig. 34.1 Computed topmographic angiogram demonstrating 3.9-cm popliteal artery aneurysm with mural thrombus.

When selecting stent sizes, we must recognize that there are no commercially available stent grafts specifically designed for PAA treatment. That said, there can be sizing difficulties when attempting to achieve seal. As with most aneurysmal pathology, 10%–20% oversizing is recommended. An average normal below-knee popliteal artery is 4–6 mm and an average normal proximal superficial femoral artery is 5–7 mm. In the setting of aneurysmal disease, it is not uncommon to have generalized arteriomegaly or borderline aneurysmal below-knee popliteal artery segments. While a traditional open bypass can overcome this with a direct anastomosis, the placement of a self-expanding, oversized stent in an already dilated below-knee popliteal artery raises concerns akin to treating large infrarenal aortic necks. With a size discrepancy between the seal zones proximally and distally, it is best to deploy the smallest stent size first so that a larger stent can be landed inside of this to avoid endoleaks. Another difference between more common lower extremity stenting performed for occlusive disease is the overlap between stents. For occlusive disease, overlap is generally minimized to avoid over-stiffening, with subsequent concern for stent fracture; but, for treating popliteal aneurysm, we need adequate overlap to ensure seal in the same way as when treating aortic aneurysms. This is especially true in very large aneurysms with minimal thrombus, which carries the risk of stent separation if insufficient overlap is used. While there is no well-defined guideline, we extrapolate from aortic aneurysm repairs and aim for at least 2–3 cm of overlap between devices to minimize this risk.

As with all aneurysms, successful repair is dependent upon proper planning and sizing of the vessel. A challenge that frequently arises is the presence of metal artifact on CT scans from prior orthopedic procedures (knee replacements, hip replacements, etc.). This can create too much artifact to evaluate the popliteal artery properly, in particular

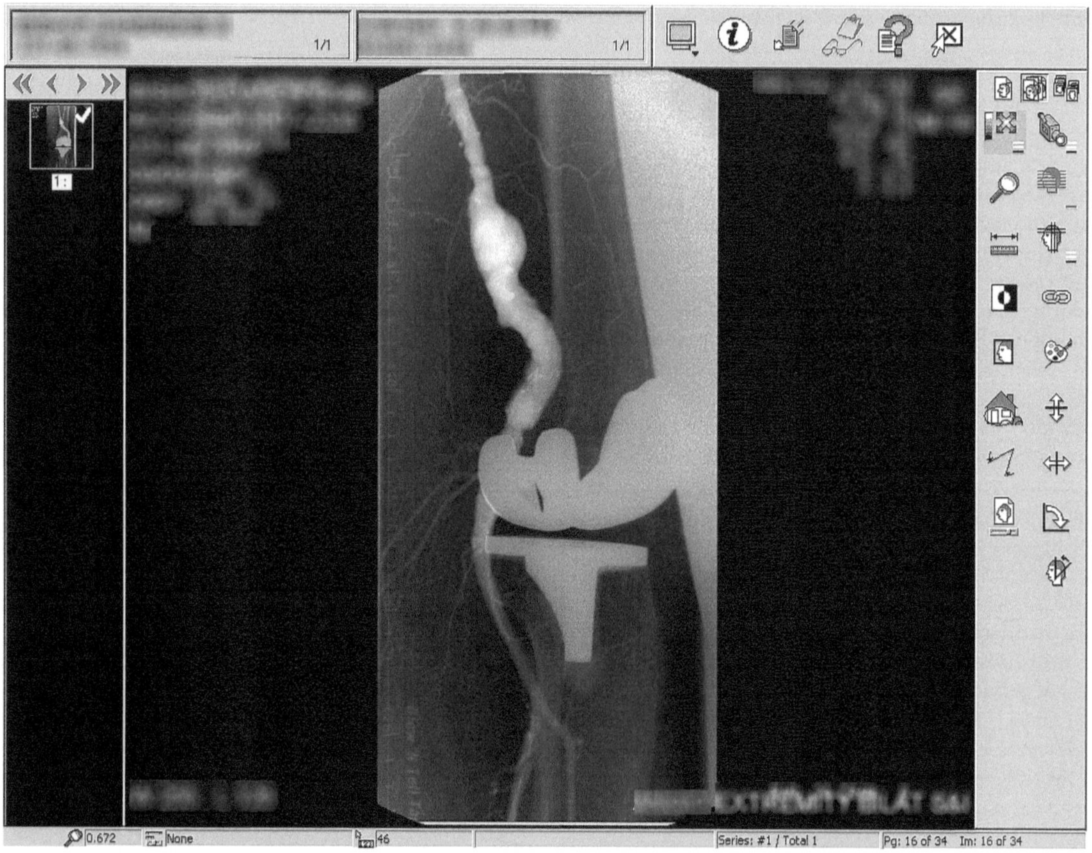

Fig. 34.2 Lateral projection arteriogram demonstrating physiologic arterial kinking proximal to anatomic knee joint, clearly depicted by prosthetic knee joint.

preoperatively. Additionally, patients with renal insufficiency may not be able to obtain CT angiograms. Angiography cannot reliably identify normal versus aneurysmal vessel because it is effectively a lumenogram. To overcome this obstacle, the best preoperative tool is ultrasound or CTA. Preoperative imaging can be used to identify segments of normal versus aneurysmal artery quite reliably and to measure the diameter of the landing zone for stent sizing (Fig. 34.1). Intra-operatively, intravascular ultrasound can be used for this identification, with the additional advantage of providing both the diameter and the location of the healthy vessel for landing.

Intra-operatively, there are concerns specific to the location of stenting and the size of the delivery systems required. Stenting across the knee joint has historically been considered an increased risk for stent fracture and/or failure. While the flexibility of the Viabahn stent graft allows it to handle the frequent bends and twists associated with being placed behind the knee, there is a tendency to find stenosis at the stent edges because of kinking at the transition from the relatively stiff metal stent to the relatively mobile native artery. This issue is related to a misunderstanding of the difference between the physiologic joint and the bony joint. The bony joint is readily seen on fluoroscopy, but identification of the physiologic joint (the position where the artery itself bends to accommodate movement of the knee), AP and steep lateral angiography must be performed, with the leg in both extension and flexion. By taking multiple views and identifying these natural arterial kinks, it is possible to extend the stents so that the ends land in a straight rather than a highly flexible segment of the artery (Fig. 34.2).

Finally, the delivery system size can provide a challenge for selecting the access site. The Viabahn stent graft requires a 7-French sheath for up to an 8-mm stent, 9-French for a 9-mm, 11-French for 10–11-mm, and 12-French for 13-mm devices. While 7-French access from the contralateral groin for traditional "up-and-over" therapy is common, larger than that, however, makes tracking a sheath over the aortic bifurcation increasingly difficult. A few options exist for overcoming this challenge. In some settings, sequentially exchanging for stiffer wires all the way up to a Stiff Lunderquist wire can at times allow routine up-and-over access to be achieved. A second option includes obtaining bilateral femoral access to snare a wire, creating through-and-through "body floss" to enable tracking of a large sheath over the aortic bifurcation. A third option includes ipsilateral antegrade puncture. The benefit of antegrade puncture is the avoidance of tracking over the aortic bifurcation, but it can be limited in the setting of obesity or a short common femoral artery. In the event of a short common femoral artery and/or obese patient, direct puncture of the superficial femoral artery is also an option. Frequently, this vessel is not small in patients with popliteal aneurysms. The potential added risks of accessing a smaller vessel or accessing too low to allow manual compression over the femur must of course be weighed, but this is an alternative in many cases, with risks minimized by use of ultrasound guidance to confirm the size of the vessel, anterior wall puncture, and compressibility should closure device failure occur. Further, many utilizing this approach will preclose, in similar fashion to percutaneous endovascular aneurysm repair. Finally, open exposure of the ipsilateral common or superficial femoral artery can be used for antegrade access to deploy the devices.

Follow-up surveillance protocols for popliteal aneurysm repair must follow for aneurysm seal and size, as with other aneurysm repairs, but they are also more subject to the concerns of infra-inguinal stenting for occlusive disease with risks of stenosis and occlusion. Seal is of less concern for popliteal aneurysms, unless there is evidence of compressive symptoms, because the majority of symptoms are from embolic or thrombotic causes. If sac growth is seen, consideration is given to angiographic evaluation for endoleak. Type I or III endoleaks may be treated with stent extension/relining or consideration of open surgical conversion if there is concern for compressive symptoms. Type II endoleaks from geniculate branches can be treated by open surgical ligation, direct embolic agent injection, and endovascular embolization if anatomy and patient condition allow. We find this to be infrequent, however, and the benefit of treating these endoleaks is unclear. When stenosis is found in surveillance, it is treated in much the same manner as any other pathology, with the caveat of ensuring that the stenosis is not being caused by kinking of the vessel. When imaging, remember again to perform AP and lateral views in both flexion and extension of the knee to ensure the distal edge of the stent is not in a kinked segment, in which case the stent should be extended rather than merely ballooning the stenotic segment. In general, patients undergoing endovascular PAA are placed on dual antiplatelet therapy with aspirin 81 mg and

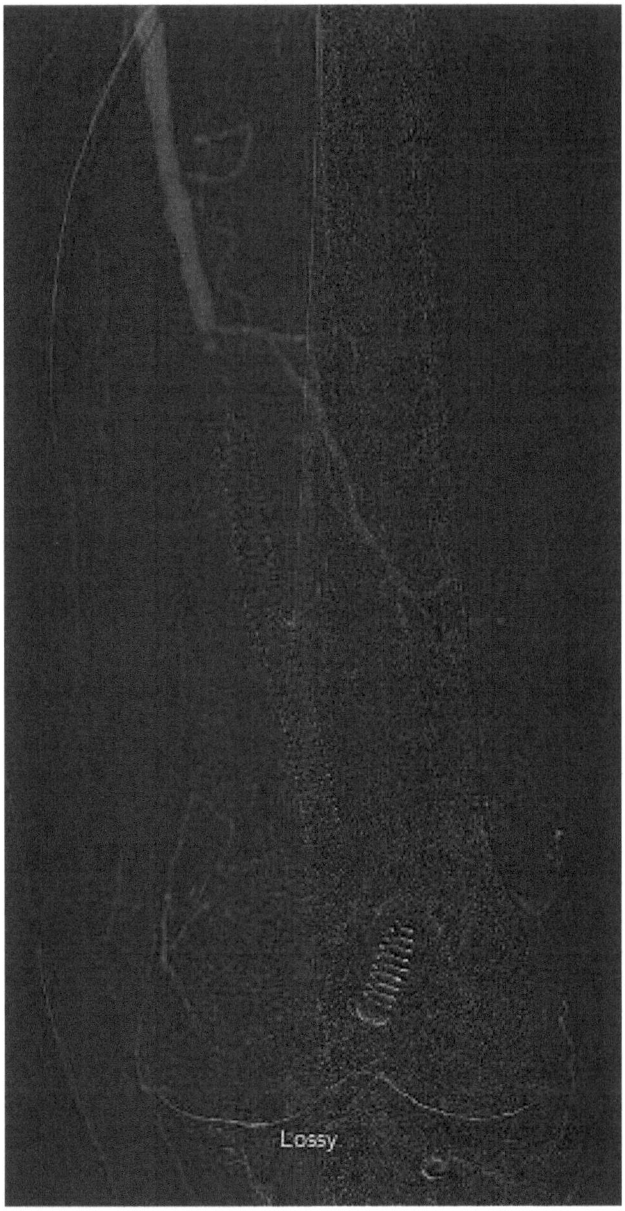

Fig. 34.3 Popliteal stent thrombosis as seen on initial CO_2 angiogram and postthrombolysis angiogram. There is a stenotic lesion distal to the stent graft, which likely contributed to the failure.

clopidogrel 75 mg daily for 60 days postoperatively, then transitioned to aspirin 81 mg daily for life. Although unsupported, patients with poor run-off or sluggish flow are often also considered for anticoagulation therapy. This is on a case-by-case basis, Duplex ultrasound velocities offer guidance with a known benefit for high-risk polytetrafluoroethylene (PTFE) bypass, with mean graft velocity less than 45 cm/s.[6]

Occlusion can be treated with a multitude of techniques, including catheter-directed thrombolysis, pharmacomechanical thrombectomy (Angiojet and Jetstream: Boston Scientific, Minneapolis, Minnesota; or Penumbra: Penumbra Inc, Alameda, California, for example), open surgical thrombectomy, or with surgical bypass. Decision for treatment of choice is based upon the urgency of revascularization (Rutherford classification), resources available, and largely surgeon preference. In general, for early or recurrent failure we would prefer conversion to open surgery, whereas for later or first time failure we would attempt an endovascular first approach to management of the occluded graft. Clearance can be performed utilizing a number of different techniques, including thrombolysis or pharmacomechanical thrombectomy (discussed in Chapter 31). Decisions regarding which mechanism to utilize will be partially guided by the run-off vessels present. Following clearance of the clot by whatever means, it is important to perform the same assessment as for primary stenosis to attempt to identify an underlying lesion (Fig. 34.3). If none is found, consideration can be given for altering the postoperative antiplatelet and anticoagulation plan. This should include testing for aspirin or Plavix resistance, and while there are no specific data to support the practice, consideration for newer antiplatelet agents or oral anticoagulants can be given.

CONCLUSION

Endovascular repair of popliteal artery aneurysms has a unique set of challenges when compared with aortic aneurysm repair or infrainguinal occlusive disease. With appropriate case planning and understanding of the nuances described here, however, excellent results can be achieved, supporting the current trend toward preferential use of an endovascular first strategy for repair.[3,5]

REFERENCES

1. Wooster M, Back M, Gaeto H, Shames M. Late longitudinal comparison of endovascular and open popliteal aneurysm repairs. *Ann Vasc Surg.* 2016; 30(c):253–257.
2. Wrede A, Wiberg F, Acosta S. Increasing the elective endovascular to open repair ratio of popliteal artery aneurysm. *Vasc Endovasc Surg.* 2018; 52(2):115–123.
3. Golchehr B, Zeebregts CJ. Reijnen MMPJ, Tielliu IFJ. Long-term outcome of endovascular popliteal artery aneurysm repair. *J Vasc Surg.* 2017;1797–1804.
4. Smialkowski AO, Huilgol RL. Percutaneous endovascular repair of popliteal artery aneurysms. *Ann Vasc Surg.* 2014;28(6):1469–1472.
5. Leake AE, Segal MA, Chaer RA, et al. Meta-analysis of open and endovascular repair of popliteal artery aneurysms. *J Vasc Surg.* 2017; 65(1):246–256.e2.
6. Brumberg RS, Back MR, Armstrong PA, et al. The relative importance of graft surveillance and warfarin therapy in infrainguinal prosthetic bypass failure. *J Vasc Surg.* 2007;46(6):1160–1166.

35

Tibial Interventions for Peripheral Arterial Disease

Patric Liang, MD, Winona Wu, MD and Marc L. Schermerhorn, MD, FACS

INTRODUCTION

Endovascular treatment for tibial arterial disease has grown in popularity through technological advancement and improvement in techniques, allowing increased success in treating difficult lesions. With growing evidence for decreased morbidity and mortality, as well as equivalent limb salvage rates following endovascular therapy when compared with open bypass surgery, tibial percutaneous transluminal angioplasty (PTA) is now commonly used as first-line treatment for infrapopliteal atherosclerotic disease.[1–3]

The Inter-Society Consensus for the Management of Peripheral Arterial Disease (TASC) guidelines provide recommendations agreed upon by multiple medical, surgical, and radiological societies in Europe and North America for the diagnosis and treatment of peripheral arterial disease. These guidelines are based on disease complexity and anatomic locality, offering treatment recommendations ranging from endovascular therapy for the least severe TASC A lesions to surgical revascularization for the most severe TASC D lesions.[4] Initially, the TASC II classification systems only included aortoiliac and femoropopliteal segment treatment recommendations, but more recently, an updated infrapopliteal classification was created to include management of tibial lesions (Fig. 35.1). However, in these updated classifications, groups such as the Society of Vascular Surgery were not represented. For many vascular specialists, endovascular treatment for TASC C or D lesions is considered because patients with chronic limb-threatening ischemia secondary to tibial disease tend to have multiple comorbidities and may benefit from a less morbid procedure rather than a tibial or pedal bypass. Proper prevention and management of complications will ensure technical success during endovascular treatment of tibial lesions when open bypass is not an option.

ARTERIAL ACCESS

Technique

The most common complication following endovascular interventions is related to arterial access. Using an appropriate technique reduces risks of arterial access complications. For lower extremity endovascular interventions, arterial entry is frequently obtained by contralateral retrograde common femoral access. This access orientation allows full evaluation of inflow aortoiliac vessels without potential visual interference from the sheath. Additionally, it provides the operator more working room, stability, and accessibility to wires and catheters along the patient's contralateral leg. However, for more severely calcified infrapopliteal lesions, ipsilateral antegrade common femoral access may prove to be beneficial, given more direct pushability of wires and catheters. High or narrow aortoiliac bifurcations can lead to difficulty in advancing sheaths up and over the bifurcation, and antegrade access can be used to avoid this anatomy. Retrograde tibial access is a useful technique for lesions that cannot be crossed in antegrade fashion. Brachial access can be considered for treatment of infrapopliteal lesions when femoral access is contra-indicated; however, for taller patients, the working length of the wires and catheters may be insufficient for treatment of distal lesions.

Retrograde Common Femoral Artery Access

Routine use of ultrasound guidance for arterial entry will help reduce access-site complications.[5] Although arterial access can be obtained with aid of direct palpation of the common femoral artery, practice with ultrasound will prove to be invaluable when more precise access is required. In our practice, we use a micropuncture technique for all arterial access, which involves the use of a 21-gauge needle and a short 0.018″ guidewire. We find this technique especially useful when obtaining access in calcified vessels by being able to place the needle tip accurately into a less diseased part of the artery. Short 21-guage micropuncture needles are also commercially available for use during retrograde tibial or pedal access. Needle entry into the vessel should be at a 45-degree angle, although a steeper angle may be required for more calcified vessels. Dilation of the skin and subcutaneous fat tract with a hemostat will aid successful deployment of the closure device at the end of the case. Please see Chapter 1 for further details regarding femoral access.

Retrograde femoral access and placement of a 4-French sheath is generally sufficient to advance a catheter into the contralateral external iliac artery for initial diagnostic imaging. However, in patients with severe peripheral arterial disease, multilevel disease burden, or poor cardiac output, injection of contrast at the external iliac level may not reach the tibial vessels for clear imaging. Therefore, the catheter will need to be advanced into the superficial femoral artery. For tibial interventions, the sheath will need to be upsized to a least a long 5-French sheath and placed into the superficial femoral artery (SFA) or popliteal artery to allow passage of tibial balloons and/or stents. Once the sheath is in place, it is always flushed and locked with heparinized saline. Alternatively, a continuous infusion of heparinized saline through the sheath may be utilized. Systemic heparinization for a diagnostic procedure is generally not necessary; however, if interventions are to be performed, a systemic bolus of heparin at 100 units/kg is given to prevent thrombosis. Activated clotting times (ACTs) are obtained every 20–30 minutes throughout the case, and heparin is redosed as needed to obtain an ACT level greater than 300 seconds. We recommend achieving these higher levels of ACT, given reported intraprocedural thromboembolism rates during tibial intervention as high as 4%.[6]

Antegrade Common Femoral Artery Access

For ipsilateral antegrade access, precision in placing the arterial puncture over the femoral head is critical in preventing access site complications. Ultrasound visualization is important, not only for arterial entry but to direct the wire into the superficial femoral artery. Upsizing to a sheath should only be done once there is confirmation of SFA selection with the wire. Direct SFA access can be performed in certain situations

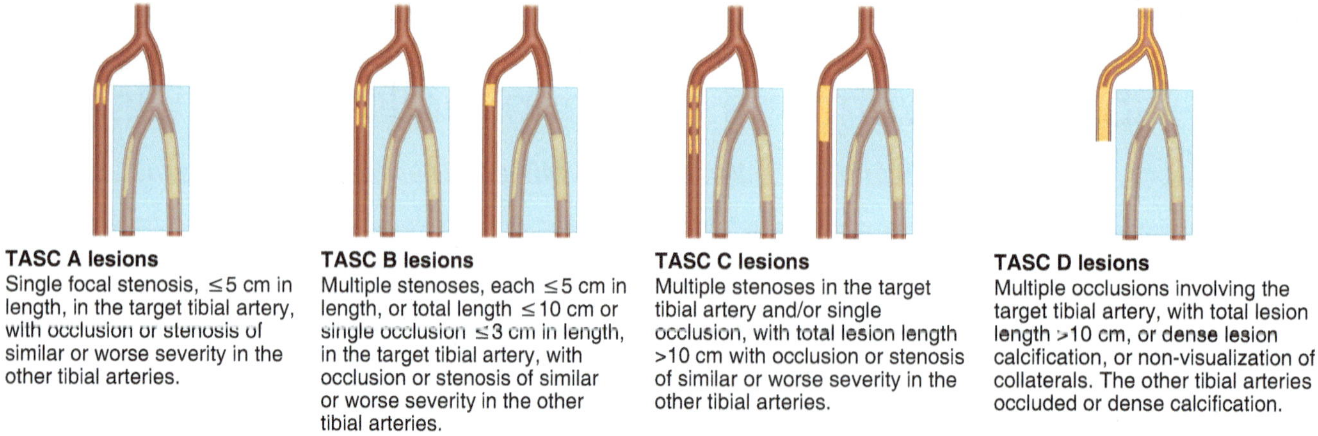

Fig. 35.1 Consensus recommendations for management of infrapopliteal lesions.
(TASC Steering Committee; Michael R Jaff et al. An Update on Methods for Revascularization and Expansion of the TASC Lesion Classification to Include Below-the-Knee Arteries: A Supplement to the Inter-Society Consensus for the Management of Peripheral Arterial Disease (TASC II). *Vasc Med.* 2015 Oct;20(5):465-78. doi:10.1177/1358863X15597877. Epub 2015 Aug 12).

where common femoral artery access is contra-indicated and the SFA is sufficient in diameter. In patients with a large obstructing pannus, it is helpful to reflect and to secure the pannus cranially with tape prior to prepping, draping, and attempting access.

Part of the difficulty of ipsilateral antegrade access is the directionality of wires toward the patient's head, resulting in workspace limitations. Using a longer sheath and arching the extracorporeal portion of the sheath to the contralateral side to direct the wires along the contralateral leg is a helpful technique. Securing the sheath to the patient or the drapes will prevent accidental sheath dislodgement. If a sheath is dislodged during a procedure, it is important to replace and reinsert the inner sheath dilator before advancing the sheath into the artery to avoid damaging the tip of the sheath and injuring the artery. Upon completion of the procedure following either retrograde or antegrade common femoral access, manual pressure is usually sufficient to obtain hemostasis, given the small sheath size required for tibial interventions. Following manual compression and hemostasis, we require patients to lie flat for 1 hour per sheath size used.

Retrograde Tibiopedal Access

Retrograde percutaneous tibiopedal access has become an important tool for treating tibial lesions that cannot be crossed from an antegrade approach. Obtaining tibiopedal access can be challenging, given the small size and extensive calcification of these vessels. Initial antegrade run-off angiography will identify the location of distal reconstitution, which will be the target for retrograde access. This arterial entry point is then identified under ultrasound visualization and accessed using a short micropuncture 21-gauge needle (Fig. 35.2A,B). If access fails following multiple attempts, the artery may go into vasospasm. Intra-arterial injection of nitroglycerin through the antegrade sheath and warming the leg can help resolve the vasospasm. Nitroglycerin can be administered intra-arterially through the sheath or catheter in 100–200 µg increments. Hypotension is rarely seen when administering nitroglycerin directly to the infrapopliteal arteries.

Alternatively, retrograde access can be obtained under direct fluoroscopy using calcification as a roadmap or handheld contrast injections from the proximal catheter. However, this exposes the interventionalist to higher doses of radiation. Occasionally, patients are unable to remain comfortable and still for these procedures while under monitored sedation, and in those cases, general anesthesia may be useful.

Following successful retrograde tibiopedal access with the micropuncture needle, the inner cannula of the micropuncture sheath is used as the tibial sheath (Fig. 35.2C). Alternatively, commercially available microsheaths can be used. However, we prefer the inner dilator alone to minimize the profile of the sheath in the tibial vessel. Following completion of the case and removal of all devices, hemostasis can be obtained via direct pressure over the tibial access point. Alternatively, inflation of a blood pressure cuff can be used for deeper accessed tibial vessels (e.g., peroneal) to achieve hemostasis. Closure devices should be avoided in these small vessels, given device-vessel size discrepancy and the risk of vessel narrowing and thrombosis.

Management of Complications

The most common complication from tibial endovascular interventions is access-site bleeding, followed by pseudoaneurysm, arteriovenous fistula, thrombosis/dissection, and distal embolization. To help triage access-site bleeding, an ACT level should be measured prior to sheath removal. For femoral access cases, bleeding following sheath removal can be controlled with direct manual pressure and reversal of heparin with protamine. Routinely, we deploy a closure device in the common femoral artery without heparin reversal. If we find continued bleeding after successful closure device deployment, we will then administer protamine. Alternatively, heparin can be allowed to wear off over 1–2 hours prior to sheath removal. As a general rule, 5 minutes of uninterrupted manual pressure per sheath size is recommended to obtain hemostasis in arteries without closure devices. If there is continued hemorrhage or hematoma expansion despite manual compression, surgical cut-down and repair of arteriotomy is indicated. In our institutional experience, the need for surgical cut-down following lower extremity access is very rare (<1%).[5]

Similarly for retrograde tibial or pedal access, bleeding is controlled by direct manual pressure over the access site. Hemostasis can be confirmed by conventional angiogram if the proximal sheath or catheter is still in place. However, heparin reversal should only be done once the proximal sheath is removed, to avoid thrombosis. If manual pressure fails or if the tibial vessel is deeper within the calf, blood pressure cuff occlusion can be attempted.

Documentation of bilateral pedal pulse examination prior to lower extremity endovascular intervention is important, especially since

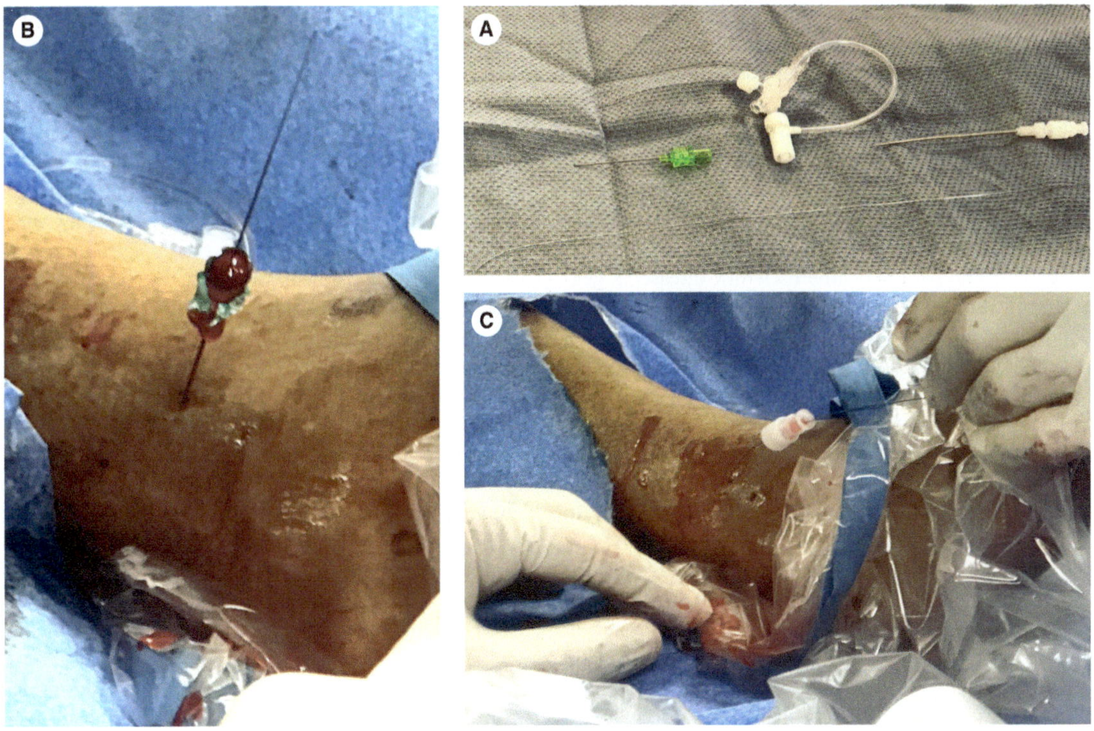

Fig. 35.2 (A) Micropuncture kit with short micropuncture needle, 0.018″ wire, and micropuncture sheath. (B) Successful peroneal artery access obtained by micropuncture needle, with evidence of back bleeding and 0.018″ wire in place. (C) Inner dilator of the micropuncture sheath acting as arterial sheath.

contralateral femoral access is commonly used. New findings of a cool, pulseless, or mottled limb at the completion of case or worsening foot pain is worrying for access site thrombosis or dissection. Access-site thrombosis is confirmed by intraoperative duplex ultrasound. If thrombosis is suspected prior to sheath removal, a contrast injection through the sheath will aid in diagnosis. However, injection through the sheath in this instance should only be performed if there is good back bleeding from the sheath side port demonstrating that the sheath itself is not thrombosed. If there is sheath thrombosis, the sheath may be removed over the wire and replaced. For femoral artery access-site thrombosis, surgical cut-down, thrombectomy, and repair of vessel are generally required. In selected cases when surgical cut-down of the groin is high risk or contra-indicated, gaining contralateral access and treatment using lysis, PTA, and stenting can be considered.

Femoral access site pseudoaneurysms can present as groin swelling, with or without an obvious hematoma or pulsatile groin mass. Retrograde tibial access-site pseudoaneurysms can present with swelling and, in very rare circumstances, can lead to compartment syndrome. Any patients with worrying findings on examination following access procedures should receive a groin or leg duplex ultrasound. Duplex ultrasound helps diagnosis and guidance for treatment options. Small pseudoaneurysms <2 cm can be observed and will usually thrombose spontaneously in the absence of systemic anticoagulation. Femoral and tibial pseudoaneurysms can be initially managed by direct manual pressure or ultrasound-guided compression, particularly if recognized immediately while the patient is sedated. Compression of a pseudoaneurysm in an unsedated patient is often not well tolerated. Open surgical repair of a pseudoaneurysm is indicated if the pseudoaneurysm is not anatomically amendable to thrombin injection or if the pseudoaneurysm is rapidly expanding, causing overlying skin necrosis, or is infected. Lower extremity fasciotomies may be required if compartment syndrome develops.

TREATMENT OF TIBIAL LESIONS

Techniques

Nonocclusive Tibial Stenosis

Angiographic evaluation of tibial vessels begins with quality arteriography. Imaging of diseased tibial vessels will often be diagnostically inadequate, with a flush catheter placed high in the aortoiliac vessels. For more detailed tibial vessel evaluation, contrast injection should be done following selective catheterization of the common femoral artery, distal superficial femoral artery, or popliteal arteries. The more distal the catheter is placed, the less contrast is required and the clearer the images become. In patients with chronic limb-threatening ischemia, contrast injection can result in a significant amount of ischemic pain. This pain is possibly caused by displacement of the limited blood supply or from the osmolarity of the contrast itself. Use of diluted isomolar nonionic contrast tends to cause the least patient discomfort.

Occasionally, patients are unable to stay still for the images under monitored sedation because of the pain, resulting in motion artifact. Placing an imaging delay following contrast injection can help reduce motion artifact. If the patient is still unable to stay still despite radiolucent restraints or increasing amounts of sedatives, the case will need to be completed with general anesthesia. To avoid these delays, it is important to assess and identify preoperatively patients who cannot tolerate an awake procedure, such as those with dementia, the elderly, or those with severe rest pain. In these patients, intervention under general anesthesia is preferred. Alternatively, cases performed with anesthesiologists can be started under monitored sedation with transition to general anesthesia during the case if needed.

It is important to remember that angiographic images are two-dimensional and lesion contours can be misrepresented when visualized in certain orientations. Imaging with different oblique projections can help clarify lesions. Obtaining tibial duplex ultrasound studies preoperatively can be helpful in identifying target lesions and for case planning. Additionally, intraoperative duplex can be performed to verify lesions that are found on outpatient imaging but not seen on arteriography and to demonstrate the presence or absence of a hemodynamically significant residual stenosis. Use of pressure wires to measure gradients across stenoses can also be performed; however, the routine use of this technique is expensive and the benefits have yet to be clearly elucidated.

Planning the sequence of tibial revascularization and selecting the number of vessels to be treated depends on indication for treatment, condition of the patient, and pattern of atherosclerotic disease. In general, for both chronic limb-threatening ischemia and claudication, revascularization of a single tibial vessel is sufficient if it provides adequate flow to the wound, either directly or through large collaterals. Based on a review from our institution, multiple-vessel tibial intervention for chronic limb-threatening ischemia, including patients with tissue loss, does not improve outcomes in terms of rates of reintervention, major amputation, or restenosis compared with single-vessel intervention.[7] In general, revascularization by angiosome does not apply to patients with chronic limb-threatening ischemia, given deviation from normal anatomy and redistribution of arterial perfusion away from the diseased vessels. We base tibial intervention instead on initial angiographic interpretation of the best vessel that will supply the lesion in question. Although in-line flow to the lesion is best, reperfusion through a collateral vessel is preferred over revascularization based on angiosome distribution, in particular when that vessel is occluded in the foot or has poor flow to the wound based on diagnostic imaging. Overall selection of the appropriate tibial vessel for revascularization is based on vessel accessibility and disease burden. Choosing a vessel that is most amenable to endovascular therapy, such as a short-segment TASC A stenosis, can result in a more durable effect than treatment of a long-segment, heavily diseased vessel.

Using an 0.014″ wire, a nonocclusive tibial lesion can be carefully crossed. Because atherosclerotic lesions are irregular, using an instrument to mold a curve onto the tip of a straight 0.014″ wire can help direct the wire to the desired direction. A large variety of wires are currently available on the market with varying stiffness, including those with tapered and weighted tips. For severe stenosis, where a lumen exists, we will choose a hydrophilic wire, such as Command 14 (Abbott Laboratories. Abbott Park, IL) or Choice PT (Boston Scientific, Malborough, MA). For chronic occlusions we will choose a weighted, tip wire such as Miracle Bros or Confianza (Asahi Intecc, Seto-shi, Japan). A torque device will help improve steerability of the wire through a lesion and 0.014″ or 0.018″ catheters, such as CXI support (Cook Medical, Bloomington, IN) or Quick-cross (Spectranetics, Colorado Springs, CO) catheters, can be fed over the wire for support and help direct the wire through an area of stenosis. Additionally, it is often helpful to use the 0.018 CXI support catheter through a 0.035″ catheter, such as Navicross (Terumo, Somerset, NJ), in a telescoping fashion to provide additional support. Additionally, a balloon catheter can be used in place of a support catheter to aid in lesion crossing by reducing the need for multiple catheter exchanges. Advancement of the sheath closer to the lesion will aid in overall stability of the system.

After crossing the stenosis, maintaining wire access is imperative to the success of the case by preventing multiple wire passes across a lesion. Multiple wire passes can result in thrombosis and dissection of the vessel. The tip of the wire should be visualized on live fluoroscopy at all times, especially during catheter exchanges, to avoid inadvertent wire advancement, causing distal vessel injury or perforation. Digital zoom can be utilized to focus on the area of interest while the wire tip is visualized simultaneously on the non-magnified image. Use of the digital zoom setting avoids the increased radiation associated with live fluoroscopic magnification.

Starting with 260–300 cm exchange length wires instead of shorter 145–180 cm length wires will ensure adequate working length for stable exchanges of balloons and catheters, especially with over-the-wire catheters and devices. Monorail catheter systems allow the wire to exit from the catheter closer to the tip of the device to facilitate quicker catheter exchanges with less wire manipulation. However, the monorail system has less pushability compared with the over-the-wire system. The Advance LP monorail balloon system (Cook Medical, Bloomington, IN) does have a longer over the wire segment (50 cm) before the wire exits the catheter, potentially allowing better pushability. When using this system through a sheath parked in the popliteal artery, most or all of the length of balloon catheter outside a sheath will be over the wire, while the monorail portion will remain within the sheath, thereby maintaining the benefits of a monorail system over long catheter lengths (170 cm). To prove intraluminal positioning of the wire once a tibial lesion is crossed, the tip of the wire should be seen freely advancing and rotating. For additional verification, a 0.014″ or 0.018″ catheter can be advanced over the wire and pass the lesion to perform a contrast injection.

Tibial balloon PTA has been widely accepted for treatment of tibial atherosclerotic disease. Prolonged balloon dilation for 2–3 minutes with gradual balloon deflation to reduce elastic recoil may help prevent intimal dissection. Balloon length and size are selected based on measurements on diagnostic arteriography. Treatment of long tibial lesions with a single long balloon instead of multiple inflations with shorter balloons may also help reduce the risk of dissection and thrombosis. Tibial PTA results in flow occlusion through the vessel. Therefore, performing multiple short balloon inflations instead of single balloon inflation will add additional ischemia time. Additionally, in small tibial vessels, the balloon catheter itself is often occlusive in the vessel without balloon inflation. To prevent thrombosis, it is important to maintain ACT levels greater than 300 during tibial PTA and remove PTA catheters promptly.

Balloon preparation is important in preventing air embolus if the balloon ruptures during PTA. This is performed by negative aspiration of air from the catheter and passively refilling the catheter shaft with diluted contrast media. Following PTA, it is important to confirm balloon deflation radiographically before removing the catheter. Having an assistant hold the sheath while walking off the balloon will prevent sheath dislodgement and help maintain wire access. Again, the tip of the wire should be visualized during the removal of the catheter. A completion angiogram is then performed to evaluate the success of the PTA treatment and to identify dissection, distal embolization, or arteriovenous (AV) fistula complications. Residual stenosis can be treated with repeat PTA or stenting.

Other adjuncts available for use in infrapopliteal lesions include drug-eluting stents (DES), drug-coated balloons (DCB), mechanical atherectomy devices, cryoplasty, cutting balloons, and laser atherectomy devices. Multiple European randomized controlled trials have shown benefit for infrapopliteal DES over PTA and bare metal stents (BMS) in terms of patency and freedom from reintervention. However, improvement in major amputations or overall mortality has been inconsistent among these trials.[8–11] There are currently no FDA approved DES for tibial vessels in the United States. Given this unavailability, DESs approved for coronary use are sometimes used off-label in tibial vessels.

The benefit of DCB therapy for infrapopliteal lesions is less clear. Whereas some studies have shown lower rates of 1-year restenosis, others found a trend toward higher amputation rates.[12,13] Regardless, there are no FDA approved DCB for tibial vessel in the United States and the smallest peripheral DCB is 4.0 mm in diameter, which is too large for use in most tibial vessels. Use of cutting balloons and atherectomy devices can lead to successful outcomes, depending on the operator's experience with these techniques. However, evidence for these devices is currently limited to smaller retrospective studies with short follow-up and conflicting outcomes.

In our practice, we do not use atherectomy devices given the risk of embolization, lack of evidence for benefit, and difficulty with successful use of distal filters in small tibial vessels. In patients who are not candidates for bypass, we occasionally use rotational atherectomy in situations where small balloon catheters will otherwise fail to pass a calcified lesion or would burst upon inflation.

Chronic Occlusions

Treatment of tibial artery occlusions can be challenging, depending on the degree of calcification and length of occlusion. Initial attempts for crossing occlusions are performed using 0.014″ or 0.018″ wires. Small back and forth movements can facilitate finding a soft spot in the occlusion. If this fails, rapidly spinning the wire like a drill with constant forward pressure can be successful. Advancing an 0.14″ or 0.18″ microcatheter over the wire and placing it directly against the occlusion will help generate more support and force for advancing the wire. Multiple wires are commercially available and designed to traverse tibial occlusions. Using a hydrophilic tipped wire or switching from a 0.14″ to a 0.35″ diameter wire can also be effective for stiffer occlusions. However, we rarely do this because of the increased risk of inadvertent vessel perforation.

Subintimal techniques are used if more traditional methods fail. If the subintimal plane is entered while trying to cross an occlusion, attempts are made to re-enter the reconstituted lumen distally. If the wire cannot be advanced any further to the reconstituted portion of the distal artery, we advance a microcatheter to the end of the wire so that progress is not lost and then switch out with a new wire and try to cross the remainder of the occlusion. If no further progress can be made, we pull the wire and catheter back to the top of the occlusion and attempt in a different plane. If the occlusive lesion is successfully crossed, subintimal PTA is then performed, and stenting may occasionally be needed.

Retrograde tibial access is very helpful in cases where antegrade crossing of the occlusion fails (Fig. 35.3). We now turn to retrograde access quickly if antegrade attempts are difficult. As described previously, a micropuncture needle is used to access the reconstituted portion of the distal tibial artery under ultrasound or live fluoroscopic guidance. Through the inner cannula of the micropuncture sheath, a long 0.14″ or 0.18″ wire is advanced through the occlusion in retrograde fashion. If there is still difficulty crossing the occlusion, the inner cannula sheath can be replaced with a 0.014″ catheter, such as a CXI catheter (Cook Medical, Bloomington, IN). Advancement of a catheter to the lesion will add additional support for the wire. Once the wire crosses through the occlusion and into true lumen proximally, the wire is then advanced into and through the antegrade sheath (Fig. 35.4A). If there is difficulty feeding the wire into the antegrade sheath, a snare device can be used to grab the wire. This technique is referred to as subintimal arterial flossing with antegrade–retrograde intervention (SAFARI). Placement of a hemostat at the retrograde access site to secure the wire will help prevent accidental wire pull-through and may be useful as a "body floss" technique to pass catheters, if there is resistance. From this point, antegrade PTA with or without stent of the tibial occlusion can be performed.

Occasionally, two different subintimal planes are created with the antegrade and retrograde wires. If this occurs, balloon PTA over the antegrade wire may disrupt the plaque adequately to allow passage of the retrograde wire into the lumen. If this is not successful, antegrade–retrograde side-by-side PTA can be performed (Fig. 35.4B). This is performed by advancing one balloon catheter over the antegrade wire and another catheter over the retrograde wire until the tips of the two catheters meet at the lesion. Following simultaneous PTA, the adjacent intimal planes will connect through a fracture in the intima. The wires can be then be advanced into the same plane and PTA/stenting performed.

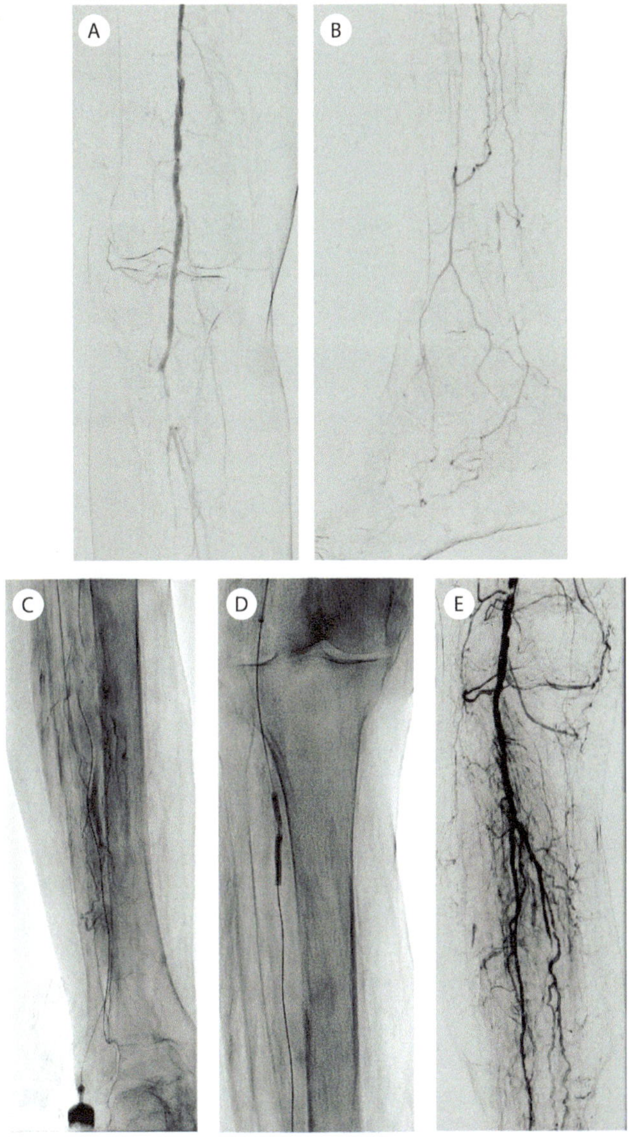

Fig. 35.3 (A) Right lower extremity arteriogram showing a tibioperoneal trunk occlusion. (B) Distal reconstitution of the peroneal artery. (C) Retrograde tibial access obtained via the distal peroneal artery. (D) Percutaneous transluminal angioplasty treatment after a retrograde wire was crossed through the occlusion and advanced into the antegrade sheath. (E) Completion angiogram showing successful treatment with improved distal run-off.

Alternatively, a retrograde balloon can be inserted and inflated while a re-entry device such as the Outback catheter (Cordis, Miami Lakes, FL) is advanced from above to puncture the retrograde balloon (Fig. 35.4C). The retrograde balloon catheter is typically inserted bare-backed with no sheath to minimize the size of the distal tibial puncture. Once the balloon is punctured, the antegrade wire is advanced into the balloon. The antegrade wire and retrograde balloon are then withdrawn simultaneously across the lesion and out through the retrograde puncture site. This maneuver is typically performed in the popliteal or tibial-peroneal trunk because of the size of the re-entry device.

Tibial Bifurcation Lesions

Lesions located at the orifice of tibial bifurcations pose a significant problem, given the risk of compromising the lumen of the neighboring

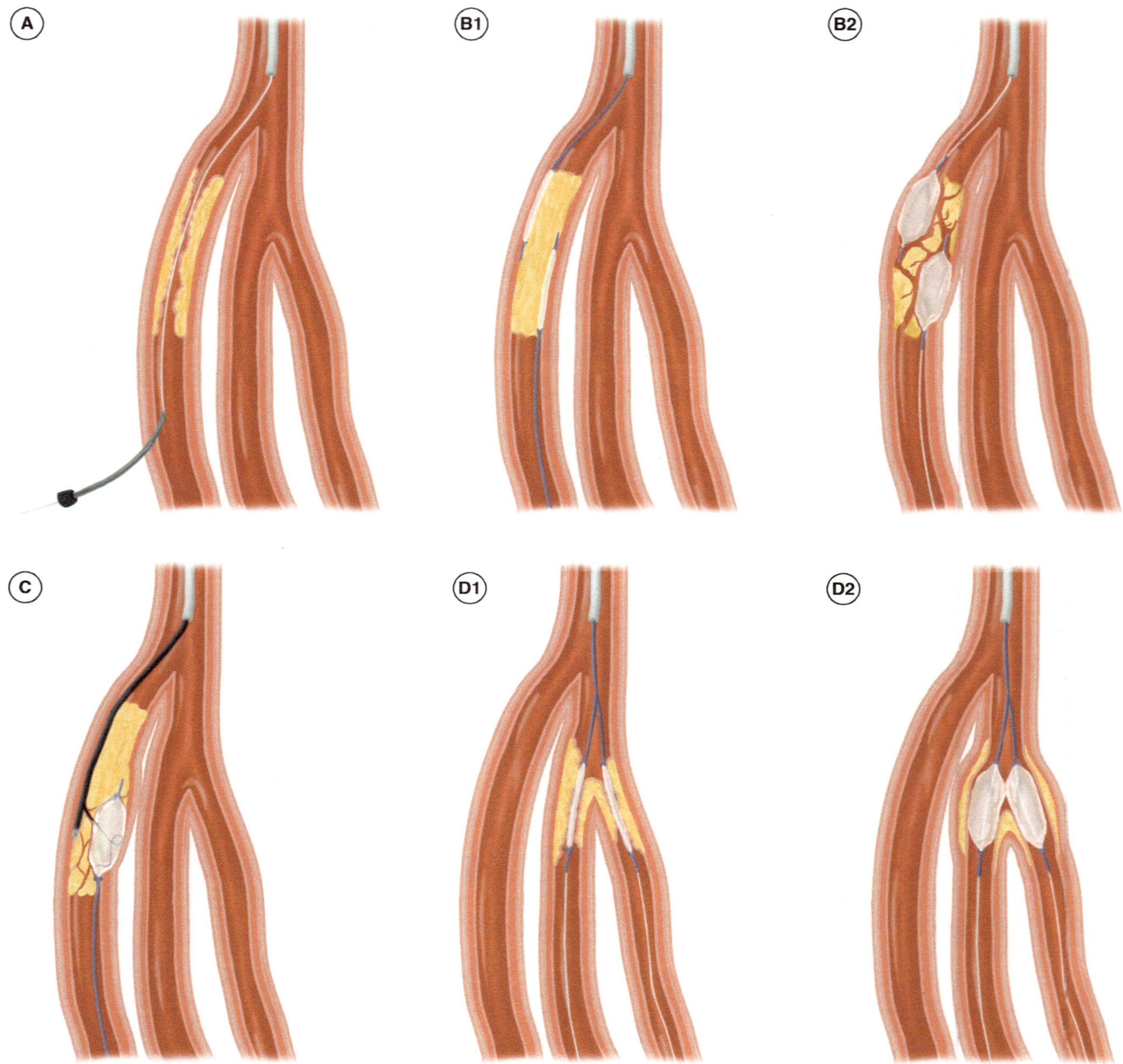

Fig. 35.4 (A) Tibial occlusion crossed in retrograde fashion and wire fed into the antegrade sheath. (B) Lumen connection through antegrade–retrograde side-by-side angioplasty. (C) Lumen connection through retrograde balloon and antegrade re-entry device. (D) Buddy-wire positioning for ostial bifurcation lesions.

vessel (Fig. 35.4D). This can occur with lesions at the anterior tibial artery and tibial-peroneal trunk bifurcation or the posterior-tibial and peroneal artery bifurcation. To prevent and to manage this complication, a buddy-wire system is helpful. This is performed by separately selecting each bifurcation vessel with a 0.14″ wire through the same antegrade sheath. If PTA of one the of the orifices leads to spillover of plaque or thrombus into the other vessel, the compromised vessel will already have a wire in place for treatment. In select situations, stents can be placed in kissing fashion for ostial lesions at a tibial bifurcation. However, it is important to realize that the buddy-system technique will often require upsizing to a larger sheath system. Therefore, it is prudent to anticipate cases where this technique may be beneficial based on initial arteriogram, to avoid needing to switch to a larger sheath over a stiffer wire mid-case. If that is the case, one of the wires may be exchanged for a stiffer 0.018″ wire and the new sheath can be introduced over both wires.

Management of Complications

Dissection

Dissections commonly occur following balloon PTA. Non-flow-limiting dissections may be left alone or retreated with PTA, focusing on a prolonged low-pressure balloon inflation and gentle deflation. For flow-limiting dissections, it is important not to lose wire access during catheter exchanges so that intraluminal access is maintained, again highlighting the need to observe the wire tip during exchanges. Typically, repeated PTA will resolve the dissection. However, if PTA fails, placement of a stent can be considered to secure the dissection. Intra-arterial boluses of nitroglycerin can be helpful if vasospasm occurs.

Vessel Perforation and Wire Fractures

Tibial artery perforations can occur when attempting to recanalize an occluded vessel. This is seen when the wire travels extraluminally on live fluoroscopy and may be confirmed with contrast injections showing extravasation. Multiple contrast injections should be avoided because the contrast will not wash away easily once outside the vessel and will lead to contrast obscuring all future efforts. When perforation occurs secondary to wire passage, it is rarely of hemodynamic significance and will usually resolve over a few minutes. If a small perforation is found, wire and catheters can be pulled back and the lesion recrossed in a different plane. However, in rare situations when the perforation results in a large arterial disruption with significant extravasation, the decision can be made to conclude the case. With continued extravasation, systemic heparinization should be reversed with protamine. Mechanical pressure with an inflated blood pressure cuff can be used if necessary. Wire fractures can occur during long calcified tibial occlusion interventions when creating too much torque and strain on the wire. This is rarely of any clinical consequence since attempts in retrieving the wire are often futile and without clinical benefit if the wire sits in an area of occlusion. This complication may be avoided by switching earlier to another tibial artery for intervention or to a retrograde tibial approach when initial efforts are unsuccessful.

Embolic Disease

Intraoperative tibial embolism can occur during tibial, femoral, or aortoiliac endovascular procedures. First, an ACT level should be checked and heparin redosed if ACT levels are subtherapeutic. If heparin-induced thrombocytopenia and thrombosis is suspected, the appropriate diagnostic tests should be made and the patient should be transitioned to a direct thrombin inhibitor, such as argatroban or bivalirudin, for the remainder of the case.

Emboli occurring during endovascular arterial manipulation can be either from atheroemboli or thromboemboli. Based on the source of embolus, these complications can be managed with various techniques, including percutaneous aspiration thrombectomy, PTA, stenting, mechanical thrombectomy, and thrombolysis. Athero-embolism occurs when atherosclerotic plaques are disrupted and small pieces of plaque break off and travel distally. Thromboembolism occurs when acute or chronic thrombus that has formed around a plaque dislodges and travels distally.

In certain cases of low-burden thromboembolic disease, aspiration using a single end-hole aspiration catheter can be attempted. However, this requires losing wire access across the lesion and may compromise further interventions if aspiration is not successful. Small volume acute thrombi are more readily removed by aspiration than large volume chronic thrombi or large calcified pieces of atheroemboli. Catheter aspiration is performed with a lure-lock syringe attached to the back end of an aspiration catheter. The larger the catheter used, the higher the chances of success. Separate monorail aspiration catheters are also available and allow maintenance of wire access but still require a 6-French sheath and have a smaller aspiration lumen than a 0.035″ or 0.038″ catheter. If the sheath in place at time of embolism is 5-French, it can be upsized without uncrossing the lesion by placing a 0.018″ buddy wire for additional wire support and exchanging the sheath carefully over the two wires together.

For athero-emboli, PTA, typically with stent placement, can be used to trap the emboli. If a wire is not already in place for intervention, careful attempts can be made to pass an 0.014″ wire around the embolized plaque. In contrast, PTA and stent should be avoided in patients with thromboemboli because of the risk of squeezing the thrombus out of the ends of the stent and causing further distal embolization.

We prefer mechanical AngioJet thrombectomy for treatment of thromboemboli. The AngioJet thrombectomy system (Boston Scientific, Malborough, MA) applies the Venturi-Bernoulli effect to create a suction force that pulls pieces of fragmented thrombus out through a catheter. Thrombectomy catheters are currently limited to use in vessels greater than 2 mm. If this method fails or treatment of a long occluded tibial segment is needed, intra-arterial injection of a thrombolytic, such as Alteplase (tPA), can be given if the patient has no bleeding contraindications. There are multiple methods of thrombolysis (see Chapter 31). Alternatively, a bolus of 2–5 mg of tPA can be directly infused at the site of occlusion through a catheter. If this fails to eliminate the thrombus, we often conclude the case and heparinize the patient, with consideration for re-imaging if the patient's ischemia worsens.

We rarely perform overnight continuous tPA infusion. tPA infusion requires placement of a catheter with multiple side holes across the thrombosed segment. These catheters may be too large to be effective for tibial vessels. For select cases where the tibial vessels are large enough for lysis catheter placement, overnight infusion can be performed using a microcatheter, such as a MicroMewi catheter (Covidien, Minneapolis, MN) or a ProStream multiple side-hole infusion 0.035″ wire (Covidien, Minneapolis, MN). However, both these devices have limited treatment lengths (12 cm maximum), and flow will still be limited around the catheter or wire. A 12- to 24-hours continuous infusion with tPA infusion rates ranging from 0.5 to 1.0 mg/h is recommended. The following day, a repeat angiogram is performed and mechanical thrombectomy can be re-attempted for any residual thrombus. Open thrombectomy via popliteal, tibial, or pedal cutdown can be considered, but success rates are generally low.

Arteriovenous (AV) Fistula

AV fistula formation following subintimal PTA is rare, with an incidence of less than 1%, and can be managed with multiple techniques, including observation, balloon tamponade, coil embolization, and stent placement.[14] Fistulas at the tibial trifurcation are most common, likely secondary to the close proximity of the tibial arteries and veins. In general, most AV fistulas created from tibial PTA are left untreated. Low-flow fistulas will probably resolve over time and can be monitored with interval lower extremity duplex studies. However, if a large high-flow fistula is created and is compromising antegrade flow to an area of ischemia, treatment of the fistula is indicated. Balloon tamponade should be attempted first by inflation of a low-pressure balloon for 3–4 minutes across the fistula. This can be repeated multiple times until the fistula resolves. The role of bare-metal stents is unclear because the open struts may not decrease the flow of the fistula sufficiently for fistula resolution. However, bare stents may provide enough pressure to cause plaque to occlude the fistula. Covered stent placement will resolve the fistula, but there are currently no readily available covered stents for tibial vessels and there is lack of evidence regarding patency of covered stents in the tibial arteries, as they tend to be bulky. Coil embolization is rarely performed for tibial AV fistula. Coiling can risk compromising tibial arterial flow and should not be performed if the arterial supply to the fistula is also the main arterial supply to the foot. Tibial AV fistulas are rarely of clinical significance and, if balloon tamponade fails, we recommend interval ultrasound surveillance to monitor for spontaneous resolution or clinical compromise of antegrade flow. We have never felt the need to perform open repair of AVF in a tibial vessel.

CONCLUSIONS

Maintaining arterial and wire access through the treated tibial lesion is vital throughout these endovascular interventions because the wire serves as a lifeline for reintervention when endovascular complications occur. An interventionalist should constantly be careful during complex endovascular interventions not to compromise a potential bypass target, as tibial or pedal bypass may prove to be a more appropriate and durable option in certain patients and, as such, we prefer to avoid sheath placement in tibial vessels. As endovascular treatment for tibial disease continues to grow and to evolve, the same attentiveness to proper technique will be required to prevent and to minimize complications. Mastering the endovascular techniques needed for treating tibial lesions will be of upmost importance for vascular specialists in the future.

REFERENCES

1. Albers M, Romiti M, Pereira CA, Antonini M, Wulkan M. Meta-analysis of allograft bypass grafting to infrapopliteal arteries. *Eur J Vasc Endovasc Surg.* 2004;28(5):462–472.
2. Romiti M, Albers M, Brochado-Neto FC, Durazzo AE, Pereira CA, De Luccia N. Meta-analysis of infrapopliteal angioplasty for chronic critical limb ischemia. *J Vasc Surg.* 2008;47(5):975–981.
3. Adam DJ, Beard JD, Cleveland T, et al. Bypass versus angioplasty in severe ischaemia of the leg (BASIL): multicentre, randomised controlled trial. *Lancet.* 2005;366(9501):1925–1934.
4. Jaff MR, White CJ, Hiatt WR, et al. An Update on methods for revascularization and expansion of the TASC lesion classification to include below-the-knee arteries: a supplement to the inter-society consensus for the management of peripheral arterial disease (TASC II): The TASC Steering Comittee(.). *Ann Vasc Dis.* 2015;8(4):343–357.
5. Lo RC, Fokkema MT, Curran T, et al. Routine use of ultrasound-guided access reduces access site-related complications after lower extremity percutaneous revascularization. *J Vasc Surg.* 2015;61(2):405–412.
6. Lo RC, Darling J, Bensley RP, et al. Outcomes following infrapopliteal angioplasty for critical limb ischemia. *J Vasc Surg.* 2013;57(6):1455–1463; discussion 1463–1464.
7. Darling JD, McCallum JC, Soden PA, et al. Clinical results of single-vessel versus multiple-vessel infrapopliteal intervention. *J Vasc Surg.* 2016; 64(6):1675–1681.
8. Bosiers M, Scheinert D, Peeters P, et al. Randomized comparison of everolimus-eluting versus bare-metal stents in patients with critical limb ischemia and infrapopliteal arterial occlusive disease. *J Vasc Surg.* 2012; 55(2):390–398.
9. Rastan A, Tepe G, Krankenberg H, et al. Sirolimus-eluting stents vs. bare-metal stents for treatment of focal lesions in infrapopliteal arteries: a double-blind, multi-centre, randomized clinical trial. *Eur Heart J.* 2011; 32(18):2274–2281.
10. Scheinert D, Katsanos K, Zeller T, et al. A prospective randomized multi-center comparison of balloon angioplasty and infrapopliteal stenting with the sirolimus-eluting stent in patients with ischemic peripheral arterial disease: 1-year results from the ACHILLES trial. *J Am Coll Cardiol.* 2012;60(22):2290–2295.
11. Siablis D, Kitrou PM, Spiliopoulos S, Katsanos K, Karnabatidis D. Paclitaxel-coated balloon angioplasty versus drug-eluting stenting for the treatment of infrapopliteal long-segment arterial occlusive disease: the IDEAS randomized controlled trial. *JACC. Cardiovasc Interv.* 2014; 7(9):1048–1056.
12. Liistro F, Porto I, Angioli P, et al. Drug-eluting balloon in peripheral intervention for below the knee angioplasty evaluation (DEBATE-BTK): a randomized trial in diabetic patients with critical limb ischemia. *Circulation.* 2013;128(6):615–621.
13. Zeller T, Baumgartner I, Scheinert D, et al. Drug-eluting balloon versus standard balloon angioplasty for infrapopliteal arterial revascularization in critical limb ischemia: 12-month results from the IN.PACT DEEP randomized trial. *J Am Coll Cardiol.* 2014;64(15):1568–1576.
14. Ananthakrishnan G, DeNunzio M, Bungay P, Pollock G, Fishwick G, Bolia A. The occurrence of arterio-venous fistula during lower limb sub-intimal angioplasty: treatment and outcome. *Eur J Vasc Endovasc Surg.* 2006;32(6):675–679.

36

Complications of Iliofemoral Thrombolysis and Stenting for Venous Disease

Linda M. Harris, MD, FACS, DFSVS, Gregory S. Cherr, MD and Brittany C. Montross, MD

INTRODUCTION

Many patients with symptomatic iliofemoral deep vein thromboses (DVTs) are now undergoing intervention to minimize thrombus burden in order to decrease venous pressures and preserve valve function. For patients with extensive and/or severely symptomatic DVT, catheter-based intervention is standard of care. Current guidelines from the Society of Vascular Surgeons and American Venous Forum for treatment are acute proximal DVT with symptoms <14 days, good functional capacity, life expectancy greater than 1 year, phlegmasia cerulea dolens, and low bleeding risk.[1]

ACCESS FOR CATHETER-DIRECTED THROMBOLYSIS

Successful catheter-directed thrombolysis (CDT) begins with access, for which preoperative assessment is helpful. Access should be obtained one level below the majority of the thrombus burden, often the ipsilateral popliteal vein with the patient in prone position. If the thrombus extends below the popliteal vein, access can be obtained in the small saphenous vein or one of the posterior tibial veins at the medial malleolus. If the thrombus is isolated to the iliac system, the ipsilateral femoral vein can be accessed with the patient in supine position. Alternatively, the contralateral femoral vein can be accessed for the up-and-over technique. Lastly, the internal jugular (IJ) can also be used; however, this is used less in acute situations, in which crossing is typically easy and thrombolysis usually necessary. One challenge with access from the contralateral femoral vein or jugular vein is that retrograde crossing of the valves can be more difficult.

Ultrasound-guided access should be obtained with a micropuncture system, with negative pressure on the attached syringe, partially filled with saline. Using ultrasound, the needle tip should be visualized entering the vein, as blood is not always seen in the syringe because of the thrombus. Multiple punctures, more likely without ultrasound guidance, can lead to hematoma and premature termination of the procedure.

An access venogram is performed via the micropuncture sheath to confirm location and visualize thrombus burden. It is important to use only gentle hand injections, not power injections, because of the risk of embolization. The microsheath is then upsized to a 6-French sheath to facilitate crossing of the thrombosed vein. Initial attempts are made with 0.035″ hydrophilic guidewire, such as a regular or stiff Angled Glidewire (Terumo, Somerset, New Jersey), along with a guiding catheter, such as a Glidecatheter (Terumo). An angled guiding catheter or wire is preferable to allow steering past the occlusions. Venograms are performed at various levels to visualize the extent of thrombus burden. Venogram is also performed once the catheter passes into the inferior vena cava (IVC) to confirm patency distal to the thrombus. If the entire thrombus burden is not treated, it is likely to fail because of continued outflow obstruction.

Once the lesion is crossed, there are several options. Thrombus removal can be achieved in one session, with pharmacomechanical thrombectomy, or in multiple sessions with thrombolysis with or without pharmacomechanical thrombectomy.

THROMBOLYSIS

After confirming appropriate position by venogram, a multi-sideport infusion lysis catheter is placed. There are several options available including: Unifuse (AngioDynamics, Latham, NY), Cragg McNamara (Medtronic, Minneapolis, MN), EkoSonic (Boston Scientific, Marlborough, MA). The length of thrombus should be measured using a marking catheter or tape, intravascular ultrasound (IVUS) pullback, or measurements based on venogram. The catheter treatment zone is based on the length of the thrombus and ranges from 5 to 50 cm. Once the infusion catheter is in place, thrombolytic therapy is initiated, typically with 0.5–2 mg/h of recombinant tissue plasminogen activator (rtPA). The optimal dose has not been established. Lower doses may result in inadequate thrombus removal and higher doses may increase the risk of major bleeds. In addition to the rtPA, heparin is infused via the sheath to maintain sheath patency. There are no studies directly assessing the optimal dose of heparin during thrombolysis. Our practice is to use subtherapeutic levels (such as 500 U/h of unfractionated heparin); however, higher levels are sometimes used with higher thrombus burdens.

Patients undergoing thrombolysis are monitored in an intensive care unit (ICU) or step down unit and kept flat, with the limb straight to prevent kinking or displacement of the catheter. Routine laboratory work is recommended, including prothrombin time, partial thromboplastin time, hemoglobin/hematocrit and fibrinogen every 4–12 hours, in addition to neurovascular checks and monitoring the puncture site for bleeding. Fibrinogen monitoring is controversial. If the fibrinogen drops below 100 mg/dL, the rtPA infusion is reduced or discontinued to decrease risk of major bleeding. While the rtPA is held, therapeutic anticoagulation is administered via the catheter and saline via the sheath and the fibrinogen level is rechecked in 2–4 hours if the patient has not undergone repeat imaging. We find that a significant reduction in fibrinogen is usually an indicator that the thrombus burden has greatly decreased, and now the lytic agent is being infused more systemically indicating more urgent follow-up is needed. Repeat imaging routinely occurs after 12–24 hours, but is done earlier if fibrinogen greatly decreases or the patient demonstrates clinical signs of significant improvement. If thrombolysis is not complete at repeat imaging and repeat fibrinogen levels have adequately rebounded, rtPA can be restarted at half the dose, with close surveillance of fibrinogen levels and for signs of bleeding. Thrombolysis >72 hours greatly increases bleeding risk. Use of retrievable IVC filters to prevent pulmonary embolus during thrombolysis is controversial. However, recommendation for consideration of an IVC filter would be the following: (1) large thrombus burden involving the iliocaval segment; (2) free-floating thrombus in the iliocaval segment; (3) patient presenting with iliofemoral DVT and pulmonary embolus (PE); and (4) patients with poor cardiopulmonary reserve. If placed, once the threat of PE is no longer an issue, the retrievable ICV filter should be removed, usually at 4–6 weeks posttreatment. In addition, and in most circumstances, there is no need to stop anticoagulation during filter retrieval. Filters can easily be placed via the popliteal access. Two filters, Optease (Cordis, Santa Clara, CA) and Optional Elite (Argon Medical Devices, Frisco, TX), have a 70-cm treatment length. If access is more distal and a filter is desired, IJ placement may be necessary prior to accessing tibial veins because the delivery system for the filter will not reach from the tibial to the correct location in the IVC.

COMPLICATIONS FROM VENOUS LYSIS

Pulmonary embolus (PE) can occur during thrombolysis. Fortunately, massive PE is extremely rare because treatment is ongoing with heparin and lytic agent infusing.

Bleeding: The most common complication from venous thrombolysis is access site hematoma, which typically does not require intervention. If a large hematoma develops, the patient may require transfusion. Hematoma evacuation and/or vein repair should be considered for patients who develop severe signs or symptoms such as skin necrosis, leg edema, or compression of adjacent structures.

Intracranial hemorrhage is a devastating, but rare, complication. It is important to obtain a head CT prior to initiation of fibrinolytic therapy in patients with concern for intracranial pathology. During thrombolysis, thrombolytic and anticoagulant medications should be immediately held if neurologic changes develop until intracranial bleed can be ruled out.

Hematuria, epistaxis, and gastrointestinal (GI) bleed can be minor or major and may require terminating thrombolysis if severe. Minor, non–life-threatening bleeding can be safely managed while continuing thrombolysis. GI bleeding typically requires cessation of lytic agent to reduce the risk for hemodynamically significant hemorrhage. If patients have a history of GI bleeding or known gastroesophageal varices, GI consultation should occur prior to initiating thrombolysis.

The CaVenT Study, a recent randomized control study looking at long-term outcomes of catheter directed thrombolysis versus standard anticoagulation for acute iliofemoral DVT, found minimal major complication in the treatment group. Of 90 patients on thrombolysis, there were 20 bleeding complications, 3 of which were major (1 abdominal wall hematoma requiring transfusion, 1 calf compartment syndrome requiring intervention, and 1 inguinal access site hematoma). There were no deaths, PE, or intracranial hemorrhage.[2] Complications are reduced with meticulous patient selection and careful access with US guidance and micropuncture kits. Patients at high risk of complications during thrombolysis include elderly patients, recent cerebrovascular event, recent childbirth, patients who underwent recent (<1–2 weeks) major surgery (abdominal, neurologic, spinal, internal eye), trauma, known conditions prone to bleeding (such as GI ulcers and varices, intracranial pathology, bladder cancer), and patients with thrombocytopenia or other bleeding disorders. For these patients, thrombolysis may be contraindicated because of the unacceptably high risk of life-threatening bleeding. Also of concern are patients who would not be able to tolerate appropriate positioning for extended lengths of time, such as those with chronic lung disease, congestive heart failure, or dementia.

PHARMACOMECHANICAL CATHETER-DIRECTED THROMBOLYSIS

Pharmacomechanical thrombectomy (PCMT) utilizes thrombolytic therapy combined with mechanical thrombectomy. PCMT is thought to macerate the thrombus, leading to improved penetration of the drug, immediate thrombus aspiration, and the potential for shorter treatment times. PCMT techniques have similar results to CDT alone in terms of thrombus removal. Advantages may include reduced dose of thrombolytic drug and shorter treatment times (with less or no ICU time), and shorter hospital stays.[3]

Initiation of PCMT is the same as CDT. Once access is obtained, the venogram is performed and the thrombus crossed. Decision regarding the type of PCMT will dictate sheath size. There are several types of pharmacomechanical devices currently available with different mechanisms of action:

1. Hydrodynamic/rheolytic effect (Venturi effect): Angiojet (Boston Scientific, Marlborough, MA): This utilizes heparinized saline or rtPA jets to break up thrombus, which is then aspirated creating a local reduction in pressure to limit embolism. Angiojet Solente Zalente DVT is specifically designed for the iliofemoral vessels (≥6 mm), and Angiojet Solente Proxi can be used in the periphery for 3–6-mm vessels. Angiojet Zalente requires an 8-French sheath over a 0.035″ wire system. The Zalente catheter is placed at the proximal end of the thrombus, power pulse mode is initiated, and then the catheter is advanced to the most distal end, delivering rtPA into the thrombus. During this mode, no thrombus or blood is aspirated. After a dwell time of ideally 30 minutes, the unit is changed out of power pulse and mechanical thrombectomy is performed. In order to maximize thrombus removal, the catheter is rotated 90 degrees following each pass because the suction ports are not multidirectional and rotation of the device allows approximation of the tip closer to the wall, thereby permitting better treatment of the thrombus.
2. Rotational devices: Arrow Trerotola Percutaneous thrombectomy device (Teleflex, Wayne, PA): These devices cause microfrag-mentation of the thrombus by rotating blades or baskets. They require a 7-French sheath with a 0.025″ wire. A handheld, battery-operated catheter rotates the 9 mm fragmentation basket at 3000 rpm macerating the thrombus into small <2-mm fragments, which are then aspirated or microembolized and cleared by the pulmonary circulation.
3. Mixing devices: Trellis Peripheral Infusion System (Medtronic, Minneapolis, MN) and Cleaner (Argon Medical Devices, Frisco, TX). These devices use oscillating sinusoidal wires, which disrupts the thrombus and have side ports for injection of the thrombolytic. Trellis is currently off the market. It used a sinusoidal wire between two balloons to localize the treatment area and prevent embolization. Cleaner XT uses a 6-French sheath for the 9-mm rotating sinusoidal wire or a 7-French sheath for the Cleaner15, with a 15-mm rotating sinusoidal wire (more suited for iliofemoral DVT). This is a battery-operated handheld device, which macerates the thrombus and allows wall contact, which facilitates removal of more chronic/adherent thrombus. The device can potentially be used with IVC filter thrombosis. It is important to note that the device is inserted "bareback" through the sheath, not over a wire. It is steerable and effective for straightforward anatomy; however, wire access is lost, which can be challenging with tortuous anatomy or with tight lesions that were initially difficult to traverse.
4. Ultrasound (US) Assisted Thrombectomy: EKOS Sonicare (Boston Scientific, Marlborough, MA). CDT assisted by high-frequency, low-energy US, which disrupts the fibrin in the thrombus to expose the underlying plasminogen, allows better

penetration and efficiency of the thrombolytic drug. Treatment times are longer than with PCMT devices, but less than standard CDT. Single-setting thrombolysis is not an option with this device. It utilizes a 6-French sheath over a 0.035″ wire. To prevent catheter thrombosis, the catheter must be immediately prepped in the angiography suite with heparin or attached to the thrombolytic drip. Kinking of the catheter can also be problematic.

5. Aspiration Catheters: Indigo System (Penumbra, Alameda, CA) and Angiovac (AngioDynamics, Latham, NY). These devices do not use mechanical thrombectomy or thrombolytic medications. A guidewire is placed through the sheath and then a thin-walled, wide lumen, nontapered catheter is placed to engage the thrombus. The thrombus is then removed with negative pressure from a 30-mL syringe or suction. Multiple passes are usually required. There is less risk of hemolysis than with PCMT, but more blood loss. Indigo uses continuous suction to remove the clot burden, and the separator within the catheter helps to break up the thrombus once retrieved to maintain patency of the catheter and prevent embolization. Angiovac is specifically designed as a venous drainage cannula for extracorporeal circulation and thrombus removal during this process. It is utilized more often to treat pulmonary emboli but can be helpful for IVC thrombus. The device is very large (22 French) and rigid, requiring a 26-French sheath, and requires general anesthesia and a perfusionist.

Data to inform the use of PCMT devices for DVT are limited. The Peripheral Use of Angiojet Rheolytic Thrombectomy with a Variety of Catheter Lengths (PEARL Registry), a multicenter study, found no difference in thrombus removal, rethrombosis, or quality of life at 1 year with Angiojet, Angiojet with thrombolysis, or thrombolysis prior to or following Angiojet thrombectomy.[4]

The Acute Venous Thrombosis: Thrombus removal with Adjunctive Catheter Directed Thrombolysis (ATTRACT) Trial comparing PCMT with anticoagulation alone found no benefit in its primary endpoint of reduced Villalta score for grading postthrombotic syndrome in the CDT/PMT group compared with anticoagulation alone at 2 years; however, secondary subgroup analysis suggested there is potential benefit in cases of acute iliofemoral DVT and those with more severe symptoms (with inadequate statistical power to assess these subgroups fully).[5]

COMPLICATIONS FOLLOWING PERCUTANEOUS PHARMACOMECHANICAL THROMBECTOMY

Patients are at risk of specific, device-related complications in addition to standard bleeding complications from CDT. Vedantham et al. found a 2.8% rate of major bleeding, 0.5% rate of symptomatic PE, and a 3.9% overall rate of major complications.[6] PCMT decreases infusion time and thrombolytic dose and can decrease or eliminate ICU stays. However, procedure times are significantly longer because of the dwell-time requirements of the thrombolytic agent. There is a potential increase in radiation exposure for the patient (which may be offset by fewer procedures) and increased cost in the angiography suite (staff and procedure room time).

The most studied devices are Angiojet (Boston Scientific, Marlborough, MA) and Trellis (Medtronic, Minneapolis, MN).

- Rheolytic (Angiojet): Because of forceful pulse spray and aspiration, hemolysis is common. This is proportional to time and volume of treatment and usually resolves within 48 hours. When severe, hemolysis can lead to hyperkalemia and renal failure. Patients should be adequately hydrated and volume and time recommendations from the manufacturer observed. Volume overload can occur as a result of fluid administered with alteplase and saline jets for maceration, and care must therefore be taken in patients with congestive heart or renal failure. Bradycardia can occur, particularly in the more central locations, but resolves with pausing the device and resuming once bradycardia disappears, typically within minutes. Incomplete thrombus dissolution and distal embolization can also occur.
- Rotational and mixing: These devices can potentially cause endothelial damage as a result of wall contact from the rotating baskets or oscillating wires, although we are not aware of any reports of this complication. Perforation in the venous system is far less catastrophic than in the arterial system and can be managed conservatively with cessation of thrombolytic, while larger perforations may require cessation of anticoagulation. More aggressive intervention is rarely necessary. If the patient is hemodynamically unstable, management options include balloon deployment at the site of rupture to tamponade the injury or covered-stent placement. Most covered stents are too small and all are off-label for the venous system. If stent-graft placement is required, IVUS should be used to prevent undersizing, which would lead to continued extravasation. These devices also have a risk of PE, especially when used without thrombolytic agents. Park et al. showed no increased incidence of PE between CDT, CDT + Trerotola, or Trerotola.[7] Trerotola (Teleflex, Wayne, PA) is a rotating, expandable basket device, designed for dialysis access. However, in this study, they placed IVC filters in 95% of patients, therefore the risk without IVC filter placement cannot be assessed.

The role of IVC filter placement during percutaneous endovenous intervention is controversial. Sharifi et al. found that among 141 patients undergoing percutaneous venous interventions, CTA or V/Q identified a reduced risk of PE in the filter group (1 PE-filter; 8 PE-control; $P = 0.048$). There were no differences in mortality or postprocedure symptoms. Identified risk factors for iatrogenic PE included PE at admission, severely symptomatic DVT (erythema, edema, pain, and induration), DVT involving two or more venous segments, venous diameter $\geq$7 mm, and normal venous anatomy.[8]

STENTING

Patients who present with acute iliofemoral DVT often have an underlying stenotic lesion. Prior to completing the procedure, venous stenosis should be evaluated using IVUS in addition to venography. The most common form of May-Thurner syndrome involves compression of the left common iliac vein by the right common iliac artery and spine, just below the iliocaval junction. There are multiple other sites of potential iliac vein compression, from crossing internal iliac arteries, as well as pathologic findings, including aneurysms, tumors, etc. In patients with swelling but without thrombosis, iliac venous compression may be suspected on duplex US if there are no respiratory variations and a lack of response to Valsalva maneuver. Patients undergoing thrombolysis or PCMT with identified compression have >70% risk of DVT recurrence without treating the venous obstruction/compression with an appropriate stent.

IVUS is critical for the diagnosis of venous stenosis. Formal venography has been shown to be inadequate to identify stenosis and compressive lesions (Fig. 36.1).

There are several available IVUS catheters, requiring differing sized sheaths. The IVUS Volcano Visions PV 0.018 (Philips, Andover, MA) on a 135-cm shaft utilizes a 6-French sheath and a 0.018″ wire and is adequate for visualizing the iliac vein, $\leq$24 mm maximal diameter. Other Volcano IVUS include the 0.035″ version, requiring an 8.5-French guiding sheath (imaging $\leq$60 mm diameter) and the 0.014″

system (imaging ≤20 mm diameter). Boston Scientific produces the Opticross 18 (0.018 system), which uses a 6-French sheath. The IVUS catheter is placed over the wire and the vein is assessed as the catheter is advanced from the femoral vein to the IVC. Measurements are taken prior to the area of stenosis, at the area of maximal stenosis, and distal to the stenosis. When the lesion is identified, it is important to mark both the proximal and distal ends with the IVUS catheter to ensure treatment of the entire lesion. It is also important to use the area measurement, not the diameter. Diameter measurements can be inaccurate depending on whether the vein is circular or oval in the area measured. The relative reduction in area is calculated to determine the significance of the stenosis. Frequently, the stenosis is so severe that the vein wall abuts the IVUS catheter in the area of maximal stenosis. The stent should be measured to the size of the vein just distal to the lesion, in an area that is circular, avoiding areas of poststenotic dilatation. Undersizing should be avoided, with risks of stent embolization, residual stenosis, and recurrent DVT (Fig. 36.2). Although the presence of the stenosis is based on area measurement by IVUS, sizing of the stent is based on the diameter of the vein in a normal region with IVUS, with 10%–20% oversizing.

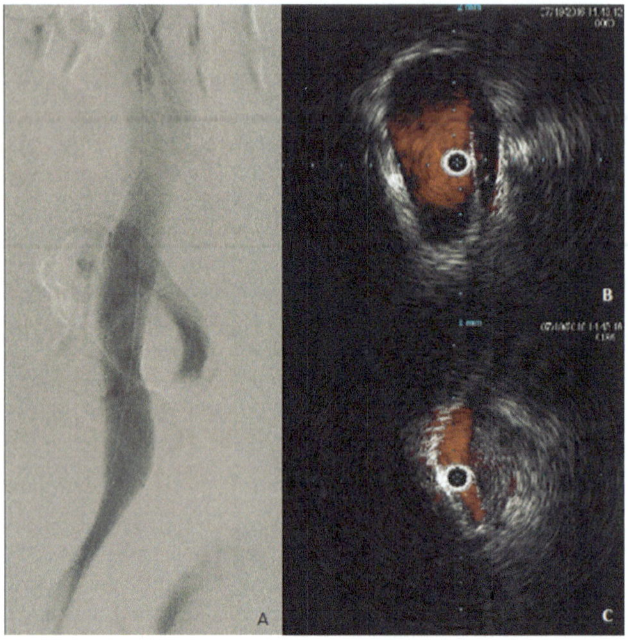

Fig. 36.1 Right iliac vein stenosis secondary to right common iliac artery aneurysm. (A) Stenosis noted on venogram. (B) Intravascular ultrasound (IVUS) within the inferior vena cava. (C) IVUS showing significantly more stenotic lesion than identified on initial venogram.

Once the decision has been made to place a stent, a 10-French sheath is placed (11 French for veins requiring ≥18-mm stent). Predilation is then performed with an 8–12 mm compliant balloon to facilitate tracking of the stent. Following predilation, the WALLSTENT (Boston Scientific, Marlborough, MA), a closed cell flexible stent, is placed, usually with diameter sizes in the range of 10–22 mm. Postdilation of the stent is then performed with appropriately sized balloons. It is important to identify the junction of the iliac veins with the IVC to avoid placing the stent too far into the IVC, putting the contralateral side at risk of thrombosis, but also to avoid falling short of the lesion, necessitating placement of a second stent. Completion IVUS is critical to ensure that the lesion is completely treated and venography is required to demonstrate restoration of normal flow through the treated region. This may require stent placement into the common femoral vein across the inguinal crease (with minimal effect on the long-term patency rates). Stents often require placement into the IVC when the lesion extends to the iliocaval confluence. Stents should be placed, ~5–10 mm, when the lesion extends to the iliocaval confluence. With tight lesions, stents are at risk of elongation (Fig. 36.3).

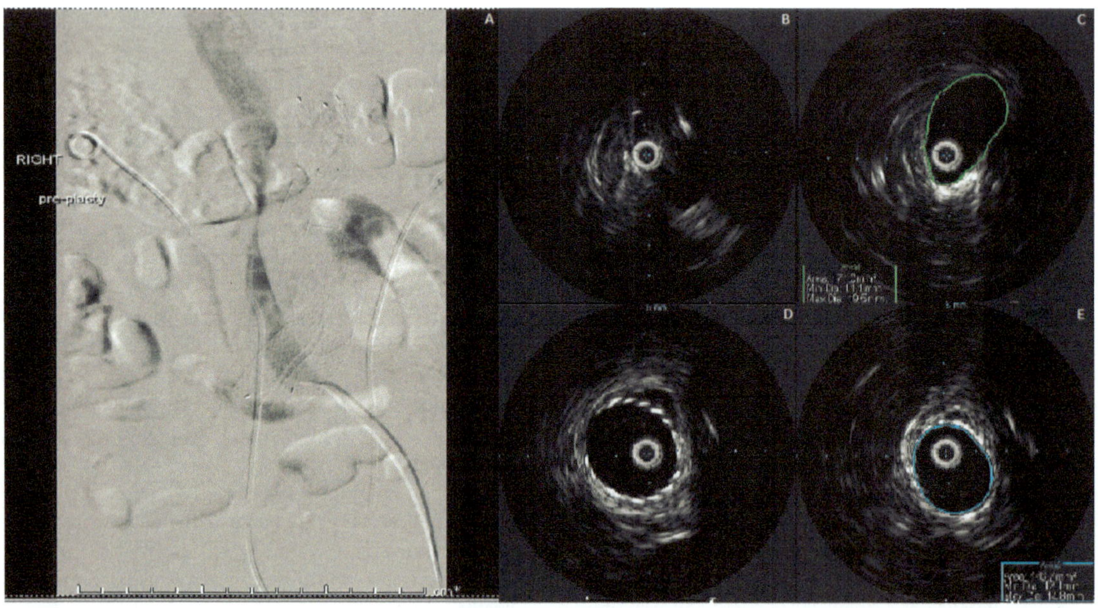

Fig. 36.2 Inferior vena cava (IVC) stenosis secondary to extrinsic compression from retroperitoneal fibrosis leading to iliofemoral deep vein thrombosis. (A) Venogram showing area of interest within the IVC. (B) Tight stenosis of the IVC. (C) Area measurement of the distal IVC to determine stent sizing. (D) Placement of 24 × 70 WALLSTENT. (E) Area measurement following stent placement and postdilation to 20 mm with good wall apposition.

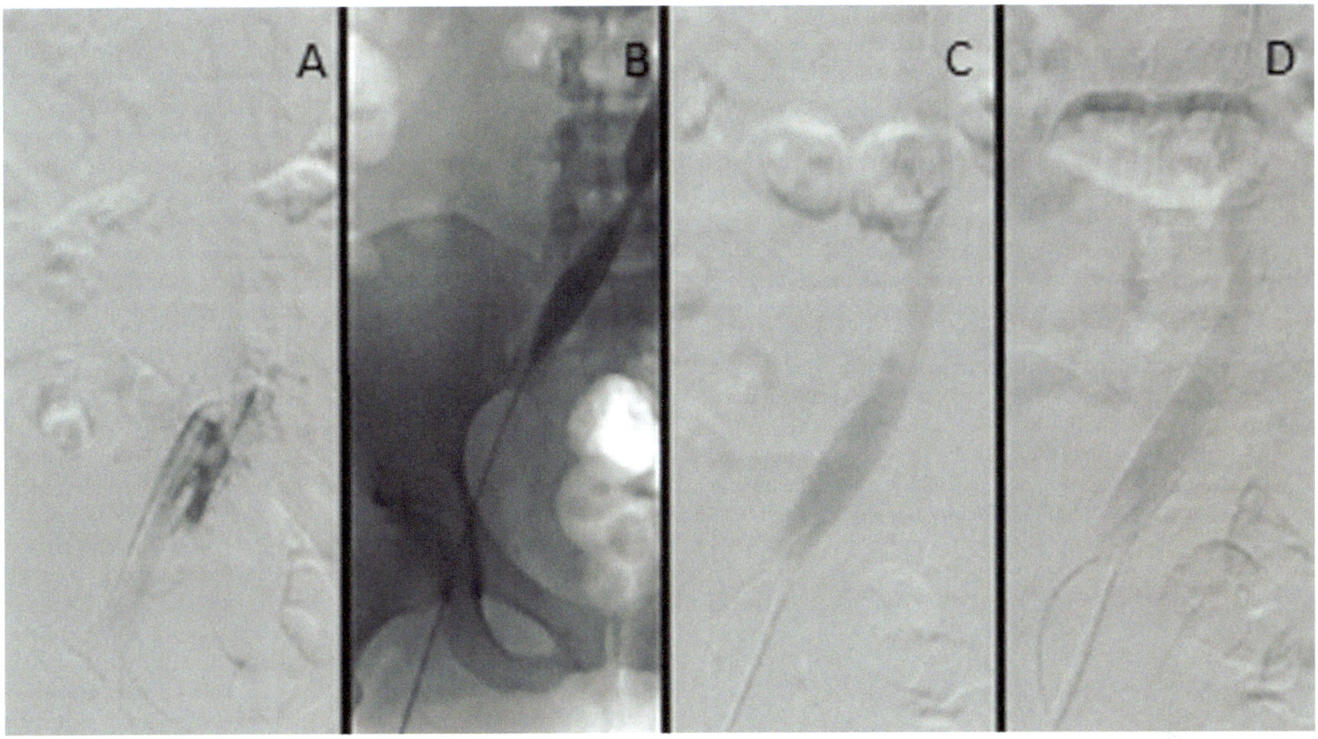

Fig. 36.3 May Thurner Syndrome. (A) Occluded left common iliac vein. (B) Venoplasty of iliac vein. (C) Improved flow following venoplasty. (D) WALLSTENT placement with slight extension into the inferior vena cava without residual stenosis.

In the United States, there are no venous stents currently on the market. WALLSTENTs have been adapted for use in dialysis access and peripheral venous interventions because of their size. Difficulties with this stent include placement accuracy and migration with tight lesions. Gianturco Z-Stent (Cook Medical, Bloomington, IN), a tracheobronchial open-cell stent, has been used proximally to help with accuracy because of increased radial force and the potential decreased risk of contralateral iliac occlusion. This stent requires a 14-French or 16-French sheath and ranges in diameter from 15 to 35 mm, with 5-cm stent length. These stents are typically only used for the most central portion, going in to the IVC. Several stents are currently being studied, both in Europe and the United States, to treat venous disease better. After intervention, patients should be treated with anticoagulation for at least 6 months to improve valve function and limit postthrombotic syndrome. Compression knee high stockings 30–40 mmHg should also be offered for patients with limb edema and symptoms and to reduce the possibility of postthrombotic syndrome.

COMPLICATIONS FOLLOWING STENT PLACEMENT

Back pain: One of the most common complications following stent placement is back pain. It is important to inform patients of this preoperatively. During angioplasty/stent placement, pain can be severe. Back pain can take 3–6 months to resolve, but typically improves within 2–3 weeks. Pain does not mean rupture of the vessel. If pain continues to worsen or is associated with limb edema, stent-associated pathology should be ruled out using duplex US or CT venogram if unable to visualize with duplex US or if pain persists despite "normal" duplex US.

Maldeployed stents: Migration and maldeployment can occur. Use of IVUS reduces the risk of stent maldeployment, both into collaterals and too far into IVC or inadequate lesion coverage. Stents that are deployed more peripherally and therefore cannot fully expand might be able to be left alone or can become "endotrash" by deploying a new stent to cage it in place, but this increases the likelihood of the segment reoccluding. Caging can also be useful for more central stent maldeployment. It is rarely necessary to remove a maldeployed stent. If a stent embolizes to the heart or lungs, retrieval with a snare, sheath, or laparoscopic forceps should be attempted immediately. Retrieval of embolized stents is usually successful and cardiac surgical intervention is rarely necessary.

Rupture/hemorrhage: Because of reduced venous pressure, venous perforation is usually not life-threatening. Thrombolysis is avoided after major perforation. Symptomatic hematomas are more frequent with prolonged thrombolysis and/or multiple large sheath exchanges.

Thrombosis: Acute venous thrombosis can occur. Wire control should have been maintained until confirmation of patency with both venography and IVUS. Treatment of the rethrombosed area with PCMT and additional stenting to treat the lesion fully are recommended. Delayed thrombosis of the contralateral side may occur if stents are placed far into the IVC, although it is rare, occurring 1%–2.4% of the time.[9,10]

CHRONIC ILIOFEMORAL VENOUS OCCLUSIONS

Some DVTs are not identified or not referred during the acute phase. Unfortunately, chronic occlusions are significantly harder to treat. In some instances, chronic venous occlusion is related to in-dwelling inferior vena cava filters. When patients present with suspected chronic venous occlusions, it is important to consider anatomic variants such as caval atresia (Fig. 36.4), left-sided IVC, and duplicated IVC, because these can complicate management.

Crossing the lesion: After gaining access as previously described, a 6-French sheath can be placed and upsized as needed. A stiff hydrophilic wire and catheter are then used to try and cross the lesions, which is difficult because of the plethora of collaterals, which the wire preferentially favors over the hard occlusion. It is important to visualize the wire tracking to avoid "crossing" the lesion only to find that the wire is in a large collateral. The wire could also potentially enter a paravertebral vein, which can cause hematoma with spinal cord compromise and neurologic symptoms if not identified. If the initial attempts at crossing the lesion are unsuccessful, different wires should be utilized (such as straight and/or soft hydrophilic wires), along with directional catheters. If this is also unsuccessful, the back end of a wire, or a heavy tipped wire, can be used in an attempt to puncture through the occlusion. Placing the directional catheter just at the occlusion enhances pushability and decreases the risk of wire perforation. If this is still unsuccessful, standard angioplasty balloon, sized to the vein, can be used to center the wire, placing the inflated balloon just below the lesion, and then attempting to cross with the aforementioned wires, preferentially directing it to the midlumen of the iliac vein. Venography is not helpful and knowledge of normal anatomy is required to follow the progress. The guidewire may pass subintimally or within vaso vasorum before reentering the intraluminal plane in the IVC, which is usually well tolerated. Retrograde crossing via the internal jugular vein can also help because of added support in difficult to cross lesions. IVUS and venography are performed to confirm intraluminal position after crossing the lesion. When standard techniques do not cross the chronic obstructive venous lesion, alternative methods should be considered.

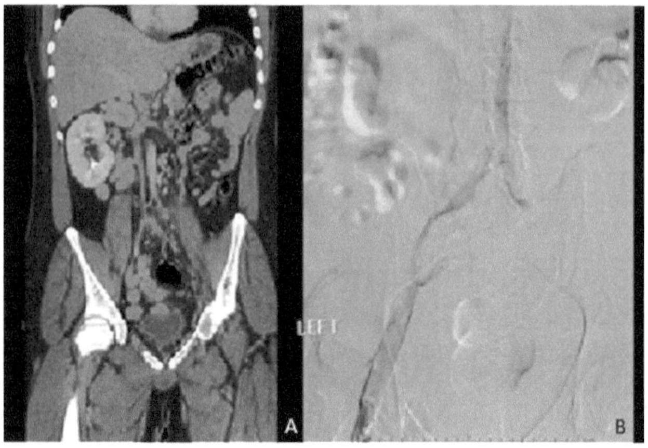

Fig. 36.4 (A) Computed tomography venogram showing inferior vena cava (IVC) atresia in a young boy with a chronically swollen left leg. (B) Venogram showing chronic atresia of the IVC and iliac veins following failed lysis attempt.

Sharp recanalization with needle or reentry devices can be attempted. These techniques are off-label. Transseptal needle set or Rosch-Uchida transjugular liver access set (Cook Medical, Bloomington, IN) allow the needle puncture into the cap of the occlusion to gain access. Standard arterial reentry devices, i.e., Outback catheter (Cordis, Santa Clara, CA), can also be used in the venous system to repuncture the occluded vein. Using the "L" on the catheter to determine the correct orientation, the needle is used to puncture the center of the vein lumen and a 0.014″ wire is advanced. Hydrophilic straight catheters can be placed over this wire Seeker (Bard Medical, Covington, GA), Quick-Cross (Philips, Andover, MA), Renegade (Boston Scientific, Marlborough, MA), and the wire then exchanged for a sturdier wire.

Another technique for difficult to cross chronic occlusions, extrapolated from dialysis access, is use of the radiofrequency wire (RF PowerWire, Baylis Medical, Mississauga, Ontario, Canada). This usually requires two access points: one side with the straight tipped radiofrequency wire and guiding catheter and the other to mark the IVC location. Short (<2 second) radiofrequency bursts should be used repetitively, with venograms if there is concern that wire is no longer within the appropriate vein. The angled catheter helps to guide away from collaterals. Once the occlusion is crossed, the wire is snared and pulled out of the alternative access to provide more sturdy traction for the catheter and to facilitate exchange to a stiffer wire, allowing balloon and stent passage. This technique can be helpful but is more successful with shorter lesions.[11] More data are needed on its use in the iliofemoral veins.

Treatment: Once the lesion is crossed, serial dilations may be required to pass the IVUS catheter, larger balloons, and the stent. Snaring the wire and providing a more rigid rail for balloons and stents are advantageous for difficult to cross lesions. High-pressure balloons should be used for venous lesions (Conquest, Atlas, or Dorado, Bard Medical, Covington, GA). Cutting balloons can also be used for tight, fibrotic lesions that do not respond to the high-pressure balloons. Stents should be oversized 2–4 mm because of recoil from the fibrotic

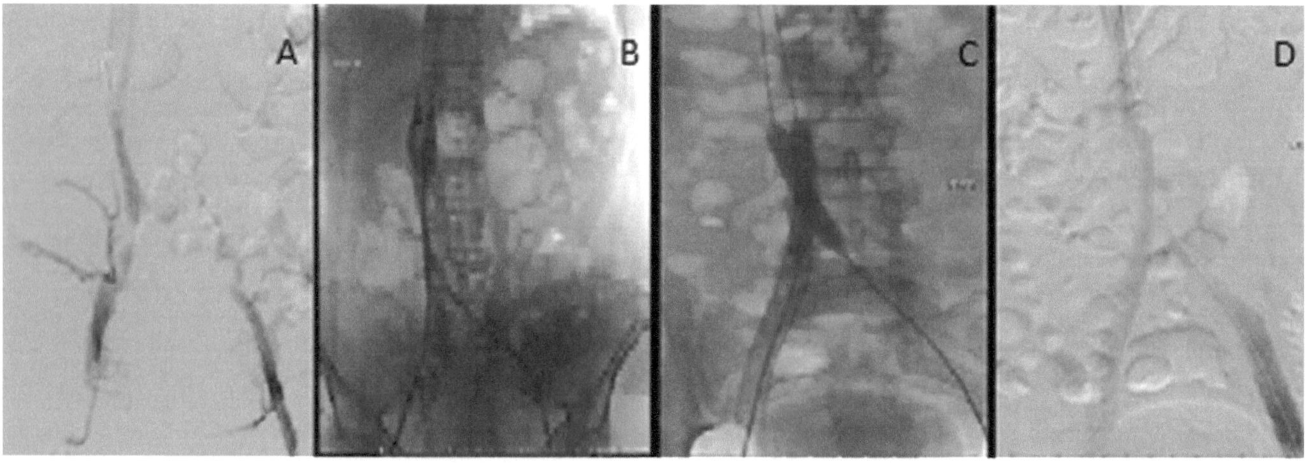

Fig. 36.5 (A) Chronic bilateral iliocaval occlusions with significant collateralization due to old maldeployed inferior vena cava (IVC) filter. (B) Serial kissing venoplasty. (C) Kissing (double barrel) stent placement at the iliocaval confluence. (D) Patent iliac veins and IVC with brisk flow and reduction of collaterals following stenting.

lesion. The goal is to achieve caliber approximating normal anatomy because residual stenosis often leads to continued symptoms and high risk of recurrent thrombosis.

Chronic iliac lesions do not require a kissing stent technique, as these lesions do not cause contralateral compression once stented. However, caution should be used as to the extent of stent placed into the IVC. When the chronic obstruction is due to a lesion that extends to the IVC, it is necessary to stent both iliac veins using "kissing stent" technique, similar to the aortoiliac system via bilateral femoral access. This can also be useful in patients with bilateral symptoms and has been shown to be the most useful technique with bilateral disease with secondary patency rates of 100%.[12] Bilateral iliocaval venoplasty is performed and then stents (16–22 mm) are placed simultaneously in double barrel fashion. The stents should fill the lumen of the IVC to prevent migration. Sizing should again be based on IVUS measurements of the normal iliac vein size. Poststenting dilation at the confluence completes the procedure with a patent bilateral outflow tract (Fig. 36.5).

CENTRAL VENOUS OCCLUSIONS ASSOCIATED WITH INTRALUMINAL DEVICES

Filter: When the occlusion is associated with an IVC filter, the filter should be retrieved (if possible) once thrombolysis has been achieved, or the IVC filter crushed and displaced by balloon dilatation and placing a large WALLSTENT, ensuring adequate outflow. If crushing the filter, it is imperative to ensure adequate flow from both iliac systems, often necessitating a kissing stent technique. If there is thrombus above the level of the filter, consideration should be given to placing a temporary filter above the in-dwelling filter during PCMT and removing both after completion.

Contralateral stent: In patients who have symptoms related to prior contralateral stenting or if the IVC is extensively involved, the only endovascular option is the inverted Y fenestration technique. The postthrombotic IVC is fibrotic and will not easily tolerate double stent placement. Although "jailing" the contralateral side is frequently well tolerated, some patients develop rapid progression of disease. One recent case report noted a pseudointima formation, which led to obstruction of the contralateral iliac vein causing unrelenting back pain and was resolved with surgical removal.[13] Once stenting across a contralateral vein and chronic obstruction of the vein has occurred, options are limited to open repair or the inverted Y fenestration.

The technique of inverted Y fenestration is achieved by placing a wire through the struts of the in-dwelling contralateral stent, with the support of a long sheath abutted to the stent. Similar techniques to crossing standard chronic occlusions can be used. Once wire access has been obtained and intraluminal location in the IVC confirmed with IVUS, it is serially dilated to 14–16 mm, beginning with low-profile balloons. Stenting is performed using the same size as the original stent, crossing into the IVC. This restores the outflow tract of the previously occluded segment and therefore should relieve the patient's symptoms.

REFERENCES

1. Meissner MH, Gloviczki P, Comerota AJ, et al. Early thrombus removal strategies for acute deep venous thrombosis: clinical practice guidelines of the Society for Vascular Surgery and the American Venous Forum. *J Vasc Surg.* 2012;55(5):1449–1462.
2. Enden T, Haig Y, Kløw NE, et al. Long-term outcome after additional catheter-directed thrombolysis versus standard treatment for acute iliofemoral deep vein thrombosis (the CaVenT study): a randomised controlled trial. *Lancet.* 2012;379(9810):31–38.
3. Lin PH, Zhou W, Dardik A, et al. Catheter-direct thrombolysis versus pharmacomechanical thrombectomy for treatment of symptomatic lower extremity deep venous thrombosis. *Am J Surg.* 2006;192(6):782–788.
4. Garcia MJ, Lookstein R, Malhotra R, et al. Endovascular management of deep vein thrombosis with rheolytic thrombectomy: final report of the prospective multicenter PEARL (Peripheral Use of AngioJet Rheolytic Thrombectomy with a Variety of Catheter Lengths) Registry. *J Vasc Interv Radiol.* 2015;26(6):777–786.
5. Vedantham S, Goldhaber SZ, Julian JA, et al. Pharmacomechanical catheter-directed thrombolysis for deep-vein thrombosis. *N Engl J Med.* 2017; 377(23):2240–2252.
6. Vedantham S, Thorpe PE, Cardella JF, et al. Quality improvement guidelines for the treatment of lower extremity deep vein thrombosis with use of endovascular thrombus removal. *J Vasc Interv Radiol.* 2009;20(7 Suppl): S227–S239.
7. Park KM, Moon IS, Kim JI, et al. Mechanical thrombectomy with Trerotola compared with catheter-directed thrombolysis for treatment of acute iliofemoral deep vein thrombosis. *Ann Vasc Surg.* 2014;28(8): 1853–1861.
8. Sharifi M, Bay C, Skrocki L, Lawson D, Mazdeh S. Role of IVC filters in endovenous therapy for deep venous thrombosis: the FILTER-PEVI (filter implantation to lower thromboembolic risk in percutaneous endovenous intervention) trial. *Cardiovasc Intervent Radiol.* 2012;35(6):1408–1413.
9. Neglén P, Hollis KC, Olivier J, Raju S. Stenting of the venous outflow in chronic venous disease: long-term stent-related outcome, clinical, and hemodynamic result. *J Vasc Surg.* 2007;46(5):979–990.
10. Caliste XA, Clark AL, Doyle AJ, Cullen JP, Gillespie DL. The incidence of contralateral iliac venous thrombosis after stenting across the iliocaval confluence in patients with acute or chronic venous outflow obstruction. *J Vasc Surg Venous Lymphat Disord.* 2014;2(3):253–259.
11. Sivananthan G, MacArthur DH, Daly KP, Allen DW, Hakham S, Halin NJ. Safety and efficacy of radiofrequency wire recanalization of chronic central venous occlusions. *J Vasc Access.* 2015;16(4):309–314.
12. Neglén P, Darcey R, Olivier J, Raju S. Bilateral stenting at the iliocaval confluence. *J Vasc Surg.* 2010;51(6):1457–1466.
13. Rathore A, Gloviczki P, Bjarnason H. Open surgical removal of iliac vein Wallstents with excision of pseudointima obstructing the contralateral iliac vein. *J Vasc Surg Venous Lymphat Disord.* 2016;4(4):525–529.

37

Complications of IVC Filters

Micheal T. Ayad, MD, RPVI, FACS and David L. Gillespie, MD, RVT, FACS

INTRODUCTION

Venous thromboembolic disease is estimated to occur in as many as 1 or 2 patients per 1000 in the United States, with about 60,000–100,000 deaths annually attributed to deep vein thrombosis (DVT) or pulmonary embolism (PE).[1] In hospitalized patients, pulmonary embolism is the third most common cause of death. Anticoagulation is the cornerstone for the treatment of DVT and PE. Inferior vena cava (IVC) filters are indicated in the uncommon occasion where there is anticoagulation treatment failure or a contraindication to anticoagulation (Table 37.1). The development of vena cava interruption in the 1970s was a critical advance in the treatment of these patients. Since the development of retrievable IVC filters, the use of IVC filters has grown rapidly. Despite their wide use, IVC filters are not without risks and complications.

The US Food and Drug Administration (FDA) developed the MAUDE (Manufacturer and User Facility Device Experience) database to enable a general device reporting system, which includes reporting on IVC filters' complications. MAUDE has its shortcomings, but it is mandatory for facilities and device manufacturers. The FDA requires manufacturers to have an established medical device reporting (MDR) certified by the FDA. On the other hand, the penalties for providers are weak and poorly enforced. An analysis by Andreoli et al. of the MAUDE database reported that the majority of IVC filter complications were associated with retrievable IVC filters (86.8%) compared with permanent IVC filters (13.2%).[2] In that same report, the authors point out that although all filters are FDA approved they are associated with various complications. The most common of these complications associated with these retrievable IVC filters are placement issues (45.1%), IVC penetration (29.9%), and IVC filter fracture (27.1%) (Table 37.2).

FILTER FRACTURE

This is defined as loss of structural integrity of the filter via break or separation. The incidence of this complication has greatly increased with the newer generations of IVC filters. Since the advent of nitinol to make filters deliverable through smaller delivery systems, the filter may not have been as durable. This especially occurs when subjected to numerous cardiac cycles. Newer generations of Nitinol filters have been developed through more robust metalloids. A review of the MAUDE database supports this in that 95% of all filter fractures reported have occurred in retrievable IVC filters. Of the potentially retrievable IVC filters reported, the highest rate of filter fractures has occurred in the Bard group (namely Recovery, G2, G2X, G2Express, Eclipse, and Meridian IVC filters) (27%).[2]

In August 2010, the FDA published a warning concerning 146 cases of filter migration and 56 filter fractures. These events occurred among a variety of filter designs, including the Bard G2. The FDA communication expressed concern that these mechanical failures may be associated with the long-term placement of retrievable filters. The FDA concluded the communication with a recommendation that

> *"implanting physicians and clinicians responsible for the ongoing care of patients with retrievable IVC filters consider removing the filter as soon as protection from PE is no longer needed."*[3]

In 2013, Morales et al. published a decision analysis to weigh the risks and benefits of retrievable IVC filter use as a function of the filter's time in situ.[4] In this study they reviewed the medical literature on patients with IVC filters and a transient risk of PE. They assigned weights reflecting relative severity to each adverse event, then defined risk scores as weight × occurrence rate, and then combined the frequency and severity for each type of adverse event. In this analysis the authors found that the net risk score reached its minimum between day 29 and 54 postimplantation. This is consistent with an increasing net risk associated with continued use of retrievable IVC filters in patients with transient, reversible risk of PE. They concluded that for patients with retrievable IVC filters in whom the transient risk of PE has passed, quantitative decision analysis suggests the benefit/risk profile begins to favor filter removal between 29 and 54 days after implantation. The FDA continues to monitor the safety of these implantable devices. Most recently the FDA sent a warning letter to manufacturers regarding deficiencies in manufacturing quality control.

In their report on long-term complications of IVC filters, Wang et al. looked at IVC filters in place for at least 4 years. They found the rate of fracture was 14%, with perforation rates higher in retrievable filters (70%) compared with permanent filters (15%).[5]

IVC FILTER MIGRATION AND/OR EMBOLIZATION

IVC filter migration is defined as movement of the filter position from its deployment site by >2 cm in either caudal or cephalad direction. IVC filter embolization refers to the movement of the filter or any of its parts to a distant anatomic location. The presence of a mega cava with IVC diameter over 28 mm is a well-known cause of migration and embolization of IVC filters. The instructions for use (IFU) for each filter specify the maximum diameter of the IVC that is suitable for the filter's use to reduce the risk of this complication. It is important for clinicians to pay attention to IVC diameter to decrease the risk of embolization or migration of the filters.

The use of Nitinol has allowed the creation of more compact IVC filters deliverable through smaller French delivery systems. There is also reduction in the amount of positive fixation in the design of retrievable filters. These factors allow option of retrieval because they are more easily compressed into a retrieval catheter and removed. An undesirable consequence of this, however, is that these filters have less radial force and less in-growth to the vena cava wall, thereby leading to their tendency to migrate or even embolize to remote locations.

From 2005 to 2010, the FDA received a total of 328 reports regarding device migration, 146 for embolization of broken device parts, and 70 for cases of IVC perforation.[3] Reports to the FDA concerning IVC filter migration using the MAUDE database involve problems with retrievable filters over three times more often than with permanent ones. In comparison with other retrievable filters, migration seems to have been reported more often with the Cordis Optease filter than others[2] (Table 37.3).

Laborada et al.[6] and Chalhoub et al.[7] reported on the dynamic nature of the IVC and how it can be a risk for IVC filter migration. Changes in the anatomy and hemodynamics of the IVC during ventilation and Valsalva maneuvers, as well as prone positioning and CPR, have all been reported as factors contributing to filter migration.

Management

Migration of IVC filter is usually best managed with retrieval and possible replacement with a new filter, or simple removal if it is no longer necessary. Fracture of the IVC filter, with embolization of the IVC filter or any of its components, can potentially be more troublesome. Struts can lodge in the heart, leading to arrhythmia and, potentially, a life-threatening cardiac perforation and tamponade.

In the event of intracardiac or intrapulmonary embolization, endovascular retrieval has been rarely attempted, and open surgical therapy has been the main stay of treatment. If endovascular retrieval is attempted, it must be done in conjunction with the cardiac surgery team because they will need to provide critical back-up if open retrieval is needed or the patient suddenly decompensates and becomes hemodynamically unstable secondary to the embolized filter components. Partnering with cardiology colleagues, who have more experience navigating the cardiac structures, is also advisable to retrieve intracardiac struts.

TABLE 37.1 Indications for inferior vena cava (IVC) filter placement.

Absolute
– Contraindication to anticoagulation
– Failure of anticoagulation (deep vein thrombosis [DVT] or pulmonary embolism [PE] while on therapeutic levels of anticoagulation)
Relative
– Free floating thrombus in the IVC or iliofemoral veins
– PE and limited cardiac reserve
– Poor compliance with anticoagulation
– As part of thrombolytic procedures for iliofemoral DVTs
– Prophylaxis in patients with severe trauma, spinal cord injury, or paraplegia

IVC THROMBOTIC OCCLUSION

All filters have been implicated in IVC thrombosis. The highest rate of IVC thrombosis has been associated with the TrapEase and OptEase IVC filters.

IVC filter thrombosis has been reported to occur with higher incidence in retrievable IVC filters compared with permanent ones.[2]

Despite reports suggesting lower risk of complications with permanent versus retrievable filters, it is the opinion of the authors that a recommendation for placement of permanent filters in all patients is not the solution, rather utilizing the retrievable IVC filter with the intent of what they are designed to be, a temporary filter. It is imperative that the vascular interventionalist make every possible effort to retrieve the IVC filter once its indication is no longer required. In cases where retrieval is not an option, a consideration for permanent IVC filter placement should be assessed and discussed by the clinician with the patient.

Management

Management of thrombotic occlusion is highly dependent on acuity of the presentation and would be very similar to managing iliofemoral DVTs, which is discussed elsewhere in greater detail.

Acute thrombotic occlusion would be managed with pharmacomechanical thrombolysis and thrombectomy. Decision to stent or not would be dependent on the clearance of the DVTs. If the thrombotic

TABLE 37.2 Comparison of complications by IVC filter type

	Bard Retrievable[a]	Cook Celect	OPTEASE	Gunther Tulip	Option	ALN
All complications	1063	157	107	51	11	5
Fracture	288 (27.1%)	31 (19.7%)	9 (8.4%)	3 (5.9%)	2 (18.2%)	1 (20%)
Migration	120 (11.3%)	15 (9.6%)	26 (24.3%)	7 (13.7%)	0 (0%)	1 (20%)
Limb embolization	131 (12.3%)	16 (10.2%)	2 (1.9%)	0 (0%)|	0 (0%)	1 (20%)
Tilt	165 (15.5%)	19 (12.1%)	6 (5.6%)	3 (5.9%)	1 (9.1%)	0 (0%)
IVC penetration	161 (15.1%)	47 (29.9%)	2 (1.9%)	3 (5.9%)	1 (9.1%)	0 (0%)
VTE/PE	15 (1.4%)	3 (1.9%)	1 (0.9%)	0 (0%)	1 (18.2%)	1 (20%)
IVC thrombus	21 (1.9%)	5 (3.2%)	7 (6.5%)	0 (0%)	0 (0%)	0 (0%)
Placement issues	144 (13.5%)	15 (9.6%)	33 (30.8%)	23 (45.1%)	2 (27.3%)	1 (20%)
Other	18 (1.7%)	6 (3.8%)	21 (19.6%)	12 (23.5%)	2 (18.2%)	0 (0%)

IVC, Inferior vena cava; *PE*, pulmonary embolism; *VTE*, venous thromboembolism. Andreoli JM, Lewandowski RJ, Vogelzang RL, Ryu RK. Comparison of complication rates associated with permanent and retrievable inferior vena cava filters: a review of the MAUDE database. *Vasc Interv Radiol*. 2014;25(8):1181–1185.

[a]Recovery, G2, G2X, G2 Express, Eclipse, and Meridian.

TABLE 37.3 Comparison of complications between permanent and retrievable IVC filters

	Total	pIVCFs (% total)	rIVCFs (% total)	P value
All complications	1606	212 (13.2%)	1394 (86.8%)	<0.0001
Fracture	350	16 (4.6%)	334 (95.4%)	<0.0001
Migration	215	46 (21.4%)	169 (78.6%)	<0.0001
Limb embolization	154	4 (2.6%)	150 (97.4%)	<0.0001
Tilt	197	3 (1.5%)	194 (98.5%)	<0.0001
IVC penetration	228	14 (6.1%)	214 (93.9%)	<0.0001
VTE/PE	30	8 (26.7%)	22 (73.3%)	<0.007
IVC thrombus	41	8 (19.5%)	33 (80.5%)	<0.001
Placement issue	318	99 (31.1%)	219 (68.9%)	<0.0001
Other	73	14 (19.2%)	59 (80.8%)	<0.0001

IVC, Inferior vena cava; *PE*, pulmonary embolism; *pIVCF*, permanent inferior vena cava filter; *rIVCF*, retrievable inferior vena cava filter; *VTE*, venous thromboembolism. Andreoli JM, Lewandowski RJ, Vogelzang RL, Ryu RK. Comparison of complication rates associated with permanent and retrievable inferior vena cava filters: a review of the MAUDE database. *Vasc Interv Radiol.* 2014;25(8):1181–1185.

disease within the IVC filter is lysed, it would be safe to retrieve the filter, decide whether further intervention is needed (venoplasty ± stenting), and whether placement of a new IVC filter is absolutely indicated. Conversely, if the filter cannot be retrieved easily, but thrombolysis has been successful, consideration can be given to stenting through the filter, thereby crushing the filter. This is typically done in a double barrel technique, with kissing stents placed from both iliac veins through the filter.

If the IVC thrombosis is chronic and unresponsive to lytic therapy, this can be treated as a CTO (chronic total occlusion) and can be crossed utilizing wire and catheter techniques (0.035″ versus 0.018″ versus 0.014″ platforms), with or without adjunct utilization of body floss method. Another technique is utilizing the Cook Triforce sheath, which is a 5-French sheath tapering to a 4-French catheter that hugs a 0.035″ diameter wire and allows the system to act as a guide for an uninterrupted transition. A tungsten-loaded tip aids pushability and adds to radiopacity as it goes through venous lesions, and the hydrophilic coating on both the CXI and the Flexor sheath enhances trackability. There are various reports for off label use of various technologies to cross venous CTO, including using the TIPS (transjugular intrahepatic portosystemic shunt) kit, using a radiofrequency guidewire, using a atherectomy device or Cordis Outback catheter to cross the occlusion before treating it with angioplasty ± stenting. Assuming success in crossing the chronic thrombotic disease within the iliac veins and IVC, the question that poses itself is what can be done to maintain patency. Angioplasty is usually an option but is unlikely to result in success by itself. IVUS-guided stenting of the occluded IVC filter from patent inflow below the filter to patent outflow above the IVC filter may be required to reestablish patency. These are difficult questions that the interventionalist must consider on a case-by-case basis and evaluate what the indication of recanalizing the IVC is and if it is worth the risk. Furthermore, the long-term outcomes of crushed IVC filters is not known.

FILTER TILT

Filter tilt is usually defined as tilting of the IVC filter axis, compared with the IVC axis, by more than 15 degrees. A consequence of the filter tilting is difficulty in IVC filter retrieval. In these cases, it is not uncommon for the filter retrieval hook to become embedded in the wall of the IVC, with tissue growth over it.

Studies have shown the insertion of IVC filters via the left or right common femoral vein have a higher tendency to tilt, as opposed to filters inserted from the right jugular approach. Other studies, however, have shown filter tilting is associated with an increased need to use advanced techniques for IVC filter removal to improve retrieval success and with a higher risk of complications.

Filter tilting has been reported to occur in nearly all retrievable IVC filters. There is a notable difference between permanent and retrievable filters (Table 37.3). Reports from the MAUDE database seem to indicate that the Optease and Gunter Tulip tilts less, with no tilting reported for the ALN filter (Table 37.2).[2]

Management

Placing the filter from the jugular can decrease the risk of tilt. Creating a slight bend in the pusher rods can also facilitate correct placement of the device when placed from a femoral approach. Filter tilt is a difficult problem to address because it is commonly associated with the apex of the filter being embedded within the wall of the IVC. Contributing factors for the success of some techniques versus others are the degree of the filter tilt and the chronicity of the involvement of the filter apex with the IVC wall.

Common techniques that are reported with varying degrees of success include loop Glidewire snaring through the filter to allow the operator to torque the filter to a more upright position to allow capturing it. Using this technique, it is important to loop near the apex of the filter to decrease the risk of bending the struts. This usually requires accessing bilateral internal jugular or bilateral femoral veins, depending on the direction of the filter retrieval. However, it can also be accomplished by upsizing the sheath, enabling a buddy wire to be placed with a catheter as well as a snare. Other methods include stiff wire or balloon venoplasty displacement techniques to dislodge the filter apex from the wall while capturing the apex of the filter simultaneously. These techniques utilize large balloons, placed either within the apex of the filter from a femoral approach and with some upward force, or against the side of the wall where the filter is embedded. Other techniques utilized to allow freeing the filter apex from being embedded in the IVC wall will be discussed in the next section.

FILTER PERFORATION

Perforation of the vena cava intima and media are required for associated hooks to embed in the adventitia of the IVC wall. Movement of the IVC hooks or struts beyond this level is referred to as a penetration. Penetration can be defined as a filter strut or anchor extending over 3 mm outside the wall of the IVC. Some reports suggest that this penetration is more common than previously estimated. Nonetheless, most of these penetrations are asymptomatic. Jia et al. reported that only 1 of 10 patients with filter penetration would present with symptoms. Their retrospective analysis identified penetration to be reported in 19% of patients (1699 of 9002). In the population identified with filter penetration, only 8% were symptomatic. The most common reported symptom was pain (77%). Major complications were reported in 83 patients (5%).[8]

Literature research showed reports of IVC filter penetration leading to symptomatic secondary pancreatitis, aortic pseudoaneurysm, symptomatic duodenal perforation, ureteral injury, retroperitoneal hematoma, and chronic pain syndrome.

One of the contributing factors to IVC filter complications that is often overlooked is the dynamic nature of the IVC. Laborada et al.

demonstrated in their retrospective review that caval morphology and its hemodynamics were affected by respiratory changes and Valsalva maneuvers leading to a reduction of the IVC cross-sectional area and was associated with higher risk of filter penetration.[6]

Although complications related to the use of IVC filters are generally low, they continue to be reported at an increasing rate. Wood et al. analyzed the MAUDE database to look for an increase in complications associated with removable IVC filters over time. They reviewed 33 adverse events of IVC filters reported in the MAUDE database from January 2000 to June 2011. Outcomes of interest were incidence of IVC perforation, type of filter, clinical presentation, and management of the perforation, including retrievability rates. The annual distribution of IVC perforation was 35 cases (9%), varying from seven (2%) to 70 (18%). A three-fold increment in the number of adverse events related to IVC filters has been noted since 2004. Wall perforation as an incidental finding was the most common presentation (n = 268, 69%). Surrounding organ involvement was found in 117 cases (30%), with the aorta being the most common in 43 cases (37%), followed by small bowel in 36 (31%). Filters were retrieved in 97 patients (83%), regardless of wall perforation. Twenty-five (26%) cases required an open procedure to remove the filter. Neither major bleeding requiring further intervention nor mortality was reported. IVC penetration by filters remains stable over the studied years despite increasing numbers of adverse events reported. The majority of filters involved in a penetration were retrievable.[9]

Management

Managing filter penetration depends primarily on the degree of penetration. A filter with penetration through the wall of the IVC that involves other vital structures should be assessed more carefully to determine whether open retrieval, cava reconstruction, and repair of other involved organs are necessary. A filter penetration that involves the cava wall partially (does not penetrate through its adventitia) can be managed with endovascular techniques, but typically requires more force than one that is not embedded. There are various reports in which biopsy forceps have been used to remove scar tissue and a portion of the inner layer of the IVC wall from the struts to allow its retrieval. Others have reported using a laser for freeing up the filter struts from tissue growth within the wall of the IVC. Both techniques carry risk of penetration, which must be weighed against the benefits of retrieval. Sandwich technique using parallel wire and dual sheath to capture tilted and partially embedded filters has been described. The guidewires are passed through a guiding catheter along either side of the filter apex. Both wires are snared and exteriorized through the opposing respective sheaths. The long catheter and sheath are advanced into snug contact against the filter, after which upward or downward force can be selectively and repetitively applied to dislodge the filter free and capture it.

FILTER RETRIEVAL

Theoretically, retrievable IVC filters provide the clinician and the patient with the advantage of cava filtration in the short term, along with the ability to retrieve the filter once the indication had subsided, to avoid long-term complications. The risk versus benefit profile tips in favor of device retrieval between 29 and 54 days postplacement, once the increased risk of pulmonary embolism subsides.

Nonetheless, as stated previously, most IVC filters are not removed. The primary hurdle to retrieving these devices is lack of patient follow-up. Multiple studies have reported on improved retrieval rate of IVC filters with the use of a dedicated IVC filter program at institutions. Kalina et al. reported an improved retrieval rate from 15.5% to 31.5% with the utilization of a "filter registry."[10] Another approach, reported by Sutphin et al., in a process to improve optional IVC filter retrieval rates was based on the DEFINE, MEASURE, ANALYZE, IMPROVE, CONTROL (DMAIC) methodology of the Six Sigma process improvement paradigm.[11] The program resulted in an improving retrieval rate from 8% to 40%.

Currently, a joint study between the Society for Vascular Surgery (SVS), Society of Interventional Radiology (SIR), and FDA was developed. PRESERVE (Predicting the safety and effectiveness of inferior vena cava filters) is a physician-initiated investigational device exemption (IDE) to understand better the current use of IVC filters and the adverse events associated with their use.[12] The PRESERVE study is a multicenter, prospective, open-label, nonrandomized investigation of commercially available IVC filters from seven manufacturers, placed in subjects for the prevention of pulmonary embolism. The primary objective of this IDE clinical investigation is to evaluate the safety and effectiveness of the commercially available IVC filters (retrievable and permanent) in subjects with a clinical need for mechanical prophylaxis of PE with an IVC filter.

CONCLUSION

Overall, filters appear to reduce the risk of subsequent PE, increase the risk of DVT, and have no significant effect on overall mortality. Reiterative process improvement has led to the evolution of these devices and an increase in their safety and efficacy. Nonetheless, they are not without their risks, which extend beyond the procedural risk of filter placement. The "out of sight, out of mind" approach to IVC filter placement, which is a trend in our practices, needs to be revised and replaced with a more diligent approach of reducing IVC filter insertion in favor of anticoagulation and an increase in IVC filter retrieval attempts.

REFERENCES

1. http://www.cdc.gov/ncbddd/dvt/data.html
2. Andreoli JM, Lewandowski RJ, Vogelzang RL, Ryu RK. Comparison of complication rates associated with permanent and retrievable inferior vena cava filters: a review of the MAUDE database. *J Vasc Interv Radiol.* 2014;25(8):1181–1185.
3. Inferior vena cava (IVC) filters: initial communication: risk of adverse events with long term use. Viewed: August 9, 2010. http://www.fda.gov/Safety/MedWatch/SafetyInformation/SafetyAlertsforHumanMedicalProducts/ucm221707.htm
4. Morales JP, Li X, Irony TZ, Ibrahim NG, Moynahan M, Cavanaugh KJ Jr. Decision analysis of retrievable inferior vena cava filters in patients without pulmonary embolism. *J Vasc Surg Venous Lymphat Disord.* 2013;1(4):376–384.
5. Wang SL, Siddiqui A, Rosenthal E. Long-term complications of inferior vena cava filters. *J Vasc Surg Venous Lymphat Disord.* 2017;5(1):33–41.
6. Laborda A, Kuo WT, Ioakeim I, et al. Respiratory-induced haemodynamic changes: a contributing factor to IVC filter penetration. *Cardiovasc Intervent Radiol.* 2015;38(5):1192–1197.
7. Chalhoub V, Richa F, Hachem K, Slaba S, Yazbeck P. Contributing factors to inferior vena cava filter migration. *Cardiovasc Intervent Radiol.* 2015;38(6):1676–1677.
8. Jia Z, Wu A, Tam M, Spain J, McKinney JM, Wang W. Caval penetration by inferior vena cava filters: a systematic literature review of clinical significance and management. *Circulation.* 2015;132(10):944–952.
9. Wood EA, Malgor R, Gasparis AP, Labropoulos N. Reporting the impact of inferior vena cava perforation by filters. *Phlebology.* 29(7):471–475.

10. Kalina M, Bartley M, Cipolle M, Tinkoff G, Stevenson S, Fulda G. Improved removal rates for retrievable inferior vena cava filters with the use of a 'filter registry'. *Am Surgeon*. 2012;78(1):94–97.
11. Sutphin PD, Reis SP, McKune A, Ravanzo M, Kalva SP, Pillai AK. Improving inferior vena cava filter retrieval rates with the define, measure, analyze, improve, control methodology. *J Vasc Interv Radiol*. 2015;26(4):491–498.
12. Predicting the safety and effectiveness of inferior vena cava filters (PRESERVE) 2015. Available from: https://clinicaltrials.gov/ct2/show/NCT02381509

38

Complications of Endovenous Treatments, Including: Thermal, Nonthermal, Sclerotherapy, and Foam Ablations

Joseph D. Raffetto, MD

INTRODUCTION

Endovenous ablation has become the treatment of choice for chronic venous disease (CVD) and chronic venous insufficiency (CVI). There are many different types of modalities to treat CVI, including thermal energy commonly with endovenous laser ablation (EVLA), radiofrequency ablation (RFA; ClosureFast, Medtronic), and less commonly with steam and cryotherapy. In addition, nonthermal ablations are effective in venous ablation and include ultrasound-guided foam sclerotherapy (USGFS), mechanical occlusive chemical ablation or mechanochemical ablation (MOCA; ClariVein, Vascular Insights, ClariVein South Jordan UT), cyanoacrylate glue (CAG; Sapheon, VenaSeal, Medtronic, VenaSeal Minneapolis MN), and liquid sclerotherapy.[1] Physician compounded foam is also used in the treatment of truncal varicose veins and tributaries, as well as recurrent varicose veins. Recently, proprietary polidocanol endovenous microfoam (PEM; Varithena, BTG International Ltd., Varithena St. Paul MN) ablation has been brought to the market in the United States, following several studies evaluating safety and efficacy and a randomized controlled trial evaluating the effectiveness in the treatment of the great saphenous vein and its tributaries.[2–4] Although both thermal and nonthermal techniques cause less pain and allow earlier return to activity and work compared with surgery, there are known complications that are both unique and common and will be the subject of this chapter.[1]

THERMAL ABLATIONS: ENDOVENOUS LASER THERAPY AND RADIOFREQUENCY ABLATION

A review of the English-language literature determined that the complications attributed to EVLA are pain, bruising, superficial burns, nerve injury, arteriovenous fistulae, deep venous thrombosis, and endothermal heat-induced thrombosis (EHIT). A large review of the world literature encompassing 12 countries, including Europe, United Kingdom, South and Central America, and the United States, reported on the top six major complications, with ecchymosis and paresthesia most commonly seen (Table 38.1).[5] There is wide variation in reporting ecchymosis, because of the lack of reporting standards. Pain is usually assessed with a visual analog scale during and immediately after the procedure and at 1 to 2 week follow-up, and pain is usually higher with EVLA at lower wavelengths (810, 940, 980, and 1064 nm, target hemoglobin), while EVLA at higher wavelengths (1320 nm and 1470 nm, target water) have reported both less pain and ecchymosis.[5–7] A randomized trial of EVLA (980 nm) and RFA demonstrated significantly less pain at 3 and 10 days, with significantly lower levels of analgesic tablets required, with patients treated with RFA.[8] However, in a recent large meta-analysis comparing EVLA and RFA, pain was similar in both treatment groups following the procedure.[9] The International Endovenous Laser Working Group (IEWG), a multicenter registry utilizing 810- and 980-nm diode laser, evaluated complications after treating more than 1000 limbs. Overall complications were 3.3% and there were no cases of motor nerve damage and no pulmonary embolisms (Pes). There was one case of third-degree skin burn (0.1%), six cases of deep venous thrombosis (DVT, 0.6%) (five at the saphenofemoral junction [SFJ] and saphenopopliteal junction [SPJ] 0.5%, and one in a gastrocnemius vein), and 27 cases of sensory nerve involvement (2.7%).[10] Burns from EVLA are a rare complication. This occurs from heat generated close to the skin when trying to treat epifascial veins or veins close to the skin (Fig. 38.1A,B), with a risk of full thickness burn. Multinational registries documented skin burn rates between 0.14% and 1.32% with EVLA. Utilizing adequate tumescent anesthetic and not treating veins close to the skin is an important method of avoiding burns.[5,11] Specific recommendations to avoid skin burns would include adequate tumescence that encircles the GSV on ultrasound, almost forming a "halo", which usually requires 300–500 ml of tumescent anesthetic in the GSV segment treated. In addition, caution should be applied when attempting EVLA of epifascial veins, or using higher wavelength EVLA or nonthermal techniques. With thermal ablations, nerve injuries can most commonly occur to the great saphenous vein (GSV, especially below the knee) and to the sural nerve when treating an incompetent small saphenous vein (SSV, especially in the distal calf) (Fig. 38.2) and are directly related to proximity of the nerve and vein. Injury leads to cutaneous paresthesia, which is usually transient but may last up to 6 months before resolving. The peroneal nerve, which is a motor and sensory nerve, is located posterior to the fibula head and in close proximity to the SPJ. Injury occurs by heat transfer, and recommendations to avoid nerve injury include careful needle entry under ultrasound guidance, large volume of tumescence (150–300 ml), and avoidance or judicious use of ablation in areas at high risk of nerve injury, specifically keeping a distance of at least 2–3 cm from the SPJ to avoid injury to the tibial nerve and not using thermal ablation below the tendinous insertion of the gastrocnemius muscle, where the sural nerve is in very close proximity to the SSV. These principles also apply to treating the GSV with either EVLA or RFA.[5] A very rare complication after thermal ablation is arteriovenous fistula (AVF, about 11 reported in the literature). AVF usually occurs during administration of tumescent anesthetic and/or thermal injury, the majority are asymptomatic, and AVF can lead to GSV recanalization. Conservative treatment is usually offered, but if the patient is symptomatic with high output cardiac failure, repair will be necessary. Reducing the risk of this rare complication can be accomplished by instilling a large volume of tumescent anesthetic

TABLE 38.1 **Complications associated with endovenous laser ablation.**

Complication	Ecchymosis	Paresthesia	Phlebitis	Burns	Deep venous thrombosis	Pulmonary embolism
Cumulative frequency	75.2%	3.1%	1.9%	0.5%	0.3%	0.02%

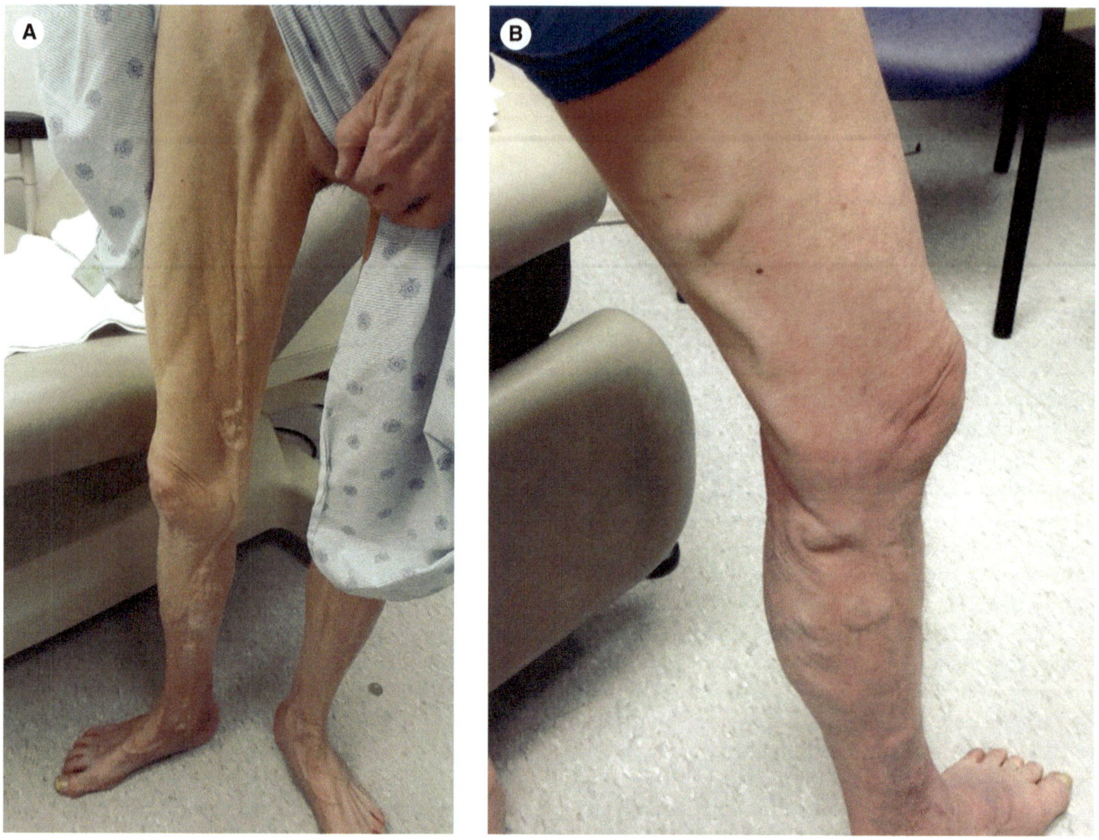

Fig. 38.1 (A) Large varicosed great saphenous vein in close proximity to the skin. (B) Epifascial great saphenous vein.

liquid (300–500 ml), proper ultrasound guidance, and injecting tumescent anesthetic /ablation 2–3 cm distal to the SFJ.[5]

EHIT is defined as propagated thrombus in the deep system. There are four stages (I: confined to the SFJ; II: extending in less than 50% of the deep venous system; III: extending in more than 50% of the deep venous system; IV: total occlusion of the deep vein). From the reported literature, venous thromboembolism (VTE) from thermal ablations ranges between 0% and 5.7%, but generally is less than 1%. Two large studies evaluated the experience of EHIT in both EVLA and RFA. In 2470 patients treated with RFA (n = 2120) or EVLA (n = 350), the incidence of EHIT II–IV was 0.28%.[12] In another large experience of 3083 patients treated with EVLA (n = 3009) or RFA (n = 74), EHIT II occurred in 1.9% of EVLA, and in 2.6% of RFA (P = 0.31).[13] Procedural attention to optimal visualization of the SFJ and increasing the distance to 2.5–3.0 cm from the SFJ to the tip of the device will reduce the event rate of EHIT. There are yet no current standards or guidelines for treating EHIT, but the consensus is that cases of EHIT II should either have follow-up evaluation and/or low molecular weight heparin (LMWH) for 2 weeks, and that cases of EHIT III–IV are treated with 3 months of anticoagulation.

RFA is also a thermal ablation and has a good safety profile. Major complications include skin pigmentation, wound problems, paresthesia, and phlebitis (Table 38.2).[14] Several large reviews have studied the rate of all EHIT following RFA. In one large series of 2470 limbs, the rate of EHIT was 0.4% and in another smaller series of 252 limbs the rate EHIT was 0%.[12,15] There are several skin complications worth mentioning since they are seen with thermal and nonthermal ablations, as well as surgery, and are derived from multimodality randomized controlled trials (RCT; Table 38.3).[16,17] The most common are thrombophlebitis, skin staining, hyperpigmentation, and skin lumpiness, of which the latter two are greatest with foam.

VENOUS THROMBOSIS PROPHYLAXIS AND LIDOCAINE TOXICITY

Two areas that are important in reducing the risk of potential complications with endovenous ablations include thromboprophylaxis and lidocaine toxicity (thermal ablations only during tumescence administration). Patients at high risk of DVT and PE are those with active malignancy, aged over 60 years, known coagulation disorders, significant medical comorbidities, female patients on estrogen-containing oral contraceptive pills or hormone replacement therapy, and previous history of phlebitis or DVT. For these selected cases, prophylactic dosing of LMWH before the endovenous treatment is recommended. There is no evidence for prolonged anticoagulation as a prophylaxis measure beyond the day of treatment. In the high-risk group, self-administration of LMWH can be suggested until the patient is fully mobile.[14] Tumescent anesthesia is very safe, but lidocaine toxicity, which is an extremely rare event during administration of tumescent anesthesia, can occur. The tumescent anesthetic solution has 0.1% lidocaine (1 mg/mL), and the usual dosing is 35 mg/kg, 70 kg person = 2450 mL of 0.1% lidocaine. Although we would not use over 2 liters of 0.1% lidocaine-containing tumescent anesthetic, it is important to note that abundant tumescent anesthetic (300–500 cc, approximately 10 cc per cm of vein treated) is encouraged to ensure that an appropriate amount of fluid has enveloped the GSV and provides analgesia, heat sink, and compressibility of the GSV. The signs and symptoms of lidocaine toxicity can be mild with light-headedness, dizziness, tinnitus, confusion, and drowsiness, to severe, including convulsions, loss of consciousness, coma, respiratory depression, and cardiac arrest. The treatment is supportive to full cardiopulmonary resuscitation and in severe situations, institution of lipid emulsion therapy.[14]

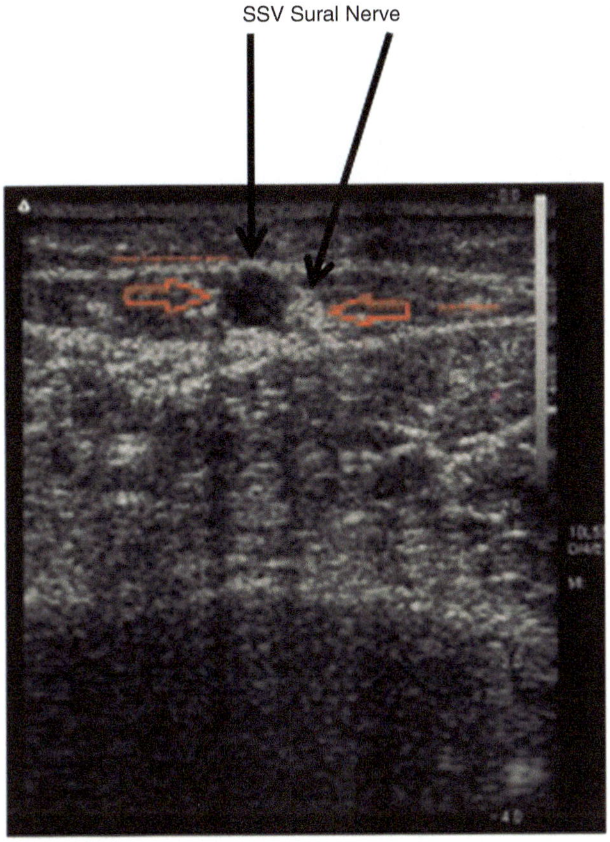

Fig. 38.2 Proximity of the small saphenous vein *(SSV)* to the sural nerve.

NONTHERMAL ABLATIONS: LIQUID AND FOAM SCLEROTHERAPY, MECHANICAL OCCLUSIVE CHEMICAL ABLATION, AND CYANOACRYLATE GLUE

The most feared complications of sclerotherapy are neurologic. A large systematic review evaluated any article with neurologic complications of sclerotherapy treating varicose veins in humans.[18] There were 41 articles reviewed (5 RCT, 18 prospective/retrospective studies, remainder case series). A total of 10,819 patients who underwent sclerotherapy with either liquid or foam sclerosants, with either sodium-tetradecyl sulfate (STS, in 5990 cases), or polidocanol (POL, in 3999 cases), were assessed for neurologic events. The majority of patients underwent physician compounded foam sclerotherapy. There were a total of 97 (0.90%) overall neurologic events, which included 12 (0.1%) cerebrovascular accidents (CVA, diagnosed based on confirmatory cerebral imaging), 9 (0.08%) transient ischemic attacks (TIA), 29 (0.27%) migraines, and the remainder consisting of speech disturbances. The neurologic events reported in the case reports consisted of CVA and TIA in 19 patients. The symptoms were documented as occurring within minutes to hours but could also be delayed by several days. In 11 of 16 CVA/TIA, the patients had a patent foramen ovale (PFO) by echocardiogram. In seven (37%) patients receiving liquid sclerotherapy, one had migraine, four had CVA, and two suffered TIA. In 12 (63%) patients receiving foam sclerotherapy, one had migraine, eight had CVA, and one suffered a TIA. The neurologic events in cohort studies and RCTs consisted of an overall 97 (0.90%) with signs and symptoms of TIA, speech, visual, and motor deficits. There were six (0.06%) TIA,

TABLE 38.2 Complications associated with radiofrequency ablation.

Complication	Phlebitis	EHIT/DVT	Skin burns	Skin pigmentations	Wound problems	Nerve injury paresthesia
Incidence	7%–9%	<0.01%	0.5%	6%–19%	6%–8%	4%–20%

DVT, Deep venous thrombosis; *EHIT*, endothermal heat-induced thrombosis.

TABLE 38.3 Skin complications associated with thermal and nonthermal ablations.

Complication/treatment modality	Thrombophlebitis	Skin staining	Hyperpigmentation	Lumpiness
EVLT	3.2%	17.4%	2.4%	13.6%
RFA	9.6%	NA	6.4%	NA
Foam	5.4%–13.7%	36.6%	6.4%	26.6%
Surgery	4.0%	10.2%	4.8%	7.2%

NA, Data not available.

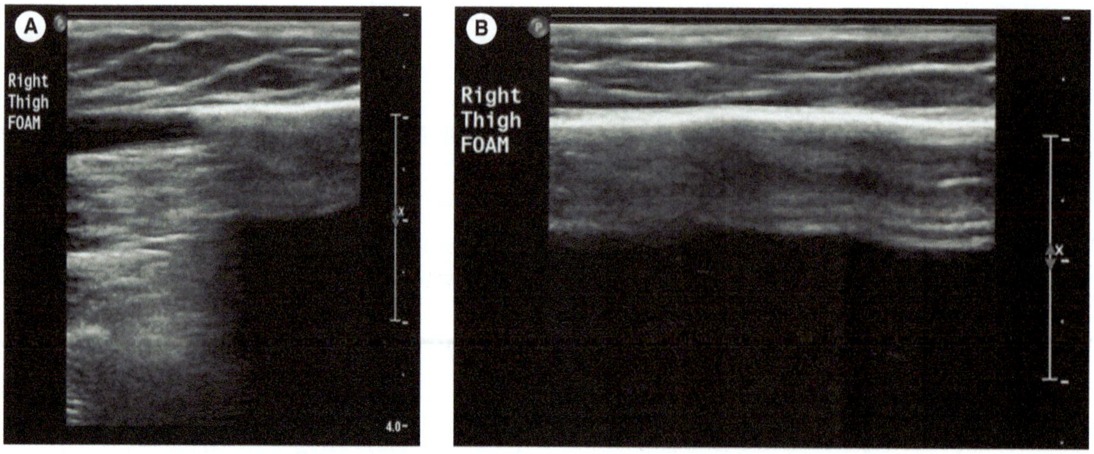

Fig. 38.3 (A) Polidocanol foam advancing in the great saphenous vein under ultrasound guidance. (B) Following polidocanol foam injection with vasospasm of the vein treated, the foam is hyperechoic.

no CVA, and only one patient had a PFO. Collectively there were 84 (0.78%) visual disturbances, 76 (0.70%) headaches, 29 (0.27%) migraine. The concentrations of sclerosant used were between 0.25% and 0.5%, and a volume of less than 20 mL was used in most instances. Air was the most common gas media in a 1:4 ratio (CO_2 in three studies and O_2 in one study, ratios 1:2 to 1:8). Importantly, there were no correlations between gas, ratio, or volume used and neurologic events.[18] There are important points to summarize with respect to liquid and foam sclerotherapy in the treatment of varicose veins. Neurologic events are rare after sclerotherapy. The majority of CVA and TIA have the presence of a PFO. Caution or avoiding sclerosants in patients with PFO is recommended. Up to 42% of patients without a PFO have foam bubbles on transcranial Doppler in the middle cerebral artery and no neurologic events, while 71.4% of patients reporting visual disturbances, migraine with aura, or chest tightness following foam treatment have a PFO. Data on replacing air with CO_2 are of low quality, but precautions and avoidance of sclerosants in either a liquid or foam in patients with a PFO and/or migraines, as well as asthma, is advised. In these patients, either thermal or nonthermal techniques should be used for treating the varicose veins (GSV, tributaries such as the AASV, SSV), and certainly microphlebectomy is an excellent alternative for the varicose vein tributaries.

Recently the FDA has approved a proprietary foam (polidocanol endovenous microfoam, PEM, Varithena) for the treatment of varicose veins (GSV, anterior accessory saphenous vein [AASV], and tributaries to the latter two veins) (Fig. 38.3A,B).[2,4] A pivotal RCT VANISH-1 study,[4] consisting of 279 patients with GSV and varicose vein insufficiency clinical class C2–C6, and five treatment groups of PEM: 0.125% (control), 0.5%, 1%, 2%, or placebo were studied. Follow-up at 8 weeks assessed quality of life, using a varicose vein symptom questionnaire (VVSymQ). PEM is a precise mixture of O_2 and CO_2 (65:35) with low N_2 of less than 0.8%. The median bubble diameter is 100 μm and no bubbles are greater than 500 μm. PEM contains 1.3 mg/mL of polidocanol and is FDA approved as 1%. The quality of life was significantly improved in the PEM groups over placebo. Of the major venous thrombosis complications there were 15 EHIT, five proximal DVT, four distal DVT, and three calf DVT, with a cumulative DVT rate of 3.3% with no PE. A total of 88% of DVT were asymptomatic and all resolved within 100 days. Minor complications included pain (21.1%), thrombophlebitis (10.5%), injection site hematoma (8.0%), headache (4.4%), transient visual impairment (0.7%), and dizziness (1.1%).[4] In the VANISH-2 study, RCT placebo controlled blind study in 232 patients with GSV or AASV varicose vein insufficiency, PEM at 0.5% or 2% was evaluated for quality of life improvement (VVSymQ). Symptoms and appearance were improved with PEM over placebo and there was a DVT rate of 5.7%, an EHIT rate of 3.9%, no PE, and no clinically important neurologic or visual adverse events were reported.[3] Skin manifestations following foam do occur, including thrombophlebitis, skin staining, lumpiness, and entry site ecchymosis/hematoma (Table 38.3; Figs. 38.4 and 38.5). Important tips are: assure entry into the vein under ultrasound (US) using a 2--05-gauge or 27-gauge needle to reduce ecchymosis, remove the coagulum within a week in the smaller varicose veins to reduce skin staining, and reduce the overall amount of foam to help in reducing events of thrombophlebitis. Thrombophlebitis is usually self-limiting and reassurance, warm compresses, and nonsteroidal anti-inflammatory medications are helpful adjuncts.

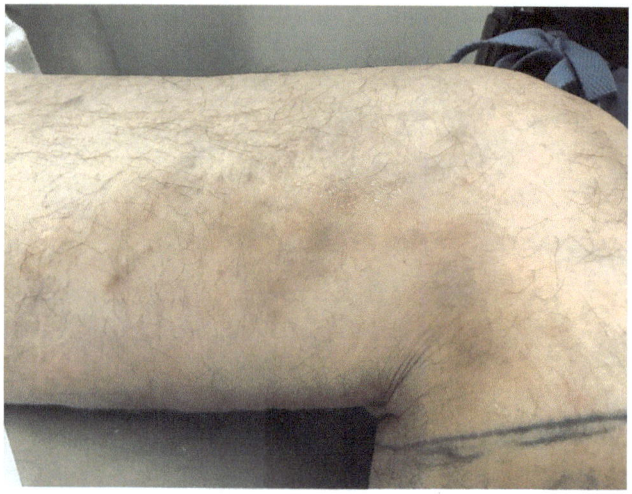

Fig. 38.4 Two weeks after polidocanol endovenous microfoam, the treated varicose veins have skin staining (brown discoloration), thrombophlebitis (red discoloration), and lumpiness.

There are newer nonthermal and nontumescent technologies for treating superficial venous insufficiency that utilize MOCA (ClariVein) or CAG (VenaSeal). MOCA is used to treat both GSV and SSV insufficiency. It involves a mechanical rotating wire at 3500 rpm, causing

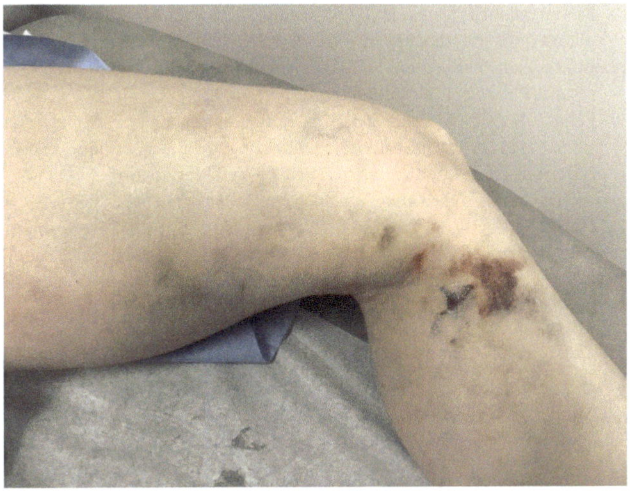

Fig. 38.5 One week following polidocanol endovenous microfoam, the treated varicose veins have skin staining (brown discoloration) and entry site ecchymosis/hematoma (red–purple discoloration).

intimal damage and a chemical sclerosant (STS or POL). Patients treated with MOCA have good 6 month to 24 month occlusion rates of greater than 90%, significantly less pain compared with thermal techniques, and no adverse events involving nerve injury or DVT.[19] In a recently published RCT, patients with symptomatic varicose veins and GSV or SSV reflux were treated with either MOCA (n = 87) or RFA (n = 83). In 74% of patients simultaneous phlebectomy was also performed. The primary outcome measurement was pain at intervention using the 100 mm visual analog scale. There was less pain with MOCA with a median of 15 mm (IQR 7–36 mm) than RFA 34 mm (IQR 16–53 mm, P = 0.003). In this study there were the following complications: phlebitis 3.4%, DVT 1.1% (which was a EHIT II), and no sensory deficits, skin necrosis, proximal DVT or PE, nerve injury, induration, hematoma, or hyperpigmentation.[20] Rotating wire entrapment was rare and caused pain and ecchymosis. It is recommended to use caution with MOCA in the presence of previous veins with thrombophlebitis, synechiae, webs, or tortuosity, to avoid the latter complication. If the wire becomes entrapped within the treated vein as a result of pre-existing luminal abnormalities, consider external massage to try to free the wire with gentle pullback. An attempt can be made to infuse saline gently on the end-port while withdrawing the wire all under US; however, if the wire does not disengage, a small cut-down over the problem area may be required to free the tip from the lumen and infusing foam sclerosant from the sheath under US guidance to complete the procedure.

CAG is also gaining popularity because of its nonthermal and nontumescent benefits. It has been utilized in over 4000 patients with CVD. A recent post-market study of 50 patients (C2–C5) demonstrated minimal pain, but 20% had phlebitis in the treatment area, which resolved in all by 1 month except in one patient. There were no DVT or PE and one EHIT I.[21] A recent RCT evaluated symptomatic varicose veins and GSV insufficiency (C2–C4b), with 108 patients treated with CAG and 114 patients treated with RFA. Pain by visual analog scale was the same (1.6 CAG versus 2.0 RFA; P = 0.13), and absence of ecchymosis was greater for CAE than RFA (68% versus 48%, P < 0.01, respectively). Phlebitis occurred in 20% of patients treated with CAG. There were no cases of DVT or EHIT in either treatment group and paresthesia in the treatment zone, access site infection, and superficial thrombophlebitis were infrequent (1%–4%) with CAG.[22,23]

CONCLUSIONS

Thermal ablations with tumescent anesthetic and the nonthermal nontumescent methods are safe and effective. Complications are usually mild and self-limiting. Ecchymosis is common after EVLA and RFA may have less postprocedure pain, but higher wavelength laser has nearly the same pain profile as RFA. Judicious use of tumescent anesthesia to avoid skin burn and nerve injury should always be used, but care should also be taken near the SFJ and a distance of at least 2–3 cm should be ensured from the junction at the femoral and popliteal regions. EHIT and DVT are very low events with thermal ablations with tumescence. Neurologic complications are rare with sclerotherapy; but practitioners should avoid sclerotherapy in patients with PFO but migraines, as well as patients with asthma. PEM has a very low incidence of neurologic events and is well tolerated with minimal pain; however, thrombophlebitis and skin staining are the most common complications, which are usually self-limiting. In addition, PEM has an acceptably low DVT/PE rate. The newer nonthermal and nontumescent methods (MOCA, CAG) are desirable, safe, and effective, with phlebitis being the most common adverse event.

REFERENCES

1. Bootun R, Lane TR, Davies AH. The advent of non-thermal, non-tumescent techniques for treatment of varicose veins. *Phlebology*. 2016;31:5–14.
2. Wright D, Gobin JP, Bradbury AW, et al., on behalf of the Varisolve European Phase III Investigators Group. VarisolveR polidocanol microfoam compared with surgery or sclerotherapy in the management of varicose veins in the presence of trunk vein incompetence: European randomized controlled trial. *Phlebology*. 2006;21:180–190.
3. Todd KL 3rd, Wright DI, VANISH-2 Investigator Group. The VANISH-2 study: a randomized, blinded, multicenter study to evaluate the efficacy and safety of polidocanol endovenous microfoam 0.5% and 1.0% compared with placebo for the treatment of saphenofemoral junction incompetence. *Phlebology*. 2014;29:608–618.
4. King JT, O'Byrne M, Vasquez M, Wright D, VANISH-1 Investigator Group. Treatment of truncal incompetence and varicose veins with a single administration of a new polidocanol endovenous microfoam preparation improves symptoms and appearance. *Eur J Vasc Endovasc Surg*. 2015;50:784–793.
5. Dexter D, Kabnick L, Berland T, et al. Complications of endovenous lasers. *Phlebology*. 2012;27(Suppl 1):40–45.
6. Spreafico G, Piccioli A, Bernardi E, et al. Endovenous laser ablation of great and small saphenous vein incompetence with a 1470-nm laser and radial fiber. *J Vasc Surg Venous Lymphat Disord*. 2014;2:403–410.
7. Lawson JA, Gauw SA, van Vlijmen CJ, et al. Prospective comparative cohort study evaluating incompetent great saphenous vein closure using radiofrequency-powered segmental ablation or 1470-nm endovenous laser ablation with radial-tip fibers (Varico 2 study). *J Vasc Surg Venous Lymphat Disord*. 2018;6:31–40.
8. Shepherd AC, Gohel MS, Brown LC, Metcalfe MJ, Hamish M, Davies AH. Randomized clinical trial of VNUS ClosureFAST radiofrequency ablation versus laser for varicose veins. *Br J Surg*. 2010;97:810–818.
9. He G, Zheng C, Yu MA, Zhang H. Comparison of ultrasound-guided endovenous laser ablation and radiofrequency for the varicose veins treatment: An updated meta-analysis. *Int J Surg*. 2017;39:267–275.
10. Spreafico G, Kabnick L, Berland TL, et al. Laser saphenous ablations in more than 1,000 limbs, with long-term duplex examination follow-up. *Ann Vasc Surg*. 2011;25:71–78.
11. Kabnick LS. Outcome of different endovenous laser wavelengths for great saphenous vein ablation. *J Vasc Surg*. 2006;43:88–93.
12. Marsh P, Price BA, Holdstock J, Harrison C, Whiteley MS. Deep vein thrombosis (DVT) after venous thermoablation techniques: rates of endovenous heat-induced thrombosis (EHIT) and classical DVT after

radiofrequency and endovenous laser ablation in a single centre. *Eur J Vasc Endovasc Surg*. 2010;40:521–527.

13. Sadek M, Kabnick LS, Rockman CB, et al. Increasing ablation distance peripheral to the saphenofemoral junction may result in a diminished rate of endothermal heat-induced thrombosis. *J Vasc Surg Venous Lymphat Disord*. 2013;1:257–262.
14. Anwar MA, Lane TR, Davies AH, Franklin IJ. Complications of radiofrequency ablation of varicose veins. *Phlebology*. 2012;27(Suppl 1): 34–39.
15. Proebstle TM, Vago B, Alm J, Göckeritz O, Lebard C, Pichot O. Treatment of the incompetent great saphenous vein by endovenous radiofrequency powered segmental thermal ablation: first clinical experience. *J Vasc Surg*. 2008;47:151–156.
16. Rasmussen LH, Bjoern L, Lawaetz M, Lawaetz B, Blemings A, Eklöf B. Randomised clinical trial comparing endovenous laser ablation with stripping of the great saphenous vein: clinical outcome and recurrence after 2 years. *Eur J Vasc Endovasc Surg*. 2010;39:630–635.
17. Brittenden J, Cotton SC, Elders A, et al. A randomized trial comparing treatments for varicose veins. *N Engl J Med*. 2014;371:1218–1227.
18. Sarvananthan T, Shepherd AC, Willenberg T, Davies AH. Neurological complications of sclerotherapy for varicose veins. *J Vasc Surg*. 2012;55:243–251.
19. Elias S, Lam YL, Wittens CH. Mechanochemical ablation: status and results. *Phlebology*. 2013;28(Suppl 1):10–14.
20. Lane T, Bootun R, Dharmarajah B, et al. A multi-centre randomised controlled trial comparing radiofrequency and mechanical occlusion chemically assisted ablation of varicose veins – final results of the Venefit versus Clarivein for varicose veins trial. *Phlebology*. 2017;32:89–98.
21. Gibson K, Ferris B. Cyanoacrylate closure of incompetent great, small, and accessory saphenous veins without the use of post-procedure compression: initial outcomes of a post-market evaluation of the VenaSeal System (the WAVES Study). *Vascular*. 2017;25:149–156.
22. Morrison N, Gibson K, McEnroe S, et al. Randomized trial comparing cyanoacrylate embolization and radiofrequency ablation for incompetent great saphenous veins (VeClose). *J Vasc Surg*. 2015;61:985–994.
23. Morrison N, Gibson K, Vasquez M, et al. VeClose trial 12-month outcomes of cyanoacrylate closure versus radiofrequency ablation for incompetent great saphenous veins. *J Vasc Surg Venous Lymphat Disord*. 2017;5:321–330.

39

Arteriovenous Access: Fistula and Graft Intervention

George H. Meier, MD

ENDOVASCULAR TREATMENT IN THE MANAGEMENT OF ARTERIOVENOUS ACCESS

Arteriovenous access surgery provides a lifeline for those patients with end-stage renal disease in need of hemodialysis. The high flow arteriovenous anastomosis results in a durable, easily accessed, reliable means of needle cannulation for high flux hemodialysis. Despite the obvious benefits of modern arteriovenous access surgery, numerous challenges make management of these accesses difficult. First and foremost, arteriovenous access is probably the most predictable situation in vascular surgery for the development of intimal hyperplasia and resultant vascular stenosis.[1] Virtually every arteriovenous access has some element of intimal hyperplasia-induced vascular stenosis.

Second, any vascular stenosis that develops because of high flow arteriovenous access can occur at any location along the course of the access. While the most predictable location for intimal hyperplasia is at the venous anastomosis of an arteriovenous graft,[2] stenoses can occur anywhere. Although it was once thought that central venous stenosis associated with arteriovenous access was mainly related to prior subclavian catheter use,[3] the current rarity of subclavian access for dialysis catheters would suggest that intimal hyperplasia in the subclavian venous out-flow may be related to anatomic flow issues unique to this location (Fig. 39.1). Although subclavian venous lines or pacemaker leads can certainly result in venous out-flow stenosis, the cause of subclavian venous out-flow stenosis is unknown in many cases and multifactorial in most (see Chapter 40). Despite this, stenosis within the central veins remains a constant issue in vascular access surgery.[4]

Endovascular treatment has revolutionized arteriovenous access management, making multiple repetitive interventions often possible.[5] While management of arteriovenous access previously necessitated repeating open operations, endovascular treatments brought a more minimally invasive option that could be done in an outpatient setting with minimal resources, often in an office-based setting. While endovascular management was initially controversial secondary to the perception of limited durability, over time it became apparent that the results of endovascular management have several advantages.[6] Nonetheless, endovascular treatment particularly with bare-metal stents may provide an impediment for subsequent treatments because of the ongoing scarring process and debris associated with placement of these devices (Fig. 39.2). The scarring process often limits further interventions as a result of the physical barrier resulting from stents or scarring within the vein.

Arteriovenous access is critical for patients requiring hemodialysis for end-stage renal disease. Continuous arteriovenous access is important in avoiding catheter use and prolonging complication-free hemodialysis. While there are both open and endovascular techniques for managing arteriovenous access, endovascular treatment has many advantages. First, any open operative revision invariably leads to loss of autogenous venous out-flow because of surgical scarring in the out-flow conduit. Every patient will need multiple accesses and revisions during the course of their dialysis lifespan, and preserving venous out-flow is therefore critical to providing adequate duration of dialysis access. Although endovascular revision of a dialysis access does not tend to be as durable as some open revisions, the fact that endovascular treatment can be repeated more than compensates for any limitation in durability. Second, open hemodialysis access revision is an operative or re-operative procedure that is inherently traumatic, painful, and requires more recovery than any endovascular treatment. Some of these open procedures may even necessitate an overnight or longer stay in the hospital. While creation of a new dialysis access often requires an open operative procedure, thrombectomy and endovascular revision are generally minimally invasive procedures that do not require overnight hospitalization and can often be performed in an outpatient setting.

CONSIDERATIONS FOR CREATION OF ACCESS

Open operative treatment is necessary to create the initial arteriovenous access. This generally involves either anastomosis of an artery to a vein or the insertion of a conduit between an artery and a vein to create a high-flow arteriovenous access that can be used repetitively for dialysis access. Once the access is established then the management necessary to maintain the access can often be provided using endovascular techniques.

What Are the Requirements for Arteriovenous Access?

In order to perform hemodialysis effectively, any arteriovenous access used will need relatively high flow. Typically, pump flows in the hemodialysis machine will be 600 to 900 mL per minute. To avoid recirculation of previously filtered blood into the hemodialysis machine, flow in the fistula or graft should generally be at least twice the pump speed. Any flow less than that will lead to recirculation and less efficient cleansing of the blood. This may result in prolonged dialysis sessions, and it is for this reason the Kt/V is (clearance) (time)/Volume is routinely measured for each dialysis session. Any trend toward decreasing dialysis efficiency would suggest a stenosis, most commonly associated with the venous out-flow.

Additionally, out-flow venous stenosis can be inferred from two aspects of the dialysis access: first, pulsatility of the access implies venous out-flow stenosis; and second, prolonged decannulation bleeding after needle removal similarly implies high venous pressures. While there are many factors that must be taken into account, in its simplest form all hemodialysis access monitoring focuses on assessment for venous out-flow stenosis.

Complications primarily related to access stenosis with or without thrombosis (Fig. 39.3) are the most common complications necessitating endovascular access treatment. Endovascular treatment is advantageous in this setting because it limits the loss of venous conduit or out-flow in the revised arteriovenous access. Although each endovascular treatment clearly increases the likelihood of restenosis, the time interval between restenosis events does not necessarily decrease.[7] If the

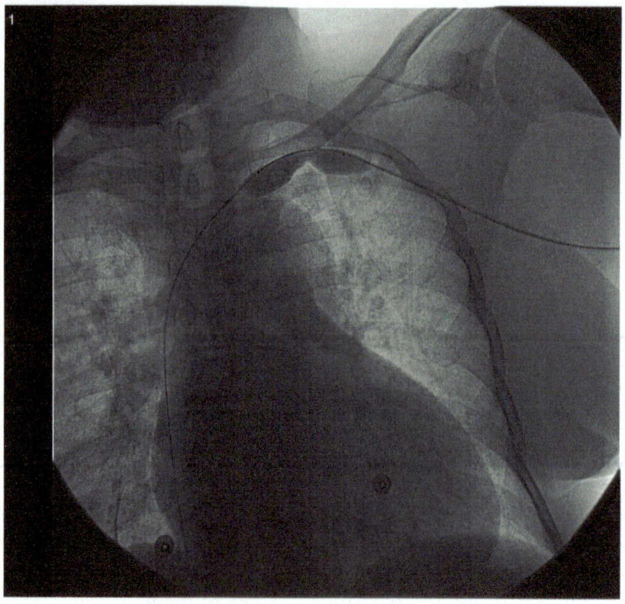

Fig. 39.1 Classic location for subclavian stenosis without prior catheter placement.

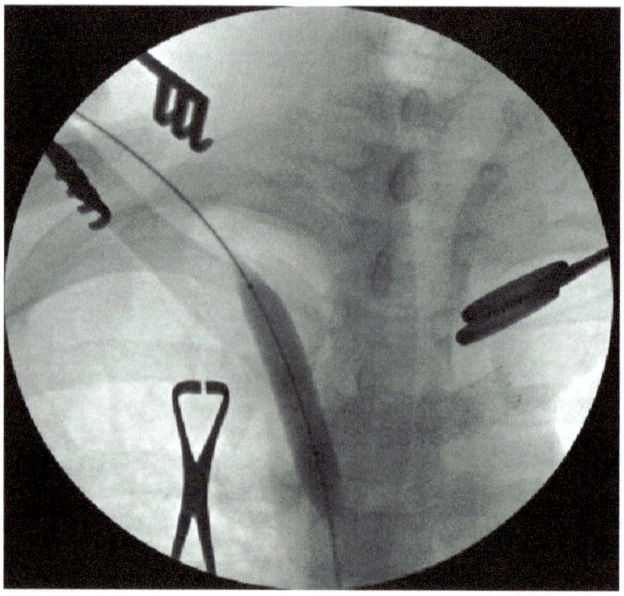

Fig. 39.2 Bare-metal stent encroaching on wire placed from opposite side.

patient suffers a restenosis after balloon angioplasty, in many cases bare-metal stenting of the venous out-flow may be appropriate. If stenosis recurs after a self-expanding bare-metal stent, covered stent or a drug-coated balloon may provide additional durability. In many cases, if not all, endovascular treatment for failure of prior endovascular treatment is the standard of care.

ENDOVASCULAR TREATMENT OF ARTERIOVENOUS ACCESS

The presence of a stenosis limiting the duration or quality of dialysis requires treatment to restore the efficiency of the dialysis session. There

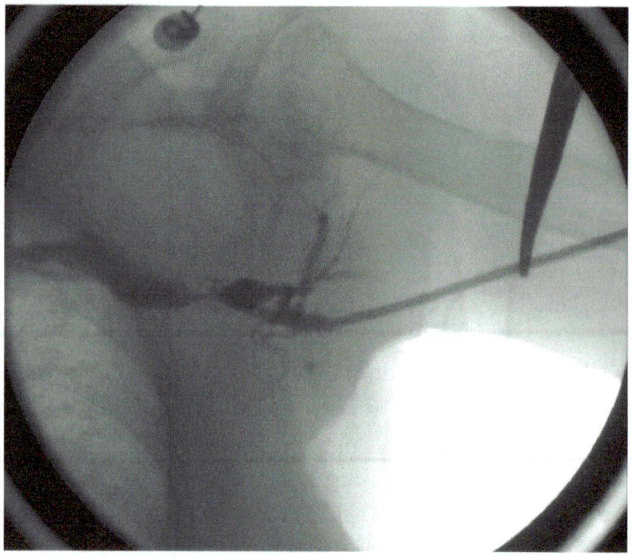

Fig. 39.3 Severe stenosis can occur without access thrombosis.

are many options for treatment of a failing or failed dialysis access to restore this efficiency. First, treatment of stenosis by balloon angioplasty can restore nearly normal flow through the conduit.[8] Second, as the stenosis recurs the scarring process may return more rapidly despite adequate venous out-flow caused by activation of the scarring process and early restenosis. In this setting, a mechanical barrier to the restenosis is sometimes needed. Bare-metal stents have been used in the setting but allow the recurrence of stenosis through the interstices of the stent.[9] After this recurrence there are two alternatives: first, mechanically altering the rate of recurrence by trying to block the in-growth of scar tissue and intimal hyperplasia; or second, by altering the scarring process using topical drug application from a drug-coated balloon. Which is chosen depends on the underlying pathophysiology in the patient's history. Longer lesions may be better treated by drug-coated balloon although this remains only a hypothesis. Mechanical recoil of a short segment may still benefit from bare-metal stent placement or, after recurrence, may necessitate a covered stent placement.

Access Stenosis versus Thrombosis

Invariably, an access becomes stenotic before it occludes (Fig. 39.4). The timing of the diagnosis of the problems with a given arteriovenous access determines whether the treatment will be management of a stenosis or an occlusion. For all practical purposes, an occlusion is simply the continuation of the process started by an arteriovenous access stenosis. As the flow becomes more restricted and the out-flow vessel more damaged, the risk of access thrombosis goes up. For this reason, treatment of an access thrombosis is often quite similar to that used for treatment of an access stenosis. In the setting of thrombosis, crossing the lesion is similar to that of a stenotic access; nonetheless, the presence of thrombus within the access requires that thrombus be removed either mechanically or pharmacologically. Both may need to be used in any given patient. Although clinically significant effects from any clot that may be embolized are rare, the clot underlying the thrombosis invariably gets released, most commonly into the pulmonary vascular bed. With a higher clot burden, thrombolysis becomes more attractive because it allows the clot to be liquefied and flow more easily out of the access.

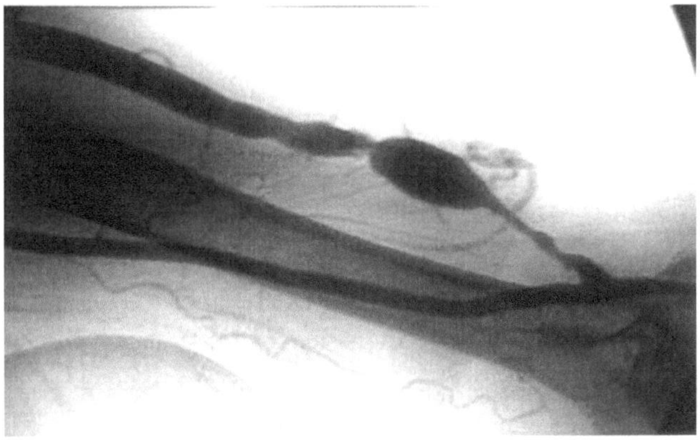

Fig. 39.4 Access stenosis generally occurs before occlusion.

Management of the Thrombosed Access Using Endovascular Techniques

Using minimally invasive techniques to reopen a thrombosed dialysis access, while feasible, is not without its complications. Generally, this technique requires injection of a thrombolytic drug such as tissue plasminogen activator (tPA), followed by treatment of the out-flow stenosis, which is commonly present. Complete arteriovenous diagnostic imaging is critical to ensuring that not only is the thrombus cleared but also that any underlying cause of the thrombosis has been adequately treated. Commonly, the lyse-and-go technique originally described by Cynamon and Pierpont[10] involves insertion of a needle or sheath and injection of 2 mg of tPA in 10 cc of volume. As this is injected, in-flow and out-flow can be occluded as needed to distribute the lytic throughout the access. Of note, manual occlusion of the venous out-flow to distribute lytic to the arterial end is usually done first to avoid inadvertently embolizing the arterial cap into the arterial out-flow as the thrombolytic drug begins to loosen the plug as it lyses, the most common major complication from this technique. With practice and experience this risk can be managed.

After or with initial lysis, heparin is often given to avoid rethrombosis while the surgeon is evaluating and treating the access. The next step is to re-establish flow within the access. In some cases, this might require passage of a Fogarty embolectomy catheter to help dislodge any arterial cap that may still be disrupting or obstructing flow; this is typically done through a minimum of a 6-French short sheath with an over-the-wire Fogarty. The Fogarty is deflated as it is brought into the sheath, frequently releasing the cap into the venous circulation. Once the access is flowing again, the focus is on preventing rethrombosis. Most commonly, a venous out-flow stenosis would be seen and treated by balloon angioplasty or stenting. In many cases an 8 mm by 80 mm Conquest balloon is inflated from the venous end back toward the proximal access to mix the lytic agent with any thrombus and to open any venous stenosis. The lytic is combined with intravenous heparin to help prevent rethrombosis. Other techniques for clot removal include pharmacomechanical thrombectomy, using devices such as the Angiojet (Boston Scientific, Marlborough, MA) or the Cleaner Rotational Thrombectomy System (Argon Medical, Frisco, TX) in conjunction with thrombolytic agents. Use of pharmacomechanical devices requires antegrade and retrograde access of the fistula or graft unless the proximal aspect is still patent.

Arteriovenous Access Stenosis versus Arteriovenous Access Occlusion

Although emotionally an occlusion seems far more advanced than a stenosis in a patent access, clinically there is often very little difference

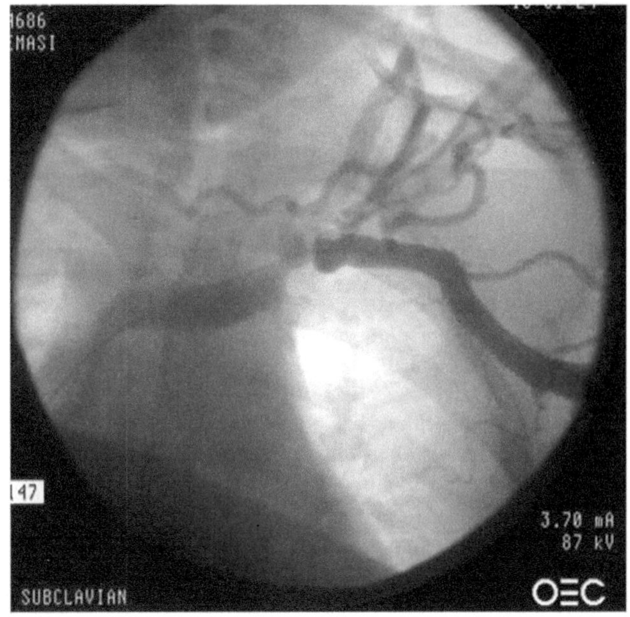

Fig. 39.5 Stenosis can lead to stagnant flow in the access and cause recirculation.

in the treatment. The presence of a stenosis will slow flow and increase venous pressures to a point where flow is virtually stopped within the access (Fig. 39.5), particularly in arteriovenous fistulas. If the conduit has a tendency toward thrombosis, then a clot will ensue. Reversal of this process requires lysis of the underlying clot followed by treatment of the underlying stenosis. Alternatively, a chronic thrombosis may require mechanical thrombectomy to move the clot out of the access. Therefore, the only difference between a clotted access and a stenotic access is the presence of thrombus within the access. If treatment is to be successful for a clotted access, lysis of the thrombus followed by intervention on the underlying cause of the clot is the key to successful treatment.

Balloon Angioplasty for Treatment of Arteriovenous Access Stenoses

In its simplest form, endovascular treatment of an access that is failing or thrombosed will require reopening any stenosis present within that access. The simplest method of reopening a stenotic access is to perform balloon angioplasty (Fig. 39.6). Although this is similar to balloon angioplasty performed in any other vascular bed, there are several features that remain unique.[11] Typically, these lesions result from intimal hyperplasia in the venous out-flow; invariably intimal hyperplasia results in a fibrous, rubbery lesion that has a high resistance to balloon angioplasty and a significant elastic recoil. Generally, treatment of these lesions requires high pressure inflations, often to more than 20 atm (Conquest, Dorado, Atlas: Bard). Balloons should start small and be gradually increased to decrease risk of rupture. The greatest worry in treating these lesions with balloons is the risk of damaging the conduit with resultant extravasation. For this reason, any lesion that requires greater than expected pressures to reach balloon profile may result in extravasation and requires completion imaging. If the area of balloon inflation is accessible for external examination, inspection of the site is usually the first option. If there is any hematoma formation, it can be noted immediately simply by examining the area of the angioplasty. If there is evidence of hematoma formation, low pressure balloon inflation is the first option to treat this. This low-pressure inflation to 2 to 4 atm is performed for 2 to 5 minutes with repeat contrast injection to evaluate the conduit again. If further treatment is needed, repeat balloon angioplasty, stenting, or covered stenting can be performed as indicated (Fig. 39.7). The key to managing this complication is to realize that extravasation might occur in the circumstances encountered. Anticipation of a complication avoids turning a minor issue into a major one.

If after the low-pressure balloon inflation there is still extravasation, generally this is going to require a covered stent (Fig. 39.8). Although the frequency of needing a covered stent is relatively low, any persistent extravasation after two low-pressure balloon inflations probably warrants covered stent placement.

Successful treatment of access lesions is identified with brisk flow throughout the access, with no hang-up of flow. A thrill should be present at completion. Measurement of pressures is not typically performed with good visual results.

STENTS FOR TREATMENT OF DIALYSIS ACCESS

Perhaps the most common complication after balloon angioplasty is elastic recoil of the lesion with persistent residual stenosis. If the stenosis remains after two treatment cycles of balloon angioplasty, a stent will probably be needed. The goal of stenting a residual stenosis is to provide persistent outward force to try to allow the stenotic vessel to remodel over time. Generally, self-expanding stents are used with post-dilatation using an appropriate sized balloon to help the stent fully expand (Fig. 39.9). Occasionally, residual stenosis within the stent persists after balloon angioplasty of the stent, and in this circumstance prolonged inflation to balloon profile may be necessary to treat the residual stenosis.[12] Balloon-expandable stents are rarely used in arteriovenous access because deformation of the stent with extremity motion or the application of force during normal extremity use may compromise the lumen created with the stent.

The bare-metal stent is generally sized to the diameter of the vessel; in a dialysis graft, this is typically 6 mm by whatever length is necessary. In a fistula, the size may need to be larger to avoid loss of contact between the stent and the wall of the proximal or distal vessel. In an arteriovenous fistula, if the stent is undersized for the vessel being treated, the risk of thrombosis will increase as a result of interference with flow by the stent itself, as well as the risk of stent embolization. Generally, oversizing the stent slightly is prudent to ensure good wall apposition.

Because the material causing the stenosis in an AV access is intimal hyperplasia, the presence of a bare-metal stent within the stenosis does little to prevent recurrent stenosis. The same hyperplastic response will be elicited by the stent, and because the interstices are widely open the stenotic hyperplastic response will simply recur within the stent. If the lesion has been treated previously with a bare-metal stent, a covered stent may be more appropriate to maintain patency and avoid early restenosis (see later). While restenosis can recur with a covered stent, there are significant advantages that limit the rapidity of recurrent stenoses and generally limit the restenosis to the areas not covered by the stent graft.

Covered Stents for Treatment of Dialysis Access

While many access-related interventions can be treated in an outpatient office-based setting, certain adjuncts must be available to use for bailout when complications occur. The most common bailout is the

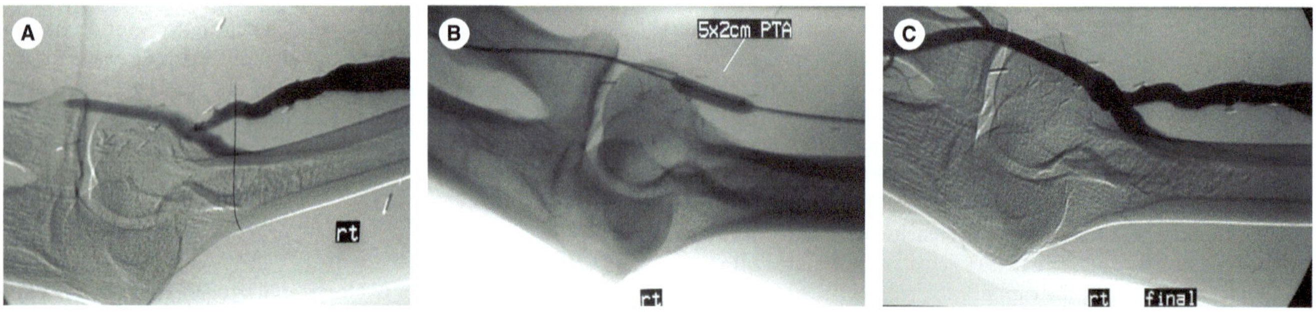

Fig. 39.6 The simplest method of reopening a stenotic access is to perform balloon angioplasty. (A) Stenosis of fistula. (B) Balloon angioplasty of fistula stenosis. (C) Postangioplasty fistula imaging.

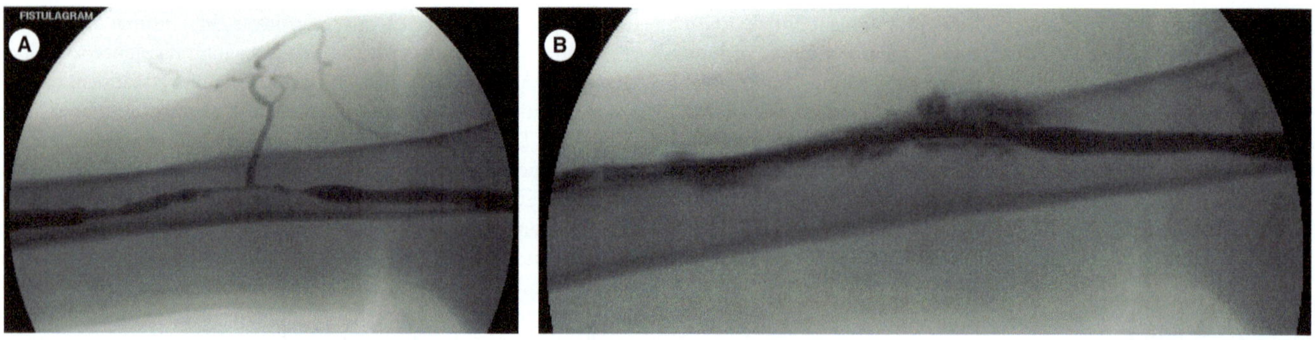

Fig. 39.7 Extravasation after balloon angioplasty of a diffuse high-grade stenosis. If further treatment is needed, repeat balloon occlusion stenting or covered stenting can be performed as indicated. (A) Severe fistula stenosis. (B) Extravasation.

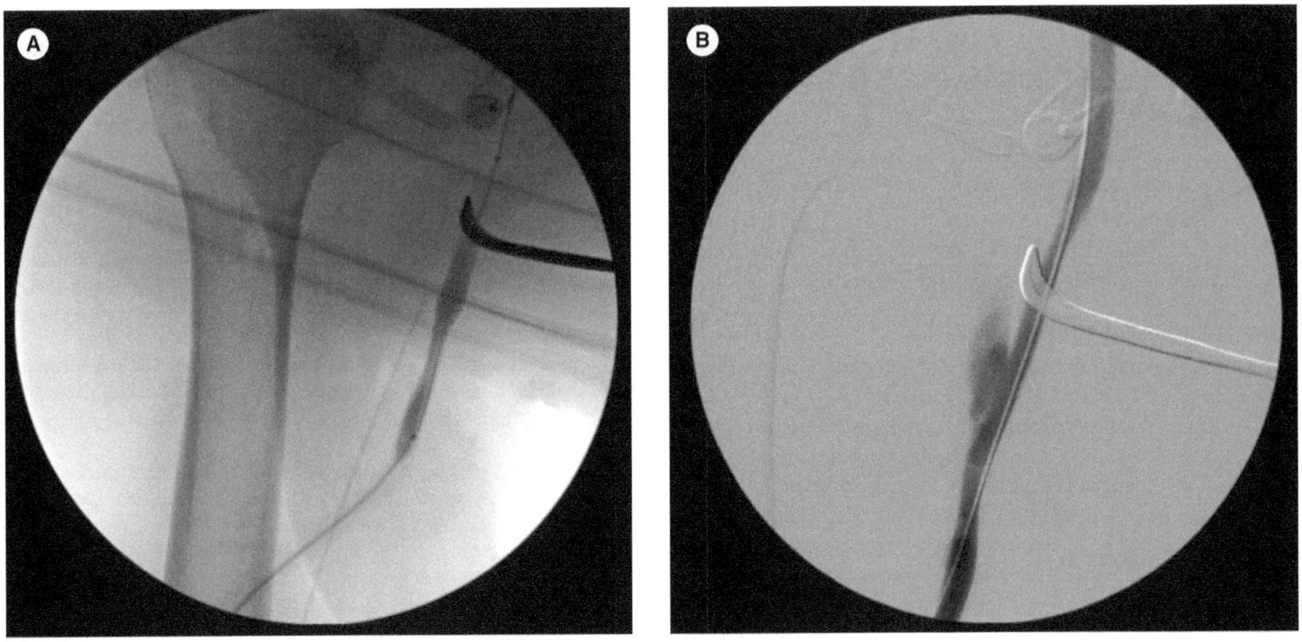

Fig. 39.8 If after repeated low-pressure balloon inflation there is still extravasation, this is generally going to require a covered stent. (A) Balloon inflated for hemorrhage control. (B) Continued extravasation.

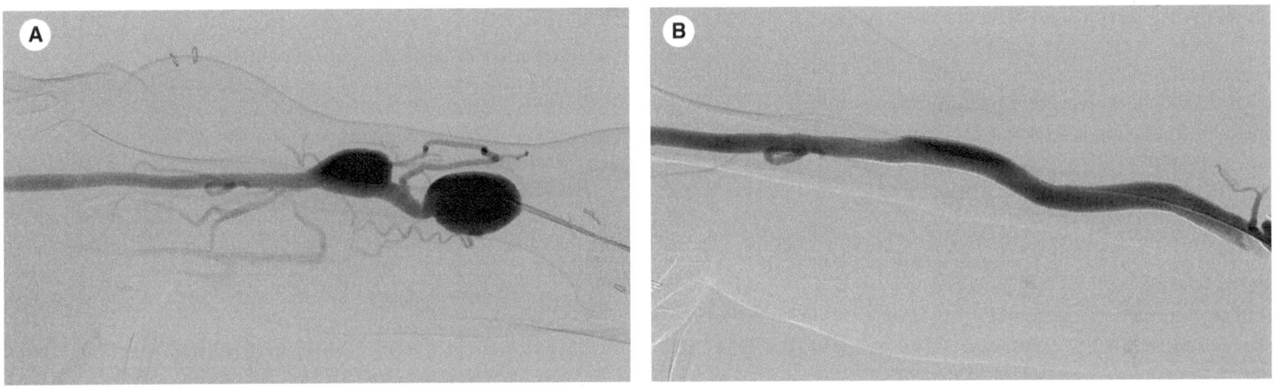

Fig. 39.9 Self-expanding covered stents used for covering aneurysms associated with access stenosis. (A) Access aneurysms. (B) Access with stent graft coverage of aneurysms.

use of a covered stent at an area of stenosis.[13] Typically, covered stents are used for one of two reasons: first, residual stenosis with recoil after balloon angioplasty in a lesion that has been treated previously may require relining of the area of the stenosis to prevent yet another recurrence; second, extravasation associated with injury suffered in the mechanical treatment of a stenosis may require a covered stent to limit the injury and allow healing. For this reason, covered stents must be available in any setting where access is treated endovascularly, including an outpatient office-based facility.

The placement of a covered stent is very similar to using a bare-metal stent with a few additional caveats. First, a covered stent may limit branch flow as a result of covering collaterals with the stent graft. Attention must be paid to all major collaterals and coverage of collaterals should be minimized, if possible. Second, the entire lesion should be covered by the covered stent to minimize the risk of recurrence. Typically, covered stents develop recurrences at the ends of the covered component, referred to as a "candy wrapper" stenosis, resembling a piece of candy with a twisted cover at the ends. Because intimal hyperplasia cannot grow through the fabric of the covered stent, the stenosis tends to occur at the ends of the cover both proximally and distally.[14] Needle access for hemodialysis can be performed through a covered stent, but access with sheaths for interventions should be done with caution, as the larger diameter of the sheath has the potential to damage the covered stent.

Drug-Coated Balloons for Treatment of Dialysis Access

More recently, the availability of drug-coated balloon technology has changed the management of access stenosis in many ways. Although initially used in lower extremity bypass grafts, the obvious place to try to utilize drug-coated balloons is an arteriovenous access because of the high likelihood of recurrence. As discussed previously, arteriovenous access is the ultimate test bed for recurrent intimal hyperplasia and progressive restenosis. Once the benefit of drug-coated balloons was demonstrated in lower extremity bypass, the next place to test it was certainly an arteriovenous access.

Initially, single-center studies[15] showed great promise with dramatically lowered incidence of restenosis after intervention using a drug-coated balloon. Not only was the patency improved versus conventional therapies, but also no residual potential inflammatory focus such as a bare-metal stent was left behind to induce inflammation and restenosis. Therefore, these single-center studies clearly suggested that drug-coated balloon technology may be the future of arteriovenous access intervention.

Subsequently, multicenter trials confirmed the potential for drug-coated balloons in arteriovenous access.[16] With some of the lowest rates of restenosis seen with any intervention, drug-coated balloons promised prolonged success. While the data for drug-coated balloons are still limited in arteriovenous access, the initial promise seems to be substantial.

Unfortunately, reimbursement for this drug delivery system remains a significant issue with drug-coated balloon angioplasty in any vascular bed. Particularly in arteriovenous access, the risk of restenosis remains high and at this point the use of drug-coated balloon technology has not been absolutely shown to be cost-effective. Nonetheless, with time, drug-coated balloon technology may indeed prove cost-effective and be beneficial, particularly in those patients who have not yet had a bare-metal stent placed. Further, the recent questions of impact on mortality may impact the use of drug-coated balloons in all vascular beds.

CONCLUSIONS

Technology has clearly improved our management of patients with dialysis access, both with graphs and with arteriovenous fistula. Nonetheless, the optimum management strategy, particularly in recurrent lesions, is still evolving as new technology is added. Current management of the failing arteriovenous access has made great strides in recent years as a result of the addition of new technologies that allow patency to be prolonged at lower cost.

REFERENCES

1. Brahmbhatt A, Misra S. The biology of hemodialysis vascular access failure. *Semin Intervent Radiol.* 2016;33:15–20.
2. Mennes PA, Gilula LA, Anderson CB, Etheredge EE, Weerts C, Harter HR. Complications associated with arteriovenous fistulas in patients undergoing chronic hemodialysis. *Arch Intern Med.* 1978;138:1117–1121.
3. Gonsalves CF, Eschelman DJ, Sullivan KL, DuBois N, Bonn J. Incidence of central vein stenosis and occlusion following upper extremity PICC and port placement. *Cardiovasc Intervent Radiol.* 2003;26:123–127.
4. Massara M, De Caridi G, Alberti A, Volpe P, Spinelli F. Symptomatic superior vena cava syndrome in hemodialysis patients: mid-term results of primary stenting. *Semin Vasc Surg.* 2016;29:186–191.
5. Miller GA, Hwang W, Preddie D, Khariton A, Savransky Y. Percutaneous salvage of thrombosed immature arteriovenous fistulas. *Semin Dial.* 2011;24:107–114.
6. Yang S, Lok C, Arnold R, Rajan D, Glickman M. Comparison of post-creation procedures and costs between surgical and an endovascular approach to arteriovenous fistula creation. *J Vasc Access.* 2017;18:8–14.
7. Greenberg JI, Suliman A, Angle N. Endovascular dialysis interventions in the era of DOQI. *Ann Vasc Surg.* 2008;22:657–662.
8. Yang HT, Yu SY, Su TW, Kao TC, Hsich HC, Ko PJ. A prospective randomized study of stent graft placement after balloon angioplasty versus balloon angioplasty alone for the treatment of hemodialysis patients with prosthetic graft outflow stenosis. *J Vasc Surg.* 2018.
9. Quaretti P, Galli F, Moramarco LP, et al. Stent grafts provided superior primary patency for central venous stenosis treatment in comparison with angioplasty and bare metal stent: a retrospective single center study on 70 hemodialysis patients. *Vasc Endovascular Surg.* 2016;50:221–230.
10. Cynamon J, Pierpont CE. Thrombolysis for the treatment of thrombosed hemodialysis access grafts. *Rev Cardiovasc Med.* 2002;3(Suppl 2): S84–S91.
11. Bittl JA, Feldman RL. Prospective assessment of hemodialysis access patency after percutaneous intervention: Cox proportional hazards analysis. *Catheter Cardiovasc Interv.* 2005;66:309–315.
12. Chan MR, Bedi S, Sanchez RJ, et al. Stent placement versus angioplasty improves patency of arteriovenous grafts and blood flow of arteriovenous fistulae. *Clin J Am Soc Nephrol.* 2008;3:699–705.
13. Peden EK. Role of stent grafts for the treatment of failing hemodialysis accesses. *Semin Vasc Surg.* 2011;24:119–127.
14. Ulloa JG, Kirkpatrick VE, Wilson SE, Williams RA. Stent salvage of arteriovenous fistulas and grafts. *Vasc Endovascular Surg.* 2014;48:234–238.
15. Swinnen JJ, Zahid A, Burgess DC. Paclitaxel drug-eluting balloons to recurrent in-stent stenoses in autogenous dialysis fistulas: a retrospective study. *J Vasc Access.* 2015;16:388–393.
16. Karnabatidis D, Kitrou P. Drug eluting balloons for resistant arteriovenous dialysis access stenosis. *J Vasc Access.* 2017;18:88–91.

40

Central Venous Stenosis Associated With Arteriovenous Access

Danielle Fontenot, MD and Karl A. Illig, MD

INTRODUCTION

Arteriovenous (AV) access for dialysis is established by connecting an artery and a vein together to create the superficial, high-flow conduit necessary for easy access and efficient dialysis. This is ideally done by connecting an anatomically or surgically superficial vein to an artery, but can also be done by interposing a prosthetic conduit between the in-flow artery and out-flow vein. For success, there must be sufficient in-flow from the artery to provide enough flow (usually at least 400–600 cc/min) and unobstructed venous out-flow to the level of the atrium. Categorized according to treatment strategy, out-flow stenosis can develop in three general areas: peripherally, defined as distal to the cannulation site, venous anastomosis in a graft, and brachial and axillary veins lateral to the thoracic outlet; centrally, veins central to the thoracic outlet; and in the thoracic outlet itself (Fig. 40.1). Endovascular interventions are the first line of therapy for both central and peripheral stenoses or occlusions as they are surrounded by soft tissue and relatively fixed bony structures. Alternatively, the veins in the thoracic outlet run in close proximity to bony structure and cross joints, and thus, surgical or hybrid techniques are a required part of the armamentarium. Stenoses can develop for several reasons. In general, the end result histologically is intimal hyperplasia which can result from intimal injury due to several factors: turbulence or high flow, a stent, indwelling catheter or pacemaker, extrinsic compression at the costoclavicular junction, thoracic outlet, or between sternum and aortic arch vessels, and/or compliance mismatch at the venous anastomosis.[1,2]

The subclavian vein enters the neck and thorax at the venous thoracic outlet. Anatomy is critical. The vein is anterior, passing by the costoclavicular junction (CCJ). The CCJ is formed by the first rib inferiorly, and clavicle, critically involving the subclavius muscle and tendon and costoclavicular ligament superiorly and anteriorly (Fig. 40.2). The anterior scalene muscle and associated phrenic nerve abut the vein posteriorly, but these do not insert on the clavicle and a true, bounded space is not present. The subclavian vein is vulnerable at this point, leading to injury and thrombosis, especially in those with muscular development and/or vocation or avocation with arms overhead. This situation, independently described in 1875 by Paget and in 1884 by Von Schroetter and officially coined Paget-Schroetter syndrome in 1934 (also termed effort thrombosis based on typical risk factors), is the venous form of thoracic outlet syndrome (VTOS).[2,3]

Although the issues surrounding VTOS have been understood for decades, it is only in the past 10 years or so that it has been recognized that those with AV access are susceptible to the same problem. The true cause of this is unknown, but it seems logical to assume that the vein is vulnerable in this location in essentially everyone. Even if only a small amount of narrowing occurs, adding the very high flow rates of liters per minute across this area would seem to predispose toward intimal hyperplasia; once this situation begins, a positive feedback loop is created (Fig. 40.3). Why does this matter? Decades of experience with conventional VTOS have definitively shown that angioplasty and stenting do not work in this situation,[4,5] and that lasting relief will not be obtained without formal decompression of the external bony compression in this area, usually by means of first rib resection.[6] It seems reasonable to extend this to patients with AV access-associated out-flow stenosis at the CCJ; for lasting relief, the bony compression must be removed.

This chapter will address complications during endovascular or hybrid treatment of central venous stenoses, defined as those occurring at the bony costoclavicular junction and centrally in the innominate vein to atrium.

PRESENTATION, DIAGNOSIS, AND TREATMENT

Any clinically relevant obstruction to out-flow will, by definition, create increased venous pressure in the arm. This increased pressure will do several things. First, it will cause swelling. AV access creation is often associated with edema of the involved extremity for the first few weeks after access creation because of the inflammatory response from surgery alone. This is usually minor. Severe or persistent swelling lasting longer than 2 to 3 weeks should raise concern for underlying central venous stenosis. If extreme, brachiocephalic or superior vena cava stenosis can be associated with facial edema, shortness of breath, difficulty swallowing, hoarseness, and headaches. Collateral veins at the shoulder and anterior chest wall are suggestive of underlying central venous stenosis. In addition, the increase in pressure can cause excessive or prolonged bleeding after decannulation, and if out-flow restriction is enough to decrease overall flow, increase recirculation as the "clean" blood "recirculates" back into the machine through the out-flow needle. In this situation, on physical examination, the access may feel pulsatile.

With experience, the diagnosis of out-flow stenosis should be extremely straightforward. A patient who presents with late, gradual arm swelling, or immediate severe swelling, has out-flow stenosis in all but extremely unusual cases. Even if swelling is not present, complaints of post-decannulation bleeding, high recirculation rates and/or inefficient dialysis, or physical findings of a pulsatile fistula and/or visible shoulder or chest wall collaterals are likely to present this problem. Out-flow stenosis in the periphery can sometimes be distinguished from more central stenosis by physical examination. "Popeye arm," massive swelling in the entire arm (Fig. 40.4), shoulder, and chest wall collaterals, and any evidence of superior vena cava syndrome suggest that the problem is more than at the venous anastomosis and probably located more centrally. Interestingly, we have seen many patients with CCJ stenoses who complain of chest wall pain, often worse with

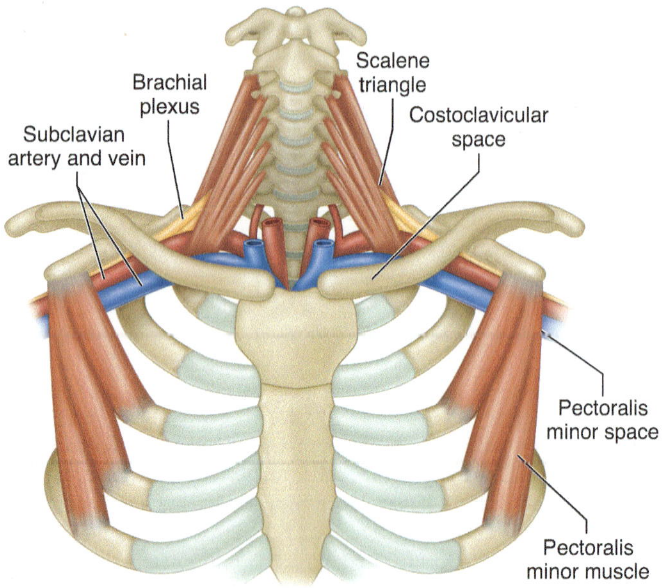

Fig. 40.1 Anterior view of the thoracic outlet. Note that the subclavian vein is anterior to the anterior scalene muscle and passes close to the anterior junction of the first rib and clavicle.

(From Illig KA, Thompson RW, Freischlag JA, Donahue D, Jordan SE, Edgelow PI, eds. *Thoracic Outlet Syndrome*. London: Springer; 2013.)

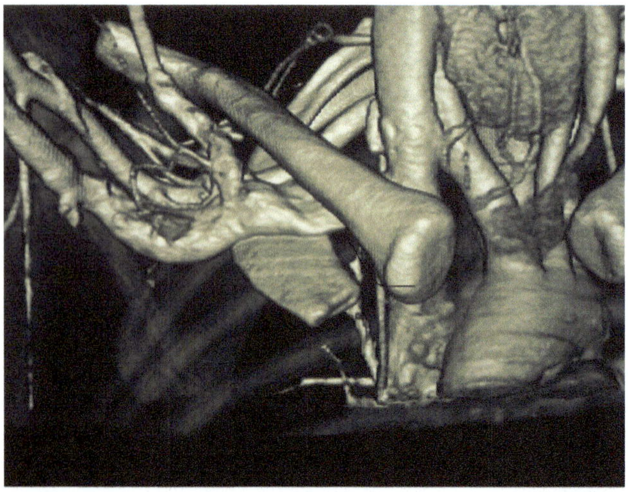

Fig. 40.2 CT scan showing the right venous thoracic outlet with the arm abducted. Note that the subclavian vein is compressed at this location, in part from the (subtracted) subclavius muscle.

(Courtesy Wallace Foster, MBBS, FRACS.)

dialysis, which is perhaps a specific, although not sensitive, marker of this problem.

The diagnosis of central venous stenosis is often clear based on physical examination alone. Ultrasound may show decreased volume flow or blunted venous waveforms but is not an accurate identifier of more central stenosis.[7] Cross-sectional magnetic resonance imaging (MRI) or computerized tomography (CT), even with modern techniques, is

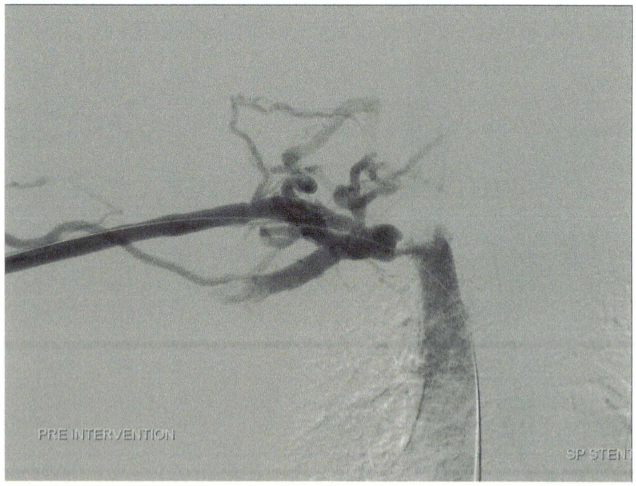

Fig. 40.3 Venogram showing severe stenosis of the right subclavian vein at the costoclavicular junction. A wire is in place across the lesion. Note extensive collaterals, pathognomonic of a hemodynamically significant stenosis.

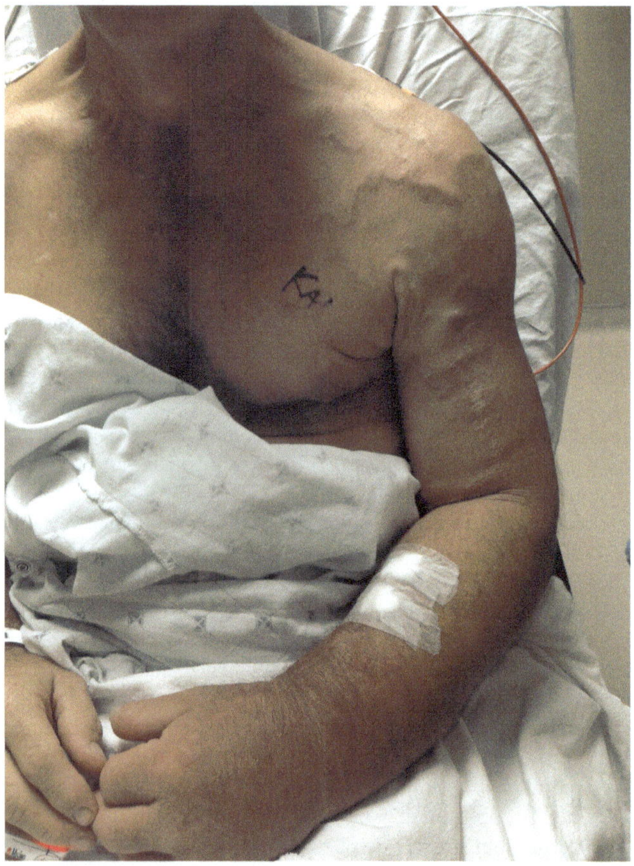

Fig. 40.4 Massively swollen "Popeye arm" in a patient with a subclavian vein stenosis. Note the extensive shoulder and chest wall collaterals.

less useful because of artifact created by the bones in this area. In addition, it is difficult to obtain images with the arm abducted. Although CT venography can diagnose central venous stenosis, it is limited by high contrast loads and expense, in addition to the problems previously mentioned. In contrast, conventional venography with fistulagram offers the opportunity to diagnose and potentially to treat an area of stenosis. We find it useful to image this area with full-strength contrast and breath-hold. If no lesion is immediately seen, repeat imaging is performed with the arm abducted. The presence of collaterals is essentially always pathognomonic (Fig. 40.5). IVUS has been shown to identify areas of stenoses or residual stenosis after venoplasty or stenting that are not evident with conventional venography,[8] although this technique may over-estimate stenoses that are probably not clinically significant.

We feel that central venous stenosis causing impending access failure, significant disability, or rapidly progressive symptoms should always warrant open or endovascular intervention. Although no data exist to support this statement, a randomized trial would not seem to be cost-effective. We believe stenosis in this area, especially if causing symptoms, predicts fistula failure and, even when failure does not immediately occur, leads to significant discomfort, at times massive cosmetic problems, and functional disability.

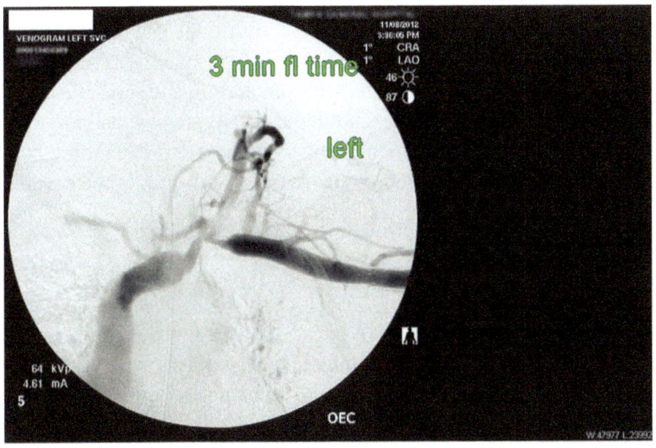

Fig. 40.5 A venogram of the left arm showing the extensive collaterals demonstrating that a hemodynamically significant lesion is present.

Treatment of central venous out-flow stenosis should be determined based on the location of the problem, specifically with regard to whether the CCJ is involved or not. In cases of venous stenosis central to the CCJ, balloon venoplasty is the first option and is associated with 70%–100% initial success rates and 1-year primary assisted patency rates of 86%.[1] While often successful, recoil is effectively and easily treated with stenting. If the problem is at the CCJ, however, decades of experience with VTOS shows that lasting relief will not be achieved without decompression of this area via removal of one of the bones constricting the vein, most often the first rib, and often combined with hybrid endovascular approaches to restore venous patency (see Fig. 40.2).

COMPLICATIONS

Based on the arguments mentioned and knowledge from decades of outcomes from treatment of venous TOS, we treat patients with symptomatic stenosis at the thoracic outlet with a combined surgical and endovascular approach: decompression of the bony thoracic outlet plus fistulagram and endovascular intervention.

Bony decompression can be performed in several ways. Most commonly, the first rib is removed. The anterior location of this compression must be kept in mind, along with the substantial role that the subclavian muscle and tendon undoubtedly play. An infraclavicular approach allows for full vascular exposure and mobilization of the subclavian vein, with resection of the muscle, and is performed with the patient supine, allowing a fistulagram and intervention at the same time. Thompson et al. have described the addition of a supraclavicular incision to allow resection of the entire vein in patients with VTOS (paraclavicular approach), but we do not feel this is necessary in the average case.[9] The transaxillary approach is cosmetically pleasing but does not allow safe vascular reconstruction and precludes concomitant endovascular intervention. The Molina approach is a medial extension of the infraclavicular incision to include a partial sternotomy involving the first interspace for full venous exposure and more central access and is very useful if surgical intervention is required (Fig. 40.6A,B).[10] If necessary for increased exposure, claviculectomy can also be performed with surprisingly little long-term morbidity.[11]

The second step in treating these patients is endovascular intervention. What can go wrong?

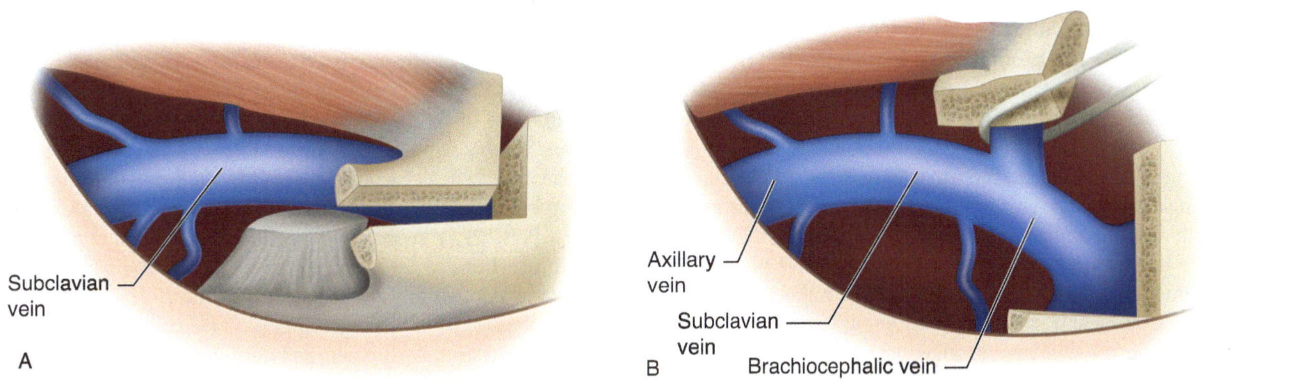

Fig. 40.6 Exposure of the subclavian and innominate veins *(on the right)* as described by Molina. (A) The anterior half of the first rib has been resected and a first interspace sternotomy performed, leaving the sternoclavicular joint intact. (B) After dissection, this structure is then rotated upward for full exposure. Closure is accomplished using two sternal wires at right angles to each other (not shown).

(From Molina JE. A new surgical approach to the innominate and subclavian vein. *J Vasc Surg.* 1998;27:576–581.)

Inability to Cross the Lesion

Obviously crossing the lesion, i.e., getting at least a wire across the area of injury and into a normal vessel centrally, is the required first step. This can be very easy even if the vessel looks occluded and can be very difficult even when it looks open. When crossing such a lesion, the first step is performed with a combination of a hydrophilic wire (e.g., Glidewire, Terumo Interventional Systems, Somerset, New Jersey) and slightly angled catheter (e.g., Hockey Stick Soft-Vu, Angiodynamics, Latham, New York). A long sheath can improve pushability and improves the logistics and quality of imaging. Attempts at crossing venous occlusions should be made with a straight Glidewire rather than curved because a curved wire has a tendency to bend at the area of occlusion rather than pass through it. If the lesion cannot be easily crossed from the upper extremity, a transfemoral approach can help. Venograms should be obtained from above and below the area of stenosis in two different projections to be used for reference.[5] These additional views can also reveal the length of the lesion to aid in determining whether more advanced techniques should be considered.

At times a wire will cross, but no catheter will follow. A very low profile catheter (e.g., Quick Cross, Spectranetics, Colorado Springs, Colorado) might pass when conventional catheters will not. Another useful technique is to snare this wire from a femoral approach; such a "body floss" technique makes dilation quite straightforward (see later section on the "inside out" technique). One technical tip that should be emphasized is that, whenever possible, the wire should be placed into the inferior vena cava and not simply be allowed to coil in the atrium when it is not treated with the body floss technique. In addition to its arrhythmogenic potential in the atrium, passage into the cava allows a much more stable system for pushability and manipulation. Finally, it should be noted that if a lesion is easily crossed or the onset of symptoms is relatively recent, acute clot may be present and mechanical thrombectomy or thrombolysis can be considered prior to angioplasty.

Some lesions cannot be crossed with any conventional techniques. In this event, and assuming transfemoral imaging suggests a short stenosis with reconstitution in a straight line from the tip of the vessel in the arm, sharp recanalization of a venous occlusion can be considered. Sharp recanalization should be performed only with both upper extremity and femoral access. Appropriately sized, covered, bare-metal stents should be immediately available in the event of rupture, and we suggest starting with a sheath large enough to place a covered stent, if needed. The first step is to use the back (i.e., stiff) end of the Glidewire. This will pass straight through most tissues; thus, such a technique should be used with great caution by an experienced operator. Great caution should also be used if the area to be traversed with this tech-$nique is not straight. A 10–15-mm looped snare is inserted from the femoral access and placed just central to the occlusion to serve as a target, with the goal being to pass the wire through the snare. To improve wire stability and to centralize the wire in the lesion, a balloon can be inflated in the peripheral vein and the wire passed through the balloon and through the target lesion. This should be performed with the assistance of multiple projections to ensure the wire remains intraluminal. Once the wire has traversed the lesion, it is snared and pulled out through the femoral access and held taught while a catheter is placed across the occlusion. Subtraction imaging should immediately be performed to ensure the wire has remained intraluminal. As soon as re-entry is established, the wire should be exchanged for a more conventional platform for any further manipulation (for example, an Amplatz wire for stiffness).

If the back end of a Guidewire is unsuccessful in crossing a lesion, needle recanalization can be used. Colapinto needles, Transseptal needles, or the needle from a Rosch-Uchida transjugular liver set (Cook Medical, Bloomington, Indiana) have all been used with some success.[12] Similar techniques of upper and lower extremity access are obtained and intervention is guided by imaging in multiple projections. It is important to direct the needle anteriorly to avoid incidental puncture of an artery (innominate or subclavian, which lie posteriorly) and to perform the sharp recanalization from the femoral direction. Theoretically, this will minimize bleeding if several punctures are made because these punctures will be against the direction of blood flow. The needle is directed toward a snare to obtain through-and-through access.

The PowerWire Radiofrequency Guidewire (Baylis Medical, Montreal, Quebec, Canada) is a 0.035″ wire with a thermal tip that has been used to cross long-segment or resistant occlusions so that stenting can be performed. The heated tip also has the ability to pass extra-luminal, and safe advancement therefore requires knowledge of the course of the vein obtained with pre-operative axial imaging. Covered stents should be used once the lesion has been crossed in case unknown extra-luminal passage has occurred.[13]

Finally, we have created an extra-anatomic endovascular bypass in two patients where the segment was short and intervention was being performed concomitant to rib resection. The wire is allowed to exit intentionally the subclavian vein peripheral to the lesion and retrieved through the open incision and, using a peel-away sheath, re-inserted into the patent vein central to the occlusion through the open surgical wound. After snaring from below to improve pushability, a long, covered stent is passed over this wire, with the ends in the subclavian and innominate vein on either side, and deployed. Aggressive balloon dilation is then used to mold this to profile. We use a self-expanding covered stent (Viabahn, Gore, Flagstaff, Arizona) but any other covered stent will probably work in this situation.

Perforation

Compromise of the vein wall can occur at any point during intervention and at any location. Extra-luminal passage during wire manipulation across difficult lesions is usually a benign complication with minimal associated bleeding, even in patients with AV access, as such perforation is of extremely small diameter and often occurs in the diseased segment. It must be kept in mind, however, that although pressure in a normal AV access is low, if high-grade stenosis or occlusion is present and the perforation is peripheral to this, pressure may indeed be high enough to cause problems. Such a situation does carry the potential for a significant amount of morbidity from excessive blood loss caused by the high-volume flow rates through the arteriovenous access. If the wire is seen or suspected to pass extra-luminally, it should be withdrawn and contrast injected to assess the situation.

Rupture of the subclavian vein during insufflation after rib resection is not unheard of. We most commonly resect the rib and image and intervene on this segment as one procedure. Using this technique, we leave the infraclavicular wound open and vein exposed, so that such a problem can be immediately recognized and treated. If rupture occurs, we hold pressure or re-inflate the balloon while obtaining a covered stent. In situations where we feel this is likely, we intervene through a sheath large enough for covered stent placement, or simply start out with this product from the beginning. We have seen no short- or long-term morbidity in this situation and consider it a relatively common (10%) variant in our conventional procedure. If a stent is needed in this situation, it should obviously be covered, and we generally oversize by approximately 20% to ensure complete wall apposition and balloon only if needed after deployment.

Rupture of the intrathoracic veins can occur during balloon venoplasty or stent deployment. Only 18 published cases could be found, and hemodynamic instability, hemothorax, or tamponade occur less often than would be expected. When these complications do occur, however, there is an associated mortality of 40%.[14] Rupture of the brachiocephalic vein or injury to the azygos vein can lead to hemothorax or mediastinal hematoma, and rupture of the superior vena cava can lead to pericardial effusion or tamponade. Recanalization of the infra-azygos portion of the SVC and cavo-atrial junction carries an increased risk of tamponade because the pericardial sac usually encases this portion of the central venous system.[12] Unfortunately, if this problem occurs, there is seldom an endovascular option because the landing zones have been disrupted and immediate thoracotomy may be the only option.

Early recognition is important, and when performing venoplasty, any changes in the patient's hemodynamics should be quickly reported to the operator. If there is any suspicion of hemodynamic compromise, the balloon should remain on the wire in close proximity to the target lesion with completion imaging performed through the sheath to evaluate immediately for extraluminal extravasation of contrast. In the event of rupture, heparin reversal should be considered. A balloon can be inflated at low pressure at the site of rupture to attempt to tamponade the perforation while clot formation occurs or to decrease blood loss while a stent is prepared to cover the site of rupture. A covered stent graft is the preferred device but a bare-metal stent may also work to re-approximate the vein walls if that is all that is available. In the event of rupture of the SVC, placement of a pericardial drain or pericardial window creation might be necessary to avoid pericardial tamponade. Chest tube placement should be used liberally if any blood is in the pleural space, although small pneumothoraces, especially if created with a small diameter wire, can be observed. Open surgical repair of a venous rupture is often not a feasible option because of the high volume blood loss that would most certainly occur through both the site of rupture while an operating room is prepared and then through the well-developed venous collaterals while surgical exposure is performed. In one report cited previously, open surgical repair by cardiac surgeons was necessary in 20% of reported SVC ruptures, and balloon tamponade was often used as a bridge while an operating room was prepared.[14] Again, if intervention is performed in the same setting as rib resection, the wound should be left open for subclavian vein intervention, and direct pressure followed by covered stent placement will solve the problem in almost all cases.

Stent Fracture

While not an acute complication of the procedures discussed here, stents placed through the CCJ are highly prone to fracture and subsequent thrombosis.[4] Stent fracture at the non-decompressed CCJ is caused by the continued external pressure created by the first rib and sternum. Stents placed more centrally can also fracture. This phenomenon may be related to increased mechanical stress on the stent because of pulsations of central arteries or respiratory and/or cardiac motions leading to a decreased space between the sternum and the aortic arch branches leading to two-point external compression.[15] Both open and closed cell stent designs have been implicated in cases of stent fracture and longer stents have an increased likelihood of fracture than shorter stents.[16]

Correction obviously depends on wire passage, which is much easier if the stent remains open. We find it useful to create a loop, passing the fractured but patent stent in this fashion, but any conventional technique can be used. Angioplasty is often used initially at that area of stent fracture, but most lesions require restenting. It cannot be overemphasized that if the fractured stent is at the CCJ, the bony compression must be corrected. Unfortunately, after any treatment for a fractured stent, restenosis seems common.[16] Repeat intervention can be attempted, but ultimately, sacrifice of the hemodialysis access or open surgical repair may be necessary.

Recoil/Lack of Success

When performing balloon venoplasty, the balloon should be 1 to 2 mm larger than the normal caliber adjacent vein. The subclavian vein is most commonly 10 to 14 mm, the brachiocephalic vein 12 to 16 mm, and the superior vena cava 14 to 20 mm.[5] The balloon should be expanded in order to eliminate the "waist," and long insufflation times of 2 to 3 min have been suggested to allow for remodeling of the stenotic area and to decrease any residual stenosis. High inflation pressures (greater than 20 atm, with noncompliant balloons, i.e., Dorado, Atlas, Conquest balloons all BD Bard, Tempe AZ) are often necessary, but caution should be used as these elevated pressures are thought to lead to vein wall trauma and the development of intimal hyperplasia and recurrent stenosis in the future.

Successful resolution of a stenosis should lead to almost immediate regression of collateral networks.[1] Nonelastic stenosis often responds well to venoplasty, and elastic stenosis is associated with a high rate of immediate recoil. In the event of residual stenosis greater than 50%, repeat venoplasty with a 2-mm larger balloon, higher inflation pressures (up to 30 or 40 atm), cutting balloons, and/or stenting can be considered.[1] Cutting balloons are too small for most venous lesions, but a second wire passed through the lesion (buddy wire technique) can serve the same function as the balloon is inflated.

Stenting is usually the next option for residual lesions after balloon dilation. Common indications are residual stenosis greater than 50% of the vein diameter, recurrent stenosis occurring less than 3 months from intervention, or dissection in the central veins or more peripherally. Data suggest that residual lesions after balloon venoplasty in patients with conventional VTOS may remodel over time and thus not always be immediately treated with stenting,[17] although the higher flow in a limb with an arteriovenous access may lead to turbulence and worsening intimal hyperplasia and stenosis. Although not directly applicable to this chapter, it should be noted that data support the use of covered stents at both the venous anastomosis of an AV graft[18] and cephalic arch.[19]

When sizing stents, the length should be adequate to land in an area of vessel that is of a normal caliber on either side of the target lesion and the stent diameter should be slightly greater than that of the normal vessel. Central veins typically require stents with a diameter of 12–20 mm. Covered stents have shown improved patency versus bare-metal stents because of a decreased rate of intimal hyperplasia,[1] while bare-metal stents have the advantage of preserving any vital in-flow veins and well-developed collateral vessels. Covered stents require precise deployment due to the risk of covering important tributaries. When stenting the brachiocephalic veins near the superior vena cava, "kissing stents" should be considered to help preserve the option of future access to the contralateral brachiocephalic vein,[1,5,6] or "intersecting/interlocking" stents placed through each other followed by aggressive balloon dilation to expand both lumens can be used. When deploying stents, the Guidewire, again, should be placed well into the inferior vena cava to prevent cardiopulmonary embolization and allow control and easier retrieval if stent migration occurs.[5]

Stent Malposition, Migration, and Embolus

Because of the inherent physiologic distensibility of the venous system, increased cardiac motion in the central venous system, large sizes needed, and potentially combined with operator inexperience, stent migration during deployment is a major potential complication of procedures in this area of the body, estimated to occur in about 3% of cases.[16] Dislodgement of a previously placed stent during a subsequent intervention can also occur, often before wire access has been secured. Migration into the right atrium or ventricle can cause conduction abnormalities, valve injury, endocarditis, cardiac perforation, chest pain, elevated troponins, acute myocardial infarction, or cardiogenic shock. Continued migration into the pulmonary vasculature can lead to pulmonary infarction.[16] To decrease the risk of this complication, stents should be over-sized by a minimum of 10%–20%. Self-expandable stents allow for more constant, uniform wall apposition with increased radial force during deployment versus balloon-expandable stents and thus have less propensity for movement. Axial shortening of 25%–50% in self-expanding stents should be anticipated when selecting the appropriate stent length, and the majority of the stent should be deployed above the lesion to increase fixation to the vessel wall. When deploying stents in the central venous system, bridging wire access between the superior and inferior vena cava should be maintained. In the event of stent migration, this will eliminate the risk of cardiopulmonary embolization and improve the ability to retrieve or "park" the stent in a benign location if fixation in the intended location does not occur.

If stent embolization into the right atrium does occur, four methods of retrieval have been described: direct snaring, balloon-assisted snaring, Guidewire-assisted snaring, and a bridging stent from the SVC to the IVC, although all in case-report format.[20] The Nitinol Amplatz Gooseneck snare (Medtronic, Minneapolis, Minnesota) is the snare used in the majority of the described cases. Direct snaring is performed by obtaining both transjugular and transfemoral wire access and then using a snare to lasso the body of the stent and constrict it. A balloon can be inserted into the stent to allow manipulation of the stent. A snare is then passed alongside the shaft of the balloon and the balloon is used to manipulate the stent so that the snare can be passed around the body of the stent to constrict it as described previously. Through-and-through Guidewire access through the stent can be obtained and an additional Guidewire can be passed through the stent. A snare is then passed along the exterior of the stent and used to snare the traversal Guidewire. This combination can then be used to withdraw the stent from the atrium. Self-expanding stents can frequently be constricted and withdrawn into a sheath and removed. Balloon-expandable stents often cannot be safely removed. Any stent that cannot be safely removed percutaneously should be repositioned to its intended location or an appropriately sized alternative location such as the iliac system. Placement of a bridging bare-metal stent is a final option for stent migration into the right atrium. This is performed again with upper and lower extremity wire access. A longer stent is deployed through the migrated stent with its proximal and distal ends secured in the SVC and IVC respectively.[10]

Completely Occluded Out-Flow

There are times when the lesion absolutely cannot be crossed using any technique. Ligation of the fistula, if present, will be effective in reducing or eliminating the arm swelling but has the obvious drawback of losing access for dialysis. Several other options can be considered. First, if the patient is being dialyzed with a catheter (i.e., has no working access), it can be used for wire access to the atrium followed by HeRO (Hemodialysis Reliable Outflow, Merit Medical Systems, South Jordan, Utah) graft placement. Obviously the catheter is removed and hence an immediate access graft (Acuseal, Gore, Flagstaff, Arizona) must be substituted for the conventional PTFE arterial component supplied. While patency rates are no better than any graft, approximately 22% at 1 year in one study, it has the advantage of maintenance of atrial access with almost infinite replaceability.[21] We have performed 11 such cases, and even though the use of the existing catheter for wire access compromises sterility, our infection rate has been zero. We emphasize use of a very stiff wire (Amplatz, Boston Scientific, Fremont, California) or even Lunderquist (Cook Medical location.) placed well into the inferior vena cava, insertion of the dilators and peel-away sheath under direct fluoroscopic vision, and predilation, if necessary, with a long 5- or 6-mm balloon. In addition, the dilator itself often blocks passage of the venous out-flow component. As long as wire access is maintained, the dilator can be removed and the venous component will often slip right in. Perforation is the major complication with this technique, which may create tamponade. If this occurs, surgical decompression is often needed as this is a large-diameter injury.

Finally, bypass can be performed across the stenotic area such as axillary to brachiocephalic or jugular vein bypasses or axillary to axillary vein crossover with reported patency rates of up to 80% at 1 year.[12,22] Some have also described a vein to right atrial bypass, creation of a superior vena cava conduit, and tunneling to the ipsilateral femoral or saphenous vein for venous decompression when all other methods to resolve central venous stenosis and thus salvage the arteriovenous access have failed.[23]

CONCLUSIONS

Central venous stenosis in the setting of hemodialysis can lead to significant patient morbidity and AV access failure as a result of inefficient dialysis or access thrombosis. We feel that stenoses occurring as the result of chronic injury at the bony costoclavicular junction should, in most cases, be treated by hybrid open bony resection and endovascular intervention. The open approach, paradoxically, makes treatment of complications that arise during the often complex endovascular portion of the procedure easily recognizable and treatable. Problems in this area are often complex and the "high-level" AV access surgeon should have a toolbox of interventions available to treat both the lesion itself and any complications that arise.

REFERENCES

1. Collin G, Jones R, Willis A. Central venous obstruction in the thorax. *Clin Radiol.* 2015;70(6):654–660.
2. Urschel HC, Pool JM, Patel AN. Anatomy and physiology of VTOS. In: Illig KA, Thompson RW, Freischlag JA, Donahue D, Jordan SE, Edgelow PI, eds. *Thoracic Outlet Syndrome.* London: Springer; 2013:339–343.
3. Moore R, Lum YW. Venous thoracic outlet syndrome. *Vasc Med.* 2015; 20(2):182–189.
4. Urschel HC, Patel AN. Paget-Schroetter syndrome therapy: failure of intravenous stents. *Ann Thor Surg.* 2003;75:1693–1696.
5. Horikawa M, Keith QB. Central venous interventions. *Tech Vasc Interv Radiol.* 2016;20(1):48–57.
6. Lugo J, Tanious A, Armstrong P, et al. Acute Paget–Schroetter syndrome: does the first rib routinely need to be removed after thrombolysis? *Ann Vasc Surg.* 2015;29(6):1073–1077.
7. Pham XD, Ihenachor EJ, Wu H, et al. Significance of blunted venous waveforms seen on upper extremity ultrasound. *Ann Vasc Surg.* 2016;34:45.
8. Graaf RD, Laanen JV, Peppelenbosch N, Loon MV, Tordoir J. The value of intravascular ultrasound in the treatment of central venous obstruction in hemodialysis patients. *J Vasc Access.* 2016;17(Suppl. 1):12–15.
9. Thompson RW. Surgical techniques: Operative decompression using the paraclavicular approach for VTOS. In: Illig KA, Thompson RW, Freischlag JA, Donahue D, Jordan SE, Edgelow PI, eds. *Thoracic Outlet Syndrome.* London: Springer; 2013:433–446.

10. Molina JE. A new surgical approach to the innominate and subclavian vein. *J Vasc Surg.* 1998;27:576–581.
11. Green RM, Waldman D, Ouriel K, Riggs P, DeWeese JA. Claviculectomy for subclavian venous repair: long-term functional results. *J Vasc Surg.* 2000;32:315–321.
12. Arabi M, Ahmed I, Mat'Hami A, Ahmed D, Aslam N. Sharp central venous recanalization in hemodialysis patients: a single-institution experience. *CardioVasc Interv Radiol.* 2015;39(6):927–934.
13. Maloney SP, Halin N, Iafrati M. Radiofrequency thermal wire: a useful adjunct to treat chronic central venous occlusions. *J Vasc Surg.* 2010; 52(4):1121.
14. Kuhn J, Kilic A, Stein E. Management of innominate vein rupture during superior vena cava angioplasty. *A & A Case Reports.* 2016;7(4):89–92.
15. Mallios A, Taubman K, Claiborne P, Blevea J. Subclavian vein stent fracture and venous motion. *Ann Vasc Surg.* 2015;29(7):1451.e1–1451.e4.
16. Bani-Hani S, Showkat A, Wall BM, Das P, Huang L, Al-Absi AI. Endovascular stent migration to the right ventricle causing myocardial injury. *Semin Dial.* 2012;25(5):562–564.
17. Freischlag J. Venous thoracic outlet syndrome: transaxillary approach. *Oper Tech Gen Surg.* 2008;10:122–130.
18. Haskal ZJ, Trerotola S, Dolmatch B, et al. Stent graft versus balloon angioplasty for failing dialysis-access grafts. *N Engl J Med.* 2010;362:494–503.
19. Miller GA, Preddie DC, Savransky Y, Spergel LM. Use of the Viabahn stent graft for the treatment of recurrent cephalic arch stenosis in hemodialysis accesses. E-pub ahead of print; available at http://www.sciencedirect.com/science/article/pii/S074152141731933X (accessed 11/1/17).
20. Taylor JD, Lehmann ED, Belli A, Nicholson AA, Kessel D, Robertson IR, Morgan RA. Strategies for the management of SVC stent migration into the right atrium. *Cardiovasc Interv Radiol.* 2007;30(5):1003–1009.
21. Gage S, Ranney D, Lawson J. The Hemodialysis Reliable Outflow (HeRO) graft. *Hemodialysis Access.* 2016;273–280.
22. Bakken AM, Protack CD, Saad WE, et al. Long-term outcomes of primary angioplasty and primary stenting of central venous stenosis in hemodialysis patients. *J Vasc Surg.* 2007;45:776–783.
23. Glass C, Maevsky V, Massey T, Illig KA. Subclavian vein to right atrial appendage bypass without sternotomy to maintain AV access in patients with complete central vein occlusion: A new approach. *Ann Vasc Surg.* 2009;23(4):465–468.

41

Catheter Issues

Karen Woo, MD, MS

INTRODUCTION

Central venous catheters can be placed for a number of indications, including hemodialysis, chemotherapy, parenteral nutrition, and antibiotics. The intended duration of the catheters can be categorized as acute or chronic. While there is no defined time frame to differentiate acute from chronic, catheters for acute use are generally intended to remain in-dwelling in the patient for 4 to 6 weeks, whereas chronic catheters can remain in place for 12 months or more. The most common acute catheters include nontunneled hemodialysis and peripherally inserted central catheters (PICC). The acute catheters are characterized by a lack of a subcutaneous cuff near the skin exit site. The most common chronic catheters include tunneled hemodialysis, Hickman, Broviac, Groshong, (CR Bard, Tempe, AZ) and port-a-cath. The chronic catheters all have a subcutaneous cuff near the skin exit site, with the exception of the port-a-cath, which is entirely subcutaneous.

Regardless of the catheter type, the initial insertion of the catheter occurs in the same manner, with the exception of the PICC. The PICC is inserted in the upper arm either through the basilic vein or through a brachial vein. The remainder of the catheters are inserted preferentially in the internal jugular or the subclavian vein, followed by the femoral vein.

The preferred access site for any central venous catheter is the right internal jugular vein. The vein takes a straight path down to the superior vena cava, providing the path of least resistance for the wire, dilators, and catheter and minimizing the risk of kinking of the catheter. The internal jugular vein is preferable to the subclavian vein because it can be visualized easily with ultrasound (US). Additionally, while there is still a risk of central venous stenosis/occlusion with internal jugular catheters, the risk is less than with subclavian vein catheters.

A recent Cochrane review demonstrated that use of US in central venous catheter insertion reduced the rate of total overall complications by 71%.[1] The number of participants with an inadvertent arterial puncture was reduced by 72%. A sterile-covered US probe should first be used to scan the course of the internal jugular vein in the neck and confirm its patency. Placing the patient in the Trendelenburg position will cause the vein to dilate, as well as reduce the risk of air embolism. The internal jugular vein is classically described as running lateral to the carotid artery and adjacent to it. However, variations in the anatomy are common and the relative position of the vein to the artery may vary through its course. The vein can be anterior, lateral posterior, or directly posterior to the artery. The course of the jugular vein in the neck should be imaged. A segment of the vein that is adjacent to the carotid artery (Fig. 41.1), and not superficial or deep to the artery (Fig. 41.2), is the preferred area for puncture.

Direct visualization of the needle entering the internal jugular vein, using US is the most effective way to avoid puncture of the carotid artery. Despite this care, the carotid artery can still be punctured through the internal jugular vein in the process of exchanging the US probe for the wire and threading the wire into the needle. During this process, the needle tip can be inadvertently advanced into the carotid artery through the jugular vein. The risk of this can be minimized by holding the needle firmly between the thumb and forefinger and stabilizing the heel of the hand and the remaining fingers against the patient. In addition, having the guidewire plastic loop secured to the drape by an Edna clamp allows rapid exchange between the US probe and wire, minimizing needle movement. After the wire has been inserted through the needle into the vein, the placement of the wire in the vein should be confirmed using US, either in the transverse or longitudinal orientation, to visualize the path of the wire. In addition, fluoroscopy can be utilized to confirm the position of the wire and that it is not crossing the midline, which would indicate possible arterial puncture. The wire should be to the right of the mediastinum, indicating access into the superior vena cava (SCV) and into the inferior vena cava (IVC).

A micropuncture 21-gauge needle and 0.018″ guidewire is recommended to make the initial puncture of the internal jugular vein. In the event that the carotid artery is inadvertently punctured with the micropuncture needle, the needle can be removed leaving a very small arteriotomy that will seal by holding pressure for 5 minutes in a patient with normal coagulation parameters. In patients who are hypotensive or poorly oxygenated, it may be unclear whether an arterial puncture was accessed, as a result of lack of return of bright red, pressurized blood. If there is concern for an arterial puncture, the 5-French coaxial sheath from the micropuncture set can be placed and the pressure can be transduced through the sheath to see whether the waveform is arterial or venous. A blood gas analysis of a sample from the sheath can also be sent to determine whether the values are consistent with an arterial or venous blood gas. Another option is to connect the sheath to a length of extension tubing and hold the tubing straight up; in patients with relatively normal hemodynamics, venous blood will not rise against gravity, whereas arterial blood will continue to rise through the tubing, eventually overflowing.

The major risk of leaving a catheter in the carotid artery is thrombus formation on the catheter and embolization of the thrombus into the brain. There are few data regarding the natural history of inadvertent catheterization of the carotid artery. In a survey of 45 vascular surgeons, most agree that if the injury is recognized in <4 hours, the catheter can be removed and pressure applied.[2] In this instance, 30 minutes of pressure is recommended, followed by close monitoring for development of a hematoma. In the same survey, most agreed that if the injury is recognized later, because of track formation and increased risk of thrombus on the catheter, the catheter should be removed in the operating room, with open repair of the artery. Other small series have been described using percutaneous closure devices.[3,4] These should be used with caution because the evidence to support their use is very limited and their use for this indication is off-label. Catheter size should also be considered when planning removal from an inadvertent arterial puncture, with larger catheters given more consideration for open surgical removal and repair.

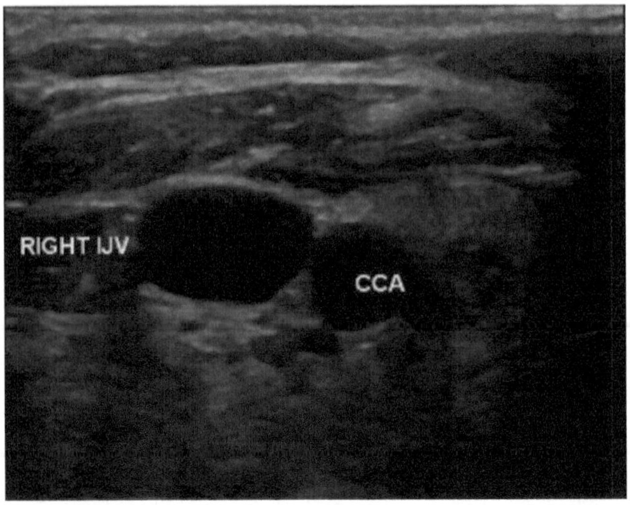

Fig. 41.1 Duplex image demonstrating internal jugular vein (*IJV*) adjacent to common carotid artery (*CCA*).

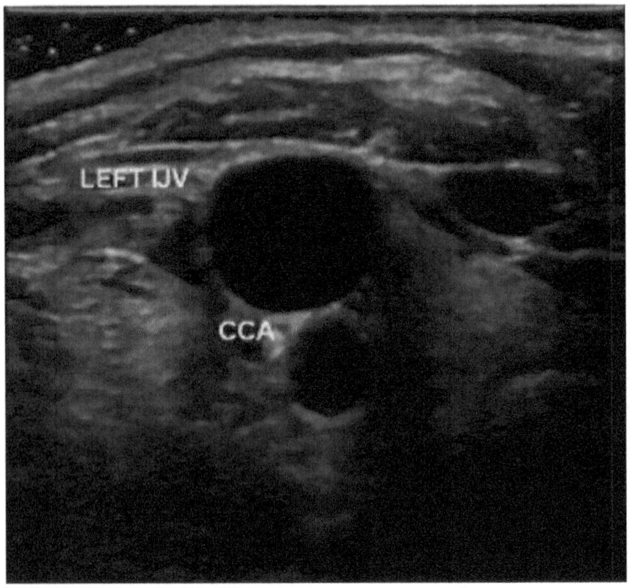

Fig. 41.2 Duplex image demonstrating internal jugular vein (*IJV*) on top of common carotid artery (*CCA*).

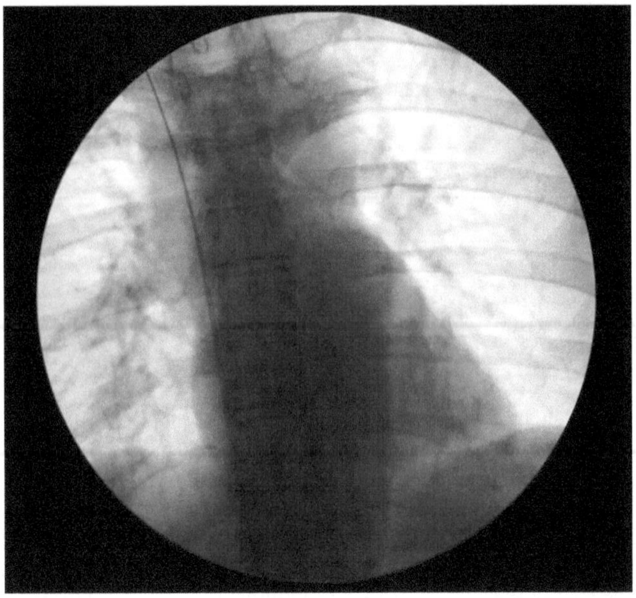

Fig. 41.3 Fluoroscopic image demonstrating wire coursing down from internal jugular vein through the superior vena cava, into the right atrium and out of the inferior vena cava.

Catheters intended for chronic use should be inserted in a procedure room under fluoroscopic guidance, for a number of reasons. The ideal position for the tip of any of these catheters is at the junction of the SVC and the right atrium. Hickman, broviac, and port-a-cath catheters are cut to the appropriate length to achieve this position. Fluoroscopic guidance is used to determine the length. Groshong and dialysis catheters are fixed lengths, and fluoroscopic guidance is used to determine the exit site for the catheter that will achieve the desired tip position.

Fluoroscopic imaging should be used to visualize wire, dilator, sheath, and catheter passage. Having the wire course through the SVC into the IVC allows extra stability of the wire without the risk of arrhythmia caused by the wire encountering the right heart chambers (Fig. 41.3). Whenever any device is passed over the wire, visualization with fluoroscopy should be utilized. This is particularly true when using the left internal jugular vein. The tortuous path of the left internal jugular to the heart makes it possible for dilators and sheaths, especially the large diameter stiff devices used in placement of hemodialysis catheters, to kink the wire and to perforate the side wall of the central vein (innominate or SVC) into the pleural cavity or the mediastinum. This is most easily avoided by visualizing the manipulation of any device over the wire in its entirety and using no more than a minimal amount of pressure when advancing the device. A stiffer wire than the one included in the catheter insertion kit can facilitate passage of devices when the course is tortuous. When placing a catheter from the left jugular, the procedure should begin with US-guided access of the left internal jugular vein, as described previously, and placement of the J-wire. If the J-wire does not pass easily through the left innominate vein into the SVC and IVC, an angled catheter can be used to guide the J-wire or a Glidewire into the correct position. The wire can then be exchanged for a stiff wire, which allows adequate stiffness to support the dilators and the peel-away sheaths. The dilator only needs to be inserted to a depth to dilate the soft tissue tract. The insertion of the peel-away sheath should be visualized in its entirety with fluoroscopy to ensure the wire is not being kinked. If any increased amount of resistance is encountered, the device should be removed and a smaller diameter device should be attempted. If this is still met with increased resistance, a contrast venogram should be performed to determine whether there is a stenosis, occlusion, or other anatomic obstruction of the vein.

If perforation of the vein occurs during catheter placement, assuming that the wire is taking a proper course into the SVC and IVC, it is imperative that the wire position be maintained. A properly sized balloon catheter can then be advanced over the wire and the balloon inflated at the area of the perforation for several minutes. For subclavian vein and innominate vein perforations, a 10–14-mm diameter balloon will be necessary, and for the SVC, an 18–22-mm balloon will be necessary. A contrast venogram can then be performed to assess for continued contrast extravasation. If there continues to be contrast extravasation, this procedure can be repeated with a longer inflation time. Because of the low pressure nature of the venous system, it is unlikely that the problem will persist after these interventions. Should the problem persist, a covered stent may be necessary to repair the injury. Diameters of covered stents required would correspond to the diameter of the balloons described previously.

If a perforation occurs and the tip of the wire is outside the vein or the wire is not following the proper course, another puncture should be performed, either in the internal jugular vein or from the ipsilateral upper extremity to introduce a wire that is following the proper course of venous anatomy. This will allow the previously described procedure to be performed.

As mentioned previously, PICC lines are generally placed at the bedside with US-guided venipuncture but without the use of fluoroscopy. Cutaneous anatomic landmarks are typically used to determine the length of the catheter and can be quite inaccurate. To assist with proper tip positioning, the catheter can be linked to an electrocardiogram (ECG) monitor. By evaluating the morphological variations of the P wave of the ECG, the appropriate tip position can be determined. In a prospective nonrandomized study of 42 patients who had PICCs placed with ECG monitoring and 48 patients who used landmarks, 25% of landmark patients did not achieve proper tip position versus only 7% in the ECG group ($P = 0.03$).[5]

Control of the wire must be maintained at all times. If wire control is lost during the procedure, the wire can become completely intravascular inside the patient. A portion of the wire can also be embolized if the wire is sheared off by the access needle during withdrawal of the wire. This can be avoided by removing the wire and needle together as a unit if any resistance is encountered during withdrawal of the wire. A Glidewire should never be used with an 18-gauge entry needle because there is a risk that the wire could be sheared off, leading to wire embolization. If wire embolism does occur, the wire or wire segment should be retrieved using a snare.[6]

If an attempt at catheter placement fails on one side, a chest X-ray should be performed to rule out a pneumothorax before attempting placement on the other side to avoid bilateral pneumothoraces. If the patient develops acute signs of a severe pneumothorax during the procedure, including shortness of breath and oxygen desaturation, fluoroscopy can be used to evaluate for a pneumothorax. If there is any suggestion of a pneumothorax on fluoroscopy in the setting of acute respiratory symptoms, a tube thoracostomy should be placed immediately.

More often, the air leak is small and the pneumothorax is not detected until later. After placement of any catheter, an end-expiratory upright chest X-ray should be performed to exclude a pneumothorax and to confirm proper tip placement. Any patient with a pneumothorax should be given supplemental oxygen, which increases the rate of pleural air reabsorption.[7] A small pneumothorax, defined as less than 2–3 cm, in an asymptomatic patient can be observed with a follow up chest X-ray in 12 to 48 hours.[7,8] If symptoms develop or there is an increase in the size of the pneumothorax on subsequent chest X-rays, tube thoracostomy should be performed. For larger pneumothoraces, a tube thoracostomy should be performed regardless of whether symptoms are present.[7,8]

Hemothoraces as complications of central line placement are rare. A hemothorax can develop when a vein and/or artery and the parietal pleura are perforated by a needle or a device. The subclavian vein or artery, the innominate vein, or the SVC can be involved. Large blood loss can occur through even a small puncture into the pleura as a result of a lack of tamponade combined with negative respiratory pressure. As with a pneumothorax, any patient who develops respiratory symptoms during central venous catheter insertion can be examined under fluoroscopy for a possible hemothorax. The post-catheter placement chest X-ray should also be examined for a hemothorax. Any hemothorax should be treated with drainage by a tube thoracostomy. If the initial volume of blood drained is over 1500 mL or there is continued bleeding of 200–300 mL/h for 2–3 hours, venography/angiography and/or surgical exploration are indicated.[8]

Air embolism is an exceedingly rare, but potentially fatal complication of central venous catheter placement. Air embolism can occur during inspiration when the intrathoracic pressure falls (negative relative to atmospheric pressure, as during normal inspiration) and subsequently the intravenous pressure falls. If a needle, catheter, dilator, or sheath is open to air during this time, air can be introduced through the device into the venous system. The resulting symptoms vary based on the amount of air introduced. The air that enters the central veins will pass to the right heart, obstructing the pulmonary circulation, and producing acute right heart failure. Symptoms can range from sudden onset dyspnea and oxygen desaturation to total circulatory collapse and death. Patients with a patent foramen ovale can suffer air embolism to the brain with stroke.

The provider should be aware of preventing air embolism throughout the catheter placement procedure. The initial maneuver prior to starting the procedure is to place the patient in the Trendelenburg position. The patient should remain in Trendelenburg until the catheter placement is completed. Avoid having any needle, catheter, sheath, or dilator open to the air by placing a finger over the opening whenever it does not have a wire in it or by using devices that have valves at the opening. For patients who are awake, they can be asked to hum when a device might be open to air, which causes a temporary positive intrathoracic pressure. This prevents the patient from taking a breath. In patients who are intubated, the anesthesiologist can perform a Valsalva to create positive intrathoracic pressure.

If an air embolism is suspected, the patient should immediately be placed in Trendelenburg position, with the feet above the level of the head and a left lateral decubitus position. This moves the air bubble away from the right ventricular outflow track.[8] At the same time, the source of the air embolism must be terminated. Aspiration can be attempted to remove the air by advancing a catheter into the right ventricle and suctioning with a large syringe. In addition, a large needle can be placed in the right ventricle directly through the chest wall and as much air as possible should be aspirated. Hyperbaric oxygen may be effective in cases of cerebral air emboli.

Another exceedingly rare complication of central venous catheter placement is cardiac perforation. This is probably caused by stiff guidewires, dilators, and sheaths. Again, prevention is of the utmost importance. As with prevention of venous perforation, visualization of any wire and device maneuvers with fluoroscopy, using only minimal forward pressure, and stopping at any sign of increased resistance will avoid cardiac perforation.[9] Acute pericardial tamponade can occur after cardiac perforation, particularly if fluid is inadvertently infused into the pericardial space. Signs and symptoms include hemodynamic collapse, cyanosis, cervical venous distention, tachycardia, and muffled heart sounds. On fluoroscopy, a large globular cardiac silhouette may be observed. If pericardial tamponade is suspected, any intravenous devices should be removed and pericardiocentesis performed or a pericardial window created. If the tamponade recurs after these interventions, open cardiac repair may be required.

Injury to the thoracic duct is an uncommon complication of central venous catheter placement.[10] This is generally not recognized during the procedure itself. Subsequent to the procedure, a lymphocele can develop in the neck. In the unlikely event that there is a communication with the pleural space, a hydrothorax or chylothorax can form. The first step in treatment is removal of the central line. Pressure should be applied in the neck. If there is lymph fluid in the pleural space, it should be aspirated. Most lymph leaks will require no further treatment.

Peripheral nerve injuries in the course of central venous catheter insertion are rare. During subclavian vein access, the brachial plexus is most at risk of injury.[11,12] If the patient complains of acute upper extremity pain during catheter placement, any devices should be withdrawn. If the symptoms occur following the procedure, the catheter should be removed. During internal jugular catheter placement, the vagus, recurrent laryngeal, and phrenic nerves are also at risk of being injured. Phrenic nerve injuries are generally not identified during the procedure. More often they are identified as incidental findings of elevated hemidiaphragm on chest X-ray.[13,14] Injury to the vagus nerve or the recurrent laryngeal nerve manifest as hoarseness after catheter placement. Injuries to the phrenic, vagus, and recurrent laryngeal nerve generally resolve. In the case of PICC lines, injury to the median nerve has been reported.[15] Again, if the patient complains of pain during the procedure, all devices should be withdrawn. Subsequent to the procedure, the catheter should be removed in the event of pain. The injury can be avoided by looking for the nerve on US imaging and avoiding an area where the target vein is near the nerve.

TIP BOX–TECHNICAL RECOMMENDATIONS

Ultrasound
Fluoroscopy
Trendelenburg position throughout
Visualize all device manipulation
Pass wire from superior vena cava to inferior vena cava

WARNING BOX–POINTS AT WHICH A COMPLICATION COULD OCCUR

Step	Potential complication
Exchanging ultrasound probe for wire after puncture	Advancing needle through vein into another structure
Advancing stiff dilator/sheath	Kinking of wire and back wall puncture of vein
Exchanging of devices	Air embolism

REFERENCES

1. Brass P, Hellmich M, Kolodziej L, et al. Ultrasound guidance versus anatomical landmarks for internal jugular vein catheterization. *Cochrane Database Syst Rev.* 2015;1: CD006962.
2. Mussa FF, Towfigh S, Rowe VL, et al. Current trends in the management of iatrogenic cervical carotid artery injuries. *Vasc Endovascular Surg.* 2006;40(5):354–361.
3. Yoon DY, Annambhotla S, Resnick SA, et al. Inadvertent arterial placement of central venous catheters: diagnostic and therapeutic strategies. *Ann Vasc Surg.* 2015;29(8):1567–1574.
4. Bechara CF, Barshes NR, Pisimisis G, et al. Management of inadvertent carotid artery sheath insertion during central venous catheter placement. *JAMA Surg.* 2013;148(11):1063–1066.
5. Baldinelli F, Capozzoli G, Pedrazzoli R, et al. Evaluation of the correct position of peripherally inserted central catheters: anatomical landmark vs. electrocardiographic technique. *J Vasc Access.* 2015;16(5):394–398.
6. Bessoud B, de Baere T, Kuoch V, et al. Experience at a single institution with endovascular treatment of mechanical complications caused by implanted central venous access devices in pediatric and adult patients. *Am J Roentgenol.* 2003;180(2):527–532.
7. Haynes D, Baumann MH. Management of pneumothorax. *Semin Respir Crit Care Med.* 2010;31(6):769–780.
8. Tabatabaie O, Kasumova GG, Eskander MF, et al. Totally implantable venous access devices: a review of complications and management strategies. *Am J Clin Oncol.* 2017;40(1):94–105.
9. Collier PE, Goodman GB. Cardiac tamponade caused by central venous catheter perforation of the heart: a preventable complication. *J Am Coll Surg.* 1995;181(5):459–463.
10. Teichgraber UK, Nibbe L, Gebauer B, et al. Inadvertent puncture of the thoracic duct during attempted central venous catheter placement. *Cardiovasc Intervent Radiol.* 2003;26(6):569–571.
11. Karakaya D, Baris S, Guldogus F, et al. Brachial plexus injury during subclavian vein catheterization for hemodialysis. *J Clin Anesth.* 2000; 12(3):220–223.
12. Ramdial P, Singh B, Moodley J, et al. Brachial plexopathy after subclavian vein catheterization. *J Trauma.* 2003;54(4):786–787.
13. Shawyer A, Chippington S, Quyam S, et al. Phrenic nerve injury after image-guided insertion of a tunnelled right internal jugular central venous catheter. *Pediatr Radiol.* 2012;42(7):875–877.
14. Takasaki Y, Arai T. Transient right phrenic nerve palsy associated with central venous catheterization. *Br J Anaesth.* 2001;87(3):510–511.
15. Alomari A, Falk A. Median nerve bisection: a morbid complication of a peripherally inserted central catheter. *J Vasc Access.* 2006;7(3):129–131.

42

Complications of ECMO and IABP

Amy B. Reed, MD, DFSVS, RPVI

INTRODUCTION

Intra-arterial devices used to assist in the management of critically ill patients with cardiopulmonary failure have become commonplace at most advanced medical centers in the past decade. Extracorporeal membrane oxygenation (ECMO) and intra-aortic balloon pumps (IABP) are two of the most commonly utilized percutaneous strategies. Temporary use of inotropic medications and IABP is successful in weaning the majority of patients from cardiopulmonary support; however, a small fraction are refractory. Similarly, only a small minority of patients with acute respiratory distress syndrome (ARDS) will not respond favorably to conventional treatment modalities (mechanical ventilation, permissive hypercapnia, positional maneuvers) and will need to go on to increased cardiopulmonary support provided by ECMO. Because these devices are often inserted from a transfemoral approach, understanding the indications, techniques, and complications that can arise from use of these devices is important for the vascular surgeon who is often called upon to manage the immediate and long-term problems that arise.

Intra-Aortic Balloon Pump

The IABP, developed as 15-French in the 1960s, is a polyethylene balloon mounted on the end of a flexible 7–9-French catheter. It is typically inserted in a percutaneous fashion via the common femoral artery or the brachial artery utilizing the Seldinger technique. In unusual circumstances where femoral or brachial access is prohibitive, such as iliac artery occlusion, upper extremity dialysis access, or occluded axillosubclavian arteries, the IABP may need to be placed via the subclavian or axillary arteries. This approach typically requires cut-down with direct arterial puncture or in some cases, the anastomosis of a short 6–8-cm prosthetic graft. IABPs can be inserted through supra-inguinal bypass grafts percutaneously or via cut-down. LaMuraglia and colleagues evaluated 19 IABPs inserted through supra-inguinal prosthetic bypass grafts and found no significant increase in complications.[1] Two patients in the analysis did require thrombectomy of occluded graft limbs and one developed a graft infection. Careful wound care and limiting catheter dwell time can help minimize risk of graft infection and bacteremia in IABPs placed through prosthetic grafts or native arteries.

The IABP is positioned in the descending thoracic aorta between the second and third intercostal space (Fig. 42.1). The balloon should be positioned in the suprarenal aorta in order to provide 85%–90% occlusion with pulsation. At the start of diastole, the balloon inflates, augmenting coronary perfusion. At the beginning of systole, the balloon deflates and blood is ejected from the left ventricle, thereby increasing cardiac output and decreasing left ventricular stroke work and myocardial oxygen requirements.

Approximately 70,000 IABPs are inserted in the United States alone representing 5%–10% of all patients undergoing cardiac surgery.[2] Complications secondary to IABP are high and reported on average in 20%–30% of cases.[3] Thrombocytopenia is currently the most common complication noted in 50% of patients followed by fever in 40% of cases.[3] Bleeding, along with aorto-iliac artery injury, dissection, thromboembolism, distal lower extremity ischemia, and balloon rupture occur less frequently.

Thrombocytopenia results from mechanical injury from the balloon to the platelets rendering them dysfunctional. Patients are typically anticoagulated systemically with unfractionated heparin during use of IABP. Thrombocytopenia in the face of full anticoagulation may precipitate spontaneous bleeding at remote sites other than the point of access. Administration of platelets, along with decreasing the level of systemic anticoagulation, can help reverse bleeding. If bleeding is significant and persistent, anticoagulation may need to be temporarily suspended.

Access site complications from IABP insertion may result in distal limb ischemia if the caliber of the brachial or femoral artery is inadequate to allow arterial flow around the sheath. Systemic anticoagulation and collateral flow around the sheath may help mitigate severe ischemia until the IABP can be removed. Arterial duplex imaging distal to the access site can be reassuring in documenting adequate distal perfusion. If profound ischemia persists, then moving access to a different site may be necessary for limb preservation. If the access is relocated, vigilance should still be maintained for possible compartment syndrome in the initial limb because of relative ischemia/reperfusion. In cases where access relocation is not possible secondary to the patient's underlying condition, a life over limb posture may be necessary. Alternately, an antegrade access to the SFA can be performed at the time of IABP insertion or if limb ischemia develops. This antegrade sheath is then connected to the pump, diverting some flow distal to the occluding catheter.

The positioning of the IABP in the descending thoracic aorta is critical for proper functioning. The balloon size is chosen by the patient's height and possible aortic diameter. By design, the IABP should provide 80%–90% aortic occlusion. Overestimating the size of the descending thoracic aorta may result in aortic dissection or rupture. Although known descending thoracic aortic dissections or aneurysms are contraindications to IABP placement, at times the balloon may have been placed in an area with atheromatous plaque. Ongoing IABP counterpulsations may lift the plaque resulting in possible atheromatous embolization or intraplaque hemorrhage and possible dissection of the aorta. Direct aortic injury can be disastrous particularly if acute intervention is necessary and the patient is unable to tolerate removal of the IABP. If the patient is stable, balloon removal can be undertaken and the aorta treated as indicated. Focal aortic injuries can be treated with endovascular means such as aortic cuffs or stent grafts if the patient is stable. Embolization can occur to the brain, spine, mesenterics, renals, or peripheral circulation and may not present itself immediately.

Occasionally the balloon may migrate or be inadvertently positioned too high or too low in the descending thoracic aorta. This can

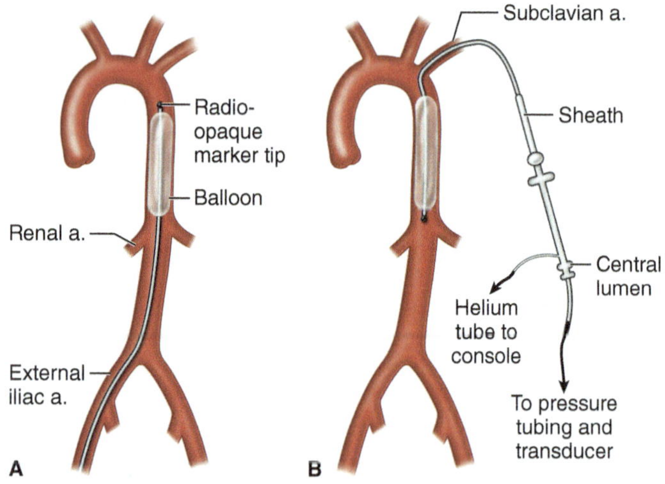

Fig. 42.1 Optimal positioning of intra-aortic balloon pump via femoral (A) and brachial (B) approaches.

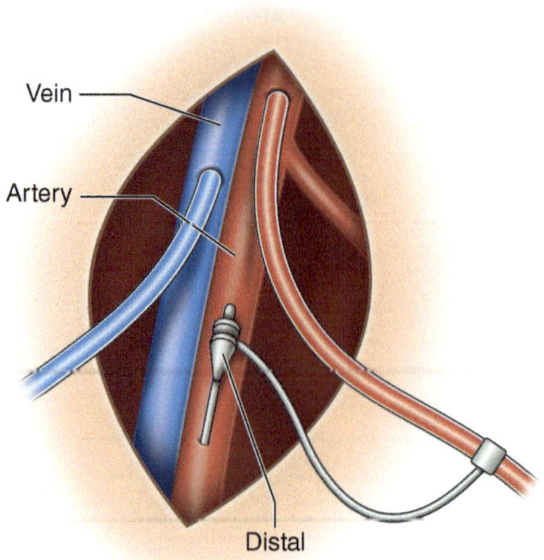

Fig. 42.2 Veno-arterial extracorporeal membrane oxygenation cannula placement with distal perfusion sheath.

result from vessel tortuosity, overestimation, or underestimation of the patient's height and aortic size, which may give rise to malpositioning. More often than not, the IABP is put in as an emergency procedure without full knowledge of aortic caliber. Arch aortography performed at the time of balloon placement should identify the left common carotid and subclavian artery origins but will not always give an accurate estimation of aortic diameter. If the IABP is placed too high, there may be occlusion of the left subclavian or carotid arteries resulting in possible cerebral ischemia, stroke, or decreased upper extremity perfusion. Migration secondary to vessel tortuosity or positioning the IABP too low may result in malperfusion to the mesenteric and renal arteries. In both cases, the IABP will need to be repositioned appropriately and in some cases a new balloon sterilely inserted.

Extracorporeal Membrane Oxygenation

Mechanical cardiopulmonary support is typically thought to be a technique utilized during cardiac surgery; however, it can be utilized in a more prolonged fashion outside of the operating room. This is referred to as extracorporeal membrane oxygenation (ECMO) and is used in conditions such as heart support after cardiac failure, pneumonia, trauma, or severe infection. ECMO has existed since the 1970s and was used primarily in severe neonatal respiratory failure. Earlier trials in adults were unsuccessful, however, because technology and protocols improved and so did outcomes. ECMO utilization has risen in the last decade in part because of the publication of the CESAR (**C**onventional versus **E**CMO for **S**evere **A**dult **R**espiratory Failure) trial in 2006, which revealed ECMO to be more effective than conventional ventilation therapy.[4] Two types of ECMO exist to provide respiratory support: venovenous (VV) and veno-arterial (VA). Only VA ECMO provides hemodynamic support in addition to respiratory support. VA ECMO has increased in popularity over the past four decades. It has been used for various cardiac diseases complicated by cardiac failure including postcardiotomy syndrome after pericardiotomy, fulminant myocarditis, acute coronary syndrome, or as a bridge to mechanical circulatory support or transplant.

The ECMO vessels cannulated depends upon the underlying clinical need. Traditional VV ECMO typically involves femoral and internal jugular vein cannulation and utilizes cannulas between 20 and 24-French. VA ECMO utilizes femoral vein and femoral artery access (Fig. 42.2). Stroke, renal failure, and sepsis (not infrequent complications seen in critically ill patients) are among the most common complications. The most frequently reported complication of VA ECMO was major hemorrhage, which led to reintervention in nearly half of patients, even in good quality studies.[5] The insult of the initial operation, systemic heparin, and heparin-coated circuits are the typical causes of bleeding and managed in the usual way.

Perhaps the most dreaded complication in VA ECMO is limb ischemia. The arterial cannulas used for VA ECMO are 15 or 17-French and are typically placed percutaneously into the common femoral artery in a retrograde fashion. A 5- or 6-French single lumen arterial sheath is positioned antegrade adjacent to the ECMO arterial cannula to improve distal perfusion. This is often done percutaneously, under ultrasound guidance or occasionally open if transcutaneous are unsuccessful. In cases of small common femoral arteries, there are options to place a temporary prosthetic limb or conduit onto the common femoral artery (Fig. 42.3).[6] When the patient is able to be decannulated, all prosthetic devices are removed and the common femoral artery patched with saphenous vein or bovine pericardium.

A meta-analysis of 1866 ECMO patients published since 2000 reported a pooled estimate rate of limb ischemia of 16.9% with a 4.7% major amputation rate.[7] By comparison, acute kidney injury (55.6%), major bleeding (40.8%), and significant infection (30.4%) were much more likely to complicate ECMO therapy in the meta-analysis. Less frequently reported vascular complications include retrograde aortic dissection (1.4%–2.2%), inferior vena cava tear (2.2%), arterial thrombus (4.2%–19%), and deep venous thrombosis (1.1%–17%).

Given the complications brought on by limb ischemia, much attention has been paid to prevention and early detection of arterial insufficiency in the lower extremity during VA ECMO. The rapid diagnosis of embolism or cannula-related vessel occlusion can be difficult in a hypotensive patient on vasoconstrictive medications. Transport for a diagnostic, contrast-enhanced scan can be life-threatening. Because of the difficulty in detecting limb ischemia, vascular consultation and noninvasive vascular studies are often used.

The distal perfusion cannula gained popularity in order to attempt to decrease limb ischemia and its complications. Varying techniques

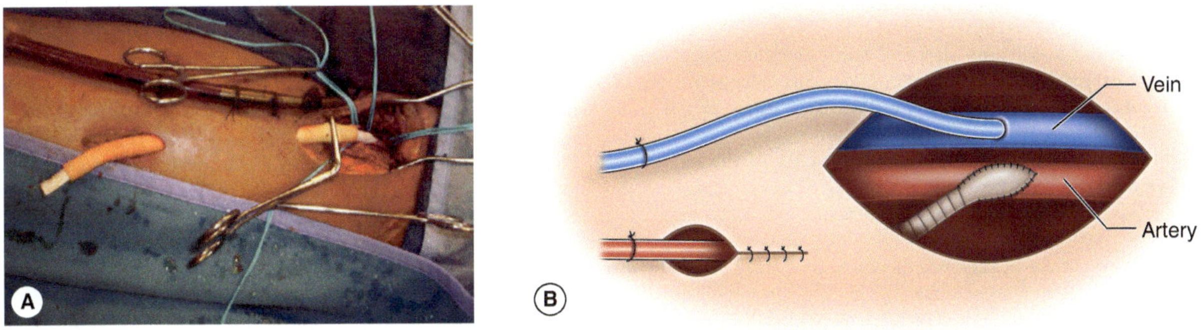

Fig. 42.3 (A) Photograph of modified T-graft for extracorporeal membrane oxygenation (ECMO) with polytetrafluoroethylene (PTFE) anastomosed to common femoral artery then tunneled through Dacron graft. (B) Arterial ECMO cannula is secured in PTFE and to skin and then overlying skin is closed over prosthetic graft material.

have been used for placing a perfusion sheath. When cannulation is being performed in an open fashion, a larger sheath (8–9 French) can provide improved flow. Some have advocated posterior tibial or dorsalis pedis artery cut-down with ligation and placement of a retrograde catheter to perfuse the distal extremity.[8] Another method to perfuse the lower extremity is cannulation through a vascular graft, which is anastomosed to the femoral artery. This requires open vessel exposure, which may be easier in selected patients with a damaged femoral artery or a limb with severe ischemia-reperfusion injury. Some have advocated a selective approach to distal perfusion cannula placement and measure the pressure in the superficial femoral artery through a 23-gauge needle after ECMO cannula insertion. If the mean pressure was below 50 mmHg, a perfusion sheath was placed.[9]

Alternative cannulation sites other than the common femoral artery have been used, including the thoracic aorta (after cardiac surgery via median sternotomy), subclavian artery, or axillary artery. These techniques are associated with equally challenging complications including pericardial effusion/tamponade, axillary artery thrombosis, and brachial plexus injury,[10] making the common femoral artery the ongoing favorite for VA ECMO access.

Vascular complications from VA ECMO access include compartment syndrome, arterial dissection, vessel laceration, pseudoaneurysm formation, thrombosis, embolism, and stenosis. The common femoral artery is the most frequent vessel injured although damage to the superficial femoral, profunda femoris, iliac arteries, and the aorta have all been described. Aziz and colleagues[11] delineated vascular complications in 17.8% of 100 patients undergoing VA ECMO. Resolution of the limb ischemia in the majority of VA ECMO patients was simply removal of the cannula. Repairs were primarily femoral endarterectomy with patch angioplasty with bovine pericardium or primary repair of the common femoral artery. No bovine pericardial patch infections occurred, consistent with recent literature of the ability to use bovine pericardium in infected fields with relatively low risk of patch infection.[12] None of the patients in the study needed distal revascularization (Table 42.1). Furthermore, the development of vascular complications did not predispose the patient to a higher risk of amputation or mortality.

Recently, Ring and colleagues compared outcomes of VA ECMO patients who had distal reperfusion catheters versus those who did not. Although there may be a sample size error, 75% (189 patients) with distal perfusion catheters and 25% (58 patients) without, no significant difference with regard to lower extremity ischemia was noted between the two groups. Limb ischemia was noted in 7% of patients with distal reperfusion catheters versus 15% in those without (P = 0.12). Of interest was the significant decrease in mortality between the two groups: 42% with reperfusion as opposed to 60% in patients without (P = 0.02).[13]

TABLE 42.1 Common vascular complications after veno-arterial extracorporeal membrane oxygenation (VA ECMO) and management.

Vascular complication	Management
Acute limb ischemia	Removal of ECMO cannula ± femoral repair
Vessel laceration	Direct repair or covered stent
Pseudoaneurysm	Direct repair or covered stent
Focal arterial dissection	Observation if nonflow limiting
Stenosis of common femoral artery	Femoral endarterectomy with patch

REFERENCES

1. LaMuraglia GM, Vlahakes GJ, Moncure AC, et al. The safety of intraaortic balloon pump catheter insertion through suprainguinal prosthetic vascular bypass grafts. *J Vasc Surg*. 1991;13:830–837.
2. Parissis H, Soo A, Al-Alao B. Intra aortic balloon pump: literature review of risk factors related to the complications of the intra aortic balloon pump. *J Cariothor Surg*. 2011;6:147.
3. Vales L, Kanei Y, Ephrem G, et al. Intra-aortic balloon pump use and outcomes with current therapies. *J Invasive Cardiol*. 2011;23(3):116–119.
4. Peek GJ, Clemens F, Elbourne D, et al. CESAR: conventional ventilator support vs extracorporeal membrane oxygenation for severe adult respiratory failure. *BMC Health Serv Res*. 2006;6:163.
5. Khorsandi M, Dougherty S, Bouamra O, et al. Extra-corporeal membrane oxygenation for refractory cardiogenic shock after adult cardiac surgery: a systemic review and meta-analysis. *J Cardio-Thoracic Surg*. 2017;12:55.

6. Calderon D, El-Banayosy A, Koerner M, et al. Modified T-graft for extracorporeal membrane oxygenation in a patient with small-caliber femoral arteries. *Tex Heart Inst J.* 2015;42(6):537–539.
7. Cheng R, Hachamovitch R, Kittleson M, et al. Complications of extracorporeal membrane oxygenation for treatment of cardiogenic shock and cardiac arrest: a meta-analysis of 1,866 adult patients. *Ann Thorac Surg.* 2014;97:610–616.
8. Haft JW, Bartlett RH. Lower extremity perfusion during VA ECMO via femoral cannulation. Presented at the 23rd annual CNMC symposium: ECMO and the advanced therapies for respiratory failure, Feb 2007, Keystone, CO.
9. Huang SC, Yu HY, Ko WJ, et al. Pressure criterion for placement of distal perfusion catheter to prevent limb ischemia during adult extracorporeal life support. *J Thorac Cardiovasc Surg.* 2004;128:776–777.
10. Mishra V, Svennevig JL, Bugge JF, et al. Cost of extracorporeal membrane oxygenation: evidence from the Rikshospitalet University Hospital, Oslo, Norway. *Eur J Cardiothorac Surg.* 2010; 37:339–342.
11. Aziz F, Brehm CE, El-Banyosy A, et al. Arterial complications in patients undergoing extracorporeal membrane oxygenation via femoral cannulation. *Ann Vasc Surg.* 2014;28:178–183.
12. McMillan WD, Leville CD, Hile CN. Bovine pericardial patch repair in infected fields. *J Vasc Surg.* 2012;55:1712–1715.
13. Ring AC, Agrawal A, Brehm CE, et al. Antegrade reperfusion catheters are associated with improved outcomes among patients who are undergoing ECMO via femoral cannulation. Presented at 41st Annual Meeting of the Vascular and Endovascular Surgery Society Meeting, San Diego, CA. June 2017.

43

Angiography

David L. Waldman, MD, PhD and Andrew J. Cantos, MD

INTRODUCTION

Angiographic procedures were first performed only months after Roentgen's discovery of X-rays. Haschek and Lindenthal injected mercury salts into an amputated hand and created one of the first recorded images of the arterial system (Fig. 43.1).[1] This showed the enormous potential of radiographic visualization of the arterial system. In 1924, Brooks reported concentrated sodium iodide arterial injection as a means of demonstrating lower extremity vessels (Fig. 43.2).[2] Over the next 50 years, multiple contrast agents were used. Iodinated compounds initially used to treat infection were soon found to be X-ray contrast agents.

Conventional angiography plays a vital role in the diagnosis and management of peripheral vascular disease. Recently, advanced, noninvasive techniques, such as computed tomography angiography (CTA), magnetic resonance angiography (MRA), and vascular ultrasound have made a significant impact on the diagnosis of vascular disease. These modalities are safe and effective in characterizing vascular disease and providing critical preprocedure planning. Despite the increased use of noninvasive measures, conventional angiography remains the gold standard.[3] Endovascular therapy is considered less invasive compared with traditional open surgery. It translates to lower cost, decreased recovery time, and fewer postprocedural complications.[4] Although catheter angiography is considered an extremely safe procedure, it is not without risk, with complications seen in 3%–5% of cases.[3] Using noninvasive modalities prior to angiography, procedure times and complication rates can be reduced.[5] We will review some of the complications encountered during and following conventional angiography.

SELECTION OF ACCESS SITE AND APPROACH

Transfemoral (TF) arterial access is widely accepted as the standard approach for angiography. It is generally well tolerated; however, alternative approaches have recently been explored, including transbrachial (TB) and transradial (TR). Preprocedure planning with CTA or MRA have simplified angiography procedures. Through creating "road maps," physicians are able to prepare appropriate access for the safest procedure to complete an intervention. TR access is found to be associated with lower complication rates compared with the TF approach.[6] However, technical success for TR is slightly lower and requires increased familiarization for improved physician's technical success. Additionally, vessel size must also be considered when planning an endovascular intervention.

ACCESS COMPLICATIONS

The most frequently encountered angiography complication is related to vascular access, with an incidence reported from 0.1% to 23%. Postvascular access groin hematomas are the most common of these complications, with an incidence ranging from 5% to 23%.[7] Groin hematomas are generally benign and self-limiting. Rarely, hematomas can become large and life-threatening, only discovered after the patient has had profound blood loss and resultant hypotension. Retroperitoneal hematomas are described in 0.1%–0.7% of the cases and are seen when femoral artery access is superior to the inguinal ligament (Fig. 43.3).

More recently, access complication rates have been reduced when utilizing real-time ultrasound (Fig. 43.4). The femoral artery access with ultrasound trial (FAUST) confirmed real-time ultrasound guidance statistically reduces the number of access attempts, time to access, and vascular complications.[8] These complications are categorized as minor or major depending on the requirement of blood transfusion.

Additional access-related complications include pseudoaneurysm, vascular dissection, and arteriovenous fistula. A pseudoaneurysm is a defect in the inner two layers of the blood vessel (tunica intima and media).[9] The incidence of pseudoaneurysms are described in 0.8%–2.2% postinterventional procedures. The likelihood increases when the superficial femoral artery or profunda femoris is accessed (Fig. 43.5). Small pseudoaneurysms can be monitored and often resolve spontaneously, but in other cases they may require treatment with ultrasound compression, thrombin injection, or surgery.

An arteriorovenous fistula (AVF) is an abnormal communication between an artery and a vein, which occurs in approximately 1% of cases.[10] AVFs occur when the access needle crosses the wall of both the femoral artery and vein (Fig. 43.6). Research suggests that at least one-third of AVFs resolve spontaneously. As such, follow-up imaging is initially suggested to avoid unnecessary interventions.[11]

Vascular dissection is uncommon. If it is to occur, it is more frequently seen with diseased and tortuous vessels or traumatic sheath insertion. The dissection can occur both at the access site and further upstream (Fig. 43.7).

In the majority of cases, a retrograde dissection is not clinically significant. If there is a symptomatic dissection, a pressure gradient should be measured across the dissection. Most pressure gradients should be treated with inflating an angioplasty balloon across the dissection and remeasuring the pressure gradient. If the dissection is not in the vicinity of a joint or osseous structure, a bare-metal stent can be placed to tamponade the false lumen. Knowing the vascular anatomy of the groin with a general awareness of the potential complications will help decrease the risk of vascular access related complications.

CONTRAST-RELATED COMPLICATIONS

Iodinated contrast agents are a fundamental component for conventional angiography. These agents are widely used in medical imaging because of their ability to opacify vascular structures. By manipulating various X-ray beam properties, a specific energy can be isolated that highlights the contrast material, optimizing vascular opacity. Reactions

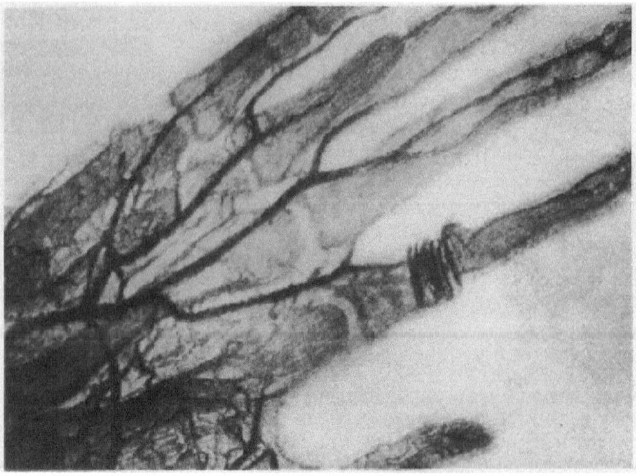

Fig. 43.1 Hasckek and Lindenthal injection into blood vessels of amputated hand.

(From Haschek E, Lindenthal O'F. A contribution to the practical use of the photography according to Röntgen. *Wien Klin Wochenschr.* 1896:9:63.)

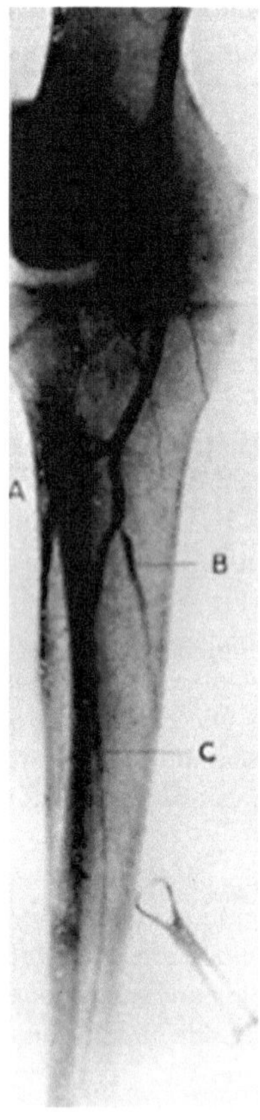

Fig. 43.2 Brooks lower extremity arterial injection using concentrated sodium iodide. (A) anterior tibial artery, (B) Posterior tibial artery, (C) Peroneal Artery.

(From Brooks B. Intra-arterial injection of sodium iodide. *J Am Med Assoc.* 1924;82:1016.)

to contrast can range from minor allergic and physiologic reactions to life-threatening ones.[12]

Iodinated contrast agents are subdivided into categories: osmolality (high, low, iso) and tonicity (ionic or nonionic). The most common combination is nonionic low osmolality with lower associated risk. In this group, reaction rates range from less than 1% for minor reactions to less than 0.1% for severe ones.[12] Risk factors include prior contrast reactions, severe allergies, asthma, cardiac or renal disease, and increasing age. It is of note that shellfish allergy is no longer considered a risk factor for contrast reactions.[13]

Acute contrast reactions are categorized into physiologic and allergic types. Physiologic reactions are thought to be related to a disruption in homeostasis. In increasing severity, physiologic reactions include flushing, warmth, nausea, vomiting, hypertension, chest pain, and seizures. Allergic reactions, on the other hand, are immunologic responses to intravenous contrast, most often type I hypersensitivity reactions. Allergic reactions, include rash, edema, nasal congestion, generalized erythema, hoarseness, throat pain, severe edema, laryngeal spasm, hypotension, and hypoxia. Contrast reactions usually occur within 1 hour, the majority within the first 5 minutes. It is critical to distinguish physiologic from allergic type reactions because treatments differ depending on etiology. Allergic reactions require premedication, but physiologic reactions do not.[12]

Management of acute contrast reactions varies depending on severity. The first step in managing acute reactions is to assess and to categorize the reaction as mild, moderate, or severe. Clinical evaluation should include overall patient appearance, ability to speak, respiratory status (i.e., use of accessory muscles), skin, and vital signs. Mild reactions usually require no intervention beyond observation, although occasional antihistamines can be administered. This can be seen in cases such as mild urticaria. Moderate and severe reactions require more aggressive treatment. Bronchospasm is treated with β-agonists as the first line along with oxygen. More severe reactions require intravenous epinephrine. Laryngeal edema is often life-threatening and is treated with intravenous epinephrine. Differentiating a vasovagal response to anaphylaxis is critical. A vasovagal reaction is treated with patient positioning and intravenous fluids. Moderate and severe reactions are treated with intravenous atropine. However, anaphylaxis is treated with intravenous epinephrine. The American College of Radiology manual[14] on contrast reactions is an excellent resource and should be required reading for physicians working with contrast agents.

Contrast induced nephropathy (CIN) is a controversial topic and the role intravascular contrast plays in its occurrence is questionable.[15] The definition of CIN varies, but according to the acute kidney injury network, CIN is an absolute or percentage increase in serum creatinine levels compared with baseline (0.3 mg/dL or 50% above baseline) or urine output less than 0.5 mL/kg for at least 6 hours within 48 hours of contrast administration.[16] For the general population with normal renal function, CIN approaches an incidence close to 0%. However, in patients with pre-existing chronic kidney disease, diabetes mellitus, or even increased age, the incidence of CIN increases to 20%–40%.[6] It is important to identify these risks factors prior to giving intravascular contrast. CIN prevention starts with identifying the at-risk patients. If CIN occurs, laboratory values start increasing 1–3 days postinjection, peaking 3–5 days, normalizing in 7–14 days. CIN is thought to be self-limiting, and the mainstay of treatment/prevention is intravenous hydration.[17] Research has been carried out to determine safe alternatives to iodinated contrast, particularly for at-risk patients. Gadolinium-based contrast agents were found to be well tolerated in patients with renal insufficiency (doses less than 0.3–0.4 mmol/kg) as well as associated with a decreased incidence of CIN.[18] Given the risk of nephrogenic systemic fibrosis, the use of gadolinium for angiography has mostly disappeared. Furthermore, while carbon dioxide may not be considered the optimal imaging agent, it can also act as an alternative for patients with CIN or allergy, given its rapid clearance through the pulmonary system (Fig. 43.8).[19]

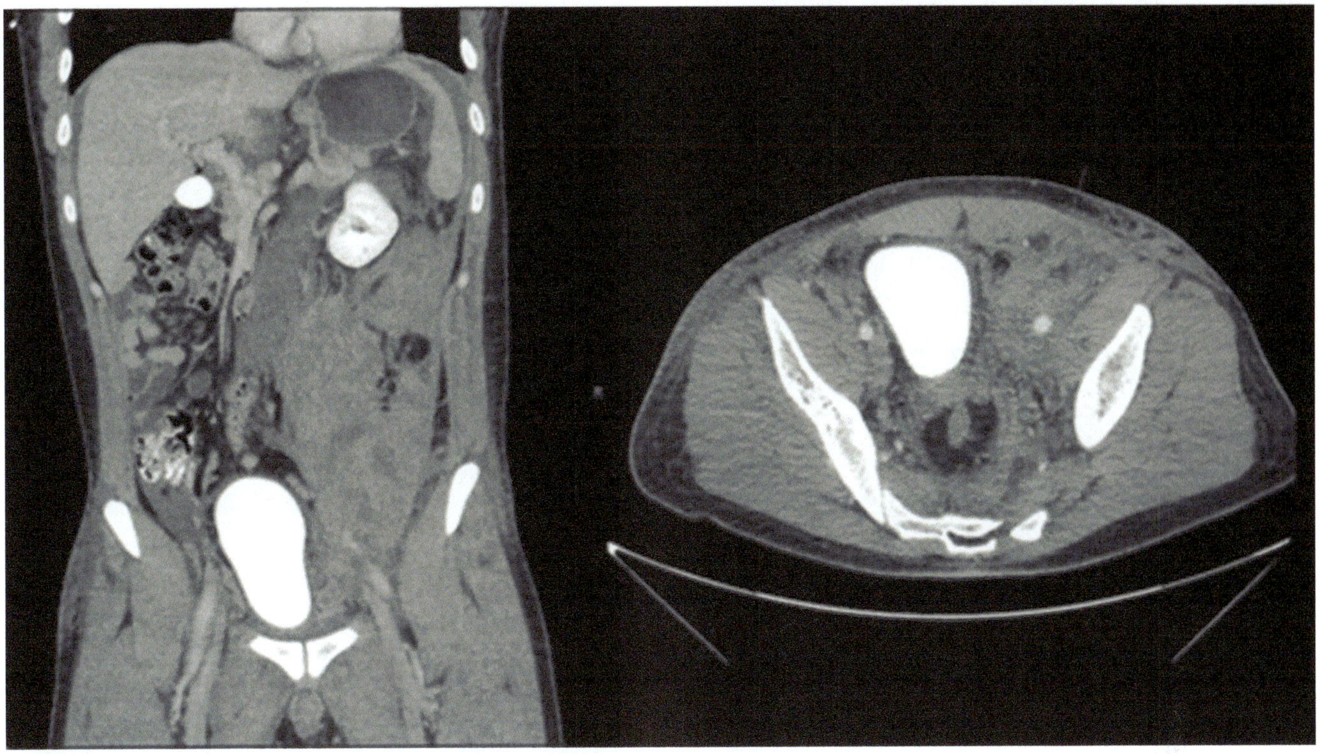

Fig. 43.3 Patient is status postcardiac catheterization from a left femoral approach. There was a high femoral puncture with a large retroperitoneal hematoma.

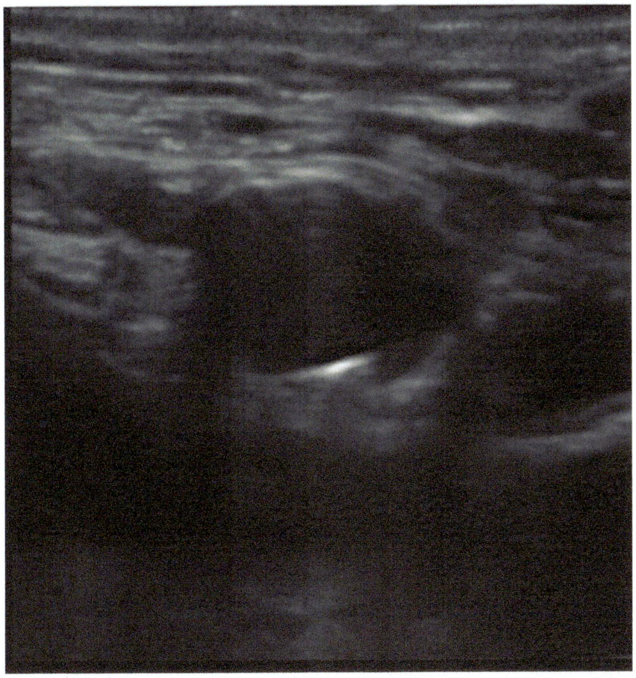

Fig. 43.4 Gray-scale ultrasound of the femoral artery and vein.

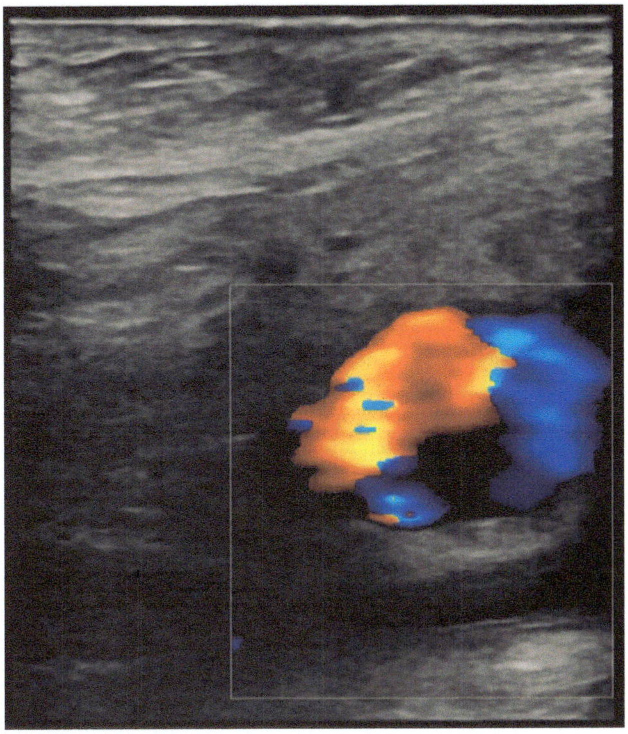

Fig. 43.5 Ultrasound of a common femoral artery pseudoaneurysm demonstrating the classic "yin-yang sign," indicating bidirectional flow.

Over the past 5–10 years, the amount of contrast administered has decreased across all modalities. For example, in most centers today, contrast dosing for CT scanning is weight based with a saline flush. Every patient no longer receives a standard dose, which in the past was 150 cc of iodinated contrast. Currently at our institution, most CT scans use less than 100 cc of contrast. For example, we have performed a cardiac CT for transcatheter aortic valve implantation (TAVI) work-ups with less than 20 cc of contrast. This principle has been carried

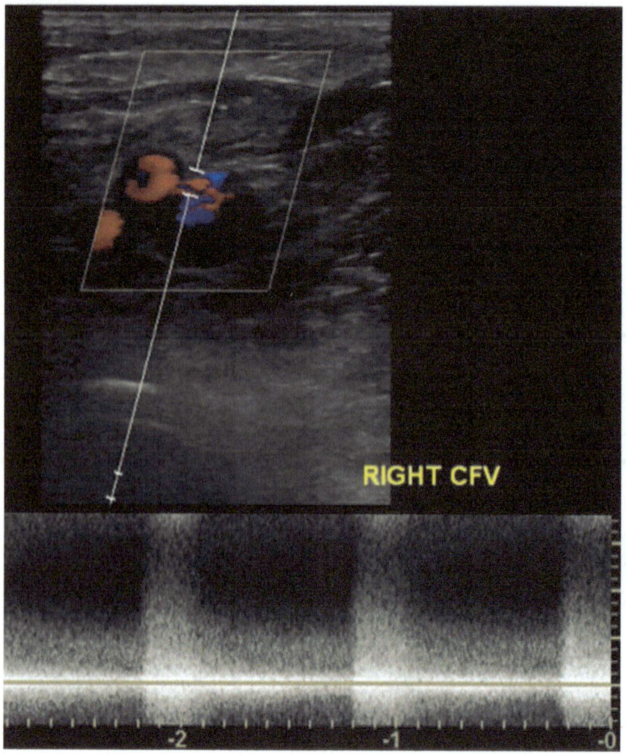

Fig. 43.6 Arteriovenous fistula of the common femoral artery and vein on ultrasound.

over to our interventional service, with pelvic angiograms being performed with as little as 10 cc of contrast as opposed to the previous 30 cc. The industry has also matured, and we have become more aggressive with changing injection parameters. Overall, the total amount of contrast has dramatically decreased, which theoretically decreases contrast-induced morbidity and mortality.

RADIATION EXPOSURE

Fluoroscopy is an imaging modality that utilizes continuous X-ray for real-time visualization and is the basis for conventional angiography. Technological advances in medical imaging have facilitated the ability to perform increasingly complex procedures using a minimally invasive approach. While fluoroscopy offers a lot to the medical field, it exposes the patient and operator to a large amount of ionizing radiation. Ionizing radiation is a carcinogen that leads to cellular damage. From 1980 to 2006, there was an approximately 600% increase in the estimated per capital radiation dose to the general population, increasing from 0.53 mSv to 3.0 mSv. Interventional procedures have contributed to 0.8 mSv of that 2.47 mSv difference, approximately 32%.[20]

The effects of radiation are well documented (Fig. 43.9) where many of the field's pioneers have succumbed to the detrimental effects of excess exposure. Marie Curie and her daughter Irene Joliot-Curie are just a few of the well-known examples who died from excess radiation exposure: Marie from aplastic anemia and Irene of leukemia. So what do we know about ionizing radiation that can cause this? The two major types of radiation effects on the human body are deterministic and stochastic effects. Deterministic effects occur above a threshold and are dose-related.[20] Stochastic effects are caused by mutations or other permanent changes and are not dose-dependent, although the incidence does increases with dose. Since stochastic effects are linear, nonthreshold with longer latency periods, deterministic effects are of

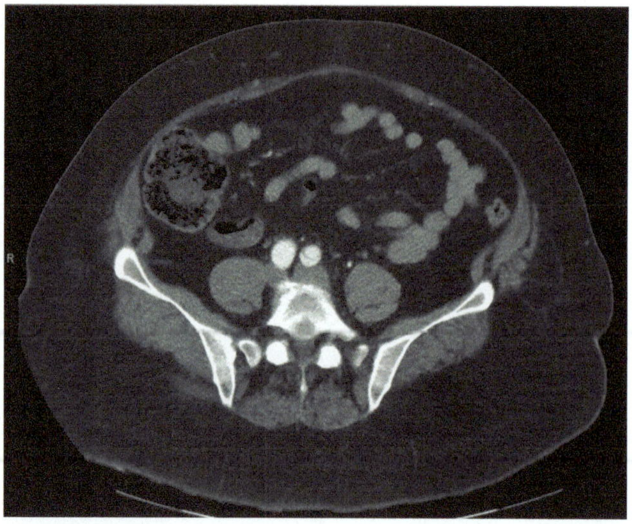

Fig. 43.7 Dissection of the left common iliac artery. Because there was no hemodynamic gradient, the lesion was not treated.

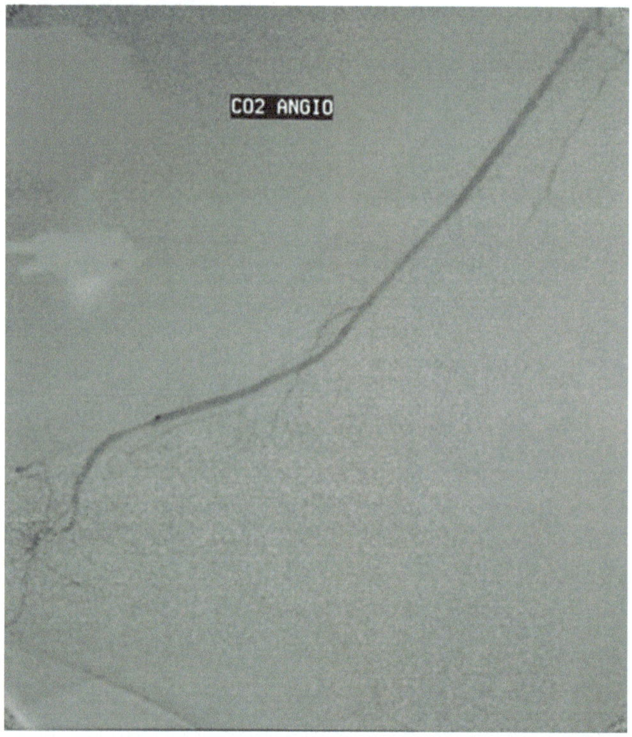

Fig. 43.8 Angiogram of the foot utilizing CO_2.

more interest for health care professionals utilizing radiation in the short term. Radiation dose is measured in dose area product (DAP), which is the total energy imparted to the patient as ionizing radiation.[21] DAP correlates well with stochastic effects. On the other hand, deterministic effects are better measured using air kerma, which is the kinetic energy per unit mass. Table 43.1 lists skin dose and their associated effect.[22]

While ionizing radiation is a considerable risk during interventional procedures, there are many new techniques that allow a significant reduction in fluoroscopy usage. First and foremost, a general

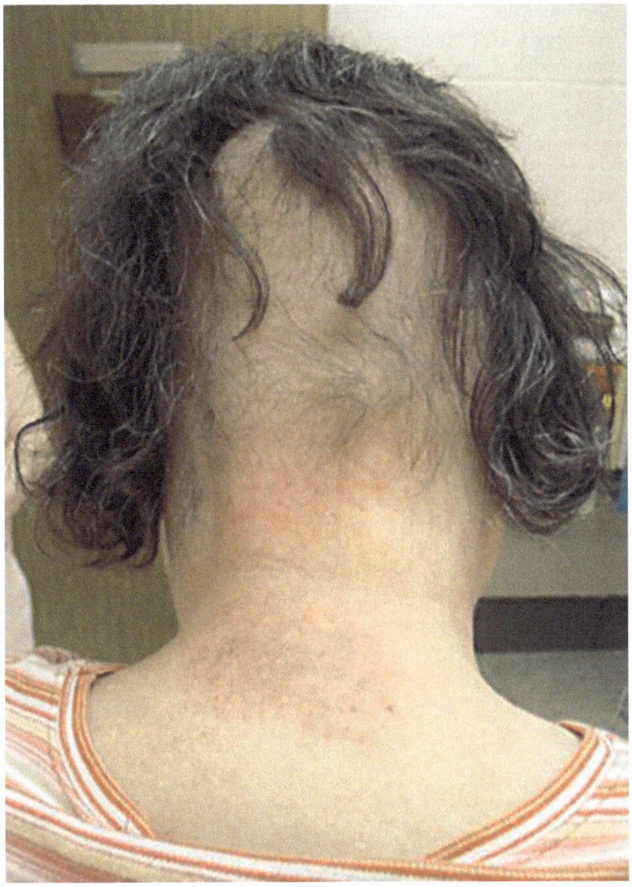

Fig. 43.9 Radiation injury in a 60-year-old woman following a successful neurointerventional procedure for the treatment of acute stroke. Estimated fluoroscopy time was more than 70 minutes; 43 imaging series were performed during the course of the procedure. The head was not shaved. Note focal epilation on scalp and skin injury on neck but not on scalp. No dose estimates were available for this case.

(From Stephen Balter, John W. Hopewell, Donald L. Miller, Louis K. Wagner, Michael J. Zelefsky, *Radiology*. 2010;254:326–341. DOI: 10.1148/radiol.2542082312.)

awareness of radiation dose and fluoroscopy time during the procedure itself leads to a reduction in radiation exposure, which is in keeping with "as low as reasonable achievable" or ALARA. In addition, strict compliance with personal protective equipment (PPE), such as lead shields, collars, and glasses, is imperative. PPE, such as lead aprons with 0.5 mm lead equivalence, reduces radiation transmission by 95%–99.5%.[23] With advancements in technology, there are features that decrease radiation dose, such as last image hold and pulsed fluoroscopy. In fact, new guidelines are implemented to increase radiation safety and awareness. For example, the US Food and Drug Administration mandates fluoroscopic units to have an alarm feature for every 4.5 to 5 minutes of "beam on time."[24] The first major dose reduction techniques included pulse fluoroscopy as opposed to continuous. This can reduce the overall dose by approximately 50%. Last Image Hold places the last image on the fluoroscopic screen so that the physician can contemplate his new sequence without patient exposure. Electronic collimation overlays a collimator blade on the last image so that field dimensions can be adjusted without exposing the patient. Road mapping is a technique to allow physicians to use fluoroscopy over a previously acquired image. Using this map greatly reduces procedure time, thus lowering overall dose.

TABLE 43.1 Skin dose, physiologic effect, and latency period.

Deterministic effect	Skin dose (Gy)	Latency period
Transient erythema	2	2–24 h
Temporary epilation	3	3 weeks
Severe erythema	6	1.5 weeks
Permanent epilation	6	3 weeks
Dry desquamation	14	4 weeks
Moist desquamation	18	4 weeks
Dermal necrosis	18	10 weeks
Secondary ulceration	24	>6 weeks
Telangiectasia	10	52 weeks

From RSNA/AAPM Physics Modules. RSNA, www.rsna.org/RSNA/AAPM_Online_Physics_Modules_.aspx.

New dose reduction algorithms, such as Philips clarity, have significantly reduced fluoroscopy dose. Philips ClarityIQ uses new technology that compensates for motion, decreasing image noise thus enhancing image quality and allowing less radiation to be used to create the image. Many studies are currently being published showing greater than 50% dose reduction.[25] Other companies also realizing the need to reduce radiation dose during procedures, are creating similar algorithms. Siemens uses Care + Clear, while GE uses a blueprint for interventional dose personalization, InnovaSense, Flourostore, and Virtual Collimation.

CONCLUSION

In this chapter we briefly reviewed some of the common and uncommon complications related to conventional angiography. The most commonly encountered complications are related to vascular access, but other complications related to the use of intravenous contrast and ionizing radiation are less common but more revered. It is imperative to have an in-depth knowledge of the potential risks prior to performing endovascular therapies, providing an efficient and safer option for the patient and operator.

REFERENCES

1. Haschek E, Lindenthal O'F. A contribution to the practical use of the photography according to Röntgen. *Wien Klin Wochenschr.* 1896;9:63.
2. Brooks B. Intra-arterial Injection of Sodium Iodide. *JAMA.* 1924;82:1016.
3. Geschwind J-F H, Dake MD. *Abrams' Angiography Interventional Radiology.* Philadelphia: Lippincott Williams & Wilkins; 2004.
4. Krajcer Z, Marcus HH. Update on endovascular treatment of peripheral vascular disease: new tools, techniques, and indications. *Texas Heart Institute Journal.* 2000;27(4):369–385.
5. Schillinger M, Minar E. *Complications in Peripheral Vascular Interventions.* Boca Raton, FL: CRC Press; 2007.
6. Jolly SS. Radial versus femoral access for coronary angiography and intervention in patients with acute coronary syndromes (RIVAL): a randomised, parallel group, multicentre trial. 2011;377(9775):1409–1420.
7. Kandarpa K, et al. *Handbook of Interventional Radiologic Procedures.* Philadelphia: Wolters Kluwer; 2016.
8. Seto AH, et al. Real-Time ultrasound guidance facilitates femoral arterial access and reduces vascular complications: FAUST (Femoral Arterial Access With Ultrasound Trial). *JACC Cardiovascular Interventions.* 2010;3(7):751–758.

9. "STATdx | Diagnostic decision support for radiology." STATdx | Diagnostic Decision Support for Radiology, my.statdx.com/.
10. Stone PA, Campbell JE. Complications related to femoral artery access for transcatheter procedures. *Vascular and Endovascular Surgery.* 2012;46 (8):617–623.
11. Toursarkissian B, et al. Spontaneous closure of selected iatrogenic pseudoaneurysms and arteriovenous fistulae. *Journal of Vascular Surgery.* 1997;25(5):803–809.
12. Beckett KR, et al. Safe use of contrast media: what the radiologist needs to know. *RadioGraphics.* 2015;35(6):1738–1750.
13. Baig M. Shellfish allergy and relation to iodinated contrast media: United Kingdom survey. *World Journal of Cardiology.* 2014; 6(3):107–114.
14. American College of Radiology. Manual on contrast media v10.3 - American College of Radiology, www.acr.org/Quality-Safety/Resources/Contrast-Manual.
15. Mcdonald RJ, et al. Controversies in contrast material–induced acute kidney injury: closing in on the truth? *Radiology.* 2015;277(3): 627–632.
16. Mehta RL, et al. Acute Kidney Injury Network: report of an initiative to improve outcomes in acute kidney injury. *Critical Care.* 2007; 11(2):R31.
17. Gupta RK, Tami JB. Prevention of Contrast-Induced Nephropathy (CIN) in Interventional Radiology Practice. *Seminars in Interventional Radiology.* 2010;27(4):348–359.
18. Spinosa DJ, et al. Gadolinium chelates in angiography and interventional radiology: a useful alternative to iodinated contrast media for angiography. *Radiology.* 2002;223(2):319–325.
19. Caridi JG, Cho KJ, Fauria C, Eghbalieh N. Carbon dioxide digital subtraction angiography (CO2 DSA): a comprehensive user guide for all operators. *Vascular Disease Management.* 2014;11(10):E221–E256.
20. Linet MS, et al. Cancer risks associated with external radiation from diagnostic imaging procedures. *CA: A Cancer Journal for Clinicians.* 2012;62(2):75–100.
21. Dendy PP. Radiation risks in interventional radiology. *The British Journal of Radiology.* 2008;81(961):1–7.
22. RSNA/AAPM Physics Modules. RSNA, www.rsna.org/RSNA/AAPM_Online_Physics_Modules_.aspx.
23. Miller DL, et al. Occupational radiation protection in interventional radiology: a joint guideline of the cardiovascular and interventional radiology society of europe and the society of interventional radiology. *CardioVascular and Interventional Radiology.* 2009;33(2):230–239.
24. Technical principles for diagnostic fluoroscopic procedures. IMAGE WISELY, 22 Dec. 2014, www.imagewisely.org/imaging-modalities/fluoroscopy/articles/pike-technical-principles. Accessed August 29, 2017.
25. Schernthaner RE, et al. A new angiographic imaging platform reduces radiation exposure for patients with liver cancer treated with transarterial chemoembolization. *European Radiology.* 2015; 25(11):3255–3262.

44

Complications Associated With Carotid Artery Stenting

Tanya R. Flohr, MD and Brajesh K. Lal, MD, FACS

INTRODUCTION

Interventionalists are especially cautious with carotid artery stenting (CAS) because complications can lead to devastating and permanent neurological sequelae, even death. Preparation for CAS can often seem excessive; however, careful and detailed planning is the key to circumvent unwanted outcomes. CAS should be used for appropriately selected patients. Knowing the fundamentals of the procedure and some tricks to adapt the procedure for the patient's anatomy and disease are important to avoid complications.

Ironically, some of the initial studies evaluating CAS were performed using stenting to treat intimal flap complications sustained during carotid angioplasty for stenosis.[1] At the time, the bailout seemed an appropriate option given the severity of the stenosis and the instability of the lesion. Unfortunately, in the earliest stages of CAS, stents and delivery systems were faulty, an appropriate antithrombotic regimen was not established, and treating physician technical competence was not ensured. Both procedural difficulties and unwanted complications led to the premature abandonment of CAS. Collaboration among neurologists, cardiologists, vascular surgeons, neurosurgeons, and interventional radiologists is crucial to select appropriate patients. The development of self-expanding stents, embolic protection devices, and a regimen of dual antiplatelet therapy led to the revival of CAS.[2]

CAS has since gone from being the believed replacement for carotid endarterectomy (CEA), to the vascular procedure subject to intense scrutiny with more than 6500 patients studied in six large randomized clinical trials.[3] Appropriate patient selection for surgical intervention and determining proper surgical intervention to treat carotid stenosis are goals of the currently ongoing Carotid Revascularization and Medical Management for Asymptomatic Carotid Stenosis Trial (CREST-2) trial.[4] Today, practitioners offering CAS do so cautiously for a select population with understanding of the complications and risks and benefits profile.

The number and sequelae of the complications associated with CAS have been highlighted with multiple clinical trials but how to avoid and treat these complications has not received as much attention. This chapter looks at the some of the most commonly encountered complications associated with CAS and methods for complication avoidance and management.

PROCEDURAL PLANNING

Simple steps can be taken prior to the procedure to help reduce the complication rate associated with CAS. A thorough history should include a detailed account of any stroke history, in addition to vascular and cardiac history. Prior use of anticoagulation or antiplatelet therapy should be noted, as well as contraindications for such therapy. Patients should have a well-documented neurologic examination performed prior to the procedure. Physical examination should also include a pulse examination of potential access sites. Antiplatelet therapy with clopidogrel should be started 5 days prior to the procedure. Patients should receive a loading dose on the day of the procedure prior to CAS if they are not already on medication. Imaging studies including a bilateral carotid arterial duplex, computed tomography angiography (CTA), or magnetic resonance angiography (MRA) of the chest, neck, and brain should be performed to assess the contralateral internal carotid artery (ICA), vertebral arteries, aortic arch, the Circle of Willis, and other pertinent anatomy. The surgical approach should be established and the appropriate length sheaths, catheters, and wires should be available. Three-dimensional imaging reconstructions can help clarify the appropriate stent, diameter, and length. The interventionalist should ensure that appropriate devices are available for the procedure. The importance of procedural planning cannot be emphasized enough.

ACCESS DIFFICULTIES

Access difficulty can present in extremely dilated aortic arches, aortic arches with severe atheroma with unrecognized ostial lesions of the common carotid or brachiocephalic arteries, and in those patients with tortuous vessels. An angled Glide catheter (Terumo, Somerset, New Jersey) and 0.035″ Glidewire (Terumo, Somerset, New Jersey) are generally the initial choices to cannulate the innominate, right common, or left common carotid arteries. In difficult arch anatomy, particularly bovine arches, a reverse curve catheter such as a JB2 (Terumo Somerset, New Jersey), Vitek (Cook Medical, Bloomington, Indiana), or Simmons-1 (Terumo, Somerset, New Jersey) can be used (or SIM select or SIM2 [Cook Medical]) (Fig. 44.1).

In the case of extremely dilated aortic arches, a sidewinder curved catheter such as a Simmons-3 (Terumo Somerset, New Jersey) can be used to access the brachiocephalic artery (Fig. 44.2). With cannulating the right common carotid artery, the stabilizing introducer sheath should not be too close to the aortic arch because this will decrease the maneuverability of the catheter used to access the right ostium.

Tortuosity in the common carotid artery can be a hindrance to sheath or guide catheter placement. Access should be accomplished by placing a stiff wire, such as an Amplatz (Boston Scientific Marlborough, Massachusetts), in the external carotid artery as far as possible. The tip of the sheath or guide catheter should be secured in the common carotid artery approximately 1 cm below the bifurcation without advancing the introducer into the bifurcation. When the lesion of interest is in the distal common carotid or the external carotid artery is occluded, an Amplatz with a J tip and short (3 cm) floppy segment can be used. Another option would be to use a telescoping guiding sheath over a slip catheter (JB2, Simmons-1, or Vitek) over a stiff Glidewire (Terumo Somerset, New Jersey) to facilitate positioning of the sheath.[5] When maneuvering the introducer sheath over the catheter to the carotid stenosis, if the sheath does not track easily over the catheter, the catheter should be removed and replaced with the sheath's inner introducer. The catheter can then be replaced once the sheath is

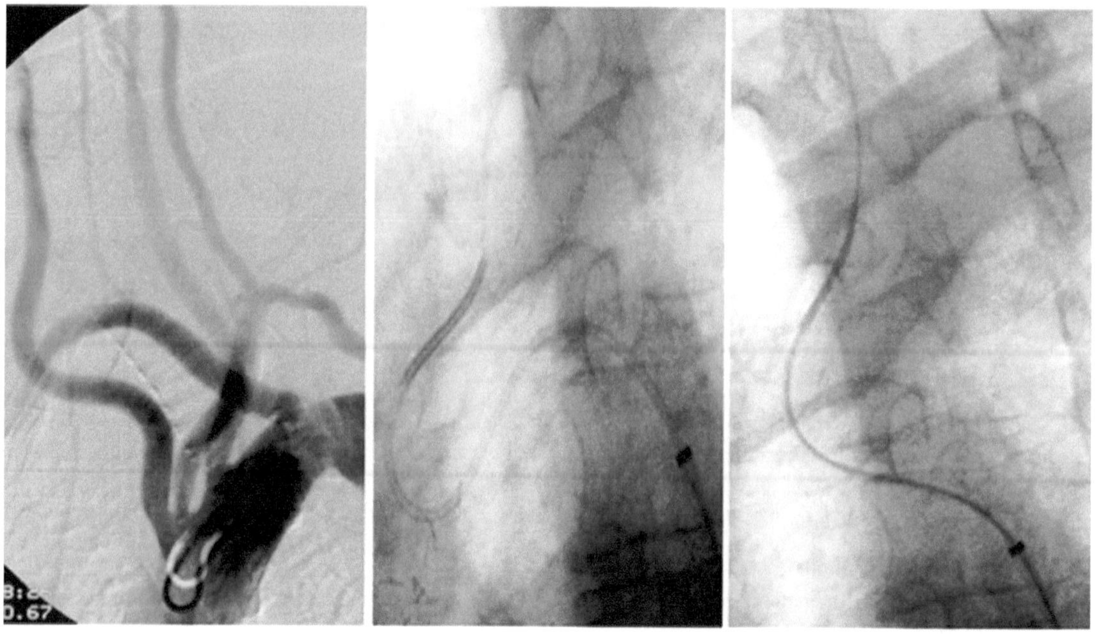

Fig. 44.1 The image on left shows a Simmons-3 catheter positioned in a type III aortic arch (difficult arch anatomy) at the orifice of the left common carotid artery. Centrally and on the right, the images are enlarged to show canalization of the left common carotid artery with wire advancement. Note the position of the stabilizing sheath. The stabilizing sheath should not be too close to the aortic arch, especially to access the right common carotid artery, because this will limit catheter maneuverability.

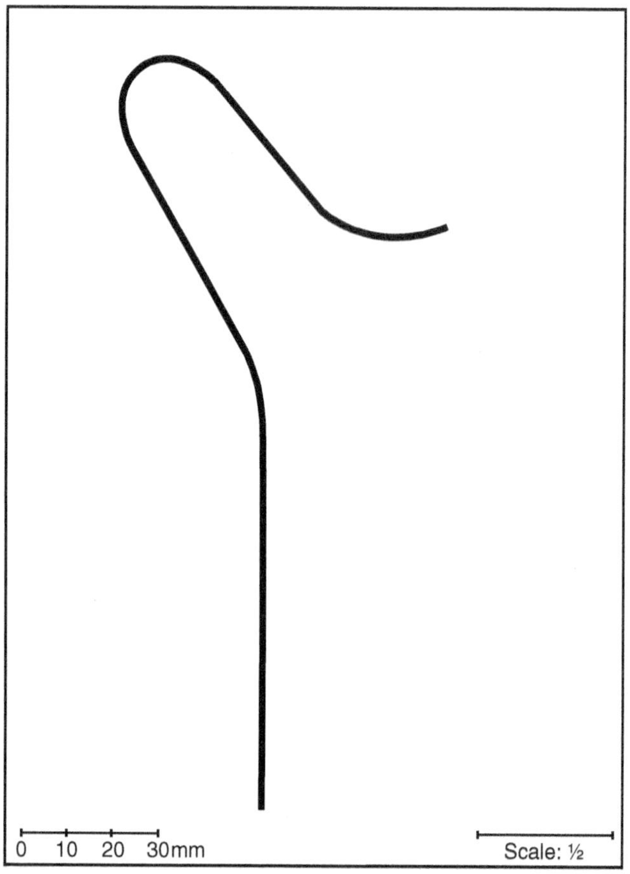

Fig. 44.2 Simmons-3 catheter with large double curvature.

moved into the appropriate position. Common carotid artery (CCA) tortuosity or a stenosis difficult to traverse can be crossed with a Glidewire and 5-French catheter. Be cognizant that when placing the introducer sheath in a long tortuous CCA, this might result in bifurcation displacement and kinking of the vessel complicating stenting. Advancement of the guide catheter or sheath should be done under fluoroscopic guidance or roadmap guidance (Fig. 44.3). ICA tortuosity can also be overcome by using a 0.014″ "buddy" guidewire to assist with straightening out the vessel and the use of a V18 wire to help aid guide catheter sturdiness.

Some anatomic limitations can impede the use of transfemoral access for CAS. Not only can diseased aortic arches and tortuous arch vessels preclude using transfemoral access, aortoiliac and femoral occlusive disease, previous vascular interventions in the groin, and obesity can make CAS with standard transfemoral access impossible. Older individuals (>70 years) have inferior outcomes with transfemoral CAS compared with CEA, probably because of the atheromatous burden leading to embolic events.[6] Careful assessment of the aortic arch is important in the elderly population and may lead to alteration in access site. In such cases, transcervical access might be preferred. In a large meta-analysis of procedures using transcervical access, Sfyroeras et al. showed a technical success rate of 96% for 579 procedures performed.[7] The incidence of transient ischemic attack (TIA), stroke, and death was 2.7%, 1.1%, and 0.41%, respectively. The transcervical approach was analyzed using both flow reversal with an arteriovenous shunt and no flow reversal for stroke incidence, and no difference was noted between the two groups.

The transcervical approach avoids having to navigate through potential atheromatous burden in the iliac arteries, aorta, and arch vessels and dislodging embolizing debris. Flow reversal creates a large arteriovenous shunt between the common carotid artery and ipsilateral jugular vein redirecting blood flow away from the internal carotid

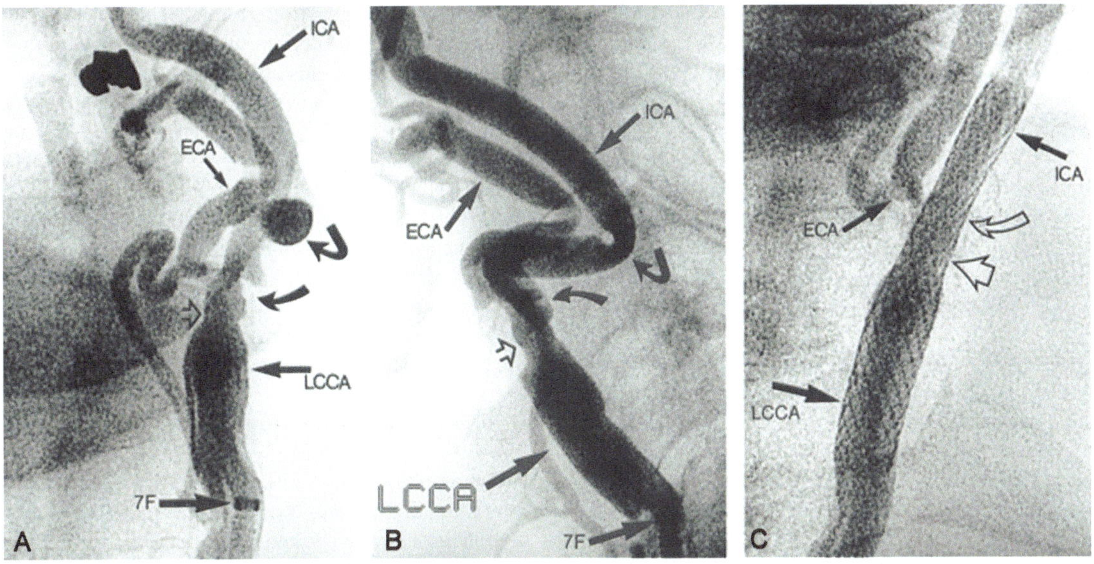

Fig. 44.3 (A) Native common carotid artery *(CCA)* and internal carotid artery *(ICA)* anatomy without the introducer sheath advanced to the distal CCA. Note vessel tortuosity at the curved arrow. (B) Carotid bifurcation displacement and increased proximal ICA tortuosity with the advancement of the introducer sheath and stent. (C) A straightened carotid artery after stent deployment. *ECA*, External carotid artery; *LCCA*, lower carotid artery.

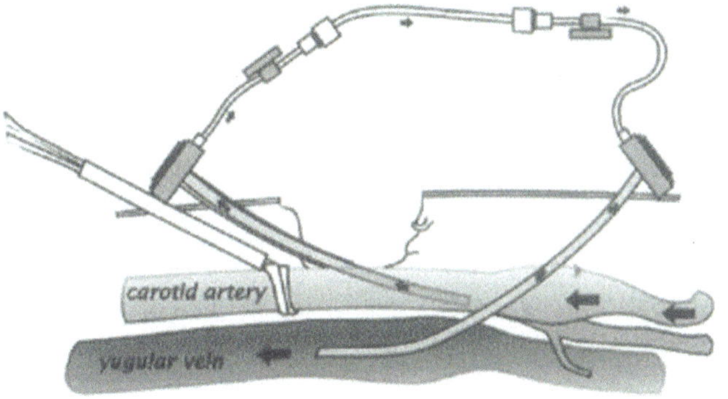

Fig. 44.4 Schematic of transcervical access with flow-reversal. Cardiac and cephalad orientation are right and left on the image, respectively. Note the orientation of the connected sheaths positioned in both the common carotid artery and internal jugular vein, as well as the Rummel tourniquet on the common carotid artery proximally. Flow is occluded in the proximal common carotid artery and directed retrograde from the internal carotid artery into the jugular vein.

artery. The procedure can in most patients be done under local anesthetic. Full details of the transcervical approach with flow reversal are described elsewhere.[8]

Alternatively, transradial approaches can be used to access the carotid artery if the femoral approach is not feasible. From the right side, this negates the need to traverse the aortic arch (Fig. 44.4).

CROSSING PREOCCLUSIVE STENOTIC LESIONS

Wire selection is of paramount importance when crossing the stenosis for CAS. Wires larger than 0.018″ should generally be avoided crossing the stenosis to decrease risk of embolization. If a smaller wire is being used to cross the stenosis, once the lesion is crossed, the wire should be exchanged for a 0.018″ wire to ensure stability and easier advancement of the device required during stenting. Wire exchanges require repeat angiography because the wire stiffness can change the anatomy and presumed stenosis location. It is important to visualize the distal placement of the wire to avoid intracranial location with increased risk of injury to the vessel. The wire needs to be advanced distally enough to allow placement of the filter or protection device.

Difficulty placing embolic protection devices distal to the stenosis is more commonly encountered with filter devices as opposed to balloon embolic protection devices. The crossing profiles for filter devices with U.S. Food and Drug Administration (FDA) approval for use in CAS are 3.4–3.9 French as opposed to balloon devices, which are closer to 3 French. Filter embolic protection devices also have an abrupt change in stiffness between the filter and wire, which can limit trackability. Such difficulties are usually circumvented with predilation of the stenosis. In a study assessing technical difficulties crossing stenotic lesions, Powell et al. reported inability to cross the lesion in 29% of CAS cases using filter embolic protection devices.[9] In 5% of those CAS cases, predilation still did not facilitate filter embolic protection devices to cross the stenosis. In all of these cases, CAS was successfully performed with balloon embolic protection devices. None of the CAS stenoses originally treated with balloon embolic protection devices was unable to be crossed or required predilation. This suggests that a tight lesion might be better treated with a balloon embolic protection as opposed to a filter device for distal protection, especially if the stenosis is narrower than 3.4 French. The MoMa device (Medtronic, Minneapolis, Minnesota) and balloon guide can allow flow reversal state instead of filter protection.

Predilation of stenoses should be performed selectively given the increased risk of periprocedural neurologic events. Nominal pressure should be used unless the lesion is heavily calcified and expected to recoil. Predilation time should be limited to a few seconds if the balloon attains its full shape quickly. Predilation time should only be prolonged (<120 seconds) if the balloon attains its full shape slowly. Preocclusive lesions might require serial predilation with a 1.5-mm or 2-mm balloon, followed by a 4-mm balloon. If the stent to be used does not pass easily through the stenosis after predilation with a 4-mm balloon, a 5-mm balloon should be used for additional predilation. Each additional predilation should be followed with an arteriogram. Only heavily calcified lesions should be postdilated and only if residual stenosis is detected by angiography or intravascular ultrasound (IVUS).

In tight lesions or severe tortuosity, embolic protection devices that are not attached to a wire and advanced independently over a wire might be preferable. Balloon embolic protection devices that advance independently over a wire, such as the GuardWire (Medtronic Minneapolis, Minnesota), have increased flexibility through highly stenotic lesion and tortuous anatomy.

PROBLEMS ASSOCIATED WITH EMBOLIC PROTECTION

It is important to evaluate distal ICA anatomy because deployment of embolic protection devices cannot be done within torturous segments (see Chapter 45). Filter embolic protection devices must be deployed in straight portions of the distal ICA so that there is adequate apposition to the vessel wall. There also needs to be adequate distance between the lesion and the embolic protection device to allow stent deployment. Balloon embolic protection devices are longer and require a greater distance from the lesion and do not allow protection after balloon deflation. If this distance is inadequate, another form of embolic protection should be used. The position of the embolic protection device must also be carefully monitored at all times. Any prolapse of the guide can allow the filter to cross the lesion while deployed.

If there is an excessive amount of embolic debris caught by the filter, a stagnant column of blood proximal to the filter can result on completion angiography. Filter clogging is an uncommon complication but should be identified with a completion angiogram, especially if post-stenting balloon dilation is to be performed. Aspiration can be performed via a catheter with side port, such as an Export AP aspiration catheter (Medtronic, Minneapolis, Minnesota) (or expressway aspiration catheter), placed proximally to the stent. Nitroglycerin can also be given after aspiration in such cases to help restore flow.

Inability to remove the filter embolic protection device is also an infrequent complication that most commonly occurs because of the inability of the capture catheter to cross the stent. This can occur especially if the stent final position is angled or if the embolic protection device wire is too close to the stent. Both can hinder the advancement of the retrieval catheter. Techniques to enable filter capture include repositioning the patient's head to straighten out the stent, external neck compression with swallowing, and advancing the stabilizing sheath into the proximal stent.

TRANSIENT INTRAOPERATIVE NEUROLOGIC COMPROMISE

Transient intraoperative neurologic compromise is a dreaded complication that can be monitored by performing the procedure with the patient awake. The patient can be asked to perform tasks, such as squeezing a squeaky toy upon command. In this way, neurologic compromise can be immediately recognized. Powell et al. reported transient neurologic compromise in 10% of CAS patients treated with balloon embolic protection occurring within several minutes of balloon inflation.[9] Neurologic symptoms were described as global. Eight of 10 patients with neurologic symptoms were successfully treated with stenting after the mean arterial pressure was increased by 20–25 mmHg for balloon insufflation for embolic protection, suggesting that the issue was one of global hypoperfusion rather than an embolic event. The remaining two patients did not tolerate balloon inflation and either required the use of a filter embolic protection device or carotid endarterectomy. Being prepared with alternative modes of embolic protection might be beneficial if the patient cannot tolerate temporary occlusion of flow.

If balloon occlusion with a balloon embolic protection device results in transient neurologic intolerance, it can often be overcome with ischemic preconditioning. If there is immediate intolerance to balloon inflation, the balloon is rapidly deflated when symptoms occur. Once neurologic function returns to normal, the balloon embolic protection is re-inflated and CAS is completed. In the experience of Chaer et al. using balloon occlusion preconditioning, symptoms completely resolved in 4–20 minutes and successful CAS was performed.[10] Balloon deflation for neurologic intolerance and hemodynamic instability should be preceded by aspiration of embolic material.

INTRAOPERATIVE HEMODYNAMIC INSTABILITY

A common physiologic response to balloon angioplasty of the carotid artery is bradycardia occurring in 27%–37% of CAS cases.[11] Hypotension is also common with the reported incidence in CAS ranging from 14% to 28%.[12] In the carotid sinus, adventitial baroreceptors are triggered with expansion leading to hemodynamic lability. Multiple researchers found that stenosis localized to the carotid bulb was an independent risk factor of procedural hemodynamic instability and required drug intervention.[11,13–15] Moreover, the aggressiveness of dilation measured as the change in stenosis severity before and after CAS has been attributed to procedural hypotension and bradycardia.[11,14]

Prolonged hypotension is also not uncommon. Defined by Gökçal et al. as a blood pressure of less than 90 mmHg for greater than 1 hour, prolonged hypotension occurred in 16.8% of patients undergoing carotid artery stenting.[16] More than 70% of those patients were reported to have a contralateral stenosis. Interestingly, prolonged intraoperative hypotension was recognized more frequently in patients who did not have a diagnosis of diabetes mellitus. The diagnosis of diabetes mellitus and history of long-term smoking were found to be protective. Both comorbid conditions are believed to be protective because they impair the carotid baroreceptor response, augmenting sympathetic tone resulting in increased heart rate and blood pressure.[13]

Hemodynamic instability during the peri-operative period in CAS patients was also evaluated by Ulley et al.[17] They defined significant hemodynamic instability as a systolic blood pressure greater than 160 mmHg or less than 90 mmHg, or heart rate less than 60 bpm lasting more than 1 h. Significant hemodynamic instability occurred in 63% of the CAS procedures performed. A predictor of hemodynamic instability during the procedure was a history of recent stroke (odds ration [OR] 5.24, 95% confidence interval [CI] 1.28–21.51, $P = 0.02$). The proposed mechanism by which recent stroke results in hemodynamic instability is impaired parasympathetic and sympathetic cardiovascular regulation that cannot make the autonomic adjustments in heart rate and vascular tone for compensation. Moreover, patients with CAS hemodynamic instability were more likely to experience a periprocedural stroke compared with other patients undergoing carotid stenting (8% versus 1%, $P = 0.03$).[12] Prolonged hypotension following CAS was associated with an increased risk of periprocedural morbidity, including minor strokes (16% versus 3%, $P = 0.003$).[18] The detrimental effects of intraoperative hypotension were also noted with higher rates of mortality at follow-up at 30 days and 6 months (4% versus 1%, $P = 0.05$ and 20% versus 4.3%, $P = 0.02$, respectively).[18]

Interventionalists and treating anesthesiologists should be prepared to treat CAS bradycardia and hypotension. Prophylactic intravenous administration of atropine (0.5–1.0 mg) or glycopyrrolate (0.4 mg) approximately 1 min prior to balloon inflation in the carotid artery is recommended for most adults undergoing CAS to mitigate the vagal

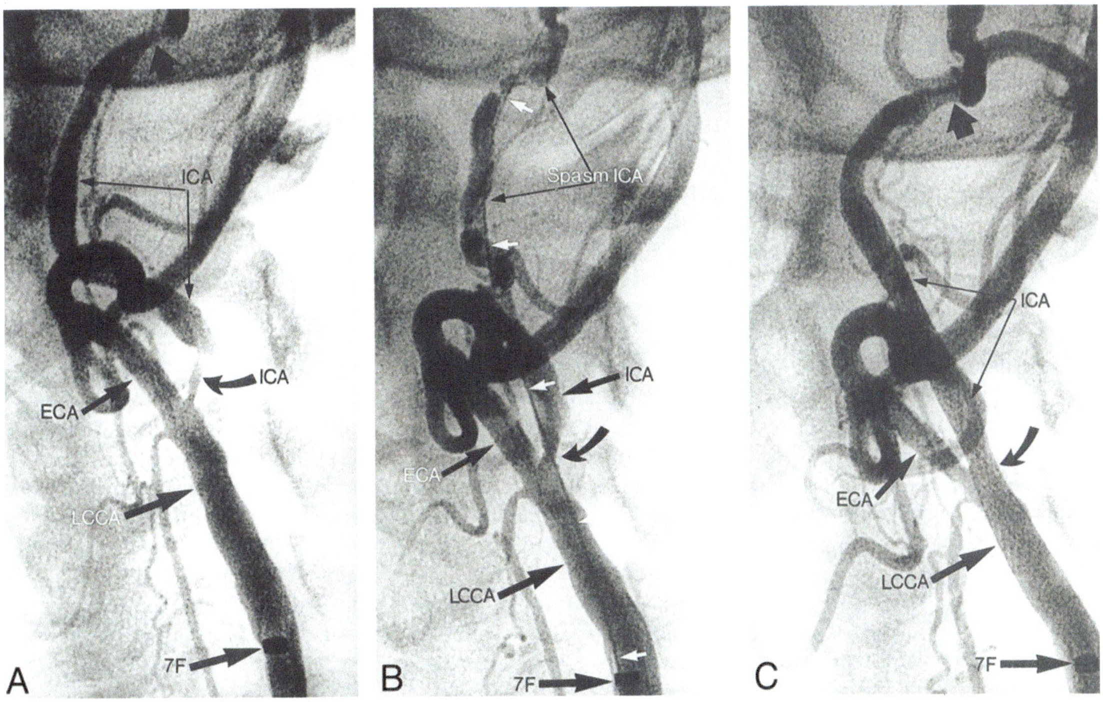

Fig. 44.5 (A) Eighty percent stenosis of the left internal carotid artery *(curved arrow)*. (B) Spasm of the distal internal carotid artery *(ICA) (thin arrows)* after predilation. (C) Minimal spasm of the distal ICA remains after carotid artery stenting is completed. *ECA*, External carotid artery; *LCCA*, lower carotid artery.

response with carotid baroreceptor stretching. Pacemaker capability should be immediately available. Patients with prior ipsilateral CEA undergoing CAS are unlikely to develop the same bradycardic response, and therefore do not require prophylactic atropine. Additional intravenous atropine can be administered to patients with bradycardia or asystole despite prophylactic dosing.

Initial treatment of hypotension should involve volume resuscitation with 500 mL increments up to 2000 mL. Asking the awake patient to cough forcefully can increase systolic pressures by providing autocardiac compression. Dopamine 3 μg/kg/min titrated to a maximum of 10 μg/kg/min can be used to treat hypotension refractory to volume resuscitation. In the absence of bradycardia, hypotension can also be treated with phenylephrine at 50–300 μg/min. Persistent hypertension can be treated with nicardipine 5–15 mg/h. The treatment goal should be a mean arterial pressure of 75–85 mmHg with systolic blood pressure 90–150 mmHg.

CAROTID ARTERY SPASM

The ICA is very sensitive to intraluminal instrumentation and manipulation. A gentle approach with insertion of the wire into the carotid bifurcation and the use of soft-tipped filter wires can, in some cases, help avoid carotid artery spasm. When a carotid artery spasm occurs in the presence of a contralateral ICA occlusion or an incomplete Circle of Willis, the results can be disastrous. Carotid artery spasm has been reported to occur in 4.0%–26.3% of CAS procedures.[19] The vasospasm in the setting of CAS most frequently occurs in the distal ICA and normally resolves with wire and filter removal.

Most of our understanding of vasospasm relates to the compensatory mechanism encountered in the setting of subarachnoid hemorrhage. The proposed mechanism of carotid artery spasm in the setting of distal protection devices suggests that the outward radial force causes endothelial irritation and possibly injury as it shifts during the procedure. First generation embolic protection devices were more likely to cause vasospasm in comparison with newer devices.[20] The frequency of vasospasm has been reported to be more common when using embolic protection filters as opposed to embolic protection balloons (12% versus 2%, P = 0.002).[9]

In a retrospective review of a single center 12-year experience with carotid artery stenting, Fanelli et al. reported ICA vasospasm in 19.4% (123 of 635) of filter-protected CAS procedures.[19] Angiograms performed prior to filter removal in 33 (27%) patients with carotid artery spasm revealed no flow in the vessel distal to the spasm. A total of two minor strokes and six TIAs occurred in the group with carotid artery spasm for a 6.5% neurologic event rate. The neurologic event rate in the population of patients with carotid artery spasm compared with those patients without was similar (P = 0.08). The vasospasm was described as self-limiting in 41 (33%) patients, resolving on its own in approximately 15 minutes with filter removal. The rest of the patients required intra-arterial injection of nitroglycerin for carotid artery spasm resolution. The researchers attributed the vasospasm to a specific stiffer embolic protection device.

If the spasm is not resolved with removal of the wire and filter, 100–400 μg of nitroglycerin in 100-μg aliquots can be infused at the carotid artery bifurcation to help with spasm resolution. Papaverine and calcium channel blockers can also be used as alternative agents. Papaverine should not be diluted in heparinized solution because precipitation can occur. A total of 300 mg papaverine (100 mL of 0.3% solution) can be administered to the affected vascular territory at a rate of 3 mL/min to relieve vasospasm.[21] An intra-arterial bolus of 1–2 mg of verapamil can also relieve vasospasm within 5–10 minutes with little to no effect on the patient's hemodynamics (Fig. 44.5).[22]

CEREBRAL HYPERPERFUSION SYNDROME

Cerebral hyperperfusion syndrome was first described by Sundt et al. after a carotid endarterectomy performed in 1981 when increased arterial blood pressure, ipsilateral headache, seizure, and transient focal neurologic deficits were observed in a patient in the absence of cerebral ischemia.[23] Prior to carotid artery revascularization, ischemic cerebral tissue loses its ability to regulate cerebral blood flow after revascularization. With a high-grade stenosis and long-lasting hypoperfusion, there is maximal vasodilation and impaired autoregulation of the cerebral tissue. High perfusion pressures after carotid artery stenting overwhelm the ability of arterioles to vasoconstrict. Although hyperperfusion, defined as an increase in cerebral blood flow, occurs in most carotid revascularizations, the presence of symptoms is essential in the diagnosis of the syndrome.

In a meta-analysis of carotid revascularization surgeries performed between 2003 and 2008, Moulakakis et al. reported the incidence of cerebral hyperperfusion syndrome after CAS and CEA were 1.16% and 1.9%, respectively.[24] Symptoms of cerebral hyperperfusion syndrome usually occur within the first few days after carotid revascularization but can present up to several weeks after the procedure. Cerebral edema is the cause of the usually transient, neurologic deficit. Hemiparesis, hemiplegia, hemianopsia, obtundation, and aphasia are cortical disturbances that have been reported as associated neurologic deficits.

The diagnosis of cerebral hyperperfusion syndrome can be made by confirming the presence of hyperperfusion on transcranial Doppler (TCD) imaging. Preoperative/baseline TCD assessing cerebral blood flow velocities in intracranial vessels are important to make such comparisons. CT angiography of the head and neck is not predictive preoperatively and can be normal postrevascularization. Conventional MRI findings in patients with cerebral hyperperfusion are not pathognomonic. Single-photon emission CT (SPECT) can detect alterations in brain perfusion and can be helpful in differentiating ischemia from hyperperfusion.

For patients with suspected cerebral hyperperfusion syndrome, initiation of appropriate treatment is important, because uncontrolled cerebral hyperperfusion can result in intracranial hemorrhage. Recommendations include hemodynamic monitoring, maintenance of systemic blood pressure at normal or slightly subnormal values, and TCD to assess cerebral blood flow. No specific antihypertensive agent is recommended.

INTRACRANIAL HEMORRHAGE

Intracranial hemorrhages (ICH), including both intracerebral and subarachnoid hemorrhages, are disastrous complications rarely associated with CAS. The incidence is reported at 0.36%–4.5% of all endovascular carotid procedures.[25,26] ICH is not uncommonly a fatal complication. Symptoms associated with increased intracerebral pressure include vomiting and altered sensorium. Risk factors for ICH include poorly controlled hypertension, intracranial aneurysms, excessive anticoagulation, and CAS in the presence of an ischemic stroke less than 3 weeks earlier. The Carotid Revascularization Endarterectomy Versus Stenting Trial (CREST) found no difference in ICH between CAS (0.3%; 4 of 1262) and CEA (0.2%; 3 of 1240).[25] The risk of ICH is increased for patients undergoing simultaneous treatment for acute stroke with intracranial thrombectomy and CAS. The operator should suspect ICH if the patient develops sudden loss of consciousness preceded by severe headaches in the absence of any intracranial artery occlusion. Anticoagulation should immediately be reversed with protamine and consideration given to reversal of antiplatelet medication. A head CT should be performed emergently.

Prior to strict postoperative blood pressure control, Xu et al. reported an ICH incidence of 1.2% after CAS in their single center experience.[27] All the CAS patients with ICH had a symptomatic ICA stenosis and 60% of them had bilateral ICA stenoses. The presentation of the ICH was generally acute within the first 7 hours after CAS. Of these ICH cases, 80% were cerebral hemorrhages occurring on the ipsilateral side of stenting. All CAS patients with ICH were treated with cessation of antiplatelet and anticoagulation therapy and decreasing systolic blood pressure 20 mmHg under preoperative blood pressure. Large ICH or ICH with midline shift was treated with surgical evacuation. Diffuse subarachnoid hemorrhage with hydrocephalus was treated with external ventricular drainage placement.

Hyperacute ICH is an early subvariant that occurs within hours of CAS following rupture of the perforating arteries in the basal ganglia. It is even more rare but usually fatal. Patient unresponsiveness without prodrome is typical. Most of the case studies describing hyperacute ICH report a highly stenotic carotid lesion and ICH on the ipsilateral side.

STROKE

The underlying pathophysiologic mechanism of stroke associated with CAS is an ischemic insult on the ipsilateral side, usually nondisabling. In a review comparing carotid revascularization techniques, periprocedural strokes associated with CAS were more likely to be nondisabling (62%) compared with CEA (42%) ($P = 0.066$).[28] Hemorrhagic strokes were less common after CAS than CEA (3% versus 18%, $P = 0.016$). With CAS, 74% of the strokes occurred on the day of the procedure, 34% occurred during the procedure, and 26% occurred between postprocedure days 1–30. It is also important to remember that contralateral strokes can occur with carotid stenting with traversal of the arch from dislodgement of atheroma. These are typically embolic and treated as such. Minimizing manipulation of wires and catheters in the aorta is of paramount importance. Also, understanding the arch type and consideration of alternate approaches in patients with diseased or anatomically more complex arch anatomy should be considered.

Age, symptomatic presentation, various anatomic factors, and technical approaches have been evaluated by numerous groups to show positive or negative correlation with stroke. Extreme age (>80 years) has been associated with increased postprocedural stroke and death rates.[6,25,29–31] The SPACE investigators suggested that the higher rate of stroke in this age group was related to manipulation through an aorta with a higher burden of atherosclerotic disease.[29,31] The CAPTURE investigators suggested arch anatomy and increased lesion calcification were the cause.[30,32]

All surgeons performing CAS would agree that symptomatic presentation is correlated with a higher periprocedural stroke rate. In a single center study looking at clinical outcomes after carotid artery stenting, AbuRahma et al. noted performing CAS for TIA was associated with an increased odds ratio of periprocedural stroke (OR 13.7, $P = 0.0114$).[33] The 30-day perioperative stroke rate for asymptomatic patients was significantly lower than for symptomatic patients (0.46% versus 4.2%, $P = 0.0144$).[33] Multiple other groups confirmed these findings.[25,31,33–35]

Interestingly, there is debate regarding whether carotid artery stenosis severity is positively correlated with periprocedural stroke rate. Mathur et al. noted carotid artery lesions with >90% stenosis were associated with a higher 30-day stroke rate compared with lesions with <90% stenosis (14.9% versus 3.5%, respectively, $P = 0.007$).[36] Others did not confirm these findings.[30,32,33] Other anatomic factors found to be correlated with higher stroke risk post-CAS include longer carotid artery lesions, highly calcified lesions, left ICA lesions, and type III aortic arches.[25,30,33,36–39] CAPTURE investigators noted an increased risk of postprocedural stroke if multiple stents were used.[32] Some have suggested the increased number of stents is a surrogate for longer lesion length.

Technical factors associated with increased postprocedural stroke rate include angioplasty prior to stenting. Angioplasty prior to stenting was associated with a 9.1% stroke rate compared with no angioplasty prior to stenting at 1.8%. A multivariate analysis showed angioplasty

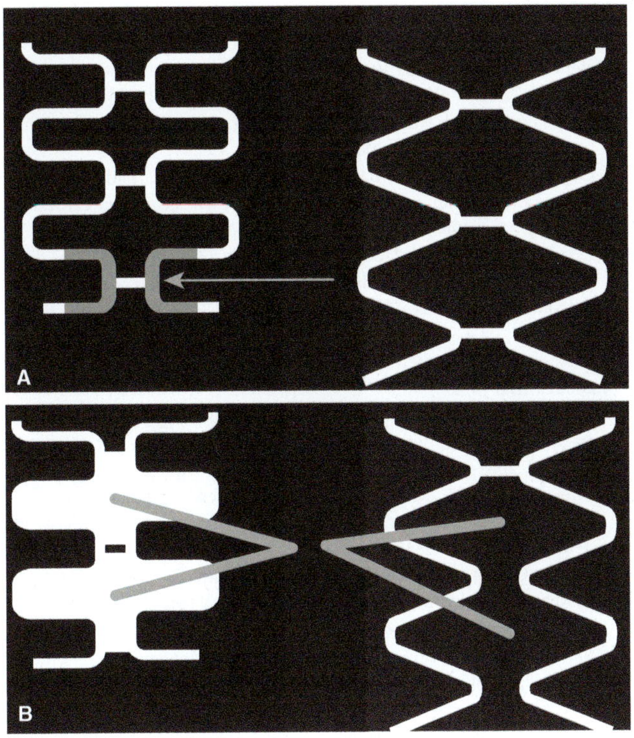

Fig. 44.6 (A) Closed-cell stent design. (B) Open-cell stent design.

prior to embolic protection device insertion had an OR 6.15 of stroke ($P = 0.062$).[33] The CAPTURE study also confirmed angioplasty prior to embolic protection or stenting was associated with a higher 30-day stroke rate.[30,32] AbuRahma et al. also showed angioplasty after stenting was associated with a higher postprocedural stroke rate, but this was not confirmed by other studies.[33] Every manipulation of the plaque, whether by crossing the lesion, angioplasty, or stent placement, can cause embolization. Unnecessary additional angioplasty can increase the risk of stroke and should be avoided. Postprocedure angioplasty places patients at risk of "cheese grating" of the plaque through the interstices of the stent. IVUS is important to assess the appearance after poststent angioplasty.

Carotid stent design continues to be controversial as certain devices in some studies have been associated with a higher stroke rate. Stents were designed with larger gaps between metallic struts (open-cell stents) to enable increased stent conformity to tortuous vessels (Fig. 44.6). These more compliable open-cell stents were found by some researchers to have higher postprocedural stroke rates compared with their stiffer, less conformable, closed-cell stent counterparts. These findings were reported by Bosiers et al. with a total (all) event rate at 30 days of 4.2% in the open cell group versus 2.3% in the closed cell group ($P < 0.005$).[40] More recent reviews and data from the EXACT and CAPTURE 2 trials did not show significant differences in stroke rates between the two stent designs.[30,32,41–43] Microemboli less than 100 μM in diameter comprise most of the emboli produced during CAS, and no current stent design can control these embolic events (see Chapters 46 and 47).

RESTENOSIS

Neurological events are typically not associated with in-stent stenosis because the process responsible is not atherosclerotic disease. In-stent stenosis that develops within 2 to 3 months can be attributed to stent misplacement and technical failure. Beyond 3 months, in-stent stenosis is attributed to smooth muscle proliferation, also known as myo-intimal hyperplasia.[44] The modern incidence of in-stent restenosis after CAS is variable with rates ranging from 2% to 8%.[45–50] In-stent stenosis can be defined as a narrowing of >50% and a peak systolic velocity >175 cm/s. An acceptable annual rate of in-stent (>50%) stenosis was determined to be 1.49% with a cumulative rate at 5 years of 6% as determined by a retrospective study of more than 3000 CAS procedures.[51] More recently, in a review of 9 years of CAS experience including 482 patients who were followed prospectively with carotid duplex ultrasound, Donas et al. reported an in-stent >80% stenosis rate of 3.3%.[45]

The clinical impact of in-stent stenosis after CAS is still uncertain. According to some, the complication rate was not increased for those with in-stent stenosis.[52–54] For others the ipsilateral stroke and death rate for those patients with in-stent stenosis was significantly greater.[55] Fortunately, a threshold for those patients requiring intervention for in-stent stenosis has been established. After a review of 14 studies evaluating for significant restenosis after CAS with CT, angiography, and diagnostic ultrasound, a suggested threshold for treatment of in-stent stenosis should occur with a diameter reduction of approximately 75%, corresponding peak systolic velocities of 300–350 cm/s, end diastolic velocities of 90–140 cm/s, and ICA/CCA ratio 3.8–4.7 on duplex ultrasound.[56] An early post-CAS duplex evaluation for comparison and repeat ultrasounds at regular intervals are suggested.

Reducing modifiable clinical risk factors including smoking cessation, statin treatment for hyperlipidemia, and good glycemic control for diabetes mellitus are the best initial steps to prevent in-stent stenosis. Continued smoking after CAS predictive of in-stent stenosis and elevated post-CAS high density lipoprotein cholesterol levels were negatively correlated with carotid stent patency at one year.[57] Good glycemic control, as measured by a lower hemoglobin A1C, were correlated with reduced major adverse cardiac events after coronary stenting in long term follow-up.[58]

Proposed treatments for in-stent stenosis include endovascular management and surgical stent removal. Whether balloon angioplasty, cutting balloon angioplasty, drug-eluting balloon angioplasty, overlap stenting, or any combination thereof, endovascular treatment is the preferred strategy for treating in-stent carotid stenosis. Moreover, in-stent stenosis, if present after CAS, is an on-going process that might require recurrent treatment and frequent surveillance. In a retrospective study of 574 patients undergoing CAS, recurrent in-stent stenosis occurred in 31% (5 of 16) patients requiring up to four treatments with balloon angioplasty.[45]

Nishihori et al. described their experience treating in-stent stenosis in six patients with overlapping self-expanding stents.[59] Their technical success rate was 100% with no procedural complications, new neurologic events, or recurrent in-stent stenosis at 12 months. The stents most commonly used were carotid Wallstents (Boston Scientific, Marlborough, Massachusetts).

Drug-eluting, balloon-expandable stent treatment for carotid artery in-stent stenosis has also been performed. Seven CAS patients with >70% in-stent stenosis, initially treated with balloon angioplasty, who developed recurrent stenosis were treated with zotarolimus-eluting coronary stents (ZES).[60] Diameter stenosis was reduced from 84.6% to 10.7% with no major periprocedural complications. At 8 and 12 months after treatment, two patients, with distal extension of their ZES beyond the previously placed carotid stent, had complications. One of the two patients suffered a TIA with ZES occlusion; the second required balloon angioplasty of the ZES for presumed crushing of the stent.

Carotid stent explantation is another option to treat in-stent stenosis that is generally reserved for poor primary stenting results and technical failures, preocclusive lesions no longer amenable to angioplasty, and primary stent thrombosis. Strategies for possible ICA reconstruction with either interposition graft or patch repair should be considered preoperatively as the associated inflammatory response to the carotid artery stent can make dissection, identification of the correct endarterectomy plane, and stent removal very difficult. Columbo et al. reviewed their experience with carotid stent explantation at three vascular surgery centers (Mayo Clinic, Dartmouth-Hitchcock Medical Center, and Beth-Israel Deaconess Medical Center).[61] The total number of carotid stents requiring removal were 8 of 971, accounting for 0.8% of carotid stents placed at these surgery centers. Most of the stents removed were Wallstents after patients had a minor stroke (four patients) or developed severe in-stent restenosis (four patients). Half of the explantations were performed urgently. Repair was accomplished with endarterectomy and patch or interposition graft.

In another study treating 41 patients with in-stent stenosis with stent removal, successful postoperative outcome was achieved for 85.4% (35 of 41) of patients.[62] Of 41 patients, 7.3% (three) required interposition graft reconstruction, 7.3% of patients developed a neck hematoma, and 7.3% of patients suffered a TIA. No recurrent restenosis occurred in long-term follow-up.

CONCLUSION

CAS is not a procedure that should be performed without careful consideration, patient selection, and surgical planning. There are many aspects of the procedure that can go awry, some which the interventionalist can control and some which cannot be controlled. Many of the technical and postprocedural complications can lead to stroke or death. While large randomized controlled trials continue to determine the patient population best suited, interventionalists performing CAS should continue to ensure detailed preoperative planning, careful intraprocedural monitoring, meticulous endovascular technique, and close postoperative monitoring to avoid potentially devastating outcomes.

REFERENCES

1. Theron JG, Payelle GG, Coskun O, Huet HF, Guimaraens L. Carotid artery stenosis: treatment with protected balloon angioplasty and stent placement. *Radiology.* 1996;201:627–636.
2. Roffi M, Mathias K. History of carotid artery stenting. *J Cardiovasc Surg.* 2013;54:1–10.
3. Noiphithak R, Liengudom A. Recent update on carotid endarterectomy versus carotid artery stenting. *Cerebrovascular Diseases.* 2017;43:68–75.
4. Mott M, Koroshetz W, Wright CB. CREST-2: Identifying the best method of stroke prevention for carotid artery stenosis. *Stroke.* 2017;48: e130–e131.
5. Malik RK, Vouyouka A, Salloum A, Marin ML, Faries PL. Tips and techniques in carotid artery stenting. *JVS.* 2009;50:216–220.
6. Voeks JH, Howard G, Roubin GS, et al. Age and outcomes after carotid stenting and endarterectomy: the carotid revascularization endarterectomy versus stenting trial. *Stroke.* 2011;42:3484–3490.
7. Sfyroeras GS, Moulakakis KG, Markatis F, et al. Results of carotid artery stenting with transcervical access. *JVS.* 2013;58:1402–1407.
8. Criado E, Boblas M, Fontcuberta J, Orgaz A, Flores A. Transcervical carotid artery angioplasty and stenting with carotid flow reversal: surgical technique. *Ann Vas Surg.* 2004;18:257–261.
9. Powell RJ, Alessi C, Nolan B, et al. Comparison of embolization protection device-specific technical difficulties during carotid artery stenting. *JVS.* 2006;44:56–61.
10. Chaer RA, Tocciola S, DeRubertis B, Lin SC, Kent C, Faries PL. Cerebral ischemia associated with PercuSurge balloon occlusion balloon during carotid stenting: incidence and possible mechanisms. *JVS.* 2006;43:946–952.
11. Lavole P, Rutledge J, Dawoud MA, Mazumdar M, Riina H, Gobin YP. Predictors and timing of hypotension and bradycardia after carotid artery stenting. *AJNR.* 2008;29:1942–1947.
12. Lin PH, Zhou W, Kougias P, El Sayed HF, Barshes NR, Huynh TT. Factors associated with hypotension and bradycardia after carotid angioplasty and stenting. *JVS.* 2007;46:846–854.
13. Gupta R, Abou-Chebi A, Bajzer CT, Schumacher HC, Yadav JS. Rate, predictors and consequences of hemodynamic depression after carotid artery stenting. *J Am Coll Cardiol.* 2006;47:1538–1543.
14. Leisch F, Kerschner K, Hofmann R, et al. Carotid sinus reactions during carotid artery stenting: predictors, incidence, and influence on clinical outcome. *Catheter Cardiovasc Interv.* 2003;58:516–523.
15. Nonaka T, Oka S, Miyata K, et al. Prediction of prolonged postprocedural hypotension after carotid artery stenting. *Neurosurgery.* 2005;57:472–477.
16. Gökçal E, Niftaliyev E, Deniz Ç, et al. Prolonged hypotension after carotid artery stenting: incidence, predictors and consequences. *Acta Neurochir.* 2017;159:2081–2087.
17. Ulley BW, Nathan DP, Shang EK, et al. Incidence, predictors and outcomes of hemodynamic instability following carotid angioplasty and stenting. *JVS.* 2013;58:917–925.
18. Dangas G, Laird JR, Satler LF, Mehran R, Mintz GS, Larrain G. Postprocedural hypotension after carotid artery stent placement: predictors and short- and long-term clinical outcomes. *Radiology.* 2000;215:677–683.
19. Fanelli F, Boatta E, Cannavale A, et al. Carotid artery stenting: analysis of a 12 year single-center experience. *Endovasc Ther.* 2012;19:749–756.
20. Vijayvergiya R, Otaal PS, Bagga S, Modi M. Symptomatic carotid vasospasm caused by a distal-protection device during stent angioplasty of the right internal carotid artery. *Texas Heart Institute Journal.* 2010;37:226–229.
21. Liu JK, Couldwell WT. Intra-arterial papaverine infusions for the treatment of cerebral vasospasm induced by aneurysmal subarachnoid hemorrhage. *Neurocritical Care.* 2005;5:124–132.
22. Feng L, Fitzsimmons BF, Young WL, Berman MF, et al. Intraarterially administered verapamil as adjunct therapy for cerebral vasospasm: safety and 2-year experience. *AJNR.* 2002;23:1284–1290.
23. Sundt TM, Sandok BA, Whisnant JP. Carotid endarterectomy: complications and preoperative assessment of risk. *Mayo Clin Proc.* 1975;50:301–306.
24. Moulakakis KG, Mylonas SN, Sfyroeras GS, Andrikopoulos V. Hyperperfusion syndrome after carotid revascularization. *JVS.* 2009;49:1060–1068.
25. Brott TG, Hobson RW, Howard G, et al. CREST Investigators. Stenting versus endarterectomy for treatment of carotid-artery stenosis. *N Engl J Med.* 2010;363:11–23.
26. Ogadswara K, Sakai N, Kuroiwa T, et al. Intracranial hemorrhage associated with cerebral hyperperfusion syndrome following carotid endarterectomy and carotid artery stenting: retrospective review of 4494 patients. *J Neurosurg.* 2007;107:1130–1136.
27. Xu Y, Wanga Y, Frng L, Miao Z, Ling F. Treatment and outcome of intracranial hemorrhage after carotid artery stenting. A 10-year single center experience. *Interv Neurorad.* 2009;15:316–324.
28. Huibers A, Calvet D, Kennedy F, et al. Mechanism of procedural stroke following carotid endarterectomy or carotid artery stenting within the international carotid stenting study (ICSS) randomized trial. *Eur J Vas and Endovas Surg.* 2015;50:281–288.
29. Kahn M, Qureshi A. Factors associated with increased rates of post-procedural stroke or death following carotid artery stent placement: a systematic review. *J Vasc Interv Neurol.* 2014;7:11–20.
30. Chaturvedi S, Matsumura JS, Gray WA, et al. CAPTURE 2 Investigators and Executive Committee. Carotid artery stenting in octogenarians: periprocedural stroke risk predictor analysis from the multicenter Carotid ACCULINK/ACCUNET Post Approval Trial to Uncover Rare Events (CAPTURE 2) clinic trial. *Stroke.* 2010;41:757–764.
31. SPACE Collaborative Group, Ringleb PA, Allenberg J, Bruckmann H, et al. 30-day results from the SPACE trial of stent-protected angioplasty versus carotid endarterectomy in symptomatic patients: a randomized non-inferiority trial. *Lancet.* 2006;368:1239–1247.

32. Gray WA, Yadav JS, Verta P, et al., CAPTURE Trial Collaborators. The CAPTURE registry: predictors of outcomes in carotid artery stenting with embolic protection for high surgical risk patients in the early post-approval setting. *Catheter Cardiovasc Interv.* 2007;70:1025–1033.
33. AbuRahma AF, DerDerian T, Hariri N, et al. Anatomical and technical predictors of perioperative clinical outcomes after carotid artery stenting. *JVS.* 2017;66:423–432.
34. Yadav JS, Wholey MH, Kuntz RE, et al. Stenting and Angioplasty with Protection in Patients at High Risk for Endarterectomy Investigators. Protected carotid artery stenting versus endarterectomy in high-risk patients. *N Engl J Med.* 2004;351:1493–1501.
35. International Carotid Stenting Study Investigators, Ederle J, Dobson J, Featherstone RL, et al. Carotid artery stenting compared with endarterectomy in patients with symptomatic carotid stenosis (International Carotid Stenting Study): an interim analysis of a randomized controlled trial. *Lancet.* 2010;375:985–997.
36. Mathur A, Roubin GS, Iyer SS, et al. Predictors of stroke complicating carotid artery stenting. *Circulation.* 1998;97:1239–1245.
37. Sayed S, Stanziale SF, Wholey MH, Makaroun MS. Angiographic lesion characteristics can predict adverse outcomes after carotid artery stenting. *JVS.* 2008;47:81–87.
38. Setacci C, Cisci E, Setacci F, Iacoponi F, de Donato G, Rosi A. Siena carotid artery stenting score: a risk modelling study for individual patients. *Stroke.* 2010;41:1259–1265.
39. Naggara O, Touze E, Beyssen B, Trinquart L, Chatellier G, Meder JF, EVA-3A Investigators. Anatomical and technical factors associated with stroke or death during carotid angioplasty and stenting: results from the endarterectomy versus angioplasty in patients with symptomatic severe carotid stenosis (EVA-3S) trial and systematic review. *Stroke.* 2011;42:380–388.
40. Bosiers M, de Donato G, Deloose K, et al. Does free cell area influence the outcome in carotid artery stenting? *Eur J Vasc Endovasc Surg.* 2007;33:135–141.
41. Schillinger M, Gschwendtner M, Reimers B, et al. Does carotid stent cell design matter? *Stroke.* 2008;39:905–909.
42. Fairman R, Gray WA, Scicli AP, et al. The CAPTURE registry: analysis of strokes resulting from carotid artery stenting in the post approval setting: timing, location, severity, and type. *Ann Surg.* 2007;246: 551–558.
43. Gray WA, Chaturvedi S, Verta P. 30–day outcomes for carotid artery stenting in 6320 patients from two prospective, multicenter, high surgical risk registries. *Circ Cardiovasc Intervent.* 2009.
44. Lal BK, Hobson RW, Goldstein J, et al. In-stent recurrent stenosis after carotid stenting: life table analysis and clinical relevance. *JVS.* 2003;38:1162–1169.
45. Donas KP, Eisenack M, Torsello G. Balloon angioplasty for in-stent stenosis after carotid artery stenting is associated with an increase in repeat interventions. *J Endovasc Ther.* 2011;18:720–725.
46. Levy EI, Hanel RA, Lau T, et al. Frequency and management of recurrent stenosis after carotid artery stent implantation. *J Neurosurg.* 2005;102:29–37.
47. Setacci C, de Donato G, Setacci F, et al. In-stent restenosis after carotid angioplasty and stenting: a challenge for the vascular surgeon. *Eur J Vasc Endovasc Surg.* 2005;29:601–607.
48. Zhou W, Lin PH, Bush RL, et al. Management of instent restenosis after carotid artery stenting in high-risk patients. *J Vasc Surg.* 2006;43:305–312.
49. Chakhtoura EY, Hobson 2nd RW, Goldstein J, et al. In-stent restenosis after carotid angioplasty stenting: incidence and management. *J Vasc Surg.* 2001;33:220–226.
50. Ogata A, Sonobe M, Kato N, et al. Carotid artery stenting without post-stenting balloon dilatation. *J Neurointerv Surg.* 2014;6:517–520.
51. Lal BK, Kaperonis EA, Cuadra S, Kapadia I, Hobson RW. Patterns of in-stent restenosis after carotid artery stenting: classification and implication for long-term outcome. *JVS.* 2007;46:833–840.
52. Eckstein HH, Ringleb P, Allenberg JR, et al. Results of the Stent-Protected Angioplasty versus Carotid Endarterectomy (SPACE) study to treat symptomatic stenoses at 2 years: a multinational, prospective, randomised trial. *Lancet Neurol.* 2008;710:893–902.
53. Arquizan C, Trinquart L, Touboul PJ, et al. Restenosis is more frequent after carotid stenting than after endarterectomy: the EVA-3S study. *Stroke.* 2011;42:1015–1020.
54. Naylor AR. Stenting versus endarterectomy: the debate continues. *Lancet Neurol.* 2008;7(10):862–864.
55. Wasser K, Schnaudigel S, Wohlfahrt J, et al. Clinical impact and predictors of carotid artery in-stent restenosis. *J Neurol.* 2012;259:1896–1902.
56. Pizzolato R, Hirsch JA, Romero JM. Imaging challenges of carotid artery in-stent restenosis. *J Neurointerv Surg.* 2014;6:32–41.
57. Topakian R, Sonnberger M, Nussbaumer K, Haring HP, Trenkler J, Aichner FT. Postprocedural high-density lipoprotein cholesterol predicts carotid stent patency at 1 year. *Eur J Neurol.* 2008;15:179–184.
58. Kassaian SE, Goodarzynejad H, Boroumand MA, et al. Glycosylated hemoglobin (HbA1c) levels and clinical outcomes in diabetic patients following coronary artery stenting. *Cardiovasc Diabetol.* 2012;11:82.
59. Nishihori M, Ohshima T, Yamamoto T, et al. Overlap stenting for in-stent restenosis after carotid artery stenting. *Nagoya J Med Sci.* 2016;78:143–149.
60. Tekieli L, Pieniazek P, Musialek P, et al. Zotarolimus-eluting stent for the treatment of recurrent, severe carotid artery in-stent stenosis in the TARGET-CAS population. *J Endovasc Ther.* 2012;19:316–324.
61. Columbo JA, McCallum JC, Goodney PP, et al. Multicenter experience of surgical explantation of carotid stents for recurrent stenosis. *Vasc & Endovasc Surg.* 2016;50:547–553.
62. Zheng J, Liu L, Cao Y, Zhang D, Wang R, Zhao J. Carotid endarterectomy with stent removal in management of in-stent restenosis: A safe, feasible, and effective technique. *Eur J Vasc Endovasc Surg.* 2014;47:8–12.

Embolic Protection Issues

Gursant S. Atwal, MD, Kunal Vakharia, MD, Vernard S. Fennell, MD, MSc and Elad I. Levy, MD, MBA, FACS, FAHA

INTRODUCTION

Stenting of supra-aortic vessels has become a reasonable alternative or sometimes the treatment of choice for cases of athero-occlusive disease of the carotid, subclavian, innominate, and vertebral arteries. Protection from distal embolic debris or thrombus remains critical while performing stenting and angioplasty. The investigators of the Stenting and Angioplasty with Protection in Patients at High Risk for Endarterectomy (SAPPHIRE) trial[1] and the Carotid Revascularization Endarterectomy versus Stent Trial (CREST)[2] demonstrated similar long-term outcomes for endovascular carotid revascularization versus surgical carotid endarterectomy (CEA). The utilization of carotid artery stenting and angioplasty (CAS) in high-risk patients has continued to increase since the publication of the CREST results.[3] The use of embolic protection devices in SAPPHIRE and CREST is thought to have led to lower stroke rates than those in earlier CAS trials. In a systematic analysis by Kastrup et al. of 2537 patients who underwent CAS procedures without protection devices versus 896 CAS procedures with protection devices, stroke rates were lower in the group with protection devices.[4] Similarly, a meta-analysis by Garg et al. reported benefit with use of embolic protection devices.[5] Technological advances continue to improve the safety and efficacy of CAS procedures with the more recent Safety and Efficacy Study for Reverse Flow Used During Carotid Artery Stenting Procedure (ROADSTER) demonstrating the lowest stroke rates of any trial.[6] With the results of these trials, performing CAS with embolic protection devices has become the standard of care.

The decision to proceed with CAS versus CEA is multifactorial. Patient comorbidities as well as anatomical high-risk criteria play a significant role. A detailed discussion on selection criteria for patients undergoing CAS is beyond the scope of this chapter; however, there are anatomical factors that are associated with higher complication rates in CAS procedures that must be taken into account. In our study of patients undergoing CAS for symptomatic disease, carotid tortuosity and difficult distal landing zones were two anatomical factors associated with higher complication rates during CAS procedures.[7] At our institution, the Buffalo Risk Assessment Scale (Table 45.1[7]) is used to aid in patient selection.

TYPES OF EMBOLIC PROTECTION: PROXIMAL, DISTAL, AND COMPLETE FLOW REVERSAL

Patient anatomy and lesion morphology are critical in selecting an embolic protection device. Embolic protection devices can be categorized into proximal embolic protection, distal embolic protection, and complete flow reversal devices or systems. (Flow reversal will be discussed in Chapter 48: Transcarotid Artery Revascularization With the ENROUTE Transcarotid Neuroprotection System). Proximal embolic protection focuses on flow arrest by inflating a balloon in the common carotid artery (CCA) and/or external carotid artery (ECA), thus limiting or arresting anterograde flow in the internal carotid artery (ICA) and preventing distal emboli. Proximal embolic protection is advantageous because it allows the surgeon to cross stenotic lesions under flow arrest, especially when these lesions may require significant guidewire manipulation. In one meta-analysis comparing distal protection with a filter device with proximal protection, proximal protection was associated with a lower incidence of diffusion restriction on magnetic resonance imaging evaluation.[8] However, the flow arrest approach for proximal protection relies on intracerebral collateral circulation, and proximal occlusion can lead to ischemic complications. Additionally, angiographic assessment cannot be performed once flow arrest has been instituted. Periodic deflation and inflation of the balloon allow intermittent anterograde flow and for angiographic assessment but can compromise distal protection.

Options for proximal protection include balloon guide catheters (Concentric or FlowGate; Stryker Neurovascular, Fremont, California) and the MoMa device (Medtronic, Minneapolis, Minnesota). These are typically 9-French systems. Balloon guide catheters are used when the lesion extends into the CCA and the plaque is considered unstable or there is concern for intraluminal thrombus. Balloon inflation allows advancement of a filter wire (0.014″) across the lesion under near flow arrest (the ECA is not occluded). Subsequently, the filter can be deployed to aid embolic protection. Intermittent inflation and deflation allows restoration of flow to prevent ischemic complications while the filter adds protection once the balloon is deflated. The MoMa device is best suited for lesions isolated to the ICA with unstable plaque or intraluminal thrombus. This is a two-balloon system that allows the lesion to be crossed under complete flow arrest (ECA occluded) with a 0.014″ wire. We prefer to use the MoMa device for symptomatic lesions. The investigators of the Proximal Protection with the MoMa Device During Carotid Stenting (ARMOUR) trial demonstrated the safety and efficacy of the MoMa device with an overall stroke rate of 1.9% with no strokes occurring in symptomatic patients.[9] Additionally, the ROADSTER investigators have shown a similar low stroke rate of 1.4%, demonstrating the safety of proximal protection and flow reversal.[6] Proximal protection is our choice when there is distal cervical ICA tortuosity that precludes safe landing of a filter device (Fig. 45.1). As stated previously, these anatomical factors can lead to higher complication rates.[7] Use of the MoMa device is limited by the fact that establishing proximal occlusion in the ECA and CCA requires that the stenotic lesion not extend into the CCA. Additionally, proximal protection relies on good intracranial collateral circulation. Ischemic complications can occur secondary to prolonged occlusion time and blood pressure management is critical while using proximal protection devices. Care must be taken when using these devices because balloon inflation can lead to dissection.

Distal embolic protection devices are filter devices. Distal occlusion of the ICA with a balloon can also be used; however, this is less common. Filter devices have become increasingly used for both

TABLE 45.1 Buffalo Risk Assessment Scale for carotid artery stenting.

Variable	Points
Carotid tortuosity (any)	2
Difficult distal landing zone	2
Concentric calcification	1
Carotid pseudo-occlusion	1
Difficult femoral access	1
NIHSS Score ≥ 10	1
Renal disease	1
Maximum scale points	9
Total score	
BRASS I (low risk)	0–2
BRASS II (moderate risk)	3–4
BRASS III (high risk)	5–9

BRASS, Buffalo Risk Assessment Scale; *NIHSS*, National Institutes of Health Stroke Scale.
With permission from Fanous AA, Natarajan SK, Jowdy PK, et al. High-risk factors in symptomatic patients undergoing carotid artery stenting with distal protection: Buffalo Risk Assessment Scale (BRASS). *Neurosurgery*. 2015;77:531–542; discussion 533–542.

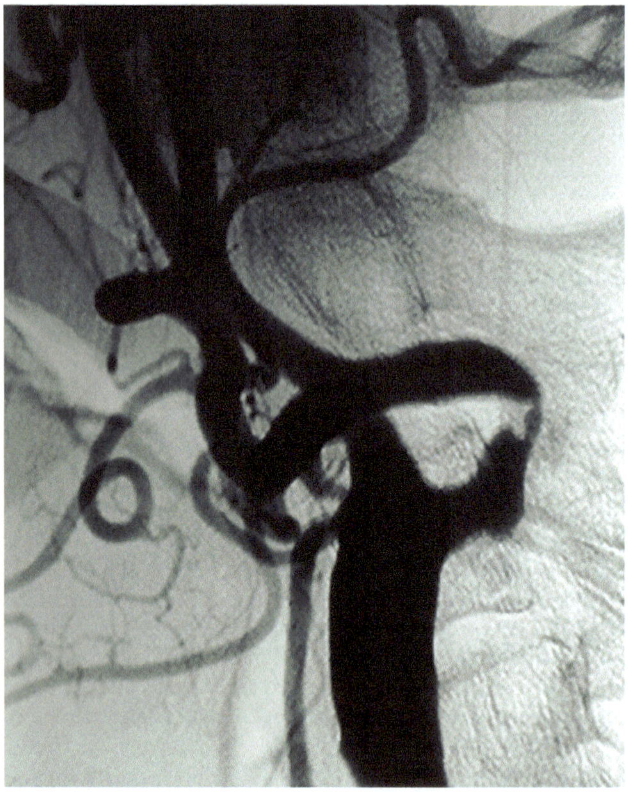

Fig. 45.1 The cervical internal carotid artery tortuosity seen on this digital subtraction angiogram presents a difficult distal landing zone for filter deployment.

symptomatic and asymptomatic carotid stenoses. Each system is based on a 0.014″ guidewire for access past the stenotic lesion. Deployment is preferred in the straight segment of the ICA, usually at the level of the C1 vertebra. Filter devices are available in different sizes (Table 45.2). The benefit of this system for the surgeon is particularly important in patients who do not have good collateral circulation and cerebrovascular reserve. In cases of insufficient collateral flow, the distal filter device allows preservation of flow during the procedure. When approaching a carotid lesion, understanding the access site is paramount for planning. Type of aortic arch, CCA/ICA tortuosity, and morphology of the lesion (isolated to the ICA versus combined CCA/ICA, plaque versus thrombus) are taken into consideration before selecting an embolic protection device. For example, type III aortic arches and tortuous proximal CCAs require more flexible catheters and devices. Proximal protection in these situations may not be feasible. Low profile, flexible filter devices allow easier maneuverability into the more distal carotid artery and safe deployment prior to angioplasty and stent deployment. In addition, surgeons must take into consideration the type of stenosis and lesion that they have to manage. Low-profile, soft-tipped flexible devices are ideal because they allow navigability without the constraint of damaging the vessel wall or disturbing the plaque burden. Moreover, these devices can be used with smaller (6-French) systems (Tip Box 45.1).

STENTING AND ANGIOPLASTY OF THE BRACHIOCEPHALIC AND SUBCLAVIAN ARTERIES

Stenting and angioplasty of the brachiocephalic (innominate) and subclavian arteries for symptomatic disease is effective. In a recent trial, patients with symptomatic subclavian or innominate stenosis undergoing stenting and angioplasty demonstrated good long-term outcomes and low periprocedural complication rates.[10] Embolic protection devices should be considered for stenting and angioplasty of the brachiocephalic (innominate), subclavian, or vertebral artery (VA). In instances of subclavian steal syndrome, flow reversal in the VA is protective from distal emboli. However, in cases where the plaque in the subclavian artery encroaches the origin of the VA or mobile thrombus is present, embolic protection must be considered. This can be accomplished with a filter, guidewire, or balloon inflation. The decision to select one of these devices is contingent upon the anatomical factors, such as size of the VA and anatomy of the stenotic segment. Balloon occlusion of the subclavian artery proximal to the lesion with a balloon guide catheter can result in flow reversal in the VA for embolic protection.[10] Additionally, distal filters can be used, as in CAS.[10]

At our institution, covered stents are preferred for subclavian and innominate arteries to prevent "cheese grating" and distal emboli during stent deployment. Additionally, we prefer combined transfemoral and transradial access to protect the VA ostia from embolic debris during subclavian artery stenting in select cases and in cases of no spontaneous flow reversal, mobile thrombus, and where the vertebral artery is the dominant or sole supply to posterior circulation and the plaque encroaches the vertebral ostia. The transfemoral route is used for stent delivery and deployment, whereas the transradial route allows access to the VA without manipulation of the plaque. An intracranial balloon mounted over a 0.014″ wire is advanced into the VA and inflated for protection. Subsequently, the transfemoral route is used to cross the lesion and deploy of the stent. This approach relies on good intracranial collateral circulation determined by preprocedure angiography. Ischemic complications can occur if the patient has poor collateral circulation or if prolonged balloon occlusion is required during the procedure. In cases of poor collateral circulations, distal filters are a better choice for embolic protection. Full heparinization with an activated coagulation time (ACT) within therapeutic range and dual antiplatelet therapy are essential, as in all stenting and angioplasty procedures. The routine use of distal embolic protection is not standard and should be considered for select cases because the use of wire and embolic

TABLE 45.2 **Specifications of stent and embolic protection device combinations approved by the U.S. Food and Drug Administration.**

Stent	Filter	Characteristics	Pore size (μm)	Lesion crossing profile (French)	Available filter diameters (mm)
Acculink[a]	Emboshield[a] NAV6	Concentric	120	2.7–3.1	5.0, 7.2
Acculink[a]	Accunet[a]	Concentric	125	3.5–3.7	4.5, 5.5, 6.5, 7.5
Precise[b]	Angioguard[b]	Concentric	100	3.2–3.9	4, 5, 6, 7, 8
Xact[a]	Emboshield[a]	Concentric, bare wire	120	2.8–3.2	Small 2.5–4.8 Large 4–7
NexStent[c]	EZ Filterwire[c]	Eccentric	110	3.2	One size fits all
Protégé[d]	SpiderRX[d]	Eccentric	Variable	3.2	3, 4, 5, 6, 7
(several)	FiberNet[e]	Occluder + filter	40	2.4–2.9	3.5–7.0

[a]Abbott Vascular (Santa Clara, California)
[b]Cordis Corporation (Bridgewater, New Jersey)
[c]Boston Scientific (Natick, Massachusetts)
[d]Medtronic (Minneapolis, Minnesota)
[e]Lumen Biomedical (Plymouth, Minnesota)
Adapted from Natarajan SK, Snyder KV, Siddiqui AH, et al. Carotid angioplasty and stenting for occlusive disease. In: Sekhar LN, Fessler RG, eds. *Atlas of Neurosurgical Techniques: Brain*, Volume 1, 2nd ed. New York: Thieme; 2016: 616–633, Table 42.2, p. 620.

TIP BOX 45.1

Evaluation of the filter landing zone is crucial in assessing proximal versus distal embolic protection.

protection devices (filters and balloons) in the vertebral artery can cause vessel injury resulting in dissection.[10]

COMMON COMPLICATIONS

For most CAS procedures, we prefer distal embolic protection with filters. Vasospasm is common because of movement of the filter wire. Severe vasospasm can lead to ischemic complications. Intra-arterial verapamil is our preferred method to treat filter-related vasospasm (10 mg of intra-arterial verapamil; repeat 1 to 2 times as needed). Care must be taken when using proximal protection devices because iatrogenic dissections can occur. Iatrogenic dissections can be treated with placement of an additional stent if flow limiting. For non-flow-limiting dissections, dual antiplatelet therapy (in which the patients are placed on for CAS) is usually the treatment of choice.

AVOIDING COMPLICATIONS

For all stenting and angioplasty procedures, systemic heparinization with an ACT >250 seconds is recommended to avoid thromboembolic complications. Additionally, we routinely check the efficacy of the dual antiplatelet regimen prior to the procedure with PY12 and aspirin assays. In our experience, ensuring responsiveness to antiplatelet therapy is associated with a lower rate of ischemic complications.[11] A complete understanding of the arch anatomy and access to the lesion enable appropriate devices to be selected prior to initiation of the procedure. It is our practice to perform a computed tomographic angiogram of the head and neck to be cognizant of anatomical considerations. Additionally, paying close attention to blood pressure control can prevent the development of reperfusion or hyperperfusion syndrome postprocedure.

TIP BOX 45.2

The use of fixed-wire distal filters can result in vasospasm. Intra-arterial verapamil is useful in treating filter-related vasospasm. Additionally, a buddy wire can be used to straighten a proximal curve, which can aid in stent deployment and capturing of the filter.

For patients with poor collateral circulation that requires proximal protection, intermittent deflation of the balloon and back bleeding by opening the stopcock are critical steps in preventing ischemic complications. For patients with significant tortuosity that requires a distal filter, the tortuous segment can be straightened with a buddy wire (typically a 0.018″ wire; preferably a V-18 wire: Boston Scientific, Massachusetts) after the deployment of the filter. This can be accomplished using the same guide catheter (minimum 6 French) without having to upsize the sheath. This can aid in deployment of the stent as well as filter retrieval (Tip Box 45.2).

GETTING OUT OF TROUBLE

Significant tortuosity can lead to difficulty deploying and, more importantly, capturing the filter. Additionally, the filter can get trapped on the stent tines. In those circumstances, we capture the filter with the guide catheter. This process can be challenging if there is significant proximal tortuosity. In such a case, a buddy wire can be used to straighten the vessel after the filter has been deployed (as mentioned previously). Also, debris can be found in the filter and/or intraluminally in the stented segment. For unstable plaques or cases involving intraluminal thrombus, intravascular ultrasound imaging can be used before capturing the filter to avoid emboli from the stented segment. If debris is confirmed in the filter after the stent deployment angiographic run, an Export catheter (Medtronic) is used for aspiration of the filter prior to capture. This helps to prevent thromboembolic complications and facilitates capture of the filter. In rare cases, there can be an intracranial large vessel occlusion. This warrants emergent mechanical thrombectomy. The occlusion can be detected by a change in the patient's neurologic status. At our institution, most extracranial stenting procedures are performed in awake patients under sedation so that frequent neurologic assessments can be performed. A change in neurologic status at the end of the procedure necessitates repeat angiographic assessment.

ACKNOWLEDGMENTS

The authors thank Paul H. Dressel BFA for preparation of the illustration and Debra J. Zimmer for editorial assistance.

REFERENCES

1. Yadav JS, Wholey MH, Kuntz RE, et al. Protected carotid-artery stenting versus endarterectomy in high-risk patients. *N Engl J Med.* 2004;351:1493–1501.
2. Brott TG, Howard G, Roubin GS, et al. Long-term results of stenting versus endarterectomy for carotid-artery stenosis. *N Engl J Med.* 2016;374:1021–1031.
3. Salzler GG, Farber A, Rybin DV, et al. The association of Carotid Revascularization Endarterectomy versus Stent Trial (CREST) and Centers for Medicare and Medicaid Services Carotid Guideline Publication on utilization and outcomes of carotid stenting among "high-risk" patients. *J Vasc Surg.* 2017;66:104–111.e1.
4. Kastrup A, Groschel K, Krapf H, et al. Early outcome of carotid angioplasty and stenting with and without cerebral protection devices: a systematic review of the literature. *Stroke.* 2003;34:813–819.
5. Garg N, Karagiorgos N, Pisimisis GT, et al. Cerebral protection devices reduce periprocedural strokes during carotid angioplasty and stenting: a systematic review of the current literature. *J Endovasc Ther.* 2009;16:412–427.
6. Kwolek CJ, Jaff MR, Leal JI, et al. Results of the ROADSTER multicenter trial of transcarotid stenting with dynamic flow reversal. *J Vasc Surg.* 2015;62:1227–1234.
7. Fanous AA, Natarajan SK, Jowdy PK, et al. High-risk factors in symptomatic patients undergoing carotid artery stenting with distal protection: Buffalo Risk Assessment Scale (BRASS). *Neurosurgery.* 2015;77:531–542; discussion 542–543.
8. Stabile E, Sannino A, Schiattarella GG, et al. Cerebral embolic lesions detected with diffusion-weighted magnetic resonance imaging following carotid artery stenting: a meta-analysis of 8 studies comparing filter cerebral protection and proximal balloon occlusion. *JACC Cardiovasc Interv.* 2014;7:1177–1183.
9. Ansel GM, Hopkins LN, Jaff MR, et al. Safety and effectiveness of the INVATEC Mo.Ma proximal cerebral protection device during carotid artery stenting: results from the ARMOUR pivotal trial. *Catheter Cardiovasc Interv.* 2010;76:1–8.
10. Przewlocki T, Wrotniak L, Kablak-Ziembicka A, et al. Determinants of long-term outcome in patients after percutaneous stent-assisted management of symptomatic subclavian or innominate artery stenosis or occlusion. *EuroIntervention.* 2017;13:1355–1364.
11. Sorkin GC, Dumont TM, Wach MM, et al. Carotid artery stenting outcomes: do they correlate with antiplatelet response assays? *J Neurointerv Surg.* 2014;6:373–378.

46

Complications Specific to Closed and Open Cell Nitinol Stents in Carotid Artery Stenting

Richard J. Powell, MD and Nikolaos Zacharias, MD, FSVS, FACS

INTRODUCTION

The use of carotid artery stenting to treat carotid bifurcation stenosis remains a topic of recent investigation and vigorous debate regarding safety and efficacy. Multiple prospective randomized controlled trials have compared carotid endarterectomy (CEA) with carotid artery stenting (CAS) and have shown comparable outcomes in asymptomatic patients.[1,2] There are certain complications that are more frequent or specific to the use of closed versus open cell nitinol carotid artery stents. This chapter focuses on clinical evidence describing the complications as well as the clinical decision making and preoperative evaluation to limit these complications.

COMPLICATIONS

Complications following CAS with closed and open cell nitinol stents can be divided into periprocedural and late. Periprocedural complications include inability to cross the lesion with the stent, severe residual stenosis, and postprocedure stroke. Late complications include stent fracture and/or deformation, restenosis, and late stroke.

Early Complications

Inability to cross the carotid stenosis has multiple etiologies that include tortuous artic arch and a tortuous common carotid artery. The flexibility of the stent can be an important determinant in successfully negotiating tortuous vessels. In general, the open cell stents such as the PRECISE (Cordis, Hialeah, FL) and ACCULINK (Abbott Laboratories, Chicago, IL) are more flexible than the closed cell XACT stent and may cross tortuous aortic arch—carotid anatomy, which the XACT (Abbott Laboratories, Chicago, IL) may not successfully track despite the use of stiffer embolic protection delivery wires.

Residual stenosis following stent placement can usually be successfully treated with poststent balloon angioplasty. However, in certain critically stenotic lesions, especially in the presence of calcification of the carotid bifurcation, residual carotid stenosis can be a problem. The higher radial force of the closed cell XACT stent may be more resistant to compressive forces at the bifurcation when compared with open cell nitinol stents and may be beneficial in limiting residual stenosis.

Postprocedure stroke severity and timing during CAS may be related to stent design. Closed cell stents have a lower cell area compared with open cell stents and may provide better coverage of the atherosclerotic lesion (Fig. 46.1). In a study by Cao and coworkers in which they reviewed 505 CAS procedures, all but one major stroke occurred during catheterization of the target vessel or crossing the lesion with the embolic protection device (EPD).[3] No major strokes occurred in the postprocedure period. Thirteen of 16 minor strokes, however, occurred within 24 hours of the CAS procedure. Minor strokes following CAS are related to embolic material extruding through the stent architecture and subsequent embolization. Theoretically, an open cell stent has a higher chance of atheromatic plaque material extruding into the arterial lumen. Although controversial, there are data suggesting that stents with the lowest stent cell area are at lower risk of postprocedure stroke.[4,5] The closed cell nitinol XACT stent has a lower cell surface area compared with the PRECISE and ACCULINK and in some studies has been shown to have a lower postprocedure incidence of stroke. However, there have been two large randomized trials comparing CAS with CEA: the CREST and ACT-1 trials.[1,2] The ACCULINK open cell stent was used in the CREST Trial and the closed cell nitinol XACT stent was used in the ACT-1 Trial. In asymptomatic patients, the primary endpoint of 30-day stroke, death, myocardial infarction, and late stroke occurred in 5.6% of patients in the CREST trial compared with 3.8% of patients in the ACT-1 trial (Table 46.1). The concept of improving coverage of the atherosclerotic plaque by lowering cell surface area has resulted in the ongoing development of stents with superimposed mesh on the stent framework to provide widespread coverage of the lesion and potentially limit postprocedure stroke.

Late Complications

Carotid stent fracture and deformation may be more common than previously thought and are related to stent design (Fig. 46.2).[6–8] Ling et al. reported a carotid stent fracture prevalence of 29% in 48 stents and also observed a higher restenosis rate of 21% in fractured stents compared with 9% in stents without fracture.[6] In contrast, Varcoe et al. described a fracture rate of 2% in 51 carotid stents and noted no clinical sequelae.[7] In a third series, which is the largest to date, the incidence of stent fracture and/or deformation following carotid bifurcation stenting approached a combined rate of 50% at 4 years. The prevalence of stent fracture was observed to be 4% and that of stent deformation to be 23%. These measurements tend to corroborate the rates noted in the two published series in which carotid stent changes were common, ranging from 13% to 29%.[6,7] The development of either stent fracture or deformation was found to be approximately six times more common in the setting of highly calcified carotid arteries, as reflected by easily visible calcification on plain films of the neck ($P = 0.003$) (Fig. 46.3). That study observed that the presence of carotid artery calcification on plain film was associated with nearly an eight-fold increase in the odds of stent fracture.[6] A correlation between extensive calcification and a higher rate of fracture had also previously been demonstrated in

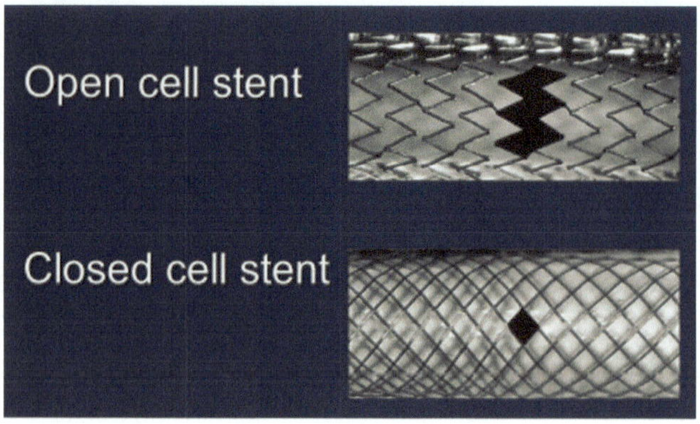

Fig. 46.1 Open and closed cell stent design.

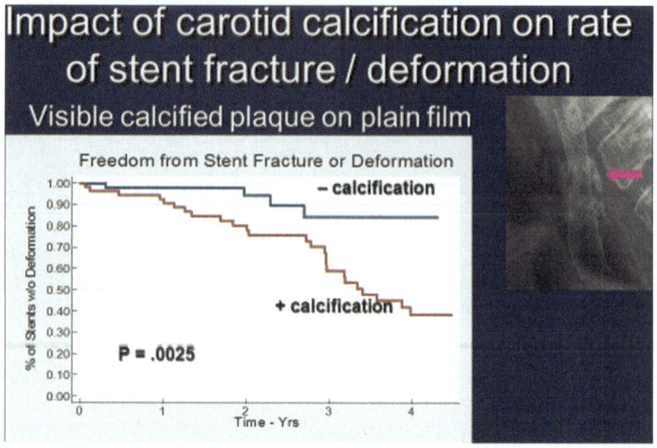

Fig. 46.3 Impact of carotid artery calcification *(pink arrow)* on freedom from stent fracture or deformation.

TABLE 46.1 Crest, ACT-1 study results for asymptomatic patients.

	CAS	CEA	P
ACT-I: Primary endpoint	3.8%	3.4%	0.11
CREST: Primary endpoint	5.6%	4.9%	0.562
ACT-I: 30 days stroke, MI, death	3.3%	2.6%	0.60
CREST: 30 days stroke, MI, death	3.5%	3.6%	0.96
ACT-I: 30 days stroke, death	2.9%	1.7%	0.33
CREST: 30 days stroke, death	2.5%	1.4%	0.15

CAS, Carotid artery stenting; *CEA*, carotid endarterectomy; *MI*, myocardial infarction.

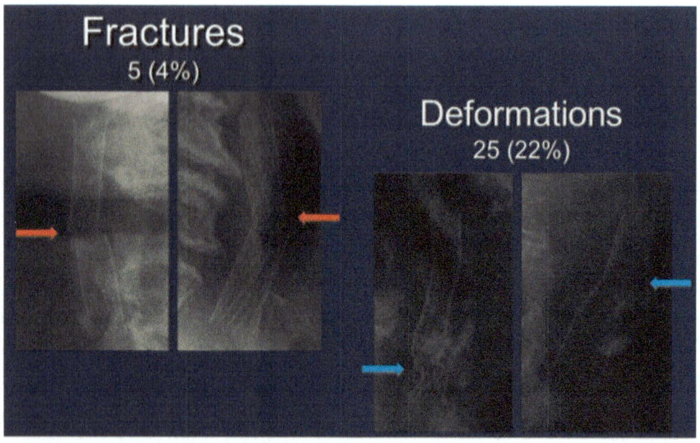

Fig. 46.2 Stent fracture *(red arrows)* and deformation *(blue arrows)*.

coronary stents. Stent fractures following CAS were significantly associated with the closed cell nitinol stent design, Xact stents, with a rate of 15% in stents older than 1 year. Ling et al. noted a similarly high Xact stent fracture rate of 24% (8 of 34).[6]

While prior studies have examined carotid stent fractures in some detail, significant stent deformation in the absence of an observed stent strut break has not been addressed. Stent deformation appear to be significantly more common in open cell stents compared with closed cell stents (hazard ratio [HR] 28, P = 0.001). This finding is consistent with the 11% stent changes "that could be confused for fracture" reported by Varcoe et al., because 92% of the stents placed in that series were open cell stents.[7] Open cell stents have a lower density of struts and generally larger free cell areas compared with closed cell stents. Thus, open cell stents are thought to be more flexible and to conform better to angulated and irregular vessels.

The impact of stent deformation and fracture on restenosis is unclear. Of the 116 stents followed in this cohort, only five stents required reintervention for restenosis of greater than 70%. None of the patients had associated neurologic symptoms. All of the recurrent stenosis occurred in open cell stents. Of the 32 stent fractures and deformations observed in this study, one deformed stent was associated with a significant restenosis that required reintervention and another was associated with late stroke (the only late stroke in the entire cohort). The remaining 30 stent changes were not associated with neurologic symptoms or restenosis. There was no evidence of significant clinical impact of stent fracture or deformation on either restenosis or neurologic complications. However, given the low rate of reintervention and stroke in this series, a less robust clinical impact cannot be accurately assessed.

Late stroke following CAS is uncommon. There is no known identifiable difference in outcome between closed and open cell nitinol stents. We have identified one case of late stroke in an open cell stent as a result of deformation of the stent struts and subsequent poor coverage of an ulcerated plaque that led to late stroke and subsequent stent explantation (Fig. 46.4).[9]

Complication Avoidance

Patient selection for CAS is the most important variable for improving CAS safety. There are several anatomic and lesion specific variables that increase the risk of CAS. Anatomic variables include a hostile aortic arch (based on tortuosity and type II–III arch anatomy), significant atherosclerosis burden in the arch, and tortuous common and/or internal carotid arteries. Unfavorable lesion characteristics include heavily calcified or circumferentially calcified internal carotid artery lesions or the presence of soft thrombus within the lesion (Fig. 46.5). These unfavorable anatomic and lesion variants can be identified prior to considering intervention through the use of three-dimensional computed tomography angiography (CTA) of the aortic arch, carotid arteries, and circle of Willis.[10]

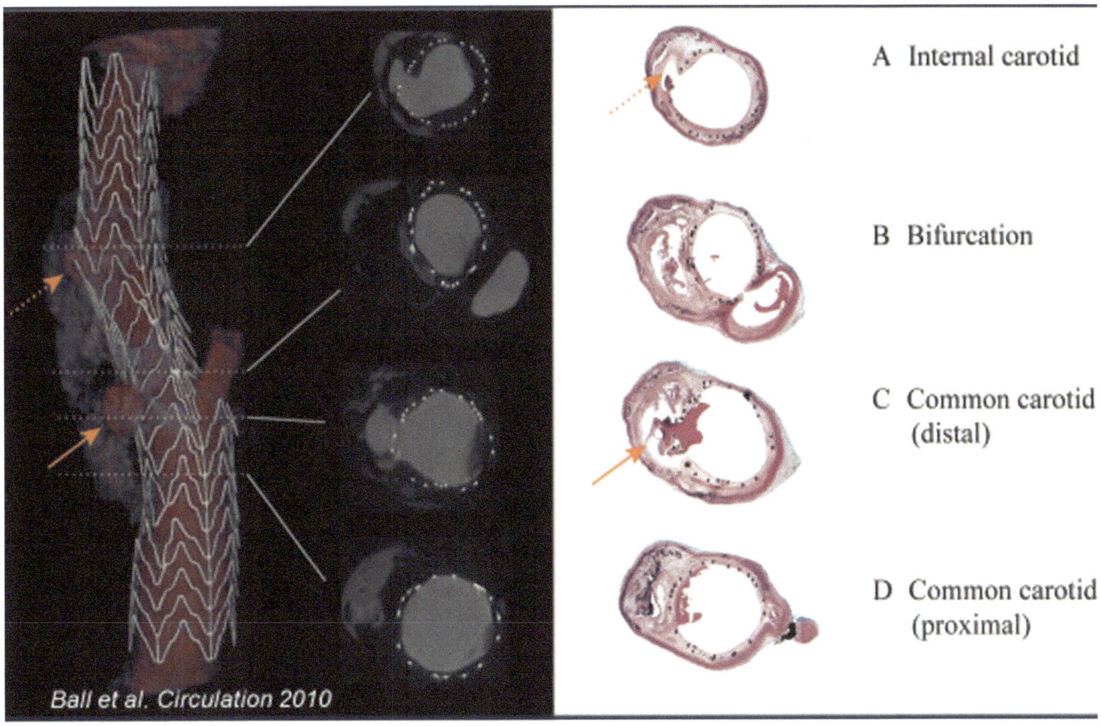

Fig. 46.4 Microcomputed tomography scan of explanted open cell nitinol stent in patient with late stroke. Note the absence of stent struts over ulcerated lesion indicated by *red arrow* in panel C.

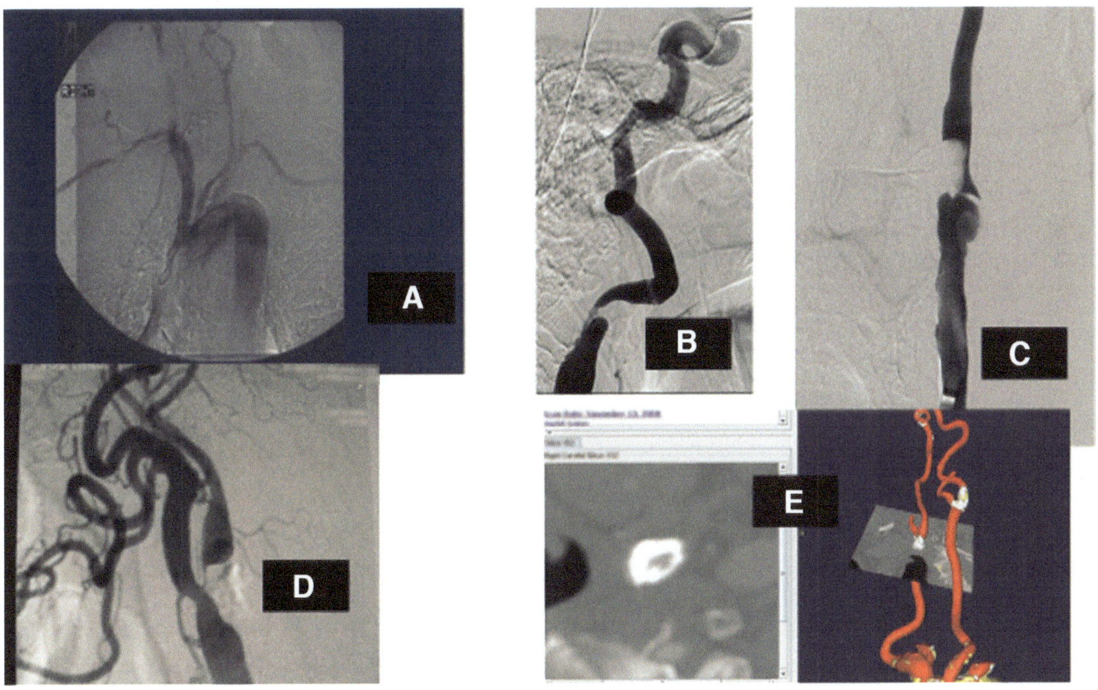

Fig. 46.5 Examples of hostile anatomy for carotid artery stenting that can be identified preprocedure on computed tomography angiography (CTA) or carotid arteries and circle of Willis. (A) Type III aortic arch. (B) Tortuous internal carotid artery. (C) Fresh thrombus in internal carotid artery. (D) Calcified complex internal carotid artery stenosis. (E) Three-dimensional CTA of internal carotid artery demonstrating circumferential calcification.

CONCLUSIONS

Both open and closed cell nitinol stents have been shown to be safe and effective in the treatment of bifurcation carotid artery stenosis. Closed cell nitinol stents tend to be less flexible but have better radial force and provide increased coverage of the atherosclerotic plaque. Both stent types are prone to fracture or deformation when placed into heavily calcified internal carotid arteries. Careful patient selection through the use of preoperative CTA can be used to select patients who would be at increased risk of CAS and use an alternative revascularization strategy.

REFERENCES

1. Brott TG, Howard G, Roubin GS, et al. Long-term results of stenting versus endarterectomy for carotid-artery stenosis. *N Engl J Med.* 2016; 374(11):1021–1031.
2. Rosenfield K, Matsumura JS, Chaturvedi S, et al., ACT investigators. Randomized trial of stent versus surgery for asymptomatic carotid stenosis. *N Engl J Med.* 2016;374(11):1011–1020.
3. Nicosia A, Nikas D, Castriota F, Biamino G, Cao P, et al. Classification for carotid artery stenting complications: manifestations, management, and prevention. *J Endovasc Ther.* 2010;17(3):275–294.
4. Bosiers M, de Donato K, Verbist J, et al. Does free cell area influence outcome in caotid artery stenting? *Eur J Vasc Endovasc Surg.* 2007;33:135–141.
5. Schillinger M, Gschwendtner M, Reimers B, Trenkler J, Stockx L, et al. Does carotid stent design matter? *Stroke.* 2008;39:905–909.
6. Ling AJ, Mwipatayi P, Gandhi T, Sieunarine K. Stenting for carotid artery stenosis: fractures, proposed etiology and the need for surveillance. *J Vasc Surg.* 2008;47:1220–1226 [discussion 6]
7. Varcoe RL, Mah J, Young N, So SS, Vicaretti M, Swinnen J. Prevalence of carotid stent fractures in a single-center experience. *J Endovasc Ther.* 2008;15:485–489.
8. Chang CK, Huded CP, Nolan BW, Powell RJ. Prevalence and clinical significance of stent fracture and deformation following carotid artery stenting. *J Vasc Surg.* 2011;54(3):685–690.
9. Ball TC, Foerst JR, Vorpahl M, Powell RJ, Virmani R, Kaplan VA. Embolic stroke after carotid stenting: microscopic computed tomography analysis of en bloc surgical specimen demonstrating ulceration. *Circulation.* 2010;121(14):1661–1663.
10. Wyers MC, Powell RJ, Fillinger MF, Nolan BW, Cronenwett JL. The value of 3D CT angiographic assessment prior to carotid stenting. *J Vasc Surg.* 2009;49:614–622.

47

Carotid Stent: Device-Specific Complications With the Wallstent

Gianluca Faggioli, MD, PhD, Rodolfo Pini, MD, PhD and Andrea Stella, MD

INTRODUCTION

The Carotid Wallstent (Boston Scientific, Marlborough, MA) is one of the most used stents in the endovascular treatment of carotid stenosis, particularly because of its design, which allows excellent plaque coverage. For that reason, it seems adequate for the treatment not only of stable uncomplicated plaques but also of dishomogenous stenosis. Although the advantages given in terms of plaque coverage are significant, as shown by the diminished rate of postprocedural events compared with open cell stents,[1] the conformability is reduced, with a higher rate of malapposition of the struts.[2] Moreover, the rigidity of the device and the interaction between the metallic struts lead to other possible problems, which are, however, extremely limited in terms of frequency and overall clinical impact as we will see in this chapter.

ENDOLUMINAL STENT COVERAGE

Because the main purpose of a carotid stent is the prevention from cerebral embolism, the endoluminal coverage of the device is crucial. De Donato et al. analyzed the interaction between carotid plaques and stents by optical coherence tomography and found that plaque prolapse was significantly lower compared with open and hybrid cell stents (23.3% versus 68.6% and 30.8% respectively; $P < 0.01$).[2]

Moreover, as shown in previous work from our group, the carotid Wallstent surface is covered by a new pseudo-intimal layer shortly after implantation. The completeness of this new layer is dependent on adequate coverage of the plaque at the proximal end of the stent where an intact intima is present[3] (Fig. 47.1).

Although the degree of neointimal coverage does not seem to be related to the number of microemboli detected by transcranial Doppler, a complete stent coverage is a potential adjunctive barrier to plaque prolapse and endoluminal fragmentation.[3]

CLASSIFICATION OF CAROTID STENT COMPLICATION

Nicosia et al. divided the carotid stent complications according to their anatomical distribution in cervical and intracranial complication.[4] Those directly related to the stent pertain to the cervical group and, although of different types, are rarely device specific. As a matter of fact, only plaque prolapse is strictly correlated with the stent design. Acute stent thrombosis, residual stenosis, and incorrect stent deployment, which are the other possible stent complications, are primarily the consequences of operator-dependent technical details, such as indication to revascularization, stent positioning and deployment, and medical management. Plaque prolapse has been defined by Clark et al. as a >0.5-mm protrusion of plaque components through the stent cells and it is considered "significant" when determining a visible lumen stenosis.[5] In addition to these morphological features, plaque prolapse is clinically relevant because it may lead to stent thrombosis or cerebral embolization,[5] and although it may be evident at completion angiography at the end of the carotid artery stenting procedure, a precise angiographic definition is lacking.[4] Intravascular ultrasound and optical coherence tomography are the most reliable methods to identify plaque prolapse, showing that the closed cell design of the Wallstent allows the greatest protection from this phenomenon.[2,6]

Incorrect stent deployment can be defined as an operator-dependent defect; however, the characteristics of the stent may play an important role in this complication. As a matter of fact, the closed cell design causes a greater degree of stiffness in the device, leading to increased risk of misalignment during deployment. This was shown by de Donato et al., who found that closed-cell design was significantly associated with a higher rate of malapposed struts compared with open cell or hybrid cell (34% versus 15% and 16%, respectively; $P < 0.01$).[2]

The use of the Wallstent in tortuous vessels should be carefully considered, because of its rigidity. It may be considered an inappropriate stent choice in these patients, rather than a complication of the stent itself. If the misplacement is minimal, within a few millimeters from the desired position, no consequences are to be expected.[7] However, in case of very tight stenosis or excessive tortuosity of the vessel, the radial forces of the stent struts may cause a watermelon effect on the stent with the stent being displaced either proximally or distally to the target zone.[7,8] As shown in Fig. 47.2, a stent may be deployed incorrectly because of the forces exerted by the struts toward a rigid calcified plaque, leading to the necessity of deploying a second more proximal stent in order to achieve complete plaque coverage. These forces may also lead to a late misplacement.[9–11] Shortening may be also aggravated by the straightening of the vessel, which is relevant when a closed-cell stent is inserted and deployed into a tortuous or stiff vessel. Part of the problem may be related to the diameter mismatch between the stent, the proximal common carotid, and the internal carotid artery. As a matter of fact, since the metal tends to distribute the force uniformly across its surface, the external energy of the widening proximal end may be transmitted as a contrary internal force at the distal end, where the lumen diameter is smaller.[12] This is particularly evident in the case of stenting of post-endarterectomy stenosis, because the decreased compliance of the artery may worsen the diameter mismatch between the stent and the artery.[12]

From a review of the literature, the reported cases of complications from the carotid Wallstent are limited to a small number (Table 47.1). Only one of these complications may be related to a structural defect, which determined the displacement of a marker ring, eventually leading to an incomplete stent expansion.[13]

OTHER TYPES OF LATE COMPLICATIONS

The late outcome of the carotid Wallstent has been analyzed by Ronchey et al. in a series of 1000 cases.[14] At a mean follow-up of 45.5 ± 9.3 months (range 3–120), they found a complete asymptomatic occlusion in six cases and a significant restenosis, with sytolic velocity at duplex >249 cm/s, in nine cases (0.9%).[14] The restenosis was treated by repeated balloon angioplasty in eight cases, of which one was with a cutting balloon, and surgical conversion was used in the remaining case.[14] Surgical conversion was also performed in one tight restenosis of a case reported by our group. The patient was referred to us from another hospital after repeated neurological symptoms resulting from a tight restenosis in a Wallstent with incomplete proximal plaque coverage.[15]

The rigidity of the stent may also lead to kinking of the distal internal carotid artery. Although the kinking may be initially benign, the hemodynamic disturbances associated with it may eventually cause a significant stenosis, as shown in the case in Fig. 47.3.

In the series of Ronchey et al.,[14] as well as in our experience of 723 Wallstents (unpublished data), no stent fracture occurred. This is consistent with the work by Sfyroeras et al., who did not report any case of Wallstent fracture in their series of 55 cases of stent fractures, suggesting that the metallic structure of the Wallstent is particularly resistant.[16]

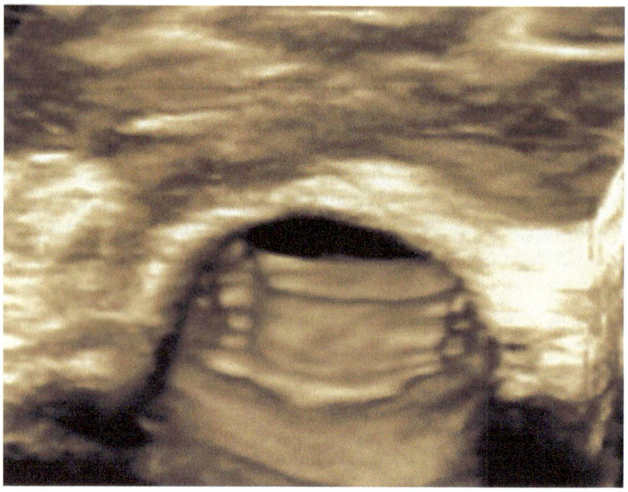

Fig. 47.1 Three-dimensional duplex reconstruction of the intimal layer in the inner surface of a carotid Wallstent 3 months after deployment. In order to achieve a complete stent coverage, the stent should be deployed with both extremities at the level of healthy arterial wall.

AVOIDING AND CORRECTING COMPLICATIONS

As with any endovascular procedure, accurate planning and material choice are the key to an uncomplicated procedure. Carotid Wallstents behave suboptimally in very tortuous vessels and, given their rigidity, proximal and distal curvature should be examined accurately before and during stent deployment, in order to prevent excessive kinking. In that sense, the length of the stent should be limited to a minimum in

TABLE 47.1 Literature review of Wallstent complications.

Author	Year	N cases	Type of complication
Akgul et al.[13]	2007	1	Displacement of marker ring
Yoon et al.[9]	2009	4	Proximal shortening
Myouchin et al.[8]	2013	2	Unsuccessful placement
Zhao et al.[10]	2013	1	Proximal shortening
Garriboli and Jannello[11]	2015	1	Proximal shortening

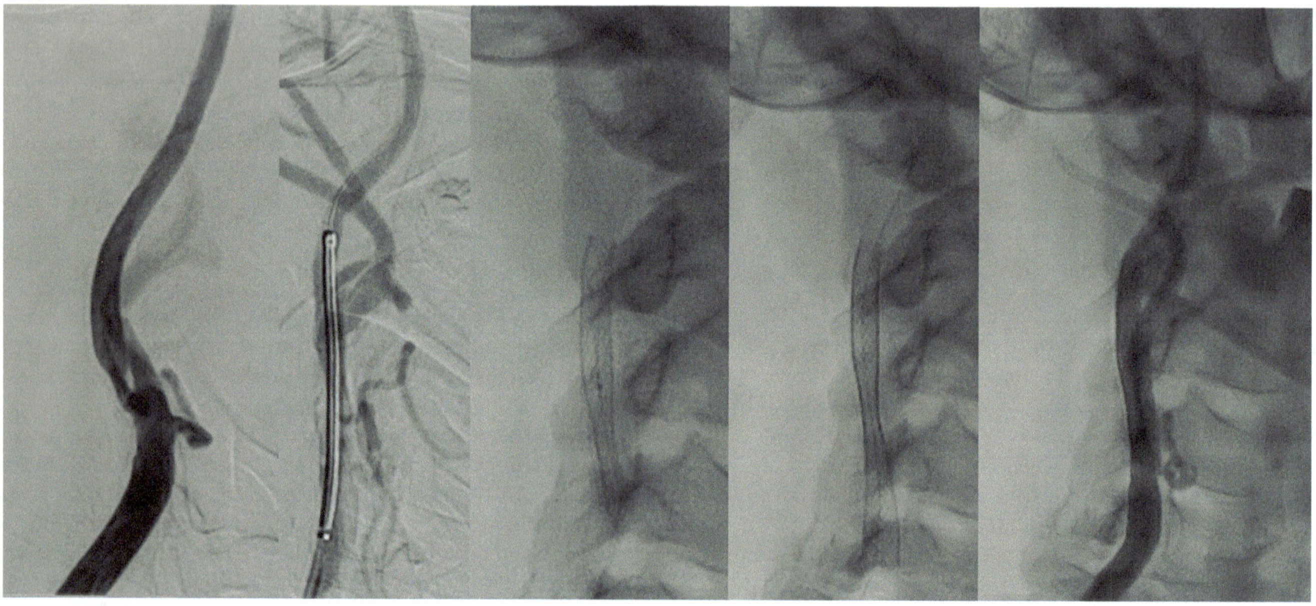

Fig. 47.2 In this sequence, the shortening of a 9 × 30 carotid Wallstent is shown. Despite accurate positioning to cover the carotid plaque completely, the stent shortened distally at deployment, leaving part of the plaque uncovered. A second, more proximal 9 × 30 Wallstent allowed precise completion of the procedure.

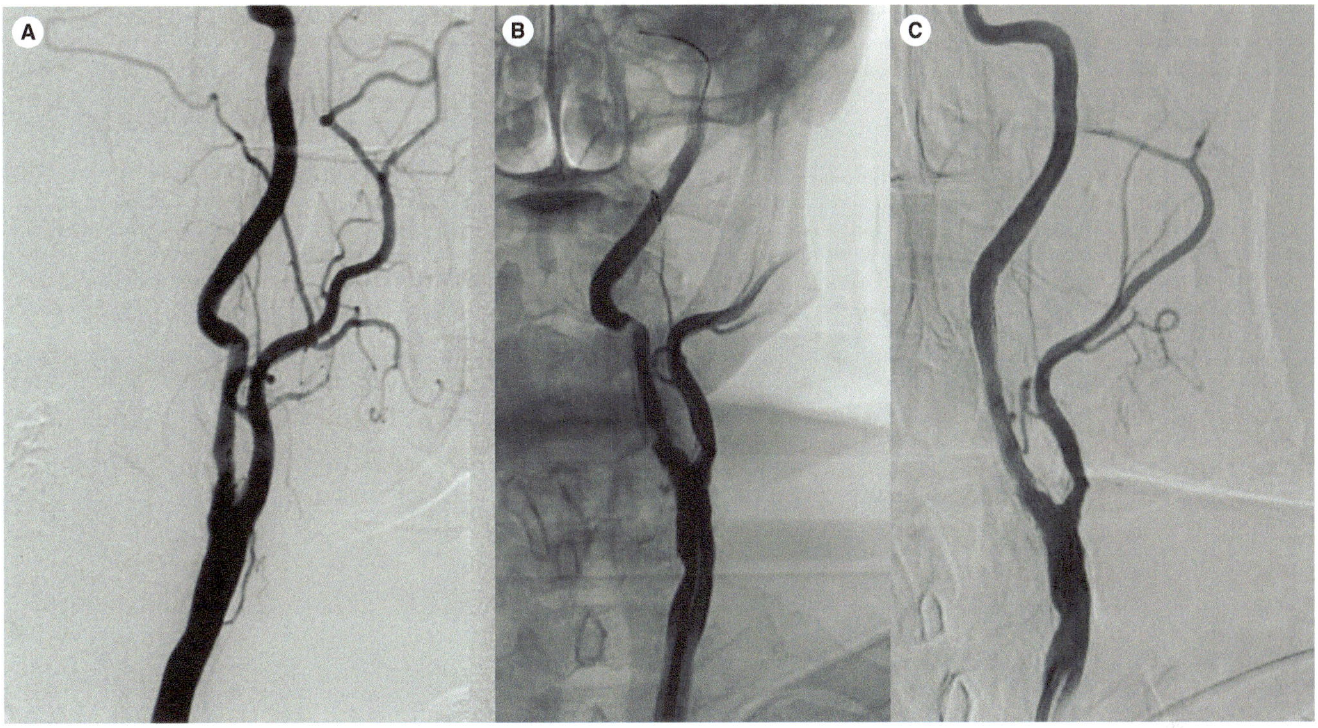

Fig. 47.3 Distal stenosis occurring 10 years after the first 9 × 30 Wallstent procedure (A). The significant, symptomatic stenosis (B) occurred as a consequence of the kinking caused by the rigidity of the stent and was corrected by a 7 × 30 distal Wallstent (C).

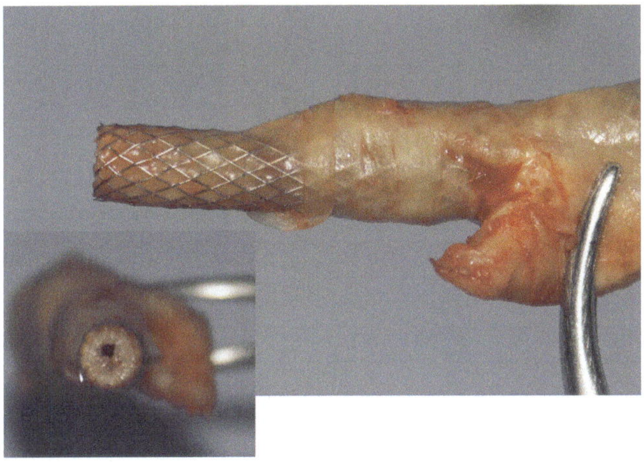

Fig. 47.4 Surgical removal of a Wallstent affected by intense, symptomatic hyperplasia. Surgical removal is a possible option in selected circumstances, particularly in the case of cerebral symptoms.

tortuous or angulated vessels. The length of the stent should, however, be calculated considering the shortening of the stent in its wider proximal end. If the shortening is greater than expected, an adjunctive proximal stent may be added because proximal plaque coverage is essential for satisfactory long-term results (Fig. 47.2).

Distal significant late restenosis may be successfully treated with distal stent extension, paying attention not to cause further distal kinking (Fig. 47.3). In rare cases, surgical stent removal together with complete carotid endarterectomy may be necessary (Fig. 47.4).[15] Please refer to the Tip and Warning boxes that follow.

TIP BOX

- Accurate planning.
- Adequate material choice.
- Possible angulation exacerbation after stent deployment should be considered.
- Careful evaluation of possible shortening of the stent, particularly in its proximal end.

WARNING BOX

- Avoid very tortuous anatomies.
- Be prepared to extend the stent either proximally or distally.
- Necessity of surgical conversion is exceptional but not impossible.

REFERENCES

1. Bosiers M, de Donato G, Deloose K, et al. Does free cell area influence the outcome in carotid artery stenting? *Eur J Vasc Endovasc Surg.* 2007;33:135–141.
2. de Donato G, Setacci F, Sirignano P, et al. Optical coherence tomography after carotid stenting: rate of stent malapposition, plaque prolapse and fibrous cap capture according to stent design. *Eur J Vasc Endovasc Surg.* 2013;45:579–587.
3. Faggioli GL, Ferri M, Serra C, et al. The residual risk of cerebral embolism after carotid stenting: the complex interplay between stent coverage and aortic arch atherosclerosis. *Eur J Vasc Endovasc Surg.* 2009;37:519–524.

4. Nicosia A, Nikas D, Castriota F, et al. Classification for carotid artery stenting complications: manifestation, management, and prevention. *J Endovasc Ther*. 2010;17:275–294.
5. Clark DJ, Lessio S, O'Donoghue M, et al. Safety and utility of intravascular ultrasound-guided carotid artery stenting. *Catheter Cardiovasc Interv*. 2004;63:355–362.
6. Clark DJ, Lessio S, O'Donoghue M, et al. Mechanisms and predictors of carotid artery stent restenosis: a serial intravascular ultrasound study. *J Am Coll Cardiol*. 2006;47:2390–2396.
7. Aikawa H, Nagata S, Onizuka M, et al. Shortening of Wallstent RP during carotid artery stenting requires appropriate stent placement. *Neurol Med Chir. (Tokyo)*. 2008;48(6):249–252; discussion 252–253.
8. Myouchin K, Takayama K, Taoka T, et al. Carotid Wallstent placement difficulties encountered in carotid artery stenting. *SpringerPlus*. 2013;2:468.
9. Yoon SM, Jo KW, Baik MW, Kim YW. Delayed carotid Wallstent shortening resulting in restenosis following successful carotid artery angioplasty and stenting. *J Korean Neurosurg Soc*. 2009;46:495–497.
10. Zhao R, Feng X-Y, Zhang M, Shen XL, Su J-J, Liu J-R. Delayed shortening and shifting of carotid Wallstent. *CNS Neuroscience & Therapeutics*. 2014;20:86–87.
11. Garriboli L, Jannello AM. Delayed carotid Wallstent shortening. *Int J Surg Case Reports*. 2015;8:68–70.
12. Yallampalli S, Zhou W, Lin PH, Bush RL, Lumsden AB. Delayed deformation of self-expanding stents after carotid artery stenting for postendarterectomy restenoses. *J Vasc Surg*. 2006;44:412–415.
13. Akgul E, Aksungur EH, Korur K, Aikimbaev K, Yaliniz H. A rare complication of carotid artery stenting: displacement of marker ring causing locking of stent and incomplete stent expansion. *Am J Neuroradiol*. 2007;28:1403–1404.
14. Ronchey S, Praquin B, Orrico M, et al. Outcomes of 1000 carotid Wallstent implantations: single-center experience. *J Endovasc Ther*. 2016;23(2):267–274.
15. Faggioli GL, Ferri M, Rossi C, Gargiulo M, Freyrie A, Stella A. Carotid stent failure: results of surgical rescue. *Eur J Vasc Endovasc Surg*. 2007;33:58–61.
16. Sfyroeras GS, Koutsiaris A, Karathanos C, Giannakopoulos A, Giannoukas AD. Clinical relevance and treatment of carotid stent fractures. *J Vasc Surg*. 2010;51:1280–1285.

48

Transcarotid Artery Revascularization With the ENROUTE Transcarotid Neuroprotection System

Zachary W. Kostun, MD and Manish Mehta, MD, MPH

Extracranial carotid artery occlusive disease is associated with the risk of stroke, disability, and death. The surgical treatment of carotid disease has undergone significant evolution from early attempts at carotid ligation to the first carotid endarterectomy by Michael Debakey in 1953.[1] Over the following decades, carotid intervention was mostly limited for symptomatic patients. There was considerable research into the treatments of carotid disease and multiple randomized prospective trials were conducted, which demonstrated a definitive benefit to carotid endarterectomy in symptomatic patients with moderate to severe disease and asymptomatic patients with severe disease. Carotid endarterectomy became the treatment of choice for disease of the carotid bifurcation.

With the expansion of endovascular interventions in the 1990s, stenting for extracranial carotid disease with cerebral protection was explored as an alternative to endarterectomy in numerous trials. Several cerebral protection devices that were based upon distal cerebral occlusion balloons versus distal embolism filters were trialed, utilizing both open and closed cell stents. Interventions were performed both with and without devices to protect against embolization during interventions. Embolic protection included distal occlusive balloons and distal embolic filters. Multiple multicentered prospective randomized and nonrandom trials further explored transfemoral carotid stenting and established it as a viable treatment option for extracranial disease.[2] These rigorous trials have also shed light on the nuances of this technique.

Based upon the results of these trials, the U.S. Food and Drug Administration granted approval for carotid artery stenting (CAS) with certain limitations. CAS from a transfemoral approach has been shown to have a significant increased risk of stroke compared with carotid endarterectomy. Factors that increase the risk include navigating tortuous anatomy, atheroma within the aortic arch, and crossing proximal common carotid lesions. The use of distal embolic protection devices improves outcome; however, these devices must be brought across the lesions in order to be deployed, which in itself can provoke embolization. Diffusion-weighted MRI studies of transfemoral CAS patients have shown an incidence of silent event as high as 40%.[4] Many of these events were contralateral to the treated side, suggesting that navigation of the aortic arch may be a frequent cause of embolization. Transcarotid artery stenting (TCAR) with flow reversal was designed to mitigate many of these risks and to prevent stroke. Accessing the common carotid artery at the base of the neck allows the operator to avoid the complexities of challenging arch anatomy. Dynamic flow reversal is designed to prevent distal embolization beyond what is possible with distal filters.

The ENROUTE Transcarotid Neuroprotection System (Silk Road Medical, Sunnydale, California) is a flow reversal circuit that connects two 8-French sheaths through a flow modulator. One sheath is placed in the common carotid artery via arterial cutdown and the other is placed percutaneously into the femoral vein. The two sheaths are connected through a flow modulator, which can regulate the rate of flow reversal between high and low. The flow modulator can also temporarily stop flow reversal. When the common carotid artery is clamped proximal to the arterial sheath, the arterial–venous pressure gradient leads to flow reversal within the external and internal carotid arteries.

The ROADSTER trial was the pivotal trial for the ENROUTE system. It was a prospective, single arm, multicenter trial to assess the safety and efficacy of the flow reversal system in carotid artery stenting. The trial enrolled 141 patients, of whom 36 were symptomatic with stenoses >50%. The asymptomatic patients all had >70% stenosis.[2] The enrolled patients were considered at high risk of endarterectomy based upon anatomic and physiologic criteria. The primary endpoint was major adverse events of death, stroke, and myocardial infarction. There were five major adverse events in the trial (two cerebrovascular accident, two deaths, and one myocardial infarction). There were also minor adverse events including eight arterial dissections, five hematomas, and one cranial nerve injury.

PROCEDURE

The patient is positioned supine as for carotid endarterectomy. The groin is prepared for placing the venous sheath. The procedure may be performed under general or local anesthesia. Patients in the ROADSTER trial were split 53% to 47% between local and general anesthesia, respectively. The common carotid artery is exposed at the base of the neck through a longitudinal or transverse incision. The sternal and clavicular heads of the sternocleidomastoid act as anatomic landmarks. The artery is found by splitting the two muscle heads and mobilizing the internal jugular vein medially. Occasionally, the vagus nerve courses anteriorly and must be avoided. Approximately 3 cm of artery should be exposed to allow proximal occlusion and sheath placement.[3] The artery should be freed circumferentially to allow proximal control with a Rummel tourniquet, silastic vessel loops, or atraumatic vascular clamp. Proximal common carotid occlusion is necessary to establish flow reversal. A silastic vessel loop or umbilical tape around the artery can facilitate control during artery access and sheath placement.

The patient is systemically anticoagulated. An adventitial U-stitch placed prior to access facilitates closure of the arteriotomy at the end of the procedure. The artery is accessed with a micro puncture needle and exchanged over a wire for a microcatheter. A stiffer wire is placed into the common carotid artery to allow placement of the 8-French flow-reversal sheath. The arterial sheath is placed over the wire up to the

2.5 cm marker. The sheath is secured to the patient externally to prevent accidental dislodging during the procedure. The venous sheath is placed in the contralateral superficial femoral vein and the arteriovenous circuit is flushed and connected. Flow reversal is established following clamping of the common carotid artery proximal to the sheath entry site.

Flow reversal should be demonstrated by arteriogram through the arterial sheath after first confirming by clearing the line with saline injection and allowing reversal of flow to be established once more. The ENROUTE Neuroprotection System allows temporary cessation of flow reversal during arteriograms for imaging purposes.

Once flow reversal has been established and the lesion is identified, it is crossed with a wire and the stent is deployed in the usual fashion. If the stenosis is particularly tight, predilation with an undersized balloon can be performed. Some surgeons advocate predilatation of all lesions. Postdilation can be performed as needed.[3] A completion cerebral angiogram is performed with cranial imaging to evaluate cerebral emboli and adequacy of stenting.

Antegrade cerebral flow is reestablished by unclamping the proximal common carotid artery. The wires and sheaths are removed and the arteriotomy is then closed with the previously placed suture.

COMPLICATIONS

The supraclavicular incision is well tolerated in patients. Ultrasound facilitates identifying an exposure site where the artery will be the most superficial and not diseased. In the pivotal trial, the incidence of cranial nerve injury was 0.7% (1/141).[2] The incidence of hematoma formation was 3.5% and the incidence of hematoma requiring surgical evacuation/exploration was less than 1%. The vast majority of carotid stent patients receive dual-antiplatelet therapy and are anticoagulated during the procedure. Care must be taken during common carotid artery cutdown and mobilization to prevent postprocedure bleeding. During closure, particular attention should be paid to the sternocleidomastoid to ensure there is no muscle bleeding provoked by mobilization and periprocedural anticoagulation.

Proximal common carotid artery dissections at the sheath entry site were seen in 2.1% of patients in the ROADSTER trial. The arterial sheath has since been modified to have more flexibility and is curved to accommodate the entry angle. To avoid carotid dissection, which probably occurs as a result of injury to the back wall, adequate sheath, dilator, and stiff wire access must be maintained. Care must be taken during arterial access and sheath placement. Proximal control of the artery during needle access, without undue tension, can help ensure single-wall access. Passage of the microcatheter and the sheath is performed over a wire to decrease the risk of dissection. Blindly passing the sheath can also lead to embolization if the plaque is engaged. An initial arteriogram through a microcatheter prior to sheath placement allows the operator to define the lesion and bifurcation more accurately. If the sheath cannot be placed over a stiff wire within the common carotid artery, the wire is advanced into the external carotid artery for additional stability. In the event of a dissection, stent placement or open surgical repair are both options for repair.

Trial results have shown that flow reversal is generally well tolerated by patients.[2–4] There may be a small subset of patients who will be intolerant to flow reversal. This effect can be mitigated in several ways. Some patients who do not tolerate prolonged high flow reversal tolerate low flow reversal, which occurred in one patient in the ROADSTER trial. Systemic blood pressure can be raised to increase cross-cerebral perfusion. If flow reversal must be abandoned, carotid stenting can still be achieved with placement of distal embolic protection through the carotid sheath. Alternatively, the procedure can be converted to endarterectomy.

Meticulous care must be taken to ensure there are no air bubbles within the contrast. A slow controlled injection of contrast allows adequate visualization without embolization.

Each exchange through the sheath has the potential to introduce air emboli. Methodical visual attention during exchanges help to ensure that no air is advanced through the sheath. If air is detected, the sheath is back bled. All balloons and stents must be carefully flushed to be free of air.

Any commercially available stent can be used with the ENROUTE Neuroprotection System. Silk Road Medical has developed a stent on a shorter (57 cm) deployment catheter to facilitate deployment from the transcarotid approach.

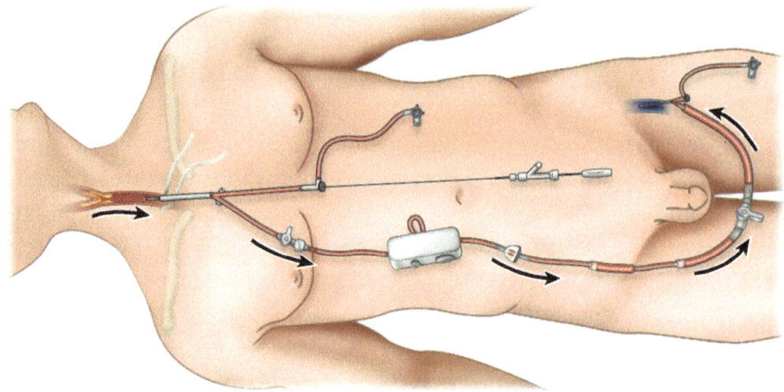

Fig. 48.1 Flow modulator device is connected between the 8-French transcarotid arterial sheath and an 8-French femoral venous sheath.

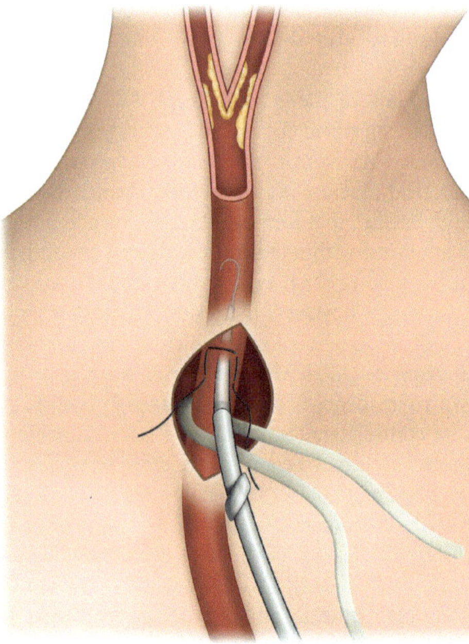

Fig. 48.2 The arterial sheath is placed through a supraclavicular incision. The sheath has an external cuff to prevent over-insertion. The intra-arterial length is 2.5 cm.

Predilatation and postdilatation can be performed as necessary. Oversized balloon and overaggressive angioplasty increase the risk of embolization and dissection.

During sheath removal, the arteriotomy should be back bled and flushed to remove any debris or stasis clot that accumulated around the sheath tip, which is a potential source of embolization.

PITFALLS

- Access: ensure sufficient artery (5 cm) from clavicle to carotid bifurcation to allow sheath placement and proximal clamp.
- Access: single-wall needle access to avoid intimal flap. All movements over wire.
- Access: a short-tipped (1 cm) stiff wire can facilitate sheath placement; alternatively the wire can be advanced into the external carotid artery for additional support.
- Access: sheath should be secured to the patient externally to avoid dislodging access during the procedure. If the artery depth is problematic, a counter incision can be made and the sheath tunneled subcutaneously.
- Flow reversal: If the use of high flow-rate reversal is not tolerated, use a stepwise approach.
- Maintain elevated systemic blood pressure
- Limited use of high flow-rate during critical steps
- Use only low flow-rate reversal for the procedure
- Discontinue flow reversal and use a standard distal embolic protection device
- Convert to carotid endarterectomy with or without shunting

REFERENCES

1. Friedman SG. The first carotid endarterectomy. *J Vasc Surg.* 2014;60(6): 1703–1708.
2. Kwolek CJ, Jaff MR, Leal JI, et al. Results of the ROADSTER multicenter trial of transcarotid stenting with dynamic flow reversal. *J Vasc Surg.* 2015;62:1227–1234.
3. Malas MB, Leal J, Kashyap V, et al. Technical aspects of transcarotid artery revascularization using the ENROUTE transcarotid neuroprotection and stent system. *J Vasc Surg.* 2017;65:916–920.
4. Moore WS, DeRubertis BG. Direct cervical carotid angioplasty with flow reversal: a single-center report from the ROADSTER Trial. *Ann Vasc Surg.* 2016;33:75–78.

49

Subclavian Steal

John F. Morrison, MD and Adnan H. Siddiqui, MD, PhD, FACS, FAHA

INTRODUCTION

Subclavian steal phenomenon (or syndrome) originates from severe stenosis or occlusion of the proximal subclavian artery resulting in the reversal of blood flow in the ipsilateral vertebral artery (VA) to perfuse the limb. Blood flows retrogradely from the brain (via blood from the contralateral VA or the circle of Willis) to the limb instead of anterogradely from the heart directly to the limb as a result of a hemodynamically significant proximal subclavian stenosis or occlusion.[1] Symptoms of subclavian steal include those associated with vertebrobasilar insufficiency or upper extremity claudication, such as cranial nerve deficits, syncope or unexplained loss of consciousness, gait and balance disturbances, ipsilateral arm pain, or a change in pallor.[2]

Noninvasive imaging modalities are useful in the initial evaluation and establishment of the diagnosis of subclavian steal. Computed tomography (CT) angiography or magnetic resonance (MR) angiography is useful for further anatomical understanding of the location of the lesion, lesion size, the location and orientation of adjacent vessels, and particularly for treatment planning. In addition, both CT-based and MR-based imaging provide information about the character of the lesion. Heavy concentric calcification, which is better seen on CT, or hypointensity on CT indicate a necrotic lipid rich core, which may impact the treatment strategy. On MR imaging, evidence of plaque hemorrhage may suggest potential fragility of the lesion and a higher risk for distal embolization. Ultrasound imaging also provides lesion information that helps treatment planning.

Treatment of symptomatic subclavian steal from subclavian stenosis may be performed via open, endovascular, or a combined/hybrid approach.[3] In this chapter, we focus on endovascular treatment, which involves percutaneous balloon angioplasty and/or subclavian stent placement, the associated complications, and prevention of these complications.[4] Patients with symptoms of subclavian steal syndrome and findings of stenosis on imaging are considered candidates for endovascular revascularization.

PROCEDURAL OVERVIEW

Meticulous review of the noninvasive vessel images aids in planning and ultimately implementing a successful procedure. This includes evaluation of the aortic arch type, identification of the stenotic lesion including its location and grade, and identification of the location and orientation of associated proximal and/or distal branching vessels, most importantly the VA.

This preprocedure plan is the key to a successful procedure and avoidance of complications. The considerations include the relationship of the lesion with the VA ostium. This is because angioplasty and stenting may result in plaque rupture, protrusion, and embolization up the VA and into the brain with devastating consequences. Although the lesion may be more proximal to the VA ostium, findings of severe plaque hemorrhage on MR imaging, severe hypoechoicity on ultrasound, or hypointensity on CT suggest high embolic potential. In these cases, a strategy to prevent VA embolization is critical. Arch anatomy also plays a key role. If the access is difficult in a severe type III arch, direct brachial access may be a better solution. Keep in mind that most balloon-mounted stents with diameters of 7 mm or greater require a 7- or 8-French sheath and that size is often too large for radial access. When using embolic protection of the VA, access is best done through a radial approach. In these cases, a second contemporary femoral access site provides a stent delivery route by means of the aorta.

We administer dual antiplatelet agents (aspirin and clopidogrel) 7 days prior to intervention. A platelet assay for clopidogrel and aspirin is obtained and evaluated to ensure efficacy prior to the procedure. If there is an inadequate response, we switch to a more effective antiplatelet agent. As noted previously, a precise strategy based on noninvasive imaging provides rationale for the access site. For this chapter, we will describe a high embolic risk proximal subclavian symptomatic plaque. For the majority of subclavian lesions, vertebral protection is not necessary, because retrograde flow is typically protective for embolization into the cerebral circulation. To achieve distal protection from embolus traveling to the neurovascular circulation, we commonly use dual access through both radial and femoral sites (Fig. 49.1). Dual access allows manipulation of the subclavian artery stenotic lesion through one catheter and protection of the VA by the placement of a balloon through the other catheter (Tip Box 49.1). Placement of the balloon in the VA ostium also allows precise marking and, therefore, avoidance of inadvertent coverage with the subclavian stent.

Following arterial access with a micropuncture kit, a sheath (6–9 French) is introduced at the femoral (radial or brachial) access site. Typically, we use a 0.035″ hydrophilic Glidewire (Terumo Interventional Systems, Somerset, New Jersey) navigated to the aortic arch. A diagnostic catheter is then advanced over the Glidewire. For interventional procedures, we routinely administer 70 units/kg of bodyweight of heparin intravenously aimed at a goal of activated clotting time of >250 seconds. In either case, the heparin is administered once access is achieved.

An angiogram of the subclavian artery from the aortic arch is performed that displays the anatomy and the pathological lesion. If needed, a 5-French pigtail catheter can be used for aortic arch angiography using an injector to opacify optimally all arch great vessels. Measurements of the stenotic segment, including the nominal vessel on either end of the stenotic segment, are obtained; and branching vessel points, particularly the VA, are noted and taken into consideration when selecting the endovascular stent or stent-angioplasty balloon endovascular construct.

Next, the stenotic segment is crossed with a 5-French diagnostic catheter, if possible. Sometimes the 0.035″ Glidewire will cross the lesion but the catheter will not. Therefore, we always use a 0.035″ exchange wire to cross and to exchange the diagnostic catheter out for a 0.035″ Quick-Cross catheter (Spectranetics, Colorado Springs,

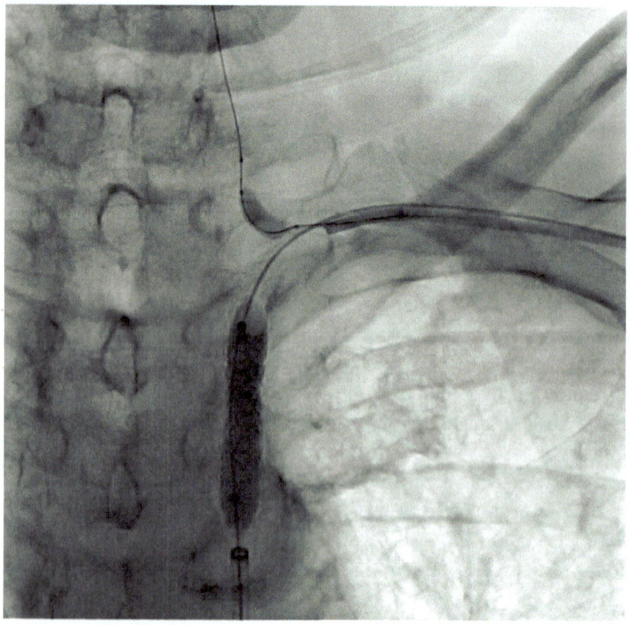

Fig. 49.1 Stent placement in the left subclavian artery with femoral and radial access. Notice the balloon in the vertebral artery origin for distal protection.

TIP BOX 49.1

Dual access is not necessary; however, it can confer increased distal protection to the neurovasculature.

Colorado) to cross the lesion. The nose cone of the Quick-Cross catheter is much smaller than a 5-French diagnostic catheter, and that helps with crossing the lesion. If the lesion is safely crossed with the wire and catheter, especially if the lesion is of high embolic risk, we prefer to use a primary balloon-mounted stent with VA protection. The delivery sheath should be advanced past the lesion to prevent dislodgment of the stent graft in the stenosis and then withdrawn over the stent graft once it is in place. This may require use of a more supportive wire, such as an Amplatz (Cook Medical, Bloomington, Indiana) or an InQwire (Merit Medical, South Jordan, Utah). However, if the lesion is more calcified, predilation with an undersized balloon may be required to cross the lesion with the aforementioned construct. The sheath can then be advanced over the balloon, as it is gradually deflated, to pass the lesion before placing the stent graft.

We have a strong preference for covered balloon-expandable stents for the subclavian artery. This artery is in a nonmobile segment of the body and therefore does not require a self-expanding stent such as would be required for the cervical carotid artery where a balloon-expandable stent will remain deformed once it has been deformed by motion or external deformation. This is because the stent graft covers the plaque and avoids intraprocedural as well as delayed plaque prolapse and distal embolization. Each stent has distinct benefits and disadvantages; however, we prefer the iCast balloon-expandable covered stent (Atrium Medical, Hudson, New Hampshire) or the VIABAHN balloon-expandable covered stent or the VBX (Gore, Newark, Delaware) for subclavian stenting. The key element and frequently the limiting factor are optimal stent size (length) to cover the lesion without obstructing the vertebral ostium or overhanging into the aorta.

Subsequent placement of additional stents may become necessary if the lesion is not covered by the initial stent. The most frequent cause for this is "watermelon-seeding" of the stent from the balloon across a high-grade heavily calcified stenosis. In such cases, it makes sense to protect the vertebral ostium with a balloon and perform predilation of the lesion. If stenosis remains following deployment of the initial stent, the ideal procedure is to bring in a higher atmospheric pressure tolerance balloon for additional angioplasty. If the lesion is longer than the initial stent, it may require tandem stent placement for additional length. However, if we feel the stent has not expanded adequately, we prefer to use high atmosphere rated balloons, which can be inflated to 24 atmospheres. For constructs with proximal overhang in the lumen of the parent vessel, we flare the proximal stent open. This is achieved with a Flash Ostial Dual-Balloon Angioplasty Catheter (Ostial Corp., Santa Clara, California). The dual balloon design of the Flash Ostial System incorporates two diameters: one diameter for dilation within the stent and the larger diameter for dilation within the parent vessel at the proximal end of the stent. Expanding the balloon causes the proximal end of the stent to dilate, or flare, and cover the ostia of the vessel in which the stenotic lesion is located. The biggest advantage of this is that re-access becomes easier because of the flared ends. This system does operate over a 0.014″ wire and therefore requires prior exchange of the 0.035″ wire to a 0.014″ wire in order to flare the end of the flash balloon.

In high-risk lesions distal protection of the VA is best done by a single- or double-lumen balloon occluding the VA ostium. Placing a filter can be problematic because the filter can snag in the subclavian stent, and therefore we do not use distal embolic filters in the VA during subclavian stenting. The balloon system can be delivered through a 5- or 6-French guide catheter through a radial approach over a 0.014″ microwire and inflated manually to assure occlusion of the ostium. This approach allows visualization of the vertebral ostium during deployment of the subclavian stent avoiding potential occlusion of the VA. However, protection of the VA is probably unnecessary in most patients if the lesion is not high risk and there is truly reversal of flow in the VA, because this reversal of flow tends to direct any embolic material to the arm, rather than the brain.

For cases where we are unable to cross the lesion in an anterograde fashion (from the aorta), we have two choices. First, we can establish brachial access and cross the lesion in a retrograde fashion with a wire and then place the stent from the brachial access site. The second option is to snare a wire from below once the lesion is crossed from the arm access site, typically with a 0.035″ wire from the distal (radial artery) access site. We then snare the 0.035″ wire with a 35-mm Amplatz GooseNeck snare (Medtronic, Minneapolis, Minnesota) delivered by way of a transfemoral approach through an appropriately sized delivery sheath, typically 8-French. Once snared, we pull the femoral sheath across the lesion in a "floss" technique (Fig. 49.2). This allows for balloon predilation of the stenotic lesion as well as the advancement of catheters proximal and distal to the lesion. We then deploy a balloon from the radial side into the VA while the stent is deployed from the femoral side. This prevents distal embolic particles from flowing into the cerebrovascular circulation during lesion manipulation and stent deployment. Although the cerebrovascular circulation is protected, the distal upper extremity remains at risk. Embolic complications to the limbs are commonly silent and considered rare.[5] Compared with ischemic emboli in the cerebrovascular circulation that may affect neurological function, the effect of small emboli would go unnoticed in the limbs. Larger emboli may affect distal perfusion of critical (eloquent) vascular territories and result in the need for further treatment via endovascular or open surgical embolectomy.

The patient will remain on dual antiplatelet agents for a minimum of 3 months.

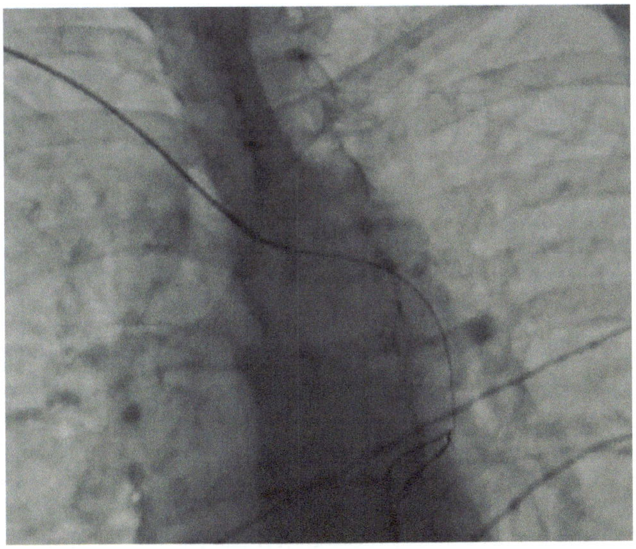

Fig. 49.2 Snare for pulling radial wire through femoral sheath. Notice the snare in the aorta from the femoral side. The radial wire is then captured and pulled through the groin.

Procedural success is determined by way of angiographic visualization of robust flow through the stenotic segment without evidence of in-stent thrombosis or vessel dissection. Likewise, absence of persistent reversal of flow from the contralateral vessel is a sign that the procedure was successful. Notably, to demonstrate physiological success of the treatment, we obtain pre- and post-treatment systolic blood pressure measurements across the stenotic lesion. A post-stenting trans-lesion differential of <5 mmHg is considered physiologically successful.

COMPLICATION AVOIDANCE AND MANAGEMENT

Treatment-related complications associated with subclavian steal are uncommon. However, possible complications include distal peripheral or neurovascular embolism, in-stent thrombosis, vessel lumen dissection with or without catastrophic pleural bleeding, stent malpositioning, and access site hematoma.

Embolism

Detection of distal vessel embolism during the procedure is difficult. At our institution, a change in neurologic examination findings in a patient who has undergone conscious sedation may signal a potential embolic event to the neurovasculature. More commonly, signs of embolism occur in the postprocedural period. This may reflect the ability of the brain to collateralize flow across the blockage immediately and mask the appearance of symptoms for minutes to hours.

Embolus to the neurovasculature may go undetected, or the patient may manifest signs of cerebral ischemia such as altered or diminished mental status, lethargy, sensory changes, cranial nerve deficit, gait disturbance, or motor weakness. However, the most common immediate symptom to be wary of is sudden onset of nausea and vomiting. This is probably related to distal embolization from the VA into the posterior inferior cerebellar artery territory and irritation and/or stimulation of the area postrema. For peripheral distal limb vessel embolism, ischemic changes may again go unnoticed or manifest silently. However, visible signs of ischemic changes include skin pallor, loss of pulses, and the extremities may be cold to touch, as well as numbness or pain. It is important to assess perfusion to the hand prior to leaving the angiography suite to allow for rapid intervention if embolic occlusion of upper extremity vessels has occurred.

On-table events should be immediately evaluated by selective vertebral angiography and full imaging of the upper extremity vasculature. If access has already been lost, initial evaluation for neurovascular embolus detection includes CT angiography with perfusion imaging or diffusion-weighted MR imaging (DWI)/fluid-attenuated inversion recovery (FLAIR) MR imaging. In the posterior fossa, the CT angiography study may be lower yield due to artifact from the surrounding bone. Larger distribution vessel emboli would be visible on the CT angiogram, but the utility of the perfusion study would be limited. Expedited MR imaging will demonstrate increased restricted diffusion on the DWI sequence in the setting of an acute infarct. The MR imaging DWI/FLAIR modality is more sensitive for small vessel perfusion deficits and is the preferred technique for detecting postprocedural embolic events. Evaluation for the detection of a peripheral distal extremity embolus includes noninvasive diagnostic imaging such as distal vessel ultrasound or CT angiography. Diminished pulsatility or vessel cut-off on contrast angiography is suggestive of larger vessel thrombi.

Management of a distal thrombus includes continued use of anticoagulation and antiplatelet agents to decrease the risk for further emboli. Likewise, administration of tissue plasminogen activator or performance of thrombectomy may be necessary to achieve reperfusion. For larger, limb-threatening lesions, an open surgical thrombectomy may be indicated.

In-Stent Thrombosis

Thrombosis of the stent after deployment may cause ischemic injury and/or embolic events. Prior to stent placement, patients receive a dual antiplatelet regimen to prevent in-stent thrombosis. We routinely initiate clopidogrel and aspirin therapy 7 days before treatment and check antiplatelet response assays prior to the procedure. In patients in whom there is clopidogrel resistance, we switch to ticagrelor. Acute in-stent thrombosis is primarily a complication of smaller diameter vessels and is proportional to higher metal density in stents. Because subclavian arteries are large arteries and these stents have low metal content, this is a rare complication.

Initial evaluation of in-stent thrombosis is based on clinical suspicion. Signs of in-stent thrombosis are recurrence of symptoms following successful stent placement, return of pulse pressure differential between limbs, and evidence of distal embolic events. The antiplatelet medication should be measured via aspirin and clopidogrel response assays. Further, obtaining vessel imaging such as CT angiography or repeat DSA is necessary.[7] This confirms the clinical suspicion of in-stent thrombosis as opposed to other possible etiologies for the signs and symptoms.

In cases with confirmed in-stent thrombosis, the initial step is to administer a loading dose of a systemic IIb/IIIa inhibitor, such as eptifibatide (Integrilin, Merck, Whitehouse Station, New Jersey) or abciximab (Reopro, Janssen, Toronto, Ontario, Canada). We always prefer to bring the patient to the angiography suite to confirm revascularization and utilize mechanical embolectomy or aspiration thrombectomy only if the lesion does not respond to pharmacologic measures. In addition, it is imperative to change the antiplatelet agent postprocedure. Careful consideration of antiplatelet agents in the setting of a complication such as in-stent thrombosis is necessary for the prevention of further complications and continued revascularization success/patency of the stent.

If the complication is partially occlusive with thrombus distal to the stent that remains after thrombolytic therapy, we will start systemic anticoagulation therapy. We typically initiate a heparin drip with a partial thromboplastin time (PTT) goal of 60–80 seconds. If there is intracranial pathology, we obtain a baseline brain CT scan prior to the initiation of anticoagulation therapy and another when the heparin is in the therapeutic range. We also obtain a CT image of the head at 6 hours and 24 hours to monitor any intracranial changes on initiation of full-dose anticoagulation therapy. To minimize spontaneous hemorrhage or exacerbation of intracranial hemorrhage, we titrate the heparin dosing and do not administer a loading dose. If the patient remains clinically and neurologically stable, we transition to an oral anticoagulant such as warfarin, with an international normalized ratio goal of 2–3.

Vessel Lumen Dissection

Dissection of the subclavian artery is a rare but potentially devastating complication. It can occur at any stage of the procedure, starting with crossing the lesion and ending up subintimal with potential dissection all the way into the pleural space and subsequent catastrophic hemorrhage Tip Box 49.2. The highest risk of this complication exists when crossing a high-grade stenosis or a chronic total occlusion, which results in a dissection around the stenosis and potentially through the adventitia. Of even greater concern is the risk of retrograde dissection of the aorta when crossing lesions from brachial or radial approaches. Glidewires should be used with extreme caution when attempting to cross lesions in this fashion because it is easy to enter the subintimal plane. This stage requires vigilance with the eyes as well as the hands. It is useful to have an arch angiogram or careful outline of the calcium in the wall to understand the subclavian ostium. If the wire progresses subintimally into the aorta, often recognized by some difficulty advancing and a loop or coiling of the wire in the wall, it should be immediately withdrawn. The catheter should not be advanced because this will enlarge the tear in the aorta. Small dissections may heal without additional intervention. If there is a catheter from the femoral access site, an aortogram should be performed to assess for the extent of the intimal flap and any compromise to branch vessels. Further efforts to cross from the arm should be aborted in this setting. CT angiography of the chest may be needed if the patient experiences any discomfort and the patient should be treated as having a standard, Type B aortic dissection.

For hemorrhage or perforation, the case immediately changes from trying to fix a stenosis to preventing a fatal hemorrhage. The next steps will depend on where the perforation is and what caused it. The anticoagulation should be reversed with protamine. If the rupture is caused by balloon or stent injury of the vessel, it is critical to maintain the wire across the lesion and then to reinflate a balloon gently to tamponade the rupture as well as to contact the operating room immediately in preparation for possible emergent open repair. If the wire has caused the perforation, it should be retracted into the healthy vessel. If the area of injury can be easily crossed, the wire is cautiously advanced and a balloon is again inflated across the lesion to tamponade the hemorrhage and allow stabilization of vital signs. As long as wire control is not lost across the area of injury, this can usually be managed by placement of additional stent grafts to cover the involved area. If endovascular repair is not feasible, but balloon tamponade is, the balloon should be left in place, inflated, while the patient is transferred to the operating room for open repair. If the lesion cannot be crossed and is not at the orifice of the artery, the orifice can be tamponaded with an inflated balloon to decrease hemorrhage. If there is dual access, a balloon can also be inflated from the brachial or radial access site to decrease hemorrhage further. Bleeding will still continue unless the lesion is able to be crossed because the multiple branches off the subclavian will continue to feed the area. If the lesion cannot be crossed, emergent transfer to the operating room is needed for open vascular surgical repair.

> **TIP BOX 49.2**
>
> Avoiding contact with the vessel wall or lesion decreases risk of dissection or embolus.

Initial evaluation for vessel lumen dissection occurs during the procedure and can be detected on angiography. Delayed dissections or dissections that were unnoticed during the procedure may remain asymptomatic; however, they can be visualized on follow-up angiography or other imaging studies. Limiting lesion manipulation is a key principle to avoid procedural dissections. Visualization is facilitated by high-quality angiography to identify the path through the stenosis, sometimes using anterograde injection through a pigtail catheter in the arch or through a guide in the subclavian ostium, and a retrograde injection through a radial or brachial guide catheter close to the lesion. Once the path is illuminated, our preference is to use a 0.035″ Glidewire to cross the lesion. However, in the case of a chronic total occlusion it is better to use a dedicated chronic total occlusion wire such as the Pilot (Abbott Vascular, Santa Clara, California) through a microcatheter followed by progressive predilation with a balloon or through insertion of the dilator over which the delivery sheath can be advanced. We always cross the lesion with the delivery sheath/guide over the wire and then unsheath the stent, rather than advance an unprotected stent or stent graft across the lesion. This greatly reduces the risk of stripping the stent off the balloon on which it is mounted. This approach may further reduce the risk of dissection.[6]

Management of vessel lumen dissection is most commonly undertaken conservatively. For early detection during the initial procedure, continuation of systemic anticoagulation for 24–48 hours after the procedure and use of antiplatelet agents help to prevent emboli from forming.

For lesions that are symptomatic in the acute or delayed setting, we often increase the dosing of the antiplatelet agent or add additional antiplatelet agents, such as ticagrelor. The addition of an anticoagulant can prevent further progression of symptoms or occurrence of embolic complications. Likewise, placement of a stent over the dissecting lesion prevents further embolic events. We reserve stenting of a dissection flap to those cases in which critical limitation of flow is angiographically evident. In lesions that result in complete occlusion of the subclavian artery or complete inability to advance a stent across the stenotic lesion, surgical transposition of the subclavian artery onto the carotid artery is indicated.

Stent Malpositioning

Inadequate positioning of subclavian stents can occur in several ways. During or after deployment, the stent may migrate distal to the stenotic segment. Likewise, the stent may be improperly sized for the vessel and cover arterial branches. Correct sizing with intravascular ultrasound imaging may be helpful prior to choosing the stent graft. Finally, placement of the stent too proximally may result in proximal overhang into the aorta. Maintaining the sheath just below the lesion will help prevent jumping of the graft into the aorta.

Retrieval with a snare may be necessary for a migrated stent.[7] Proper stent size selection before the intervention prevents covering branching vessels. Using a balloon to dilate the stent cells that cover the vessel allows maintained flow; however, proper stent sizing is key. Finally, we use a balloon to flare the ends of the stent to correct proximal overhang (Fig. 49.3). We may intentionally leave proximal overhang and balloon dilate, or flare, specifically to allow a longer construct and better anchor against the parent vessel wall. This also diminishes the risk of distal stent migration resulting from the proximal end being flared and unable to fit into the narrower vessel lumen.

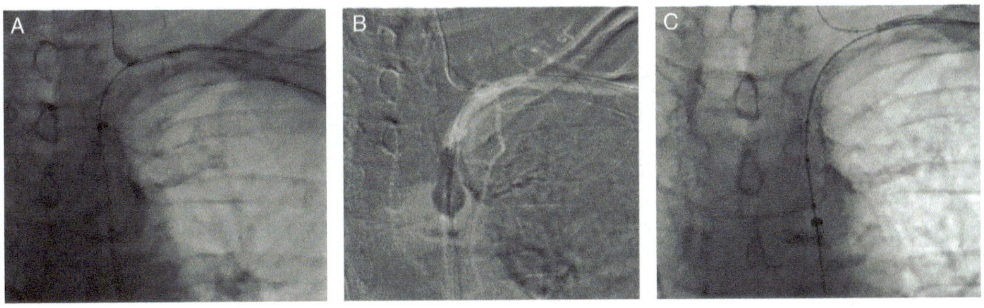

Fig. 49.3 Stent placement with proximal overhang and remodeling. (A) Pre-remodeling angiogram. (B) Flash Ostial dual diameter balloon (Ostial, Santa Clara, California) angioplasty of proximal stent. (C) Post-stenting and remodeling angiogram.

CONCLUSION

Stenting for subclavian steal is a common procedure. Using the aforementioned procedural advice and protection allows successful and safe treatment with a decreased risk of associated complications.

ACKNOWLEDGMENTS

The authors thank Paul H. Dressel, BFA for preparation of the illustrations and Elaine C. Mosher, MLS for editorial assistance.

REFERENCES

1. Liu Y, Zhang J, Gu Y, et al. Clinical effectiveness of endovascular therapy for total occlusion of the subclavian arteries: A study of 67 patients. *Ann Vasc Surg.* 2016;35:189–196.
2. Cua B, Mamdani N, Halpin D, et al. Review of coronary subclavian steal syndrome. *J Cardiol.* 2017;70:432–437.
3. Lu X, Ma Y, Yang B, et al. Hybrid technique for the treatment of refractory vertebrobasilar insufficiencies. *World Neurosurg.* 2017;107:e13–e17.
4. Chatterjee S, Nerella N, Chakravarty S, et al. Angioplasty alone versus angioplasty and stenting for subclavian artery stenosis—a systematic review and meta-analysis. *Am J Ther.* 2013;20:520–523.
5. Levy EI, Turk AS, Albuquerque FC, et al. Wingspan in-stent restenosis and thrombosis: incidence, clinical presentation, and management. *Neurosurgery.* 2007;61:644–650; discussion 50–1.
6. Tang X, Long WA, Hu C, et al. The modified "no touch" technique in the antegrade endovascular approach for left common carotid artery ostial stenosis stenting. *J Neurointerv Surg.* 2017;9:137–141.
7. Acar G, Fidan S, Alici G, et al. Retrieval of a malpositioned left subclavian artery stent from the ascending aorta: combined percutaneous and surgical management. *Herz.* 2015;40:325–328.
8. Alkhouli M, Porter J, Waits B, et al. Distal embolization during percutaneous subclavian artery intervention. *Vasc Endovascular Surg.* 2016;50: 175–179.

50

Complications in the Endovascular Treatment of Intracranial Arteriovenous Malformations

Vernard S. Fennell, MD, MSc, Gursant S. Atwal, MD, Kunal Vakharia, MD and Kenneth V. Snyder, MD, PhD, FACS, FAANS

INTRODUCTION

Intracranial arteriovenous malformations (AVM) are a demanding pathology to treat. There is ample discussion about which single modality or which amalgam of modalities is the most optimal, i.e., endovascular embolization, microsurgical resection, or radiosurgery. The discussion also extends to not only how but also whether to treat. Several grading scales for AVMs exist, while classically the relative morbidity of the open microsurgical approach has been previously outlined in the Spetzler-Martin (SM) grading scale.[1] The microsurgical morbidity has been tied largely to specific anatomical and physiological characteristics that may make microsurgical resection more challenging. The SM grading scale specifically highlights the size of the AVM nidus, the presence of deep venous drainage, and the relative eloquence of the surrounding cortical tissue as crucial factors to consider in the microsurgical treatment of these complex lesions (Table 50.1). This grading system is widely in use and wonderfully outlines the surgical morbidity.[1] Although many interventionists have superimposed the relative risk of surgical treatment of SM-graded AVMs onto that of endovascular treatment, the SM scheme does not adequately reflect the unique determinants of risk associated with endovascular treatment of AVMs.[2–6]

As endovascular techniques have briskly evolved as part of single modality and multimodality treatment, additional grading measures have been outlined.[2,3,7] In this chapter, we focus on the technical aspects of endovascular treatment of intracranial AVMs, common complications, and how to avoid them.

COMMON COMPLICATIONS

Endovascular treatment of AVMs involves superselective microcatheterization of pathologic arterial feeding vessels (pedicles) and the infusion of embolic material with the goal of reducing or eliminating arterial supply to the AVM nidus.[8] Common intracranial complications associated with endovascular treatment of intracranial AVMs are largely hemorrhagic or ischemic in nature.[4,8–13] Hemorrhagic complications can be further viewed as immediate or delayed.[14] Meanwhile, ischemic complications occur most commonly as a result of arterial embolization to vessels supplying normal cortex. In their review of AVM embolization performed in 153 patients, Kim et al. noted outcomes in 508 embolized vessels during 203 sessions.[4] Those authors noted increasing neurological deficit with increasing number of branches embolized per session. The periprocedural complication rate was 11.8% in the short term and the rate of permanent disability (modified Rankin scale score [mRS] >2) was 2%. They also noted increasing neurologic deficit with increasing SM grade at rates of 0%, 5%, 7%, 10%, and 18% for grades I–V, respectively. Using a grading system germane to the endovascular treatment of AVMs, Dumont et al. stratified AVM treatment risk based on the number of arterial pedicles, the diameter of arterial pedicles, and eloquence of the surrounding cortex.[3] Their scale, similar to the SM system, purports increasing morbidity with increasing grade (Table 50.2). Others have added further hemodynamic parameters with respect to possible endovascular grading of AVMs.[2] Bell et al. included the number of feeding arteries and the region of cortical eloquence as part of their analysis.[2] Those authors also added the additional hemodynamic factor of the presence of an arteriovenous fistulous component as a crucial hemodynamic component. They noted that their grading scheme was useful in determining the multimodal outcomes of AVM treatment.

The most common hemorrhagic complication is associated with arterial perforation secondary to wire manipulation.[14] However, the most deleterious hemorrhagic complication is associated with delayed postprocedural hemorrhage, which is commonly attributed to premature venous outflow opacification.

The choice of embolic material can have an effect on radiographic and clinical outcomes.[8,11] Elsenousi et al. reviewed 103 studies of AVMs treated with n-butyl cyanoacrylate (NBCA) and a more recent and widely used liquid embolic agent, ethylene-vinyl alcohol co-polymer (EVOH).[11] Poor neurological outcome occurred in 5.2% of NBCA cases and 6.8% of EVOH cases, although the difference was not statistically significant. However, complete obliteration rates were 13.7% in the NBCA cohort and 24% in the EVOH group, which did exhibit statistical significance. As a result, the common consensus is that although NBCA may provide a more pronounced radiographic treatment response, the use of EVOH is associated with fewer treatment-related complications.

AVOIDING COMPLICATIONS

With respect to avoiding complications, a meticulous review of the imaging studies to obtain a thorough understanding of the complex angioarchitecture of the lesion is critical preprocedurally as well as intraprocedurally. Identification of high-risk components is of paramount importance; these include intranidal aneurysms, high-flow arteriovenous shunts, venous stenosis, deep venous drainage, number and size of feeding pedicles, and relative eloquence of adjacent cortical structures. Eloquent location can be assessed with pretreatment magnetic resonance imaging of the brain. Any portion of the AVM nidus noted to be in the primary motor or sensory cortex, including language and vision areas, as well as the hypothalamus, thalamus, midbrain, pons, medulla, and the cerebellar peduncles, is considered to be in an eloquent location (Table 50.3).[1] The relative goals for treatment should be clear and apparent and will differ for patients who present with hemorrhage, with other nonhemorrhagic neurologic sequelae, or with no apparent neurologic symptoms.

The selection of access via a transradial or a transfemoral route depends on the location of the lesion. Lesions with primary right

TABLE 50.1 Spetzler-Martin arteriovenous malformation (AVM) grading scale.

Feature		Points
Size		
	Small (<3 cm)	1
	Medium (3–6 cm)	2
	Large (>6 cm)	3
Eloquence of adjacent brain		
	Noneloquent	0
	Eloquent	1
Venous drainage pattern		
	Superficial only	0
	Deep	1

AVM Grade = [size] + [eloquence] + [venous drainage pattern]; that is [1, 2, or 3] + [0 or 1] + [0 or 1].
Adapted from Spetzler RF, Martin NA. A proposed grading system for arteriovenous malformations. *J Neurosurg.* 1986;65:478.

TABLE 50.2 Buffalo endovascular grading score.

Angiographic feature		Points
Number of arterial pedicles		
	1 or 2	1
	3 or 4	2
	5 or more	3
Diameter of arterial pedicles		
	Most >1 mm	0
	Most ≤1 mm	1
Nidus location		
	Noneloquent	0
	Eloquent	1

AVM grade = [number] + [diameter] + [nidus location] AVM, Arteriovenous malformation.
From Dumont TM, Kan P, Snyder KV, et al. A proposed grading system for endovascular treatment of cerebral arteriovenous malformations: Buffalo score. *Surg Neurol Int.* 2015;6:3 [open-access article].

vertebral artery feeding branches or difficult to navigate aortic arches may be well suited for transradial or transbrachial access. However, we most commonly utilize transfemoral access. We most often begin our approach with 6-French sheath access and may upsize to 8-French access if additional stability necessitates triaxial access and the use of an intermediate or distal access catheter. Proper assessment with respect for the need for biaxial versus triaxial support is crucial in eliminating issues related to navigation and support. Biaxial systems are used most frequently because they offer the ability to perform injections from the guide catheter while having access to a microcatheter to select the arterial feeders to an AVM. Triaxial systems are effective when trying to reach very distal lesions that may need support from an intermediate catheter to allow the microcatheter to gain distal access or may need an intermediate catheter to help remove the microcatheter if reflux occurs during the procedure.

TABLE 50.3 Eloquent cortex by Spetzler-Martin criteria.

1. Primary motor cortex
2. Sensory cortex
Language Visual cortex
3. Hypothalamus
4. Thalamus
5. Midbrain
6. Pons
7. Medulla
8. Cerebellar peduncle

Created from data presented in Spetzler RF, Martin NA. A proposed grading system for arteriovenous malformations. *J Neurosurg.* 1986;65:478.

TIP BOX 50.1

Although an Allen test may be useful, a failed Allen test does not necessarily correlate with an ischemic hand following radial catheterization. If the patient fails the Allen text, we may consider using a transfemoral approach instead.

TIP BOX 50.2

Address intranidal aneurysms first.
Avoid premature venous opacification: If premature venous opacification occurs, the surgeon must be prepared to treat the AVM completely because this may change the hemodynamic flow patterns, leading to higher risk of rupture.
Avoid over-embolization in a single session: <35% of total AVM volume per session.

The preintervention plan should also include assessment of the relative size of the feeding arteries. Vessels with diameters <1 mm should either be avoided or traversed with a 0.010″ microwire and a smaller flow-directed microcatheter. Larger feeding arteries may be more robust and able to accommodate a 0.014″ wire system.

TREATMENT PARADIGM

Our general treatment paradigm is as follows:

1. Selection of 6-French short (10 cm) sheath for transfemoral access.
   a. 6-French slender sheath may be utilized for patient-appropriate transradial access (Tip Box 50.1).
2. Benchmark 6-French outer diameter (OD), 0.071″ inner diameter (ID) guide catheter (Penumbra, Alameda, California) or Envoy DA/XB 6 F OD, 0.070 ID guide catheter (Codman, Raynham, Massachusetts) for standard coaxial access.
   a. NeuronMax catheter OD 8.5 French, ID 0.088″ ID (Penumbra) with intermediate catheter for triaxial access.
3. Microcatheter and wire selection based on perceived navigability of arterial feeders and dimethyl sulfoxide (DMSO) compatibility.

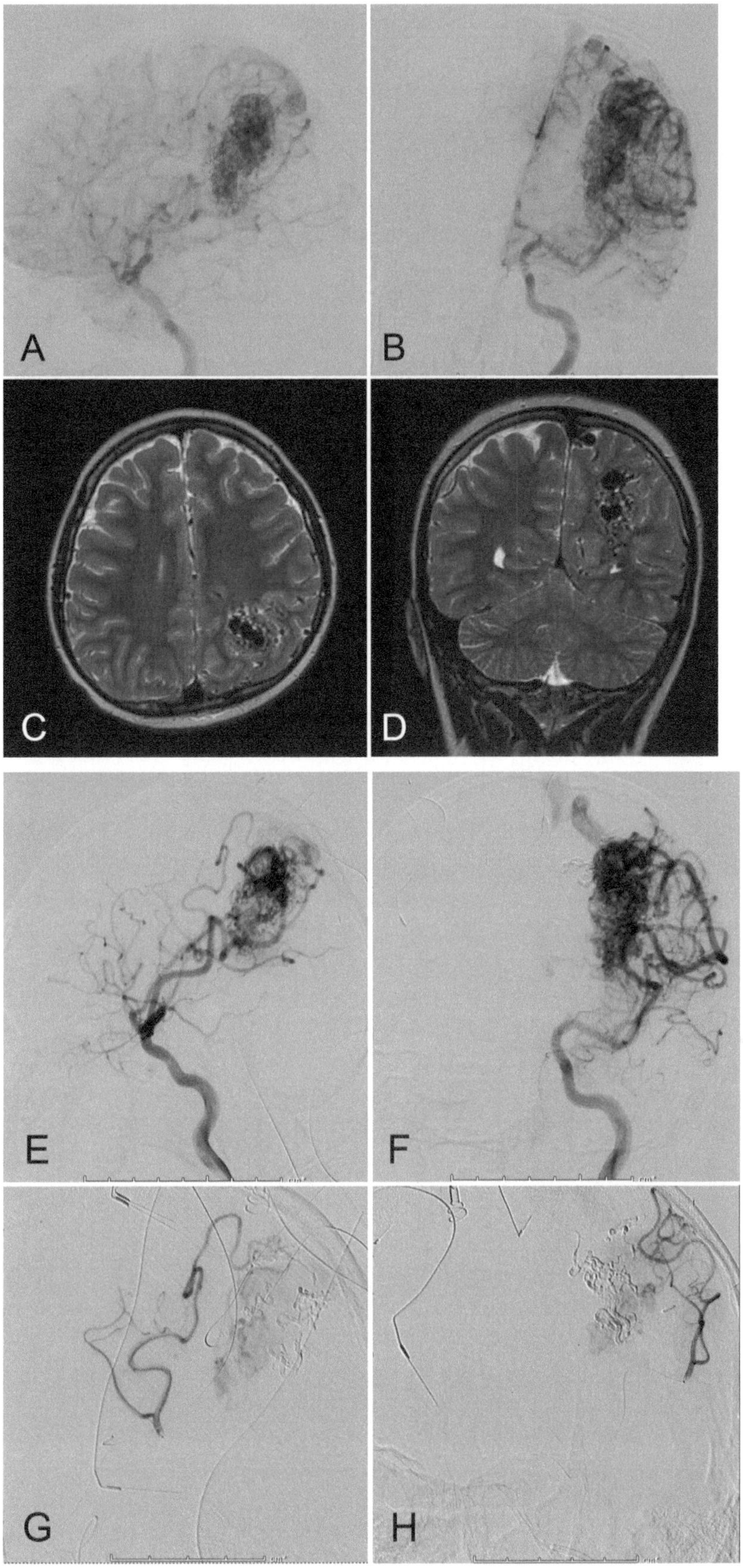

Fig. 50.1 An 11-year-old boy initially presented with a small hemorrhage and was noted to have a Spetzler-Martin grade 3 arteriovenous malformation (AVM) (size 3, eloquence 0, venous drainage 0). Images at presentation include anteroposterior (A) and lateral (B) diagnostic cerebral angiogram and axial (C) and coronal (D) T2-weighted magnetic resonance images and show a left parietal AVM. The patient underwent multiple endovascular embolizations. Prior to his final embolization treatment, persistent AVM supplied by early draining veins was noted on digital subtraction angiography (E, F). Anteroposterior (G) and lateral (H) projection microcatheterizations indicate the high degree of tortuosity. Microangiographic examination after long and tortuous micronavigation shows extravasation of contrast material (I–N). Control of the hemorrhage was assumed by keeping the microcatheter in place, purging with DMSO, and then administering Onyx (Medtronic, Minneapolis, Minnesota) while slowly pulling the catheter back into the vessel. Absence of extravasation is noted on a follow-up run through the guide catheter (O). Postprocedural axial (P) and coronal (Q) computed tomography images of the head demonstrate intra- and extraparenchymal contrast material. After microsurgical resection, no residual AVM is seen on the final digital subtraction angiogram (R, S).

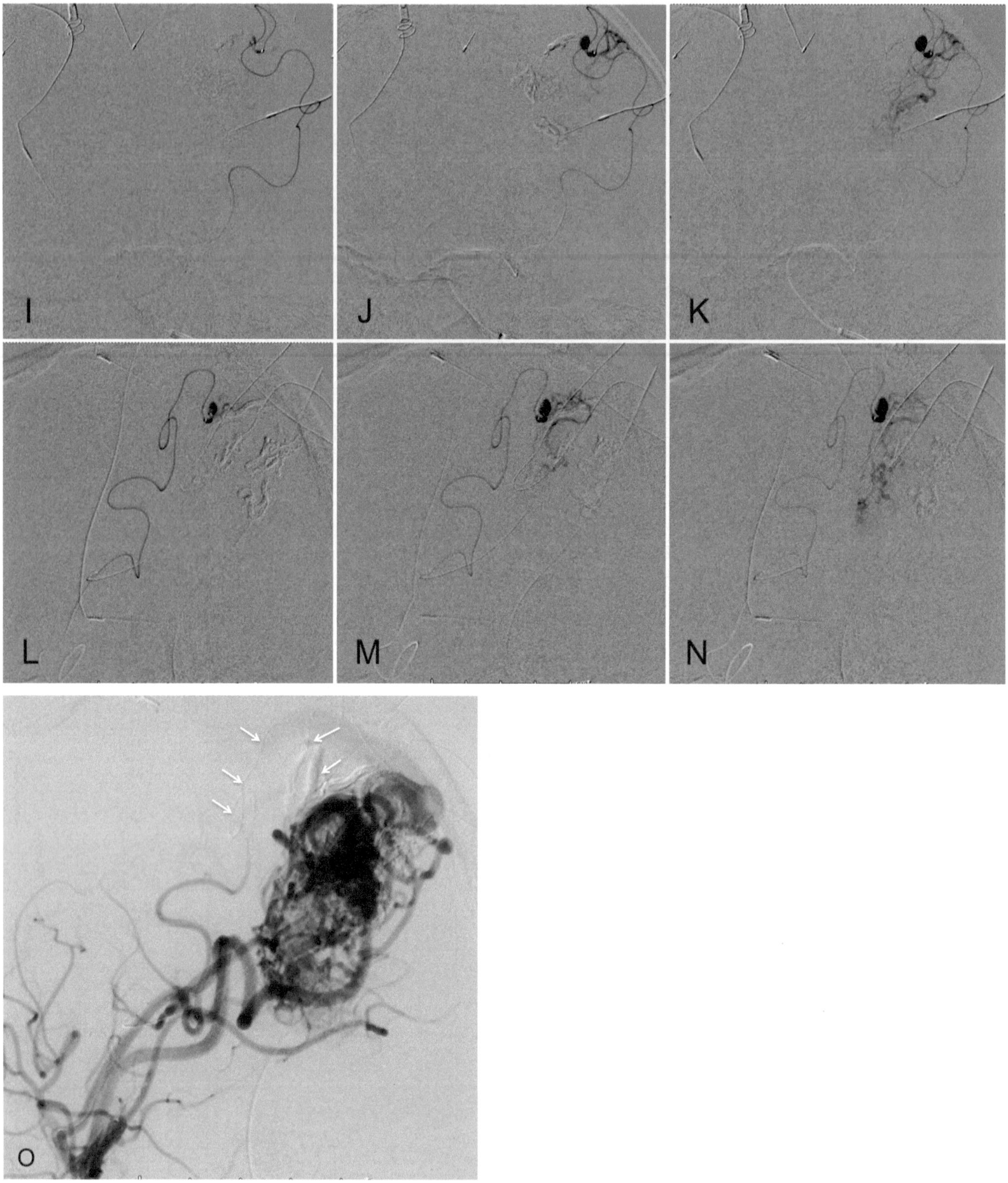

Fig. 50.1 (Continued).

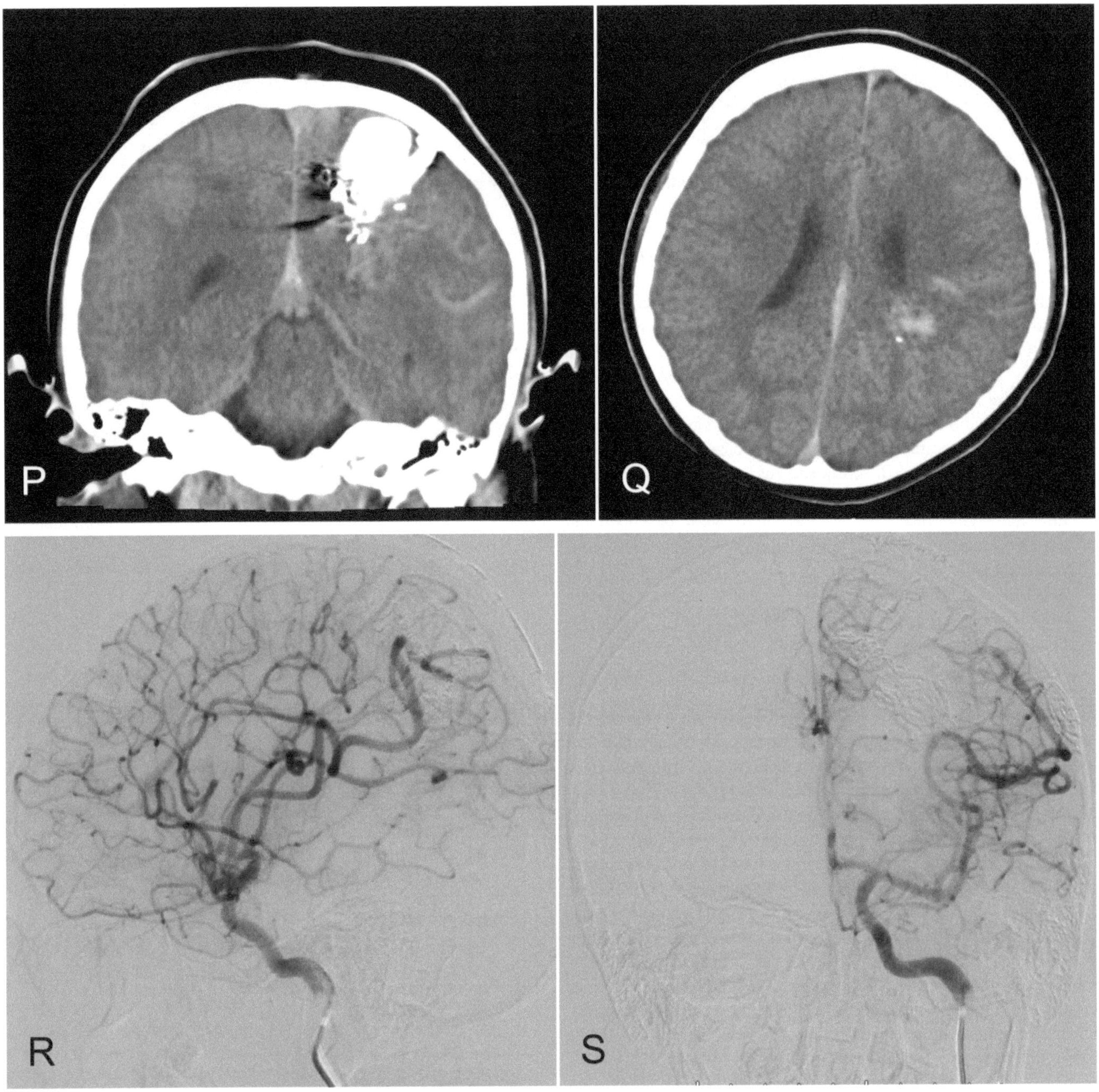

Fig. 50.1 (Continued).

a. Headway duo 156 cm OD 2.1 French, ID 0.016″ microwire (MicroVention, Aliso Viejo, California)
b. Headway duo 167 cm OD 2.1 French, ID 0.013″ (MicroVention)
c. Marathon 165 cm OD 2.7 French, ID 0.013″ microwire (Medtronic, Minneapolis, Minnesota)

4. Once arterial access (femoral) achieved, intravenous heparin bolus (50 units/kg) delivered.
   a. Radial access requires radial artery cocktail: heparin, nitroglycerin, verapamil, lidocaine, and bicarbonate.
5. Activated clotting time (ACT) obtained from transarterial sample prior to microcatheterization. Goal ACT >300 seconds.
6. Achieve secondary access to intracranial vasculature with standard speed 6 frames per second and high speed 12 frames per second.
7. We routinely obtain three-dimensional rotational spin angiography to visualize the angiographic architecture completely.
8. Working views obtained from rotational angiography.
9. Navigate most accessible feeding arteries with microwire and microcatheter, getting as close to the nidus as possible.
10. Microangiographic assessment with first 3-cc syringe with 100% contrast material, followed by a 1-cc syringe of contrast material if inadequate.
11. Once vessel has been selected, while the patient is on the angiography table, a Wada test is performed with a 1.5 mL infusion of sodium amobarbital, followed by 1.5 mL of lidocaine.
12. Clinical examination on the table (conscious sedation), specific to region of cortex involved in AVM. (Baseline examination should be known prior to on-table Wada test.)

a. Assess changes in neurophysiological monitoring with somatosensory evoked potentials (SSEP) or motor-evoked potentials (MEP). Compare with baseline findings.
13. Changes from baseline clinical examination or in SSEP or MEP should result in alternative artery selection or advancement of catheter to closest distance to AVM nidus and repeat Wada testing.
14. Microcatheter purged with DMSO titrated to dead space of DMSO-compatible microcatheter at a rate of 0.1 mL/min.
15. Ensure no microbubbles are present when connecting with liquid embolic syringe.
16. Infuse Onyx liquid embolic agent (Medtronic) at a rate similar to that for DMSO.
17. Obtain reverse roadmap imaging at 75% volume of microcatheter dead space and infuse under fluoroscopic guidance.
18. Careful assessment of nidal penetration and observance of liquid emboli reflux around microcatheter and monitoring for any premature venous penetration.
19. Frequent follow-up angiographic examination after embolization.
20. Use one microcatheter per vessel embolized; once adequate embolization is achieved, "break seal" of liquid embolic and exert negative pressure on syringe with aspiration from guide catheter.
21. Re-acquire additional feeding vessel and repeat or obtain de-magnified angiographic run to assess for any spurious or unintended vessel occlusion.
22. Assessment of secondary access (vertebral artery, common carotid artery) for potential catheter-related injury.
23. Postprocedure transfer to intensive care unit (Tip Box 50.2).

GETTING OUT OF TROUBLE

Getting out of trouble is most commonly associated with staying out of trouble. With respect to hemorrhagic complications, wire perforations can be addressed with timely embolization of the perforated vessel segment and reversal of the therapeutic effect of the intravenous heparin if appropriate (Fig. 50.1). Postprocedural hemorrhage can be addressed with control of blood pressure and induced hypotension (systolic blood pressure <120 mmHg) and monitored with serial neurologic examinations and C scans. Aminocaproic acid (Amicar, Xanodyne Pharmaceuticals, Newport, Kentucky) has been administered in these cases, but that is not our common practice. A microcatheter that is retained after liquid embolic delivery can be navigated by applying persistent negative syringe pressure with intermittent infusion of DMSO back down the microcatheter. If a long unencumbered feeding artery is anticipated, a detachable microcatheter (e.g., Apollo, Medtronic) may also be prophylactically used.

CONCLUSION

AVM treatment has evolved into multimodal treatment that involves, in part, endovascular embolization. Keeping complications in any sole treatment modality to a minimum is crucial to effective and safe treatment of these challenging lesions.

ACKNOWLEDGMENTS

The authors thank Paul H. Dressel, BFA for preparation of the images and Debra J. Zimmer for editorial assistance.

REFERENCES

1. Spetzler RF, Martin NA. A proposed grading system for arteriovenous malformations. *J Neurosurg.* 1986;65:476–483.
2. Bell DL, Leslie-Mazwi TM, Yoo AJ, et al. Application of a novel brain arteriovenous malformation endovascular grading scale for transarterial embolization. *Am J Neuroradiol.* 2015;36:1303–1309.
3. Dumont TM, Kan P, Snyder KV, et al. A proposed grading system for endovascular treatment of cerebral arteriovenous malformations: Buffalo score. *Surg Neurol Int.* 2015;6:3.
4. Kim LJ, Albuquerque FC, Spetzler RF, et al. Postembolization neurological deficits in cerebral arteriovenous malformations: stratification by arteriovenous malformation grade. *Neurosurgery.* 2006;59:53–59.
5. Mokin M, Dumont TM, Levy EI. Novel multimodality imaging techniques for diagnosis and evaluation of arteriovenous malformations. *Neurol Clin.* 2014;32:225–236.
6. Pollock BE, Flickinger JC. A proposed radiosurgery-based grading system for arteriovenous malformations. *J Neurosurg.* 2002; 96:79–85.
7. Spetzler RF, Ponce FA. A 3-tier classification of cerebral arteriovenous malformations. Clinical article. *J Neurosurg.* 2011;114:842–849.
8. Conger A, Kulwin C, Lawton MT, et al. Endovascular and microsurgical treatment of cerebral arteriovenous malformations: Current recommendations. *Surg Neurol Int.* 2015;6:39.
9. Asadi H, Kok HK, Looby S, et al. Outcomes and complications after endovascular treatment of brain arteriovenous malformations: a prognostication attempt using artificial intelligence. *World Neurosurg.* 2016;96:562–569.e1.
10. Cagnazzo F, Brinjikji W, Lanzino G. Arterial aneurysms associated with arteriovenous malformations of the brain: classification, incidence, risk of hemorrhage, and treatment—a systematic review. *Acta Neurochir (Wien).* 2016;158:2095–2104.
11. Elsenousi A, Aletich VA, Alaraj A. Neurological outcomes and cure rates of embolization of brain arteriovenous malformations with n-butyl cyanoacrylate or Onyx: a meta-analysis. *J Neurointerv Surg.* 2016;8:265–272.
12. Parsaee M, Saedi S, Emami S, et al. Detection of a rare complication of endovascular treatment for brain arteriovenous malformation with echocardiography. *World Neurosurg.* 2017;98(869):e13–e15.
13. Pierot L, Januel AC, Herbreteau D, et al. Endovascular treatment of brain arteriovenous malformations using Onyx: preliminary results of a prospective multicenter study. *Interv Neuroradiol.* 2005;11:159–164.
14. Baharvahdat H, Blanc R, Termechi R, et al. Hemorrhagic complications after endovascular treatment of cerebral arteriovenous malformations. *Am J Neuroradiol.* 2014;35:978–983.

51

Complication of Endovascular Treatment of Intracranial Stenosis

Fucheng Tian, MD, Mithun G. Sattur, MD, MBBS, MCh, FEBNS, Devi P. Patra, MBBS, MCh, MRCSED, Matthew E. Welz, MS, Chandan Krishna, MD, Karl Abi-Aad, MD, Joseph B. Farnsworth, PA-C MMS, MBMS and Bernard R. Bendok, MD, MSCI

INTRODUCTION

Intracranial atherosclerotic disease (ICAD) is defined as atherosclerosis of the large intracranial arteries, namely the intracranial internal carotid artery (ICA), intracranial vertebral and basilar arteries, middle, anterior and posterior cerebral arteries, and their cortical branches (up to M3, A3, or P3 segments). Atherosclerotic disease of the small perforator and penetrating arteries is termed as small vessel (or small artery) disease. The term intracranial stenosis (ICS) usually denotes atherosclerotic narrowing of the main segments of the intracranial arteries involving the intracranial ICA, proximal segments of middle cerebral artery (MCA) (M1), anterior cerebral artery (ACA) (A1), posterior cerebral artery (PCA) (P1), basilar artery (BA), and the distal segment of vertebral artery (V4).

ICAD is a major cause of ischemic stroke accounting for up to 10% of strokes in the United States and as many as 30% in Asian, Hispanic, and African American communities.[1] After one symptomatic event, the risk of recurrent stroke may be as high as 15% per year. Treatment with aspirin (or warfarin) in addition to other risk factor modification reduces the risk but the risk may still be as high as 22% at 2 years despite therapy.[2] Multiple randomized clinical trials including SAMMPRIS (Stenting and Aggressive Medical Management for Preventing Recurrent Stroke in Intracranial Stenosis) and VISSIT (The Vitesse Intracranial Stent Study for Ischemic Stroke Therapy) have evaluated the outcome after medical management alone and with percutaneous angioplasty and stenting. In spite of all efforts, management of ICAD is still challenging and optimal treatment modality is still unclear.

PATHOPHYSIOLOGY OF STROKES IN INTRACRANIAL STENOSIS

It is imperative to understand the pathophysiology of strokes in ICAD patients to perceive the complications associated with its treatment. ICS can produce symptoms through the following mechanisms[3,4]:

- artery-to-artery emboli
- hemodynamic insufficiency
- acute thrombotic occlusion (unstable plaque)
- branch (perforator) occlusive disease

The literature tends to be unclear regarding in-depth descriptions of these pathophysiologic mechanisms in individual patients. This is particularly relevant in the case of branch occlusive disease (BOD). This entity is often mistakenly identified as small vessel disease while in reality it is ICAD that incorporates the perforator origins. The plaques in these cases have been identified on high resolution MRI to be unstable, despite a relatively smaller extent of luminal stenosis.[3] This has potential implications in interpreting data from stenting trials. MRI in such cases shows small deep "lacunar" infarcts. The phenomenon of hypoperfusion from severe stenosis is well described and occurs as a result of exhausted cerebrovascular reserve in the affected vascular territory. Patients typically develop orthostatic or exercise/stress-related ischemic symptoms. MRI reveals multiple watershed cortical infarcts in the affected arterial territory. Patients with ICS who have hypoperfusion symptoms have a higher recurrent stroke risk than those without.[5] Although SAMMPRIS failed to identify these patients as benefiting from stenting, well-designed prospective single center studies have shown impressive reduction in recurrent ischemic events in such patients following extracranial–intracranial (EC–IC) bypass.[6] Finally, one of the important causes of stroke in ICAD patients is the artery-to-artery embolism in which small emboli formed de novo because of relative stasis or plaque rupture may travel along the gradient to smaller distal territories to produce focal strokes.

All three of these pathomechanisms produce distinct stroke patterns and have different therapeutic and prognostic implications. For example, perforator related strokes are usually located in the subcortical or basal ganglia region, hypoperfusion strokes affect the water-shed areas, and artery-to-artery embolic strokes affect distal small vascular territories. Hypoperfusion related border-zone infarct was the most common pattern observed in the SAMMPRIS trial in contrast to the territorial strokes from artery-to-artery emboli seen in the WASID (Warfarin Aspirin Symptomatic Intracranial Disease) trial. Nevertheless, the stroke pattern in ICAD patients can be mixed, involving more than one pathomechanism.

TREATMENT

The optimal treatment protocol of ICAD is still evolving and is subject to great controversy especially after multiple randomized trials published variable results. However, the SAMMPRIS trial and its subsequent post hoc analysis studies, along with the VISSIT trial, have supported the role of medical management as the first line therapy to be instituted in all patients of ICAD with a significant risk of stroke.[7] Surgical/endovascular management is now reserved for patients who develop recurrent transient ischemic attack (TIA) or strokes despite aggressive medical management. Although the protocol for maximal medical management is poorly defined, broadly it includes smoking cessation, antiplatelet therapy such as aspirin, clopidogrel, or dual antiplatelet therapy (DAPT), hyperlipidemia management with statins, hypertension control, and lifestyle modification with diet and activity.

Up to 12% of patients with medical management may fail therapy at 1 year, which may increase to 14%–22% at 2 years, and keep experiencing recurrent stroke/TIA symptoms. These patients are the focus of potential endovascular neurosurgical intervention. It is reiterated that based on studies to date it is advisable to prove failure of full medical therapy and, where indicated, demonstrate hemodynamic insufficiency before embarking on the endovascular path.

Endovascular Procedures

Since the 1980s, endovascular angioplasty has emerged as a successful minimally invasive treatment option for intracranial stenosis. Multiple retrospective and non-randomized studies published successful treatment with balloon angioplasty with or without stenting with a technical success rate of around 97% and complication rates ranging from 10% to 50%.[8,9] The landmark SAMMPRIS trial was designed to evaluate the role of stenting in patients with severe stenosis with the Wingspan stent (Stryker Inc., Fremont, California). Interestingly, the trial concluded that intracranial stenting carried a higher 30-day and 2-year primary end-point of stroke, TIA, or death from vascular cause than best medical therapy. Similarly, the VISSIT trial enrolled 112 patients with symptomatic intracranial stenosis (70%—99%) into medical management and balloon-expandable stent group; however, the trial was prematurely halted because the interim analysis showed clear increased 30-day risk of any stroke in the stented group.

There is appreciation in the neurovascular world that there is most likely a distinct subset of patients with ICAD who may benefit from endovascular luminal restoration techniques in addition to medical therapy. This is especially relevant as technology rapidly evolves making devices much safer and more user-friendly than those used in SAMMPRIS. The high periprocedural stroke rate related to intracranial stenting in select locations in SAMMPRIS, which used a first-generation device, has led to a resurgence of interest in balloon angioplasty.[10] The technique of submaximal angioplasty has been described in prospective studies to be feasible and safe, with periprocedural complication rates of around 5% as opposed to the nearly 15% rate in SAMMPRIS.[11,12] The technique has been described using Gateway or Maverick (Boston Scientific, Fremont, California) or Mini-trek (Abbott, Abbott Park, Illinois) balloon catheters. The latter two are semi-compliant coronary balloons. The actual surgical technique involves using a standard access system with a sheath and an intermediate guide catheter. A 0.014″ microwire is navigated across the stenosis and the balloon is navigated either as an exchange technique with a microcatheter or directly delivered over the wire. The balloon is 50%—80% undersized for the luminal diameter. Inflation is gradually performed and held at nominal pressure for up to a minute. Total flow arrest times are thus negligible and only one inflation usually suffices. The angiographic end-point that is aimed for is restoration of luminal diameter of more than 50% instead of a perfect-appearing result.

Complications with Endovascular Therapy of ICS

Although many of the prospective and retrospective individual case series have reported an acceptable complication rate, the main reason for negativisms for angioplasty and stenting from the SAMMPRIS and VISSIT trial is the higher periprocedural and 30 days event rates. It should be noted that these trials did not stratify lesions based on morphology, which probably influenced the trial results. A detailed understanding of complications of endovascular therapy is needed to advise patients. Overall, these complications can be categorized into two types:

General complications associated with cerebral angiography.

Specific complications related to angioplasty and/or stenting.

1. **General complications associated with cerebral angiography**

   These are dealt with in detail elsewhere in this book. Briefly, they mostly relate to access site hematoma, pseudoaneurysm, or contrast nephropathy (Table 51.1). The important complications related to catheterization of cervicocerebral arteries are thromboembolism and spasm or dissection. These important adverse events can be catastrophic and may be caused by poor technique, challenging vessel anatomy, and underlying vasculopathy related to atherosclerosis. There was a higher than expected angiographic stroke rate in the SAMMPRIS trial. Tortuous arch anatomy with a high burden of aortic arch/carotid artery atherosclerosis, improper technique, prolonged intravascular time, inadequate preparation with antiplatelets, or anticoagulation are potential risk factors. Transradial access has been described as a means of reducing complications from catheterizing across the arch.[13] Clot formation in the catheter with distal embolism in the catheterized vessel is a very common yet partially avoidable complication. Use of pressurized flush lines, use of periprocedural anticoagulation with heparin and/or antiplatelet agents, and proper cleaning of guidewires before reinsertion are potentially helpful toward reducing complications. Dissection is a feared complication but can be minimized with over-the-wire and proper techniques.

2. **Specific periprocedural complications related to angioplasty and/or stenting**

   These complications are seen in any cerebrovascular endovascular procedures; however, they are more common during angioplasty and/or stenting because of the presence of diseased vessel and atherosclerotic plaques.

   a. ***Microwire perforation***

      This potentially catastrophic complication can result in intracerebral and subarachnoid hemorrhage. The risk increases as smaller vessels are catheterized. Use of stiff wires may increase the risk, which is greater in tortuous vessels. Performing multiple steps over an exchange length wire may increase the risk. Keeping the distal wire in a straight segment of a larger vessel with a J tip configuration may reduce this complication. Therefore, the use of highly navigable balloons in rapid-exchange or monorail fashion would be desirable features of future devices. Vessel perforation caused by the microwire or microcatheter can also be the result of sudden movement of the wire/catheter tip during manipulation with less than adequate proximal guide catheter support. Advances in guide catheter technology have partially mitigated this risk, but tortuosity remains a challenge in many cases. Studying vessel anatomy preoperatively may allow the surgeon to weigh the potential risk and to plan access and support strategies. Microwire perforation caused half of the intraprocedural hemorrhages in the SAMMPRIS trial.[14] Significant advances have occurred since SAMMPRIS in guide catheter, microcatheter, and microwire technology. A post hoc analysis of the trial showed that a higher degree of vessel stenosis, a poor modified Rankin score, and a clopidogrel load are associated with a higher risk of intraprocedural hemorrhage.[15] Vessel perforation usually manifests as subarachnoid hemorrhage and may be seen as contrast extravasation. The bleeding is usually less brisk compared with vessel rupture and can spontaneously seal off due to vessel spasm. In these cases, active contrast extravasation may not be evident because of slow leak and can be detected on the postoperative CT scans. However, in patients with ICAD, a significant subarachnoid hemorrhage can theoretically result because of stiff and sclerosed vessels, which does not allow spontaneous spasm of the vessel. Perforation in larger vessels such as the ICA, BA, and VA can be potentially salvaged with balloon tamponade ideally for no longer than 10 minutes at a time and/or flow diversion stenting. Smaller vessels, however, such as the MCA or ACA may require permanent occlusion with coils or glue.

TABLE 51.1 Important complications and their preventive measures.

Type	Complication	Preventive measures
Access related	Groin hematoma	• Arterial puncture over the femoral head that allows appropriate application of manual pressure after the procedure • Use of USG for vessel localization that avoids multiple punctures • Appropriate use of closure devices • Manual pressure application as indicated
	Retroperitoneal hematoma	• Arterial puncture along the extraperitoneal course of femoral artery • Arterial puncture at an angle of 45 degrees • Arterial puncture over the femoral head that allows appropriate application of manual pressure after the procedure
	Femoral artery dissection	• Arterial puncture at angle of 45 degrees • Use of soft Glidewire after vessel puncture • Avoidance of forceful insertion of guide sheath or catheters • Use of longer sheaths that avoid vessel trauma from multiple insertion of catheters • Careful insertion of sheath or catheters in presence of massive atherosclerotic or calcified femoral artery
	Pseudoaneurysm	• Minimize vessel trauma during puncture by using USG • Appropriate use of closure devices • Manual pressure to seal the puncture site in case of bleeding • Serial USG monitoring for vessel diameter in case of groin hematoma
	Thrombosis	• Avoidance of larger guide sheath or catheters in narrowed femoral vessel • Use of pressurized flush lines using heparinized saline • Appropriate anticoagulation during procedure • Avoid kinking of guide sheath
	Infection	• Use of appropriate sterile precautions during procedure • Use of prophylactic antibiotics not recommended
Renal	Contrast-induced nephropathy	• Preoperative documentation of kidney disease, previous contrast induced nephropathy • Adequate periprocedural hydration • Minimal possible use of intravenous contrast • Maximum suggested contrast dose = (5 mL × body weight [kg])/baseline serum creatinine (mg/dL) • Consider dilution of contrast during injection if kidney function is marginal and/or volumes of contrast become high
Intracranial	Vasospasm	• Use of appropriate sized catheter • Smooth and slow navigation of catheter • Appropriate use of balloon catheter and inflation at nominal pressure
	Dissection	• Smooth and slow navigation of catheter • Use of appropriate sized catheter • Avoid navigation through acute kinks and tortuous vessel • Avoid forceful navigation • Placement of catheter tip along the curve of the vessel before contrast injection • Avoid stiffer wires or catheters
	Thrombosis and embolism	• Appropriate use of pressurized flush lines with heparinized saline • Avoid exchange wires if possible. If necessary, wipe the wire properly before insertion of catheter over the wire • Follow safe contrast injection techniques to avoid air embolism • Periprocedural anticoagulation and antiplatelets • Maximize procedural time efficiency without compromising techniques
	Vessel perforation	• Use of soft wires and catheters • Avoid forceful navigation through kinks and tortuous vessels • Careful navigation through atherosclerotic plaques

USG, Ultrasonography.

b. ***Balloon-related complications***

The main problems with balloon inflation are vessel rupture and dissection. Undersizing the balloon by 0.25–0.5 mm diameter of the normal vessel segment, inflating strictly to the nominal pressure, and a slow inflation time (up to 60 seconds for every atm) may reduce these risks. Vessel rupture diagnosed on the examination table may necessitate occlusion of the ruptured vessel by coiling to prevent a massive intracerebral hemorrhage but it comes at the risk of major infarction of the vascular territory. Vessel rupture in the cavernous segment of the ICA presents with carotid-cavernous fistula and is usually contained. In such cases an attempt with pipeline deployment should be made, which can seal the perforation site. Dissection of the arterial wall after angioplasty is again an important complication, usually related to over-inflation of the balloon or less than ideal catheter/microwire navigation. Mild dissections without flow limitation (Table 51.1) can be carefully observed for progression and some may arrest without luminal compromise, especially with the anticoagulation that is already on board. Some dissections need endothelial reinforcement with stent placement.

c. ***Stent-related complications***

Sizing a stent correctly for the stenosis is important because it helps achieve a smooth procedure. A rule of thumb is choosing a stent diameter that is at least equal to or greater than (next size up) the largest vessel diameter. Length is chosen to be equal to stenosis length plus 2–3 mm on either side. Incorrect wall apposition is always a concern when deploying intravascular stents particularly across tortuous segments. A post-stent placement angioplasty may be necessary to ensure proper wall apposition of the stent and to dilate the stenosis further, but we typically try to avoid this because of stent migration or over-aggressive disruption of the underlying plaque. Again, using a balloon with a diameter smaller than the normal parent artery is important. A semi-compliant balloon is used for this indication, although a noncompliant balloon may be necessary in very calcified lesions. A second stent can be used strategically to overcome deficiencies of deployment with the first stent but potentially added risks. Acute in-stent thrombosis is a dreaded complication. Proper platelet inhibition and anticoagulation may reduce this risk. Immediate recanalization is the goal and may be achieved by intra-arterial thrombolysis with tPA (tissue plasminogen activator) or glycoprotein IIb/IIIa inhibitors such as abciximab or eptifibatide. Ensuring that patients are on dual antiplatelet therapy before and after the procedure is very important in minimizing this risk. Some centers routinely perform platelet inhibition testing to screen potential nonresponders. Nonresponders are at high risk of ischemic complications and are therefore switched to alternative medications. The use of heparin-coated stents to prevent in-stent thrombosis and restenosis in ICS has been reported to be effective, but these stents are currently unavailable. This is an area of potential development with improvements in device and drug technology.[16]

A more medium-term problem that has been described in up to 30% of patients is in-stent restenosis or chronic occlusion on follow-up angiography, but fortunately only about 14% of these are symptomatic. A recent analysis by SAMMPRIS investigators found that one in every seven patients undergoing stenting develops symptomatic restenosis by 3 years.[17] Diagnosing in-stent restenosis is difficult with CT or MR angiography alone because of metal artifact and therefore catheter angiography is the gold standard. But given that most are asymptomatic, noninvasive perfusion techniques such as MR perfusion can serve as useful adjuncts to detect in-stent stenosis.[18] Treatment when indicated is best performed with balloon angioplasty. Rarely, a second stent may be required.

d. ***Periprocedural ischemic strokes***

Multiple mechanisms can contribute to ischemic events during intervention including thrombosis, embolism from proximal segments, occlusion of the parent vessel during stent/balloon placement, etc. However, occlusion of the perforators is a mechanism of ischemic events that is more specifically seen in stenting of ICAD patients. In fact, this was presumed to be the most common mechanism of ischemic events after percutaneous angioplasty and stenting in the SAMMPRIS trial.[15] The post hoc analysis identified older age, nonsmokers, and old infarcts in the baseline imaging and basilar stenosis as the factors associated with increased risk of perforator infarcts. The pathomechanism suggested for this complication includes displacement of atherosclerotic debris during stenting, "snow plowing" of the perforators during angioplasty. An interesting finding to note in SAMMPRIS is the lower incidence of stroke involving MCA stenosis, which is a perforator-rich segment. A recent study has identified higher risk of symptomatic stroke with angioplasty and stenting in perforator-bearing arteries of the posterior circulation compared with the anterior circulation.[19] In this study, the risk of stroke with angioplasty alone did not differ from angioplasty and stent placement, which suggests perforator occlusion secondary to plaque movement rather than stent microthrombosis per se. In this regard, a high-resolution MRI with detailed evaluation of the plaque properties in relation to the vessel wall and perforator origins have been suggested in a few studies to select high risk patients.[20,21]

e. ***Cerebral hyperperfusion syndrome***

Although cerebral hyperperfusion syndrome (HPS) is not a direct complication of endovascular treatment, it is an important and serious complication after revascularization of chronically hypoperfused brain. This is essentially a hemodynamic instability of cerebral autoregulation that can produce a myriad of clinical presentation. In its milder form, it can cause headache, hypertension, and asymptomatic edema of ipsilateral cerebral hemisphere. However, it can also cause seizures, neurological deficits that are reversible with time. In more serious instances, it can cause acute intracerebral hemorrhage. In a retrospective study of 178 patients, HPS occurred in six patients (3.4%) after revascularization.[22] The most important predictive factors identified were inadequate control of blood pressure, less than 3-week interval between operation and last ischemic symptoms, and poor collateral circulation. Treatment is usually supportive with control of blood pressure. Avoidance of intraprocedural vasodilators is one of the important preventive measures and should be strictly followed in patients with chronic ischemia and poor collateral supply.

CURRENT AND FUTURE DIRECTIONS

The role of endovascular balloon angioplasty with or without stenting is still debatable. Although the WASID trial is relatively recent, SAMMRIS has been rigorously analyzed and investigated for possible confounding factors that prevented the true estimation of treatment benefit of angioplasty and stenting. For instance, the use of exchange length wire in SAMMPRIS has been criticized because it predisposes to periprocedural strokes. Critics believe modern balloon and stent systems that utilize rapid-exchange or monorail techniques may circumvent many stroke events with stenting. Another important point to note is that recognition of lesion characteristics according to the Mori classification, which has a known association with angioplasty outcomes with lesion morphology, was also not rigorously followed in SAMMPRIS.[23] Mori et al. in their original paper classified intracranial stenosis based on their morphology into three types with increasing complexity (Fig. 51.1). In their series the clinical success rate for simple (type A) lesions was high (92% versus 86% and 33% in type B and type C lesions) because of favorable anatomy that gives easy access to the lesion so that a balloon-mounted stent can easily be deployed. In contrast, the type C lesions were associated with high incidence of fatal or nonfatal strokes (87% versus 8% and 26% in type A and type B lesions) because of their complex morphology and associated vessel anatomy

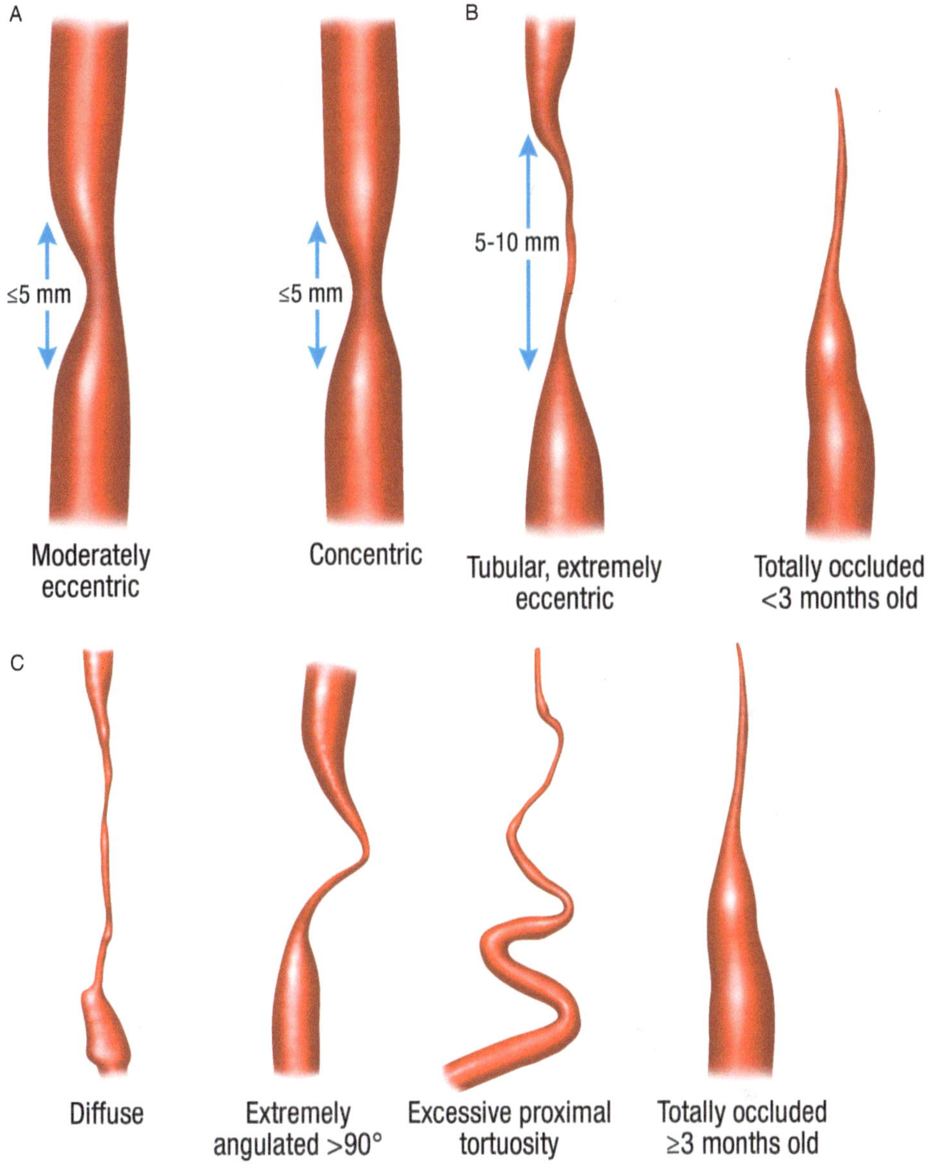

Fig. 51.1 Mori classification: A, B, C.

that need complex navigation with a polyaxial system. Therefore, endovascular angioplasty and stenting is more suitably indicated in type A lesions and should be avoided in type C lesions. Miao et al. have proposed that with an individual treatment with angioplasty and stenting based on the vessel tortuosity and MORI type may result in improved outcome compared with angioplasty alone in patients with symptomatic stroke caused by hypoperfusion.[24] As discussed previously, the major mechanism of periprocedural strokes in patients undergoing angioplasty or stenting is perforator occlusion. Therefore, stenosis involving high perforator burden, e.g., basilar trunk, basilar bifurcation, ICA terminus, M1 segment of MCA, should have a high threshold for angioplasty and stenting. In particular, the posterior circulation stenoses have a high tendency for perforator occlusion and therefore should be carefully selected for intervention.

Identification of the suitable patient who might benefit from endovascular intervention is the key for successful outcome. At present, indications are less clearly defined and therefore it is an area that needs further exploration. The central tenet is to identify patients who continue to have TIA/mild stroke symptoms despite maximal medical management in the affected vascular territory and do not have disabling stroke or high stroke burden on MRI (ideally, they should not be allowed to progress to this stage in the first place). Patients with corresponding hypoperfusion symptoms are usually good candidates for revascularization. Other factors to be noted diligently are the status of extracranial atherosclerotic disease and issues with navigation. Subgroup analyses have been carried out after SAMMPRIS to define selective groups who might benefit from endovascular management. For example, Fiorella et al. analyzed the periprocedural strokes in patients undergoing stenting in SAMMPRIS trial and found that patients with plaques near perforator origins are at high risk of post-stenting strokes.[15] However, another study analyzing the patient and stenosis variables of SAMMPRIS enrolled patients did not identify any subgroup who did better with stenting than medical management.[25]

Despite the negative results from trials, neurointerventionists are still optimistic about the promising role of endovascular therapy, which can benefit these critical patients.[26,27] Many potential avenues are being explored to improve the safety profile of angioplasty and stenting. For instance, looking into plaque characteristics with high resolution MRI, pattern of disease about branch (perforator) occlusion, and greater use of physiological hemodynamic data are potential directions that might improve patient selection. Additionally, rapid technological advancement in endovascular hardware and stent materials will exponentially increase the safety and reliability of intracranial recanalization strategies for ICS. As mentioned previously, the use of rapid exchange or monorail systems for balloon catheter and stent delivery is user-friendly and convenient and has improved the safety of angioplasty and stent deployment. Bioresorbable stents are another promising advancement that needs further study to explore their applicability.[28] Drug-eluting balloons such as paclitaxel-eluting balloons are an attractive borrow from the coronary world and have been reported in a few studies.[29] The concept of submaximal angioplasty is attractive and therefore should be investigated with prospective trials.

CONCLUSIONS

Intracranial stenosis is an important cause of strokes and therefore needs treatment, especially when symptomatic. Although the overwhelming majority of patients with ICS should be treated with best medical therapy, a subset of patients with recurrent strokes require endovascular revascularization by angioplasty with or without stenting. In addition to the general complications of angiography, important complications with angioplasty and stenting for intracranial stenosis are vessel rupture, stent thrombosis, and restenosis. Most of the acute complications are caused by improper technique and inadequate platelet inhibition. Technical advances and improved stent delivery systems have substantially reduced the complication rates. Submaximal angioplasty appears to be a valid strategy that is equally effective with reduced complication rates.

REFERENCES

1. Al Kasab S, Derdeyn CP, Guerrero WR, Limaye K, Shaban A, Adams Jr. HP. Intracranial large and medium artery atherosclerotic disease and stroke. *J Stroke Cerebrovasc Dis*. 2018;27(7):1723–1732.
2. Chimowitz MI, Lynn MJ, Howlett-Smith H, et al. Comparison of warfarin and aspirin for symptomatic intracranial arterial stenosis. *N Engl J Med*. 2005;352(13):1305–1316.
3. Ryoo S, Park JH, Kim SJ, et al. Branch occlusive disease: clinical and magnetic resonance angiography findings. *Neurology*. 2012;78(12):888–896.
4. Bang OY. Intracranial atherosclerosis: current understanding and perspectives. *J Stroke*. 2014;16(1):27–35.
5. Mazighi M, Tanasescu R, Ducrocq X, et al. Prospective study of symptomatic atherothrombotic intracranial stenoses: the GESICA study. *Neurology*. 2006;66(8):1187–1191.
6. Low SW, Teo K, Lwin S, et al. Improvement in cerebral hemodynamic parameters and outcomes after superficial temporal artery-middle cerebral artery bypass in patients with severe stenoocclusive disease of the intracranial internal carotid or middle cerebral arteries. *J Neurosurg*. 2015;123(3):662–669.
7. Chimowitz MI, Lynn MJ, Derdeyn CP, et al. Stenting versus aggressive medical therapy for intracranial arterial stenosis. *N Engl J Med*. 2011;365(11):993–1003.
8. Marks MP, Wojak JC, Al-Ali F, et al. Angioplasty for symptomatic intracranial stenosis: clinical outcome. *Stroke*. 2006;37(4):1016–1020.
9. Nguyen TN, Zaidat OO, Gupta R, et al. Balloon angioplasty for intracranial atherosclerotic disease: periprocedural risks and short-term outcomes in a multicenter study. *Stroke*. 2011;42(1):107–111.
10. Dumont TM, Kan P, Snyder KV, Hopkins LN, Siddiqui AH, Levy EI. Revisiting angioplasty without stenting for symptomatic intracranial atherosclerotic stenosis after the stenting and aggressive medical management for preventing recurrent stroke in intracranial stenosis (SAMMPRIS) study. *Neurosurgery*. 2012;71(6):1103–1110.
11. Dumont TM, Sonig A, Mokin M, et al. Submaximal angioplasty for symptomatic intracranial atherosclerosis: a prospective Phase I study. *J Neurosurg*. 2016;125(4):964–971.
12. Lee KY, Chen DY, Hsu HL, Chen CJ, Tseng YC. Undersized angioplasty and stenting of symptomatic intracranial tight stenosis with Enterprise: Evaluation of clinical and vascular outcome. *Interv Neuroradiol*. 2016;22(2):187–195.
13. Bendok BR, Przybylo JH, Parkinson R, Hu Y, Awad IA, Batjer HH. Neuroendovascular interventions for intracranial posterior circulation disease via the transradial approach: technical case report. *Neurosurgery*. 2005;56(3):E626; discussion E626.
14. Derdeyn CP, Fiorella D, Lynn MJ, et al. Mechanisms of stroke after intracranial angioplasty and stenting in the SAMMPRIS trial. *Neurosurgery*. 2013;72(5):777–795; discussion 795.
15. Fiorella D, Derdeyn CP, Lynn MJ, et al. Detailed analysis of periprocedural strokes in patients undergoing intracranial stenting in Stenting and Aggressive Medical Management for Preventing Recurrent Stroke in Intracranial Stenosis (SAMMPRIS). *Stroke*. 2012;43(10):2682–2688.
16. Parkinson RJ, Demers CP, Adel JG, et al. Use of heparin-coated stents in neurovascular interventional procedures: preliminary experience with 10 patients. *Neurosurgery*. 2006;59(4):812–821; discussion 821.
17. Derdeyn CP, Fiorella D, Lynn MJ, et al. Nonprocedural Symptomatic Infarction and In-Stent Restenosis After Intracranial Angioplasty and Stenting in the SAMMPRIS Trial (Stenting and Aggressive Medical Management for the Prevention of Recurrent Stroke in Intracranial Stenosis). *Stroke*. 2017;48(6):1501–1506.
18. Bendok BR, Sherma AK, Hage ZA, et al. Periprocedural MRI perfusion imaging to assess and monitor the hemodynamic impact of intracranial angioplasty and stenting for symptomatic atherosclerotic stenosis. *J Clin Neurosci*. 2010;17(1):54–58.
19. Nordmeyer H, Chapot R, Aycil A, et al. Angioplasty and stenting of intracranial arterial stenosis in perforator-bearing segments: a comparison between the anterior and the posterior circulation. *Front Neurol*. 2018;9:533.
20. Jiang WJ, Yu W, Ma N, Du B, Lou X, Rasmussen PA. High resolution MRI guided endovascular intervention of basilar artery disease. *J Neurointerv Surg*. 2011;3(4):375–378.
21. Shi M, Wang S, Zhou H, Cheng Y, Feng J, Wu J. Wingspan stenting of symptomatic middle cerebral artery stenosis and perioperative evaluation using high-resolution 3 Tesla MRI. *J Clin Neurosci*. 2012;19(6):912–914.
22. Xu S, Wu P, Shi H, Ji Z, Dai J. Hyperperfusion syndrome after stenting for intracranial artery stenosis. *Cell Biochem Biophys*. 2015;71(3):1537–1542.
23. Mori T, Fukuoka M, Kazita K, Mori K. Follow-up study after intracranial percutaneous transluminal cerebral balloon angioplasty. *Am J Neuroradiol*. 1998;19(8):1525–1533.
24. Miao Z, Song L, Liebeskind DS, et al. Outcomes of tailored angioplasty and/or stenting for symptomatic intracranial atherosclerosis: a prospective cohort study after SAMMPRIS. *J Neurointerv Surg*. 2015;7(5):331–335.
25. Lutsep HL, Lynn MJ, Cotsonis GA, et al. Does the stenting versus aggressive medical therapy trial support stenting for subgroups with intracranial stenosis? *Stroke*. 2015;46(11):3282–3284.
26. Ringer AJ, Khalessi AA, Mocco J, et al. Intervention for intracranial atherosclerosis after SAMMPRIS. *World Neurosurg*. 2012;78(5):409–412.
27. Mokin M, Khalessi AA, Mocco J, et al. Endovascular treatment of acute ischemic stroke: the end or just the beginning? *Neurosurg Focus*. 2014;36(1):E5.
28. Aoun RJ, Sattur MG, Panchanathan RS, Bendok BR. The ABSORB III Trial: potential new concepts for intracranial atherosclerosis in the Post-SAMMPRIS era. *Neurosurgery*. 2016;78(2):N19–N20.
29. Qureshi AI, Kirmani JF, Hussein HM, et al. Early and intermediate-term outcomes with drug-eluting stents in high-risk patients with symptomatic intracranial stenosis. *Neurosurgery*. 2006;59(5):1044–1051; discussion 51.

Complications in the Endovascular Treatment of Intracranial Aneurysms

Kunal Vakharia, MD, Jaims Lim, MD, Jeffrey S. Beecher, DO and Adnan H. Siddiqui, MD, PhD, FACS, FAHA

INTRODUCTION

Since the initial introduction of endovascular coiling techniques by G uglielmi in 1991,[1] endovascular therapies for intracranial aneurysms have evolved. Initially, intrasaccular coiling and parent vessel occlusion with coils after balloon test occlusion were the mainstays of treatment. At the turn of the 21st century, intracranial stents were designed as support and scaffolding for coils to treat wide-necked and unruptured aneurysms. With more advanced catheter and microcatheter technology in addition to balloon-assisted and stent-assisted techniques, endovascular therapy for intracranial aneurysms has significantly diversified the management options for ruptured and unruptured intracranial aneurysms. Although these techniques now represent the forefront of endovascular therapies, the past decade has seen the advent of flow diversion as a significant aid in treating broad-based aneurysms as well as aneurysms in difficult locations. In 2011, a flow diverter, the Pipeline embolization device (PED, Medtronic, Minneapolis, Minnesota), received approval from the U.S. Food and Drug Administration (FDA) for the treatment of large and giant wide-necked aneurysms from the petrous to superior hypophyseal segments of the internal carotid artery (ICA).[2]

Complications may occur during different phases of treatment for intracranial aneurysms. These events may be related to general issues associated with endovascular treatment including access site hematomas, retroperitoneal hematomas, femoral artery dissections, and nephrotoxic and contrast-related complications, the details of which are outside the scope of this chapter. The most common complications and plans associated with endovascular intracranial aneurysm treatment will be discussed here.

COILING

Complications related to intrasaccular coiling can be divided into thromboembolic or hemorrhagic complications. Thromboembolic complications commonly arise as a result of coil extrusion from the aneurysm into the parent vessel in addition to the thromboembolic risk associated with the neuroangiographic procedure itself. Hemorrhagic complications are primarily associated with entry of the microcatheter into the aneurysm dome and initial placement of the framing coil.

Thromboembolic Complications

As with any neuroangiographic procedure, embolic material can materialize on catheters and guidewires. In addition, during coiling procedures, coil mesh in contact with blood or stagnation from near-occlusive guide catheters or prolonged arterial vasospasm can increase the chance of embolic material causing ischemia. In addition, arterial dissection and vasospasm caused by the guide catheter prior to microcatheter and microwire manipulation can be associated with thromboemboli. The rate of thromboembolic complications in unruptured aneurysm series ranges from 3.7% to 6.9%.[3] The investigators of the Analysis of Treatment by Endovascular approach of Nonruptured Aneurysms (ATENA) study demonstrated an overall thromboembolic complication rate of 7.1% in 700 procedures.[4] Among patients who suffered from thromboembolic complications in the study, 4.1% died and 24.5% had permanent neurological deficits. It is difficult to identify the etiology of thromboembolic complications based on aneurysm location and morphology. Although aneurysm neck morphology may alter management plans, the use of intrasaccular coiling itself does not seem to be associated with high-risk features. In addition, the ATENA investigators have shown that the safety of the remodeling technique in unruptured aneurysms is similar to that of conventional coiling procedures.[4]

The rate of thromboembolic complications during intrasaccular coiling of ruptured aneurysms ranges between 4.7% and 6%.[3] The investigators of the Clinical and Anatomic Results in the Treatment of Ruptured Intracranial Aneurysms (CLARITY) study demonstrated a higher thromboembolic complication rate of nearly 12.5% for ruptured aneurysm treatment.[3] This study evaluated 782 ruptured aneurysms, and 3.8% of patients with thromboembolic complications had permanent neurological deficits or died. In another study, van Rooij et al. described a higher rate of thromboembolic complications for aneurysms >10 mm in diameter, with aneurysm necks larger than 4 mm, and in patients who were smokers.[5]

Thromboembolic complications are associated with high morbidity and mortality, and precautionary steps are taken to prevent such events. Full heparinization with a goal for activated coagulation time (ACT) between 250 and 300 seconds during unruptured aneurysm treatment is suggested. Heparinization helps reduce rates of thromboemboli but presents a clinically significant challenge while treating ruptured aneurysms. Our experience has shown that half heparinization prior to coiling and full heparinization after the aneurysm has been secured is a good protocol and approach to limit thromboemboli formation. If there is concern for iatrogenic vasospasm from the guide catheter, verapamil can be locally administered proximally to the vessel concerning for spasm at a dose ranging from 10 to 20 mg. Surgeons should be keenly aware of the different physiological and biological factors associated with vasospasm in the setting of ruptured aneurysms in addition to other variables that may predispose patients with ruptured aneurysms to altered states of coagulation.

Iatrogenic arterial dissection is another possible cause of thromboembolic complications and should be carefully monitored throughout the procedure. During removal of the microcatheter and guide catheter, final angiographic runs should be performed to confirm no signs of arterial dissection, flow limitation, or blood stagnation.

Either intraprocedurally or during final angiographic runs, acute intraprocedural thrombus formation is usually identified if a vessel branch is not seen or if there is delayed filling of the branches surrounding and distal to the site of occlusion. If coil extrusion near the aneurysm neck or into the parent vessel is observed, the surgeon can find the cause of the flow reduction. Thrombus formation is caused by platelet aggregation in these acute settings and is treated with intra-arterial or intravenous thrombolytic therapy including glycoprotein IIb/IIIa inhibitors. Cronqvist et al. performed superselective intra-arterial therapy with urokinase for thromboemboli occurring during endovascular intracranial aneurysm therapy in 19 patients with resultant complete recanalization in ten patients and partial recanalization in nine.[6] Furthermore, abciximab, a monoclonal antibody to the glycoprotein IIb/IIIa complex, has also been used for thrombolytic therapy. Brinjikji et al. reported higher mortality in patients receiving glycoprotein IIb/IIIa inhibitors alone.[7] In their meta-analysis, those authors found that patients who received glycoprotein IIb/IIIa inhibitors had statistically significantly lower perioperative morbidity than patients treated with fibrinolytic therapy.

Hemorrhagic Complications/Intraprocedural Aneurysm Rupture

The risk of intraprocedural rupture with intrasaccular treatment of cerebral aneurysms is greatest during initial catheterization of the aneurysm and ranges between 2% and 8.8%. Cloft et al. conducted a meta-analysis and evaluated 1248 ruptured aneurysms and revealed that rupture occurred in 4.1% of treated aneurysms during coil embolization.[8] These results demonstrated that there is a slightly higher risk of intraprocedural rupture in cases where the aneurysm has already ruptured. This higher risk is attributable to the fragility of the vessel wall in previously ruptured aneurysms. The most common causes include perforation from the microwire and microcatheter or perforation during coil deployment. Some authors have noted that dense packing of the aneurysm with coils can predispose aneurysms to delayed hemorrhagic complications.

Often during micronavigation of the carotid siphon, a significant amount of force can build up within the microwire and microcatheter. This potential energy can convert to kinetic energy during advancement of the microcatheter or removal of the microwire. When this occurs, either the microwire or microcatheter will begin to advance by itself. Meticulous control of the microwire–microcatheter system is imperative during these procedures; however, there are methods for minimizing the risk of the progression of a wire or catheter that could potentially go through the wall of the aneurysm.

Reducing the energy built up in the system can be performed by simply backing off the microcatheter until the tip marker is seen to move slightly prior to entering the aneurysm sac. However, this technique requires the catheter then to be advanced into the aneurysm, which may reproduce the forces that were just reduced. Our favored method is to advance the microwire past the ostia of the aneurysm and then follow it with the microcatheter. The whole system can then be withdrawn until the catheter either falls into the aneurysm sac or is in a perfect position for the microwire to be advanced into the aneurysm. This completely reduces the tension in the system prior to aneurysm catheterization and permits one-to-one movement of the devices for optimal control.

If intraprocedural rupture occurs while the catheter is within the aneurysm, the next best move is to deploy a slightly oversized, very long coil. Ideally, a coil around 20–30 cm in length (depending on the aneurysm dome size) is deployed in the hopes of achieving the greatest amount of occlusion of the aneurysm with a single coil. Prior to detachment of the coil, an injection of contrast material should be performed via the catheter, and frames should be captured into the late venous phase to evaluate for any continued extravasation. If continued extravasation is evident, standard management of elevated intracranial pressures (i.e., releasing cerebrospinal fluid if a ventriculostomy catheter is in place) should be simultaneously performed. The anesthesiologist should be informed and the coil can be detached after simultaneously using standard management of elevated intracranial pressure, such as releasing cerebrospinal fluid if a ventriculostomy is in place. A small compliant balloon could then be brought up to occlude the parent vessel temporarily to decrease the pressure head further and to allow for hemostasis. However, it may take precious minutes to introduce an exchange length microwire and bring it up a small, compliant balloon in a fully heparinized patient with a ruptured aneurysm. Rather, opening and inserting a long coil into the parent vessel without detaching it to occlude the vessel temporarily in the same fashion as a balloon is a more timely and quicker option. Protamine should be administered to reverse the heparin effect. If the patient is intubated, having the anesthesiologist induce "burst suppression" with sedation can possibly help reduce cerebral metabolism to decrease risk of ischemic injury. If the patient is under conscious sedation, a neurologic examination should be performed as soon as possible. If the patient is lethargic or has a concerning neurological change on examination, intubation and sedation are warranted. It may also be pertinent to place a ventriculostomy if one is not already in place. Alternatively, some interventionists may advocate simply coiling the aneurysm as quickly as possible until extravasation is no longer seen. However, this can lead to the catheter being pushed out of the aneurysm, poor placement of coils with prolapse into parent or branch vessels, and it may be ineffective in resulting in hemostasis. It is imperative that the interventionist remain calm when encountering an intraprocedural rupture as hastily made decisions and treatment attempts can result in devastating injury, bleeding, and permanent neurologic deficits for the patient.

Early Hemorrhagic Complications

Risk factors associated with early hemorrhagic complications other than intraprocedural rupture are not well understood. The greatest risk of hemorrhagic complications tends to be in the first 48 hours. In a study by Zheng et al., 1764 aneurysms were treated with 13 patients suffering from early hemorrhagic complications, more commonly seen with ruptured aneurysms.[9]

It is believed that the risk of rebleeding after coiling is 1.1% for ruptured aneurysms with an associated mortality of 31%.[9] Anticoagulation during microcatheter manipulation and aneurysm coiling as well as antiplatelet therapy have been suggested to be the cause of delayed aneurysm rupture not caused by perforation, although these have not been observed at our institution. Hemodynamic changes secondary to subarachnoid blood may elicit dynamic changes postprocedurally and may be additional causes of delayed hemorrhagic events.

Coil Migration

Migration of detached coils is a serious complication. Coil masses in contact with blood are highly thrombogenic. The thrombogenicity is proportionate to the surface area in contact with blood. Coil migration has been noted to have an incidence of 2.4% to 2.8% with significant morbidity and mortality related from parent vessel occlusion.[9] Henkes et al. reported a 2.5% rate of coil migration in the treatment of 1811 aneurysms, with no significant difference between unruptured and ruptured aneurysms.[10] Cases with large aneurysms >10 mm and broad-based aneurysm necks >4 mm tend to be associated with higher rates of coil migration. Surgeons must pay particular attention to sizing coils in these cases because the first framing coil will play a major role in the frame set for the remaining coils. Henkes et al. reported only a 0.1% risk of arterial thrombosis with coil migration into the parent vessel.[10]

Endovascular management of coil migration has not been standardized. Many patients with coil protrusion or prolapse can be treated with anticoagulation and antiplatelet therapy. Coil protrusion with noted thrombus formation can be treated within 24 to 48 hours of anticoagulation therapy with a stroke protocol heparin drip with a goal-activated partial thromboplastin time (aPTT) of 50 to 70 seconds without a heparin bolus. This can be followed with antiplatelet therapy for 6 months (Fig. 52.1). If flow limitation secondary to coil fracture, stretching, or migration occurs, there are methods to extract these coils including goose neck snares, stent retrieval devices, and trapping the coil mass against the arterial wall with an intracranial stent. To date, there are no defined or standardized methods to retrieve problematic coils. Snares and stent retriever devices are interchangeably used among surgeons based on comfort level and, if unsuccessful, interventionists may resort to trapping the coil mass via stenting.

STENT-ASSISTED/BALLOON-ASSISTED COILING

Stent-assisted coiling poses many potential technical challenges. Decisions regarding the use of open-cell stents (e.g., Neuroform [Stryker Neurovascular, Fremont, California]) versus closed-cell stents (e.g., Low-profile Visualized Intraluminal Support [LVIS] Junior [MicroVention, Aliso Viejo, California], LVIS Blue [MicroVention], and Enterprise [Codman Neuro, Raynham, Massachusetts]) allow the use of dual catheter access for jailing the coiling catheter or approaching coiling across the cells (i.e., trans-cell) in open-cell stents, which allows the interventionist to reaccess the aneurysm dome. Chalouhi et al. reported the results of stent-assisted coiling in 508 patients and reported a 6.8% complication rate.[11] Those authors noted that stent delivery before coil deployment reduces the risk of procedural complications.

Other factors when planning to treat broad-based intracranial aneurysms include electively administering a loading dose of antiplatelet agents to patients for stent placement to minimize risk of thromboembolic complications rather than planning the use of balloon-assisted coiling and then reverting to stenting. In addition, staging the procedure with stent placement followed by coiling does not improve procedural safety. Planning the use of open-cell versus closed-cell stents is important for the approach in addition to whether (or not) a vessel needs to be recanalized. Open-cell stents are more flexible and are better at conforming to the vessel wall as opposed to closed-cell stents that are more rigid but offer more radial force within the vessel as well as plaque coverage.[12] A closed-cell stent has better scaffolding properties and may be a great option for thick carotid plaques, limiting the amount of plaque that can penetrate the stent and travel distally and potentially causing a thromboembolic crisis.[13] Chalouhi et al. found that closed-cell stents were associated with significantly lower recanalization rates.[11] On the other hand, open-cell stents have increased conformability and may be particularly beneficial when

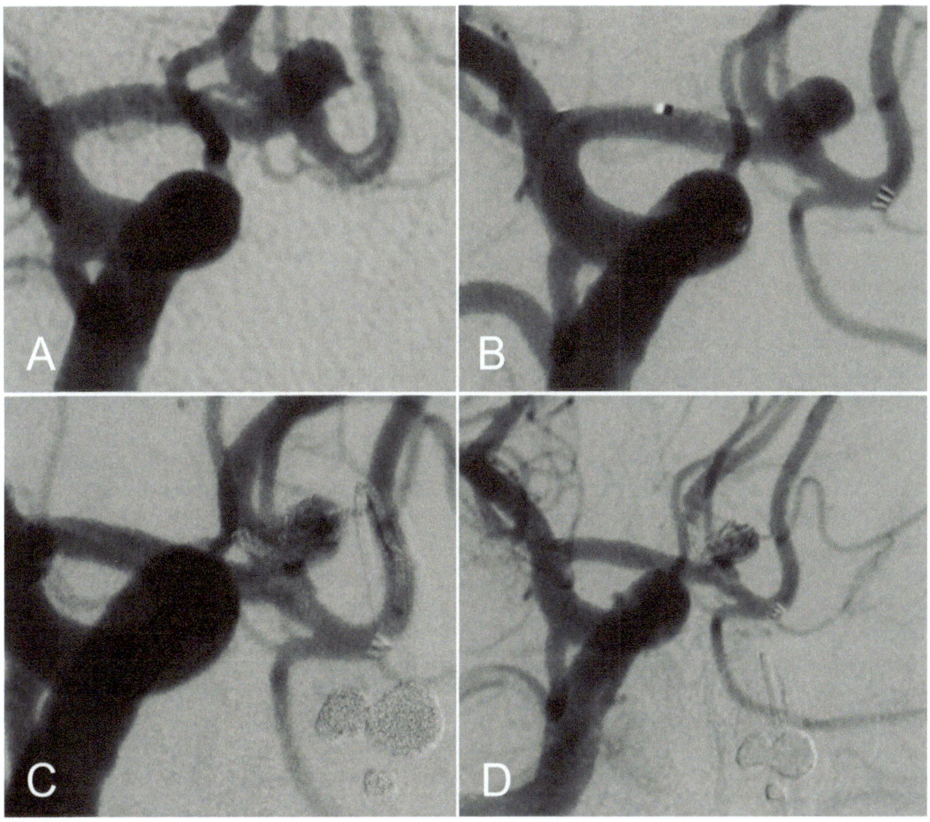

Fig. 52.1 Stent-assisted coiling of a 5-mm anterior communicating artery aneurysm. (A) Anteroposterior (AP) angiographic image (working view) of the anterior communicating artery aneurysm. The aneurysm appears to be broad based and fed primarily from the right A1 segment vessel. (B) AP working view after stent placement shows initial jailing of the coiling catheter within the aneurysmal dome. (C) Angiographic run after the initial frame coil deployment with protrusion into the A2 segment. (D) Delayed filling of the right A2 segment. The patient had significant collateral flow and did not suffer any ischemic symptoms postprocedure.

stenting a vessel with great tortuosity and difficult angles. Furthermore, open-cell stents allow for possible trans-cell coiling, as mentioned previously.[14] The tortuosity of the vessel and need for recanalization may be considerations when deciding between open-cell and closed-cell stents.

Thromboembolic Complications

In-stent thrombosis with stenosis is a real concern for stent-assisted coiling. Confirming that patients are responsive to antiplatelet therapy is crucial prior to planning such procedures. Patients are typically premedicated with aspirin and clopidogrel. Aspirin resistance is seen in 5% to 60% of patients and clopidogrel resistance is seen in 4% to 30% of patients. The appropriate dosing of antiplatelet agents and suitable alternative agents for patients with aspirin and clopidogrel resistance is continuously being studied and evaluated. One possible alternative antiplatelet agent is ticagrelor. Although no trials have specifically looked at ticagrelor's efficacy compared with aspirin and clopidogrel, a post-trial subgroup analysis of the Acute Stroke Or Transient IsChaemic Attack TReated With Aspirin or Ticagrelor and Patient OutcomES (SOCRATES) trial demonstrated that ticagrelor was more effective than aspirin in preventing a recurrent stroke and myocardial infarction within 90 days post-stroke.[15] Therefore, given the sizeable chance of a patient being resistant to aspirin, confirming responsiveness with P2Y12 inhibition levels and obtaining aspirin inhibition levels prior to stent placement is important in avoiding thromboembolic complications.[16] As mentioned for other platelet-related thromboembolic complications, glycoprotein IIb/IIIa can be administered intraprocedurally for acute thrombus formation and in-stent thrombus formation. In addition, leaving the microwire in the stent after deployment until confirmation that the stent has fully opened is the best protection for avoidance of failure of stent deployment and associated thrombus formation.

During balloon-assisted coiling, heparinization is the key to complication avoidance. In addition, confirming the size of balloons based on angiographic runs and determining use of compliant versus noncompliant balloons to assist in coiling procedures are important. Understanding the limitations of certain balloons and benefits of other balloons can play a critical role in coiling procedures. Based on location, different balloon types may be more suitable. Classically, balloon-assisted coiling utilized single-lumen low-compliance balloons that were ideal for aneurysms present on a single distinct vessel as an outpouching with clear boundaries. Using such a low-compliance balloon for coiling can be challenging for aneurysms at vessel bifurcations. Thus balloons with a higher degree of compliance such as the HyperForm (Medtronic) may result in more successful coiling of bifurcation aneurysms as well as those with wide necks in which coiling would have previously been discouraged. Such compliant balloons may be ineffective in distinct sidewall aneurysms. Balloons with double lumens such as the Scepter (MicroVention) that have two lumens providing one opening for the coil and another for navigation of the coil or other microstents[17] are also a viable alternative. Furthermore, use of a Scepter balloon also allows the surgeon to maintain distal access and potentially coil aneurysms through the balloon catheter. This can serve as a salvage maneuver to stent a vessel if deflation of the balloon promotes unwanted coil protrusion (Fig. 52.2).

Coil Stretching

Coil stretching is unpredictable. This can lead to thromboembolic events in addition to parent vessel occlusion. There are several rescue methods that can be used by surgeons to avoid and manage such issues. Although single loops of coils or mild stretching with appropriate detachment of the coil can be managed with anticoagulation and antiplatelet therapy, stretching with significant coil extrusion can lead to thrombus formation. The Amplatz gooseneck microsnare (Medtronic) and the Merci retriever (Stryker Neurovascular) have been used to retrieve extruded coils.

Technical factors that should be taken into account include whether the coil should be extracted, whether stenting the coil to the vessel wall is an option, and how distal the coil has migrated. If portions of the stretched coil still reside within the coil delivery microcatheter, the stretched coil can most probably be removed safely without complications. Otherwise, aforementioned devices such as the microsnare and retrievers should be used to attempt retrieval. If all attempts are unsuccessful, final resort measures include creating a stent construct to fix stretched coil fragments to vessel walls.[18] Stent retrievers have been used in vessels with <2 mm into the M2 and A2 segments. The goal of these maneuvers is to unsheath the stent retriever 5 mm distal to the coil.[19] After the stent has integrated with the coil mass, an attempt should be made to partially resheath the stent retriever by advancing the microcatheter back over the device. Once the coil is engaged, the entire system can be withdrawn into the guide catheter and removed from the circulation.

FLOW DIVERSION

Hemorrhagic Complications

Intraprocedural rupture during flow diversion is extraordinarily rare. This is mostly because the aneurysm sac is not directly involved. However, postprocedure rupture has been described after flow diversion. Unfortunately, this is a devastating, often unsurvivable complication because the patient is placed on dual antiplatelet therapy, which exacerbates the hemorrhage. The literature demonstrates a poor outcome in 80% of patients with a delayed hemorrhage after flow diversion, and approximately 80% of these hemorrhages transpire within 30 days of the procedure (Fig. 52.3).[20] Giant cerebral aneurysms account for 50% of delayed aneurysm ruptures, but the etiology remains unclear. This remains controversial, but theories regarding hemodynamic and biologic changes within the aneurysm are often at the center of such debate.[21]

Endovascular salvage techniques for active hemorrhage include temporary balloon occlusion, parent vessel sacrifice, or the placement of additional flow diverting stents. Temporary balloon occlusion of the parent vessel can be performed in the hope of achieving thrombosis at the site of extravasation. However, this can lead to further complications and may waste precious time. In our experience, placing an additional flow diverter can achieve thrombosis of the aneurysm. If these methods are unsuccessful, parent vessel sacrifice must be considered.

Cases of delayed hemorrhage after flow diversion are particularly complicated because of the dual antiplatelet regimen prescribed for a patient who will probably require a ventriculostomy. A fine line must be navigated between the antiplatelet medications and this surgical procedure.

Endoleak

This is a specific problem with flow diversion and it occurs when the flow-diverting stent is not appropriately sized to the vessel lumen proximally. To avoid this problem, it is imperative that the stent size is based on the most proximal aspect of the parent vessel, otherwise blood will continue to flow on the outside of the stent and into the aneurysm. This phenomenon could result in aneurysm rupture because there is inflow directly into the aneurysm as well as reduced outflow through the flow

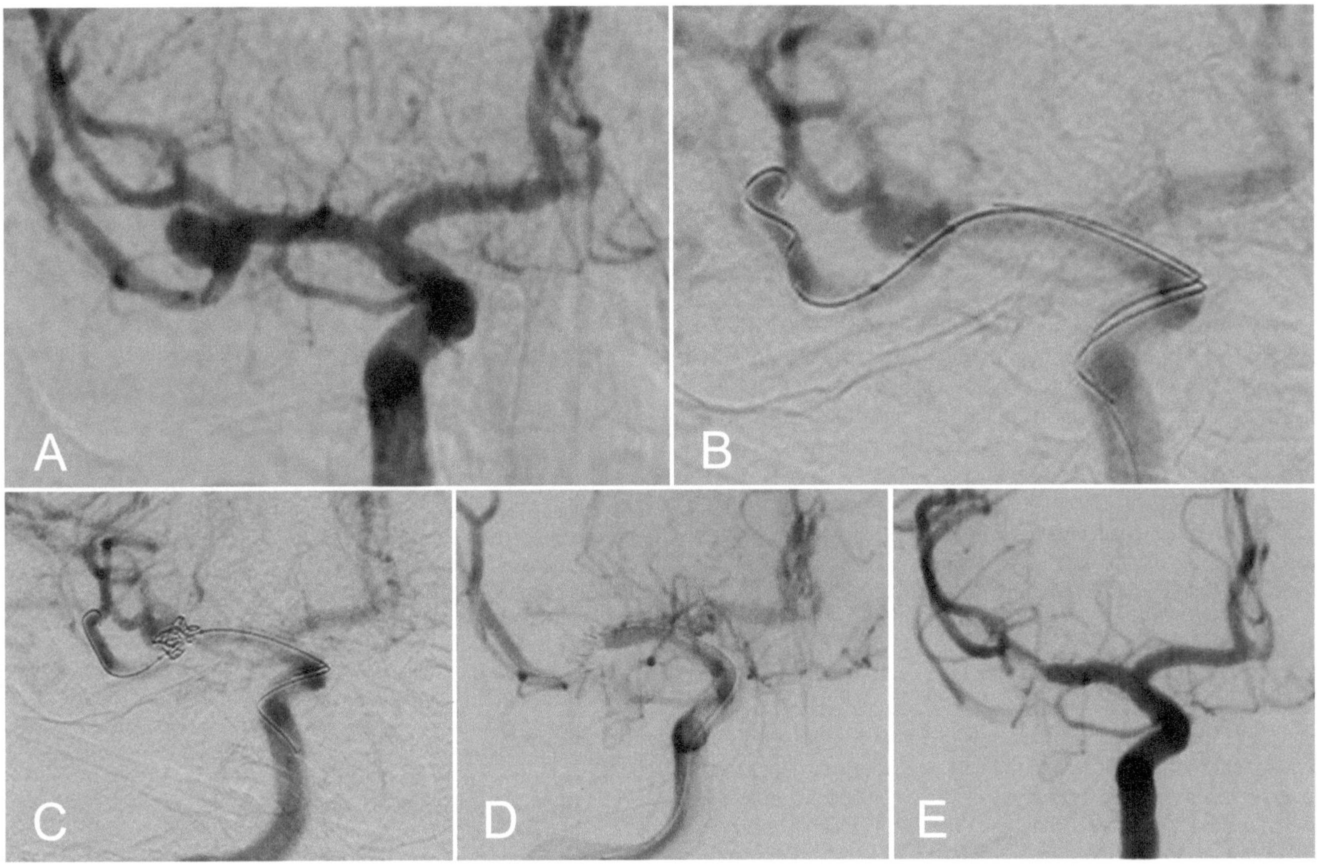

Fig. 52.2 Balloon-assisted coiling of a ruptured middle cerebral artery (MCA) bifurcation aneurysm. (A) The broad-based aneurysm seen on a diagnostic angiogram in the anteroposterior (AP) plane. (B) A Scepter C balloon (MicroVention) placed at the base of the aneurysm with the coiling catheter jailed into the aneurysmal dome. (C) AP view shows coil protrusion into the parent vessel on deflation of the balloon. (D) AP view demonstrates occlusion of the superior M2 branch of the MCA. At this point, a loading dose of dual antiplatelet therapy was administered urgently to the patient. (E) AP view after stent deployment into the superior M2 branch to recanalize the MCA branches. The patient remained neurologically intact postprocedure.

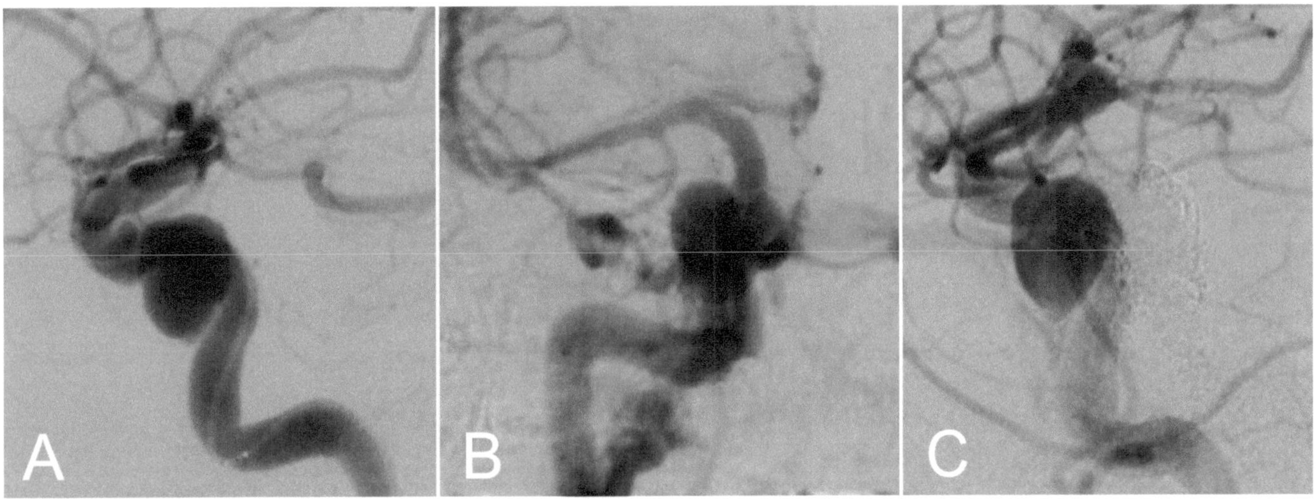

Fig. 52.3 Pipeline embolization for flow diversion treatment of a right cavernous carotid aneurysm. (A) Lateral angiographic run showing a microcatheter past the aneurysm neck in preparation for deployment of a Pipeline embolization device (PED; Medtronic, Minneapolis, Minnesota). (B) AP view 1 month after PED placement when the patient presented with a "whooshing" sound in her right ear and was found to have a direct carotid cavernous fistula. (C) Lateral view after transvenous embolization of the cavernous sinus and circular sinus and occlusion of the fistula. The treatment was complicated because the previously placed PED limited direct access to the aneurysm.

> **TIP BOX 52.1**
>
> A Pipeline embolization device should be sized to the nominal diameter of the parent vessel, with the understanding that it might expand by 0.25 mm in width.

diverter. A PED can expand to 0.25 mm greater than its nominal diameter, but this should not be relied upon because the PED should still be sized to the nominal diameter of the parent vessel.[21] Balloon angioplasty can be used to correct size mismatch; however, if the mismatch is too great, damage can be caused to the stent or flow-diversion properties can be lost. Ideally, an additional flow-diverting stent should be placed at the proximal aspect ensuring that there is good apposition to the vessel wall. This may result in rapid thrombosis of the aneurysm, which may be combatted with medications such as anticoagulation medication that carry a bleeding risk or steroids if there is a concern for inflammation during thrombosis of nearby structures. Furthermore, care should be taken not to cover small, critical vessels such as the anterior choroidal artery with more than one flow diverter because this can result in occlusion of the vessel and a devastating stroke (Box 52.1).

CONCLUSION

Endovascular coiling and endovascular therapy for intracranial aneurysms have had significant advances with stent- and balloon-assisted coiling and flow diversion. The ultimate goal is to stop flow into the aneurysmal dome while preserving all parent and branching vessels. Complications may occur throughout different stages of the procedure and thorough knowledge of anatomy and physiology, and preparation of technique are needed to manage these situations effectively and creatively. Complication management is crucial in delivering the best available care to patients.

ACKNOWLEDGMENTS

The authors thank Paul H. Dressel, BFA for preparation of the illustrations and Debra J. Zimmer for editorial assistance.

REFERENCES

1. Guglielmi G, et al. Electrothrombosis of saccular aneurysms via endovascular approach: part 1: electrochemical basis, technique, and experimental results. *J Neurosurg.* 1991;75(1):1–7.
2. Brinjikji W, Murad MH, Lanzino G, et al. Endovascular treatment of intracranial aneurysms with flow diverters: a meta-analysis. *Stroke.* 2013;44:442–447.
3. Orru E, Roccatagliata L, Cester G, et al. Complications of endovascular treatment of cerebral aneurysms. *Eur J Radiol.* 2013;82:1653–1658.
4. Pierot L, Spelle L, Vitry F, et al. Immediate clinical outcome of patients harboring unruptured intracranial aneurysms treated by endovascular approach: results of the ATENA study. *Stroke.* 2008;39:2497–2504.
5. van Rooij WJ, Sluzewski M, Beute GN, et al. Procedural complications of coiling of ruptured intracranial aneurysms: incidence and risk factors in a consecutive series of 681 patients. *Am J Neuroradiol.* 2006;27:1498–1501.
6. Cronqvist M, Pierot L, Boulin A, et al. Local intraarterial fibrinolysis of thromboemboli occurring during endovascular treatment of intracerebral aneurysm: a comparison of anatomic results and clinical outcome. *Am J Neuroradiol.* 1998;19:157–165.
7. Brinjikji W, Morales-Valero SF, Murad MH, et al. Rescue treatment of thromboembolic complications during endovascular treatment of cerebral aneurysms: a meta-analysis. *Am J Neuroradiol.* 2015;36:121–125.
8. Cloft HJ, Kallmes DF. Cerebral aneurysm perforations complicating therapy with Guglielmi detachable coils: a meta-analysis. *Am J Neuroradiol.* 2002;23:1706–1709.
9. Zheng Y, Liu Y, Leng B, et al. Periprocedural complications associated with endovascular treatment of intracranial aneurysms in 1764 cases. *J Neurointerv Surg.* 2016;8:152–157.
10. Henkes H, Fischer S, Weber W, et al. Endovascular coil occlusion of 1811 intracranial aneurysms: early angiographic and clinical results. *Neurosurgery.* 2004;54:268–280; discussion 280–285.
11. Chalouhi N, Jabbour P, Singhal S, et al. Stent-assisted coiling of intracranial aneurysms: predictors of complications, recanalization, and outcome in 508 cases. *Stroke.* 2013;44:1348–1353.
12. Eller JL, Dumont TM, Sorkin GC, et al. Endovascular advances for extracranial carotid stenosis. *Neurosurgery.* 2014;74(Suppl 1):S92–S101.
13. Eller JL, Siddiqui AH. Stent design choice based on anatomy. In: Gonzalez LF, Albuquerque FC, McDougall C, eds. *Neurointerventional Techniques: Tricks of the Trade.* New York: Thieme; 2015.
14. Yahia AM, Gordon V, Whapham J, et al. Complications of Neuroform stent in endovascular treatment of intracranial aneurysms. *Neurocrit Care.* 2008;8:19–30.
15. Amarenco P, Albers GW, Denison H, et al. Efficacy and safety of ticagrelor versus aspirin in acute stroke or transient ischaemic attack of atherosclerotic origin: a subgroup analysis of SOCRATES, a randomised, double-blind, controlled trial. *Lancet Neurol.* 2017;16:301–310.
16. Delgado Almandoz JE, Kadkhodayan Y, Crandall BM, et al. Variability in initial response to standard clopidogrel therapy, delayed conversion to clopidogrel hyper-response, and associated thromboembolic and hemorrhagic complications in patients undergoing endovascular treatment of unruptured cerebral aneurysms. *J Neurointerv Surg.* 2014;6:767–773.
17. Piotin M, Blanc R. Balloons and stents in the endovascular treatment of cerebral aneurysms: vascular anatomy remodeled. *Front Neurol.* 2014;5:41.
18. Ding D, Liu KC. Management strategies for intraprocedural coil migration during endovascular treatment of intracranial aneurysms. *J Neurointerv Surg.* 2014;6:428–431.
19. Leslie-Mazwi TM, Heddier M, Nordmeyer H, et al. Stent retriever use for retrieval of displaced microcoils: a consecutive case series. *Am J Neuroradiol.* 2013;34:1996–1999.
20. Rouchaud A, Brinjikji W, Lanzino G, et al. Delayed hemorrhagic complications after flow diversion for intracranial aneurysms: a literature overview. *Neuroradiology.* 2016;58:171–177.
21. Cebral JR, Mut F, Raschi M, et al. Aneurysm rupture following treatment with flow-diverting stents: computational hemodynamics analysis of treatment. *Am J Neuroradiol.* 2011;32:27–33.

53

Acute Ischemic Stroke

Hakeem J. Shakir, MD and Elad I. Levy, MD, MBA, FACS, FAHA

INTRODUCTION

Accounting for 87% of all types of stroke, ischemic stroke has both fatal and disabling consequences for affected patients.[1] Ischemic stroke remains the leading cause of long-term disability; however, technologic and therapeutic advances made in the past decade offer significant potential to change this. Recent randomized controlled clinical trials have demonstrated the efficacy of endovascular intervention over tissue plasminogen activator (tPA) alone and have catalyzed the treatment of ischemic stroke, affording patients much more favorable outcomes than before. Landmark studies such as Solitaire With the Intention For Thrombectomy as Primary Endovascular Treatment (SWIFT PRIME) demonstrated that patients who suffered large-vessel anterior circulation occlusions treated with intravenous tPA in conjunction with the Solitaire stent retriever (Medtronic, Minneapolis, Minnesota) saw reductions in post-stroke disability.[2] Alongside the diffusion-weighted imaging (DWI) or computed tomography perfusion (CTP) assessment with Clinical Mismatch in the Triage of Wake-Up and Late Presenting Strokes Undergoing Neurointervention with Trevo (Stryker Neurovascular, Fremont, California) (DAWN) trial,[3] acute ischemic stroke (AIS) treatment underwent a shift leaning toward early and aggressive endovascular intervention. Newer stent retrievers have been introduced by various neurovascular companies offering providers different tools with the hope of improved recanalization rates and times and, ultimately, improved patient outcomes.

In addition to the proven efficacy of stent retrievers, a method known as a direct aspiration first pass technique (ADAPT) has emerged as an alternative technique for mechanical thrombectomy (MT) without the use of a stent retriever.[4] This technique relies heavily on large-bore aspiration catheters.

Although clinical care and intervention for ischemic stroke have undeniably advanced in a positive direction, stroke intervention remains a high-risk, high-reward process. Regardless of extra effort taken to prevent complications, complications from vessel access to recanalization of affected vessels occur along various junctures during the stroke intervention. According to the results of recent randomized controlled trials, the risk of complications with sequelae for patients with MT is 15%.[5] Here we discuss specific approaches in the endovascular treatment of AIS, focusing on common complications, tips for avoidance, and strategies to apply when complications do occur.

ACCESS-RELATED COMPLICATIONS

Seemingly simple to some and often overlooked by neophyte interventionists, arterial access is the basis by which intervention may be undertaken and the source of disastrous complications during thrombectomy. For stroke interventions, the femoral artery remains the standard for gaining access. However, novel techniques have emerged using the radial or brachial artery and, in rare instances, the carotid artery. In patients with intracranial vascular disease, co-existing peripheral vascular disease may render access difficult. Prior to intervention, vessel tortuosity and age-related changes to vessels may pose difficulties. Access-related groin and retroperitoneal hematomas can negatively alter the outcome of stroke intervention. Inadequate closure of the vessel at the end of the procedure can result in substantial blood loss, especially in instances where larger sheaths are used. In AIS intervention, time is of the essence.[6] Groin access-to-vessel recanalization times are key; therefore, time lost in attempting to gain access can prolong the ischemic period and potentially alter clinical outcomes. If access is difficult to obtain within 2–3 minutes, ultrasound imaging should be used for assistance in gaining vascular access. If the standard transfemoral routes are deemed inappropriate or tenuous, quick adjustments should be made to use radial, brachial, or even direct carotid access. Misplaced sheaths may be temporarily left in place while proceeding with the thrombectomy. Close attention should be paid to preprocedure computed tomography angiography (CTA). CTA of the head and neck or CT stroke studies reveal arch anatomy, anatomical variations of large vessels, and possible vascular tortuosities that may hinder intracranial lesion access. Complications pertaining to access are avoidable if the neurointerventionist adequately anticipates the aforementioned factors prior to the procedure (Box 53.1).

THROMBOEMBOLIC COMPLICATIONS

From beginning to end, neurointerventional procedures predispose patients to having thromboembolic complications. There is an inherent risk of embolic material forming on catheters and guidewires introduced into the vasculature. Cleanliness and the organization of catheters and wires as they are introduced and removed can reduce risk. In addition, arterial dissection and vasospasm caused by the guide catheter prior to microcatheter and microwire manipulation can be associated with thromboemboli. Systematic heparinization of the patient is a strategy used to minimize thromboemboli alongside intra-arterial administration of verapamil in select instances of severe catheter-induced vasospasm.

More concerning for the neurointerventionist is the possibility of pre-existing clot fragments dislodging and leading to embolization of new territory resulting from manipulation of an endovascular device. Distal embolization is a legitimate concern that can be handled with different approaches. The use of stent retrievers of any kind mandates that a lesion be crossed with a microwire for facilitating the unsheathing of the stent retriever device. The sole act of crossing a lesion can dislodge clot debris downstream. Companies in the neurovascular sector sell varying components of their stent retriever devices including stent length, cell size, radial force, and other factors that may allow for better clot engagement. A plethora of devices ranging from stent retrievers to balloon guide catheters (BGCs) fill the toolbox of neurointerventionists and should be used based on their comfort and experience level with the understanding that no device is devoid of complications. Table 53.1 shows several of these devices, some of which are approved for use in MT by the U.S. Food and Drug Administration.

The role of direct aspiration versus stent retrievers is an ongoing debate in stroke and also the subject of recent trials such as COMPASS (https://clinicaltrials.gov/ct2/show/NCT02466893). The Contact Aspiration versus Stent Retriever for Successful Revascularization (ASTER) trial[7] showed no statistically significant differences between stent retriever and ADAPT in procedural complications such as symptomatic intracranial hemorrhage (sICH) and embolization in a new territory. Overall, each device has its unique benefits; however, there is no clear discrepancy with regard to embolization to new territory. Newer generation devices attempt to account for clot fragmentation in their design.

EMBOLIZATION OF NEW TERRITORIES

MT opens the door for a previously unaffected territory proximal to a lesion to be affected or for distal migration within the target artery. The mechanism by which previously unaffected territories proximal to a lesion can be affected during MT occurs when a clot is dragged from a distal location and thrombus fragments. An example of this occurs commonly in the distal middle cerebral artery where a clot may be lodged. Removal of the clot requires proximal navigation of the retrieval device; in the midst of retrieving the clot, fragmentation may occur that allows thrombus to migrate into proximal lenticulostriate vessels or even to the anterior cerebral artery circulation. In distal embolization to new territory, the migrated clot can remain in the same vessel or break up and dissipate into many multiple tiny branches and possibly affect other surrounding vessel territories.[8] The risk of distal embolization has been shown to be reduced with the use of BGCs in conjunction with aspiration as the inflation of the balloon minimizes anterograde blood flow during clot retrieval, preventing clot fragments from travelling distally.[9] (Our preferred BGC is the Merci Balloon Guide Catheter; Stryker Neurovascular, Fremont, CA.)

As MT technologies evolve, the correct instruments should be selected. Considering embolization to new territory, BGCs may be advantageous because the inflated balloon prevents anterograde flow during the thrombectomy, potentially reducing the opportunity for small emboli to travel forward during the "pull." Having experience with a volume of cases is the best way to avoid common complications.

TIP BOX 53.1

If access is difficult to obtain within 2–3 minutes, ultrasound imaging should be used for assistance in gaining vascular access.

REPERFUSION INJURY/REPERFUSION HEMORRHAGE/HEMORRHAGIC CONVERSION

The current literature suggests that if treated successfully, large vessel occlusion (LVO) can improve patient outcomes. The restoration of blood flow to viable brain tissue permits salvage of the penumbra while opening the door for a process known as cerebral reperfusion injury, which is defined as deterioration of salvageable brain tissue that was initially ischemic after reperfusion.[10] Although research of the mechanisms of injury is ongoing, several studies have demonstrated various mechanisms that are involved. Inflammatory response and release of free radicals to injured tissue by restored blood flow is one process in addition to the involvement of leukocyte infiltration and breakdown of the blood–brain barrier. Reperfusion injury occurs on a microvascular or cellular level but is certainly related to the more overt and conspicuous phenomenon of reperfusion hemorrhage or hemorrhagic transformation.

sICH after ischemic stroke is not an uncommon consequence of recanalization of LVO by either tPA or MT.[11] Hao et al. determined that a number of factors may predispose patients to sICH following thrombectomy.[11] These factors include cardio-embolic stroke, poor collateral circulation, delayed endovascular treatment (delay from

TABLE 53.1 Device approvals and indications for cerebrovascular procedures.

Device	FDA approved	FDA-approved indication	Supporting evidence for FDA approval
MicroVention ERIC	No	NA[a]	NA
Neuravi EmboTrap II	No	NA[a]	Prospective, single-arm, multicenter—ongoing
Stryker Baby Trevo	Yes	Thrombectomy	Substantially equivalent
Medtronic Mindframe Capture	Yes	Thrombectomy	Substantially equivalent
Penumbra ACE68, Aspiration System	Yes	Thrombectomy	Prospective, single-arm, multicenter—completed
Walk Vascular ClearLumen	No	NA[b]	Substantially equivalent
Stryker AXS Catalyst 6	Yes	Intracranial access	Substantially equivalent
MicroVention Sofia Plus	Yes	Intracranial access	Substantially equivalent
Medtronic Arc	Yes	Intracranial access	Substantially equivalent
MIVI Neuroscience Mi-Axus	Yes	Intracranial access	Substantially equivalent
DePuy Synthes Envoy DA	Yes	Intracranial access	Substantially equivalent
BGCs	Yes	Intracranial access	Substantially equivalent
Medtronic Lazarus Effect Cover	No	NA	NA

BGCs, Balloon guide catheters; *FDA,* U.S. Food and Drug Administration; *NA,* not applicable.

Reproduced with permission from Chartrain AG, Awad AJ, Mascitelli JR, et al. Novel and emerging technologies for endovascular thrombectomy. *Neurosurg Focus.* 2017;42:E12.

[a]Approved for cerebrovascular thrombectomy in Europe.

[b]FDA-approved for thrombectomy in the coronary vasculature.

symptoms onset to groin puncture >270 minutes), multiple passes with a stent retriever device (>3 passes with retriever), lower pretreatment Alberta Stroke Program Early Computed Tomography Score (ASPECTS), and a high baseline neutrophil ratio. sICH has potentially devastating ramifications for patients depending on the severity of the bleed. The potential worsening of a patient's poor clinical examination findings or increasing their postprocedure National Institutes of Health Stroke Scale (NIHSS) score is a known risk. Therefore, patient selection and evaluation of the risk–benefit profile is imperative. Of the modifiable factors studied by Hao et al.,[11] the neurointerventionist should pay close attention to the time at which endovascular treatment is rendered with regard to the onset of stroke symptoms and the number of passes attempted with the stent retriever because these can directly impact the outcome. However, delays in treatment are modifiable only to a certain extent. Expediting door-to-groin times and streamlining the process by which patients receive interventions is a constant effort by providers to prevent treatment delays. With the introduction of ADAPT, intervention may not require the use of stent retrievers. Stent retrievers may have the deleterious effect of endothelial damage and weakening of diseased atherosclerotic vessel lumens. New clinical trials, such as the DAWN trial,[3] demonstrate that the 6-hour therapeutic window may be extended for intervention while still providing benefit to patients. However, with longer periods of ischemia, cerebral tissue may be exposed to a higher risk of injury and potential sICH.

COMPLICATION AVOIDANCE

Careful selection of patients for stroke intervention with adherence to recent evidence-based guidelines is the first step in avoiding pitfalls. Imaging modalities such as CT or magnetic resonance imaging perfusion remain a mainstay for determining the salvageability of penumbra, but significant attention is paid to the control of hypertension to prevent reperfusion injury and hemorrhage in patients who undergo stroke intervention. Blood pressure control is an integral component in avoiding post-recanalization injury or sICH even in normotensive patients because delayed hypertension can occur.[12] The use and titration of antihypertensive medications such as nicardipine before, during, and after recanalization reduce potential for both reperfusion injury and reperfusion hemorrhage. Nicardipine is a preferred medication because it does not increase cerebral blood flow, nor does it promote vasodilation features of other, less-favored antihypertensive agents. Target systolic blood pressure after recanalization should be kept <140 mmHg.

VASOSPASM, DISSECTION, AND ARTERIAL PERFORATION

Vasospasm

Vasospasm, arterial perforation, and dissection are well-known complications in AIS intervention. Vasospasm has rare clinical significance in AIS intervention. Most vasospasm seen in stroke intervention is a result of mechanical stimulation of a vessel when it comes in contact with a catheter. Depending on severity, vasospasm may have deleterious effects locally at the site or distal to the site if not managed appropriately. In inexperienced hands, vasospasm is likely to occur within the cervical internal carotid artery and beyond as the interventionist hastily attempts to advance a larger bore catheter in preparation for MT. Although pre-existing atherosclerosis and underlying unhealthy vasculature may predispose vessels to vasospasm, these complications can occur in nondiseased vessels even with the gentlest of manipulations.

Vasospasm Avoidance and Management

It is imperative for the interventionist to use the utmost care when performing a stroke intervention. Appropriate preprocedure planning should be undertaken to anticipate vessel diameters and calibers that might change the selection of a guide catheter or wire. A preoperative review of the patient's CTA might dissuade the use of an 8- or 9-French system as the guiding catheter. If vasospasm occurs, simple maneuvers may alleviate the local irritation. Pulling the catheter back more proximally (in essence, allowing the affected vessel to "cool down") seems to be one effective approach. However, as time is of the essence in stroke intervention, when this event occurs, local intra-arterial verapamil can be of great use in relaxing the vessel and allowing the procedure to proceed without further delay. Typical dosing of verapamil ranges from 5 mg intra-arterial to 20 mg intra-arterial, which is diluted with saline (Box 53.2).

Dissection

Dissection can involve an extracranial or an intracranial vessel. Aggressive manipulation of a catheter or wire can cause damage to the intima of the vessel and create a dissection flap. It is incumbent upon interventionists to select guide catheters with which they are comfortable and softer wires to minimize the potential for dissection. Dissections increase the risk of occlusive or thromboembolic complications and may lead to severe neurological deficits if not dealt with appropriately. Common sites for dissection are most notably seen in the cervical carotid artery and petrocavernous segments of the internal carotid artery. Dissection can appear as an intimal flap on digital subtraction angiography and as a double lumen on CTA. Although sometimes asymptomatic, the effects of dissection are naturally thromboembolic and may put the patient at further risk of stroke.

Dissection Avoidance and Management

Even in the most skilled hands, dissection can occur when advancing a catheter over a wire in an already diseased vessel. The decision to treat a dissection is based on severity, i.e., if the dissection limits blood flow. Balloon angioplasty or stenting of the vessel may be needed to treat a flow-limiting dissection. If the dissection flap is treated by stenting, dual antiplatelet therapy is required and may increase the risk of bleeding (Box 53.3).

Perforation

Vessel perforation caused by wire penetration through a vessel lumen can have catastrophic effects even in straightforward thrombectomy cases. Albeit rare, this complication, if dealt with in a timely fashion, does not preclude a good outcome for the patient. Mokin et al.

> **TIP BOX 53.2**
>
> If vasospasm occurs, simple maneuvers may alleviate the local irritation. Pulling the catheter back more proximally (in essence, allowing the affected vessel to "cool down") seems to be one effective approach.

> **WARNING BOX 53.3**
>
> If the dissection flap is treated by stenting, dual antiplatelet therapy is required and may increase the risk of bleeding.

concluded that intraprocedural perforations during stent retriever thrombectomy were rare; but when they occurred, they were associated with high mortality.[13] In their multicenter retrospective study, perforations were most commonly found to occur at distal occlusion sites and were often characterized by difficulty traversing the occlusion with a microcatheter, microwire, or while withdrawing the stent retriever. A history of intracranial atherosclerotic disease may predispose a patient to vessel injury and perforation, especially if a microwire is used to cross either a stenotic or an occlusive lesion or if a stent retriever is deployed in a vessel.

Perforation Avoidance and Management

In the rare event that vessel perforation occurs, immediate verification must first be made. Initial measures include reducing blood pressure and, if necessary, reversal of anticoagulation to lessen the severity of the bleed. Several techniques have been described in the literature for handling acute vessel perforation, one of which is temporary inflation of a balloon proximal to the perforation. This technique allows temporary occlusion of the vessel and a chance for platelet aggregation preventing further extravasation. To avoid prolonged ischemia to already at-risk tissue, we recommend the use of balloon occlusion for 5–10 minutes at a time.

CONCLUSION

Because thrombectomy has gained more traction and indications for treatment of AIS have expanded, the volume of complications will invariably increase. Complications are often unavoidable; however, anticipation and preparation for complications can improve outcomes. Stroke intervention should be performed by experts at high-volume centers if possible. This ensures that patients receive treatment from teams who have seen and performed an adequate number of stroke cases. Recognition of potential risk factors can help prevent complications; but in rare cases, complications do occur. Understanding the reasons they occur and knowing how to handle them can directly influence clinical outcomes. There are no significant evidence-based guidelines for the management of complications that occur in AIS intervention. The complications are well known and documented in the literature, but most management is based heavily on anecdotal evidence. The field of stroke intervention continues to grow and evolve. As newer technologies emerge, complication avoidance and management are necessary for optimal patient outcomes.

ACKNOWLEDGMENTS

The authors thank W. Fawn Dorr, BA and Debra J. Zimmer for editorial assistance.

REFERENCES

1. Sacco RL, Adams R, Albers G, et al. Guidelines for prevention of stroke in patients with ischemic stroke or transient ischemic attack: a statement for healthcare professionals from the American Heart Association/American Stroke Association Council on Stroke: co-sponsored by the Council on Cardiovascular Radiology and Intervention: the American Academy of Neurology affirms the value of this guideline. *Circulation*. 2006;113:e409–e449.
2. Saver JL, Goyal M, Bonafe A, et al. Stent-retriever thrombectomy after intravenous t-PA vs. t-PA alone in stroke. *N Engl J Med*. 2015;372:2285–2295.
3. Nogueira RG, Jadhav AP, Haussen DC, et al. Thrombectomy 6 to 24 hours after stroke with a mismatch between deficit and infarct. *N Engl J Med*. 2018;378:11–21.
4. Turk AS, Spiotta A, Frei D, et al. Initial clinical experience with the ADAPT technique: a direct aspiration first pass technique for stroke thrombectomy. *J Neurointerv Surg*. 2014;6:231–237.
5. Balami JS, White PM, McMeekin PJ, et al. Complications of endovascular treatment for acute ischemic stroke: prevention and management. *Int J Stroke*. 2018;13(4):348–361.
6. Saver JL. Time is brain—quantified. *Stroke*. 2006;37:263–266.
7. Lapergue B, Blanc R, Gory B, et al. Effect of endovascular contact aspiration vs. stent retriever on revascularization in patients with acute ischemic stroke and large vessel occlusion: the ASTER randomized clinical trial. *JAMA*. 2017;318:443–452.
8. Papanagiotou P, White CJ. Endovascular reperfusion strategies for acute stroke. *JACC Cardiovasc Interv*. 2016;9:307–317.
9. Stampfl S, Pfaff J, Herweh C, et al. Combined proximal balloon occlusion and distal aspiration: a new approach to prevent distal embolization during neurothrombectomy. *J Neurointerv Surg*. 2017;9:346–351.
10. Pan J, Konstas AA, Bateman B, et al. Reperfusion injury following cerebral ischemia: pathophysiology, MR imaging, and potential therapies. *Neuroradiology*. 2007;49:93–102.
11. Hao Y, Yang D, Wang H, et al. Predictors for symptomatic intracranial hemorrhage after endovascular treatment of acute ischemic stroke. *Stroke*. 2017;48:1203–1209.
12. Coutts SB, Hill MD, Hu WY. Hyperperfusion syndrome: toward a stricter definition. *Neurosurgery*. 2003;53:1053–1058; discussion 1058–1060.
13. Mokin M, Fargen KM, Primiani CT, et al. Vessel perforation during stent retriever thrombectomy for acute ischemic stroke: technical details and clinical outcomes. *J Neurointerv Surg*. 2017;9:922–928.

INDEX

Note: Page numbers followed by "b", "f", and "t" indicate boxes, figures, and tables respectively.